Practical
Urogynecology

Practical Urogynecology

L. Lewis Wall, M.D., D.Phil.
Department of Gynecology and Obstetrics
Emory University School of Medicine
Atlanta, Georgia

Peggy A. Norton, M.D.
Department of Obstetrics and Gynecology
University of Utah Medical Center
Salt Lake City, Utah

John O.L. DeLancey, M.D.
Department of Obstetrics and Gynecology
University of Michigan Medical Center
Ann Arbor, Michigan

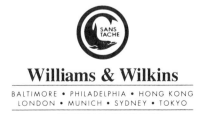

Williams & Wilkins

BALTIMORE • PHILADELPHIA • HONG KONG
LONDON • MUNICH • SYDNEY • TOKYO

A WAVERLY COMPANY

Editor: Charles W. Mitchell
Project Manager: Raymond E. Reter
Copy Editor: Richard H. Adin
Designer: Norman W. Och
Illustration Planner: Ray Lowman
Cover Designer: Norman W. Och

Copyright © 1993
Williams & Wilkins
428 East Preston Street
Baltimore, Maryland 21202 U.S.A.

Accurate indications, adverse reactions, and dosage schedules for drugs are provided in this book, but it is possible that they may change. The reader is urged to review the package information data of the manufacturers of the medications mentioned.

Printed in the United States of America.

Chapter reprints are available from the publisher.

Library of Congress Cataloging-in-Publication Data

Wall, L. Lewis, 1950–
    Practical urogynecology / L. Lewis Wall, Peggy A. Norton, John O.L. Delancey.
        p. cm.
    Includes bibliographical references and index.
    ISBN 0-683-08645-6
    1. Urogynecology. I. Norton, Peggy A. II. DeLancey, John O.L.
III. Title.
    [DNLM: 1. Genital Diseases, Female. 2. Urologic Diseases. WJ
190 W187p 1993]
RG484.W34 1993
616.6—dc20
DNLM/DLC
for Library of Congress   93-9416
                                                         CIP

93 94 95 96 97
1 2 3 4 5 6 7 8 9 10

To
Helen, Kevin, and Barb

Foreword

Oriented to the general clinician and resident-in-training, this volume discusses the lower urinary tract problems of the adult female. Although major emphasis is given to stress urinary incontinence (SUI), other symptomatic difficulties are not neglected. It is a much-needed textbook that fills a niche both in resident training and as a source of catalogued information for the busy gynecologist. In some areas, where physiologic activity and anatomy do not always jibe, the authors have not hesitated to state their opinion, even though the complicated coordination of all of the activities involved in the retention and voluntary expulsion of urine from the bladder are still not entirely understood. Such controversies simply point out the need for additional basic research in the field of adult female urinary control. As the authors state, "urodynamic testing is an adjunct to, and not a substitute for, a thorough history and physical examination." SUI is still a clinical problem!

Sometimes the important details of a patient's history are not easily analyzed. I recall a patient referred by an expert gynecologist from Texas because of a "failed" retropubic urethropexy operation. Metallic bead-chain lateral urethrocystograms disclosed excellent and secure elevation of the urethrovesical junction. Direct electronic urethrocystometry demonstrated no detrusor dysfunction. Yet, she demonstrated distressing SUI when erect. No reason for the operative failure was apparent until on rounds the resident said, "Did you know she eliminated nearly 9000 ml of urine yesterday, and that her intake was over 8000 ml?" We jumped at the conclusion she had diabetes insipidus. The endocrinologist was consulted. Two days later, he reported no diabetes insipidus. We elicited additional history. On being asked why she drank so much fluid, she responded, "The doctor in Texas told me that drinking as much water as possible was my best medicine." Her intake was limited to less than 2500 ml and her incontinence was cured!

Our concepts of lower urinary tract function in adult women need to be based on research *done* on adult women. Many concepts of female lower urinary tract function have been improperly carried over from studies done on males. Bladder capacity is not necessarily approximated most accurately by cystoscopy. The way the bladder is filled has a dramatic effect on how capacity is determined. Too hot or too cold or too rapid retrograde filling of the bladder can all cause artifacts in determining bladder capacity. On the other hand, if the bladder is filled to maximum capacity by diuresis after it has been emptied by catheterization, different results are obtained. In such a study, we showed that patients with SUI often had much larger bladder capacities than patients without SUI. (Hodgkinson CP, Dirghangi J, Salako O. The physiologic capacity of the urinary bladder of the adult female subject. Trans AGOS 1984;2:192–199.) Uncontrolled, unstandardized retrograde cystometry was discredited as a reliable, reproducible test of bladder function many years ago, but Lapides later championed retrograde water cystometry as a valuable urologic test provided it was performed properly. He emphasized standardization and uniformity in performing the test procedure, and emphasized the need to control subjective influences. He emphasized that the test should be performed by the physician involved, and not by a harassed nurse. More physiologic filling techniques may give even better results. Direct electronic urethrocystometry using natural filling by diuresis is probably more accurate than retrograde techniques, and is about as free of subjective and objective adverse influences as is presently possible.

It is the function of the urogynecologist to bring order to this newly arrived specialty. The term "urogynecology" implies the creation of a specialty under the combined umbrella of urology and gynecology; not the "either/or" situation that is sometimes presented. This book should be basic for all those interested in this specialty.

The authors are to be complimented upon the thoroughness with which they have undertaken this project. I am pleased to have had the opportunity to add my humble remarks.

C. Paul Hodgkinson, M.D.

Preface

Lower urinary tract disorders are among the most common—and among the most neglected—health care problems faced by women. Urinary incontinence in particular has remained an embarrasing problem which has been neglected by the medical community for far too long. This situation is slowly changing. The American Board of Obstetrics and Gynecology, along with other specialty bodies, has called for more intensive resident training in this field; however, this encouraging process has been hampered by a lack of suitable educational resources.

Practical Urogynecology is an attempt to help remedy this situation by providing a clear, concise, and *practical* clinical introduction to the evaluation and treatment of lower urinary tract problems in women. It is oriented to the needs of residents-in-training and those of the busy general obstetrician-gynecologist, but it also contains substantial information which we hope will be of use to urologists, internists, geriatricians, and family practitioners. Our goal has not been to write a comprehensive reference work, but rather to write a practical and *readable* book which covers the core material on those lower urinary tract disorders likely to be encountered in the routine clinical practice of gynecology. Like other subspecialties, urogynecology has its areas of controversy. In such cases we have attempted to present one reasonable approach to the problem rather than a catalogue of competing views. Our intent has been to be pragmatic rather than dogmatic; we realize that there may be many other acceptable ways of achieving similar clinical ends and hope that we (as well as our readers) will remain receptive to new developments in this field.

This book has been written in at least six countries on three different continents, often in airport waiting rooms. To acknowledge everyone to whom we are indebted for help, assistance, or insight would be impratical, but certain individuals merit our special thanks: Dr. Al Addison at Duke University; Dr. Niall Galloway and Dr. Anne Wiskind at Emory University; Dr. Leon Speroff at the University of Oregon; Dr. James Scott at the University of Utah; and Dr. George Morley, Dr. Tom Elkins, and Dr. Ed McGuire at the University of Michigan. In England we owe special thanks to Mr. Stuart Stanton of St. George's Hospital in London, and to Dr. David Warrell of St. Mary's Hospital for Women and Children, Manchester. Most of all, we thank our patients, who have taught us most of what we know.

Our largest debts of gratitude, however, go to Helen, Kevin, and Barb, who put up with the three of us throughout this entire process, even when it was getting pretty deep.

L. Lewis Wall
Peggy A. Norton
John O.L. DeLancey

Contents

1

"Unspeakable Women's Problems"

"There is no more distressing lesion than urinary incontinence—a constant dribbling of the repulsive urine soaking the clothes which cling wet and cold to the thighs making the patient offensive to herself and her family and ostracising her from society."

—Howard A. Kelly, 1928

The long line outside the women's restroom during any intermission is testimony to the impact of urinary continence on our daily lives. To stand in such a line means that the woman has been able to suppress urgency and other bladder sensations until intermission, and despite a full bladder, the close proximity of the toilet and the sound of running water, she nonetheless is able to wait patiently in line. Of course, some of these individuals are in the line as a matter of habit; but women who are unable to control their bladder function will stay at home and avoid such situations. The ability to choose when and where to urinate, to be free from the clinging smell of urine so reminiscent of infant diapers, to be able to sleep through the night unawakened by the disruptive demands of bladder sensation, these are all functions which are taken for granted by many adults who have forgotten that bladder control of this kind is not present at birth but develops as a complex, learned behavior. Generations of parents in every society take upon themselves the task of teaching their young children the rules of bladder control appropriate for their culture. "Potty training" of some kind is a universal phenomenon. These seemingly straightforward rules about bladder control actually involve developing a complex biofeedback system which regulates the interaction of the bladder and the autonomic nervous system—imagine controlling blood pressure or bowel motility to such a degree!

Because of this, patient education is one of the most important points in the evaluation and treatment of women with loss of bladder control. Many women are greatly relieved to discover that urinary incontinence is common, since many of them have hidden their problem for many years, to the detriment of relationships with their family, spouse, and friends. But providing adequate patient information means that physicians themselves must know enough to answer some basic questions: How common is urinary incontinence? Why don't people talk about it? How can health care workers talk to patients about these problems? How should it be evaluated? And what can be done about it?

Hiding the Problem

Loss of urinary continence implies a loss of adulthood, of control over bodily function. Many women cannot discuss their loss of bladder control with their family or friends. Often family members may have already suspected that something is wrong when mom needs to stop the car every half hour on the family vacation; when she is teased about this, mom may begin to make excuses as to why she does not wish to go on a trip next year. A bladder accident while laughing with friends at lunch may be hidden by wearing bulky pads or dark clothing; but they may later wonder why their friend had to leave early. Women are used to hiding menstrual flow with absorbent pads. It is a simple step to use menstrual pads to hide the problem of urinary incontinence as well, a fact that is not lost on the paper products industry. Probably 30% of menstrual pads are really used by women for urinary incontinence. This practice has allowed women to temporize, to hide the problem of incontinence, and to avoid discussing it with their physician. One British study found that over half of women who delayed seeking treatment for significant urinary incontinence did so because they were too embarrassed to discuss the problem with their general practitioner or any other health worker. Although the women in this study reported significant shame and distress associated with their symptoms, more than half of these women had waited more than a year before seeking medical attention, and one-quarter had delayed seeking help for more than five years. This was especially true of elderly women. Overall, less than half of patients with significant urinary incontinence have sought help for their condition. Despite increasing attention to the problem of incontinence in both the lay press and the medical literature, it seems that health workers must still question patients actively regarding urinary symptoms if they are going to find those patients who need help.

Acknowledging the Problem

Half of young, nulliparous women without other urinary complaints will experience occasional loss of urine with coughing or sneezing. Does this mean that urinary incontinence is "normal" in women? Of course not. Urinary incontinence is never "normal"; but it develops at different thresholds in different patients. The important question is: How much does urine loss affect daily life? Most women are not particularly troubled by the occasional loss of small amounts of urine while exercising vigorously with a full bladder, or sneezing violently when they have a cold. This is just one of life's nuisances. On the other hand, recurrent daily urine loss can be devastating. Imagine what it is like for the woman with chronic pulmonary disease who soaks her clothing every time she coughs. Imagine how frustrating it is for the woman with urinary urgency who loses control of her bladder every time she rushes home and fumbles with her keys to open the door of her house. The International Continence Society, a multidisciplinary body concerned with this problem, defines urinary incontinence as the involuntary loss of urine which is severe enough to be a social or hygienic problem, and which is objectively demonstrable. This means that even infrequent urine loss can produce clinically significant incontinence. Consider the plight of a professional tennis player who only loses urine while serving or returning a cross-court volley, or the businesswoman who cannot suppress bladder contractions while sitting through an extended meeting over contract negotiations. These women have significant problems irrespective of the amount of urine they lose. A demented patient may lose large amounts of urine and not be the slightest bit concerned about it. Incontinence does not present a social problem for her, but skin breakdown from constant maceration by urine does present a significant hygienic problem for her and for her caretakers. Finally, there are other bladder problems which do not necessarily involve incontinence. The woman who must empty her bladder every 20 or 30 minutes will find herself criticized at work for wasting time, and the woman with interstitial cystitis may be totally preoccupied with seeking relief from tormenting bladder pain.

The definition of incontinence given above is a technical one for use by the medical profession in clinical encounters with patients. An epidemiologic definition that would allow us to define the prevalence of urinary incontinence in different populations is more difficult because of the broad social factors involved which often cloud the true situation. The prevalence of urinary incontinence varies widely in different cultures depending on how the information is obtained and the way in which the questions are asked. Depending on the definition and on the method of questioning, the prevalence of urinary incontinence in the United States and Britain is 10% to 25% of the general female population and 20% to 40% of community-dwelling (as opposed to institutionalized) women over sixty-five. Half of all nursing home patients have incontinent episodes at least once per day. For many years the Japanese believed that female urinary incontinence was a negligible problem in their culture until it was realized that social stigma prevented women from admitting the problem to male physicians. Studies from Britain and New Zealand have found the same reluctance to discuss urinary incontinence because of embarrassment, fear of needing surgery, or the belief that incontinence was a normal part of aging.

In 1988, the National Institutes of Health held a consensus development conference to assess the impact of urinary incontinence and to recommend strategies for addressing this problem in the United States. The conference concluded that:

- Urinary incontinence is very common among older Americans and is epidemic in nursing homes.
- Urinary incontinence costs Americans more than $10 billion each year.
- Urinary incontinence is not part of normal aging, but age-related changes predispose to its occurrence.
- Urinary incontinence leads to stigmatization and social isolation.
- Of the 10 million Americans with urinary incontinence more than half have had no evaluation or treatment.
- Contrary to popular opinion, most cases of urinary incontinence can be cured or improved.
- Every person with urinary incontinence is entitled to evaluation and consideration for treatment.
- Most health care professionals ignore urinary incontinence and do not provide adequate diagnosis and treatment.
- Inadequate nursing home staffing prohibits proper treatment and contributes to the neglect of nursing home residents.
- Medical and nursing education neglects urinary incontinence. Curriculum development is urgent.
- A major research initiative is required to improve assessment and treatment for Americans with urinary incontinence.

Overcoming Medical Neglect

Patients need to understand that incontinence is not "normal" and that help is available. This is one reason why labels have been placed on the packages of absorbent incontinence pads advising patients that they should seek medical evaluation of bladder control problems. But while increased public knowledge about urinary incontinence is needed to reduce the vast under-reporting of this problem and to bring it into the arena of public discussion, the health profession itself also needs more information about how to diagnose and treat it. The unfortunate fact is that the medical profession, as a whole, is woefully ignorant of the nature and scope of the problem of incontinence and how to deal with it. Vastly more education needs to be directed at physicians in training as well as physicians in practice, particularly in the fields of gynecology and obstetrics, urology, general medicine, geriatrics, and family practice. The subject of urinary (not to mention fecal) incontinence is poorly taught in almost all medical schools, perhaps because incontinence is usually not life threatening and is therefore not seen as a "real disease." Many practicing physicians feel uncomfortable when a patient brings the subject up because they are uncertain how to evaluate or treat urinary incontinence. For the patient who has summoned up all her courage to broach the subject with her physician in the first place, to be brushed off with an ignorant reply like "What do you expect at your age?," is devastating and may end her attempts to seek help. As the American population ages, and as the stigma attached to incontinence is gradually removed, many more women will go to their doctors with urinary incontinence. Those physicians who are reluctant or unwilling to learn more about this problem will soon find themselves losing patients to physicians who are well versed in the subject.

Actually, the truth is that taking care of incontinent patients is usually quite rewarding. Although this condition is rarely life-threatening, the reduction in quality of life experienced by these patients cannot be overstated. Few conditions in medicine are associated with such a sense of suffering and isolation from society as urinary incontinence—and yet incontinent women are usually otherwise healthy and are highly motivated to comply with therapeutic regimens. These patients are truly grateful when their problem is improved or cured! How many patients with hypertension or hypercholesterolemia know when they have improved with medical treatment? Or experience similar daily satisfaction with their progress?

Treating the "Whole" Pelvis

Unlike an infectious disease such as smallpox, which has been eradicated by an intensive worldwide public health campaign, incontinence will always be a medical problem. It is bound up with the trauma of childbirth, medical illness,

Figure 1.1 Territorial imperatives at work on the pelvic floor. A gynecologist, a urologist, and a colorectal surgeon quarrel with each other while ignoring the common ground on which they all stand. (Wall and DeLancey 1991 Perspec Biol Med 34: 486–96, University of Chicago Press, with permission.)

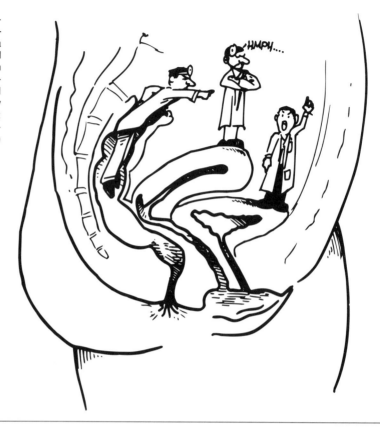

neurologic disease, and the consequences of aging, which together predispose some people to lose urinary control. Urinary incontinence will continue to be a significant health problem in the United States, especially among the elderly and the institutionalized, and it will increase as the average age of the American population shifts upwards. The goal for clinicians, therefore, is not a Quixotic quest to eradicate incontinence, but rather a quest to make possible the diagnosis and treatment of incontinence for all patients with a significant clinical problem. The goals for each patient will be different, and treatment must be individualized. For some women this may mean being dry enough so that they can simply sit through a church service and not have to change an incontinence pad or rush to the toilet. For others this may mean absolute dryness through obstructive surgery which then requires lifelong self-catheterization to achieve bladder emptying. Ultimately we may be able to identify those women at risk for developing incontinence and learn how to prevent it from developing in many patients the first place.

How do we begin? It has become increasingly obvious over the past few years that female urinary incontinence is only a subset of a wider range of problems involving the entire pelvic floor. Appreciation of this fact has been obscured by the territoriality of medical specialization which has resulted in gynecologists, urologists, gastroenterologists, and colorectal surgeons practicing within millimeters of each other but without significant interaction regarding the problems that they treat. This has led to a compartmentalization of the pelvic floor into three separate "holes," each with its own specialty, its own distinctive point of view, and its own territorial imperative to defend its field of practice (Fig. 1.1). The urethra and bladder "belong" to the urologist. The vagina and female genitalia "belong" to the gynecologist. The colon and rectum "belong" to the GI specialist and his surgical counterpart. This approach ignores not only the foundations common to all of these organs, but also overlooks the treatment of concurrent pathology in other organ systems. For example, a surprising number of women who have suffered obstetric trauma have urinary and fecal incontinence as well as genital prolapse, and an enormous number of women with irritable bowel syndrome have detrusor instability as well.

Who should treat these women? The term "urogynecology" has come to represent the field of special interest which deals with the interrelationships of the bladder and the rest of the female pelvic floor. However, this term should not necessarily imply that these women are best treated by a gynecologist with an interest in urology. What is needed, rather, is a closer interaction between gynecologists and their colleagues in other specialties: urologists, neurologists, gastroenterologists, colorectal surgeons, and geriatricians. The "hole" pelvis with its separate isolated compartments needs to be replaced by a multidisciplinary viewpoint which seeks to treat the "whole" pelvis instead. Each specialty has something of value to teach the others where these problems are concerned. Gynecologists need to have a greater understanding of the neurologic diseases which may be involved in pelvic floor dysfunction and of the potential for upper urinary tract damage which may exist under certain circumstances. Urologists need a greater understanding of the relationship between incontinence and genito-urinary prolapse, particularly the consequences of performing only bladder neck suspension surgery on patients with other pelvic floor defects. Both urologic and gynecologic surgeons need a greater appreciation of the role of conservative, nonsurgical behavioral management and exercise therapy in the treatment of pelvic floor problems and urinary incontinence. And *all* specialties must begin to pay more attention to the problem of fecal incontinence, which remains the most hidden, most stigmatizing, and least understood of all these distressing conditions. Wherever possible we advocate a multidisciplinary approach to treating these patients. Clinicians who adopt this attitude will find that their practices are both busier and more interesting. Since somewhere between 10 and 20 million adult Americans have a problem with urinary incontinence, there certainly is no dearth of patients!

SUGGESTED READING

Diokno A, Brock B, Brown M, Herzog A. Prevalence of urinary incontinence and other urological symptoms in the noninstituionalized elderly. J Urol 1986; 136:1022–25.

Eriksen B, Eik-Nes S. Long-term electrostimulation of the pelvic floor: Primary therapy in female stress incontinence? Urol Int 1989; 49:90.

Holst K, Wilson PD. The prevalence of female urinary incontinence and reasons for not seeking treatment. Aust NZ Med J 1988; 101:756–58.

Hu T, Igou J, Kaltreider D. A clinical trial of a behavioral therapy to reduce urinary incontinence in nursing home: Outcome and implications. JAMA 1989; 261:2656–62.

Kato K, Dondo A, Okamura K, Takaba H. Prevalence of urinary incontinence in working women. Nippon-Hinyokika Gakkai-Zassh 1986; 77:1501–05.

Madoff RD, Williams JG, Caushaj PF. Fecal incontinence. N Engl J Med 1992; 326:1002–07.

National Center for Health Statistics. The national nursing home survey: 1977 summary for the United States by Van Nostrand J, et al. (DHEW Publication No. 79-1794.) Vital and Health Statistics. Series 13, No. 43. Washington, DC.: Health Resources Administration, U.S. Government Printing Office.

Nemir A, Middleton R. Stress incontinence in young nulliparous women. Am J Obstet Gynecol 1954; 68: 1166–68.

Norton P, MacDonald L, Stanton S, Sedgwick D. Distress and delay associated with female urinary complaints. Br Med J 1988; 297:1187–89.

Nygaard I, DeLancey JOL, Arnsdorf L, Murphy C. Exercise and incontinence. Obstet Gynecol 1990; 75:848–51.

Takai K, Miyashita A, Mochizuki K. Actual conditions of female stress incontinence. Jpn J Clin Urol 1987; 41: 393–96.

Thomas T, Plymat K, Blannin J, Meade T. Prevalence of urinary incontinence. Br Med J 1980; 281:1243–45.

Urinary Incontinence Consensus Development Panel. Urinary incontinence in adults. JAMA 1989; 261:2685–50.

Urinary Incontinence Guideline Panel. Urinary Incontinence in Adults: Clinical Practice Guideline. AHCPR Pub. No. 92-0038. Rockville, MD: Agency for Health Care Policy and Research, Public Health Service, U.S. Department of Health and Human Services. March 1992.

Wall LL, DeLancey JOL. The politics of prolapse: A revisionist approach to disorders of the pelvic floor in women. Perspec Biol Med 1991; 34:486–96.

Whorwell PJ, Lupton EW, Erduran D, Wilson K. Bladder smooth muscle dysfunction in patients with irritable bowel syndrome. Gut 1986; 27:1014–17.

Wyman J, Choi S, Harkins S, Wilson M, Fantl J. Psychosocial impact of urinary incontinence in women. Obstet Gynecol 1987; 70(3):378–81.

Yarnell J, Voyle G, Richards C, et al. The prevalence and severity of urinary incontinence in women. J Epid Comm Health 1981; 35:71–77.

2

Pelvic Anatomy and the Physiology of the Lower Urinary Tract

Pelvic Anatomy
General Embryology

The details of the embryologic development of the lower urinary tract are complex, yet the overall pattern of its development is relatively simple. During the first three to seven weeks of embryonic life, each kidney develops from a ridge which forms on the dorsal body wall lateral to the midline. These raised areas are composed of intermediate mesoderm and are called the nephrogenic ridges.

Developmental changes within the nephrogenic ridge begin at its cranial end and progress caudally. Three major stages occur, culminating in the development of the kidney. First a series of tubules and a duct (the pronephros) form in the uppermost portion. During the second stage of kidney development, the pronephros regresses and is replaced by the mesonephros. The mesonephric duct and tubules form just caudal to the pronephros. Finally, the metanephros (which is destined to become the adult kidney and collecting system) develops in the most caudal portion of the nephrogenic ridge. This structure arises from two primordial antecedents: a metanephric blastema which will form the kidney, and the ureteric bud which becomes the calyces, renal pelvis, and ureter.

The primitive gut forms the cloaca, out of which the bladder and urethra ultimately develop. The cloaca is separated from the amniotic cavity by the cloacal membrane. The cloaca has two parts: a dorsal hindgut and an anterior sausage-shaped allantois which extends into the body stalk. The wedge of tissue called the urorectal septum grows caudally until it reaches the cloacal membrane and divides the cloaca into an anterior urogenital sinus and posterior anorectum. The urorectal septum also divides the cloacal membrane into the urogenital membrane and anal membrane. The urorectal septum ultimately becomes the perineal body in the adult. The portion of the urogenital sinus lying above the mesonephric ducts is continuous with the allantois and is called the vesicourethral canal. It will form the urethra and bladder in the adult. The sinus below the mesonephric ducts is destined to become the vaginal vestibule.

There are four different embryologic primordia within the urogenital sinus which develop into the female bladder and urethra. These are the smooth muscle of the detrusor, the trigone, and the urethra; and the primordial striated muscle of the urethra (Fig. 2.1). Although the urethra and bladder appear to form a single continuous structure on gross inspection, there are actually important microscopic and functional differences in the musculature of different regions. These differences are the result of the different embryologic origins of each region. In both males and females there is a fifth (prostatic) primordium, but this does not develop into any significant structure in the adult female.

Anatomy of the Lower Urinary Tract
Subdivisions of the Lower Urinary Tract

Clinicians have traditionally divided the lower urinary tract into the bladder, the vesical neck, and the urethra (Fig. 2.2). The bladder consists of the detrusor muscle and its interior epithelium, and the trigone (an embryologically separate structure lying on the dorsal wall of the bladder). The urethra is a multilayered muscular tube which extends below the bladder. It has its own specialized mucosal and vascular lining. The vesical neck is the region of the bladder base where the urethra enters the bladder. Because it has special characteristics and

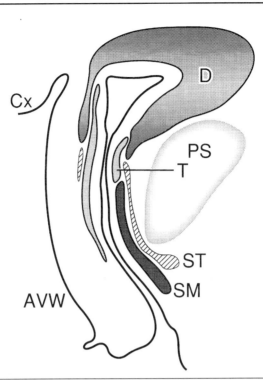

Figure 2.1 Schematic drawing of the vesicourethral primordia in a 20 cm fetus. *AVW*, anterior vaginal wall; *CX*, cervix; *D*, detrusor primordium; *PS*, pubic symphysis; *SM*, smooth muscle primordium; *ST*, striated primordium; *T*, trigonal primordium.

because the urethral lumen is actually surrounded by the bladder as it traverses the bladder wall, the vesical neck will be considered separately.

Bladder.   The bladder is a hollow viscus with a wall made of coarse bundles of smooth muscle. It is lined by transitional epithelium resting upon a loose submucosa. The bladder can be subdivided further into the dome and the base, roughly at the level of the ureteric orifices. The bladder dome is relatively thin and quite distensible, while the bladder base has thicker musculature and is less distensible during filling.

Detrusor Muscle.   Although separate layers of the detrusor muscle have sometimes been described, these are not nearly so well defined as the separate layers of other muscular organs such as the gut. This reflects the fact that the bladder only needs to contract periodically, and when it does contract it only needs to raise its internal pressure enough to evacuate the bladder contents. The gut, on the other hand, must contract in a sequential, repetitive, and coordinated manner to move its contents forward. The smooth muscle layers in the dome of the bladder are relatively indistinct, but near the bladder base they become better defined. The outermost muscle layer is predominantly oriented longitudinally. Longitudinal fibers on the anterior surface of the bladder continue past the vesical neck into the pubovesical muscles and insert into the tissues of the pelvic wall near the pubic symphysis (see below). An intermediate layer of oblique and circular fibers lies within this outer longitudinal layer. The actual directions of the muscle fibers in this portion of the dome are less well defined than those in the outer layer. The innermost layer of muscle fibers is plexiform. This arrangement of muscle fibers is responsible for the trabeculated pattern which is often seen during cystoscopy. Although the arrangement of muscle fibers in the innermost layer is often described as being longitudinal, this pattern is not particularly striking when the bladder is viewed from its lumen.

There are two ''U''-shaped bands of fibers in the region of the vesical neck. Each ''U'' opens in the opposite direction. The more prominent of these (Heiss's loop or the detrusor loop) passes anterior to the internal meatus. The end of this loop opens posteriorly. The second loop consists of intermediate circular detrusor

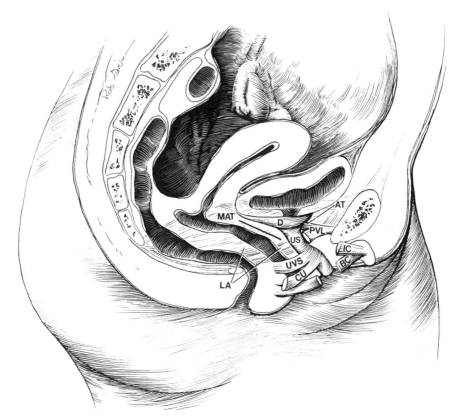

Figure 2.2   Interrelationships and approximate location of paraurethral structures. Levator ani muscles are shown as light lines running deep to the pelvic viscera. *AT*, arcus tendineus fasciae pelvis; *BC*, bulbocavernosus muscle; *CU*, compressor urethrae; *D*, detrusor loop; *IC*, ischiocavernous muscle; *LA*, levator ani muscles; *MAT*, muscular attachment of the urethral supports; *PVL*, pubovesical ligament (muscle); *US*, urethral sphincter; *UVS*, urethrovaginal sphincter. Reprinted with the permission of the American College of Obstetricians and Gynecologists, from Obstet Gynecol 1986; 68:91.

muscle fibers lying under the trigone. This loop opens anteriorly. Some authors, noting that the urethral lumen passes through the middle of these two U-shaped bundles of muscle, have speculated that this arrangement creates a sphincteric mechanism which closes the urethra by pulling in opposite directions. However, this concept is not logical since these are the very detrusor fibers that contract during micturition. This kind of arrangement would close the internal meatus and would lead to inefficient bladder emptying. The only way an arrangement of this kind could work would be if the autonomic innervation in this area were different from that of the bladder dome. This might allow for a synergistic interaction between the bladder dome and bladder base during bladder emptying to alleviate this problem. The bladder base is comprised of these bundles of fibers together with the urinary trigone.

Trigonal Muscle.   As previously mentioned, the trigone has a separate embryologic origin from the rest of the bladder. The trigonal muscle is a specialized smooth muscle located in the bladder base and the vesical neck, and extending into the urethra. It has three portions; the urinary trigone, the trigonal ring, and the trigonal plate. The superficial urinary trigone is a triangular body of smooth muscle arranged so that its corners lie at the internal urinary meatus and the two ureteric orifices (Fig. 2.3). It is elevated slightly above the rest of the detrusor musculature and is easily seen during cystoscopic examination. This fact helps locate the ureteric orifices. The trigonal musculature spreads out to form a ring

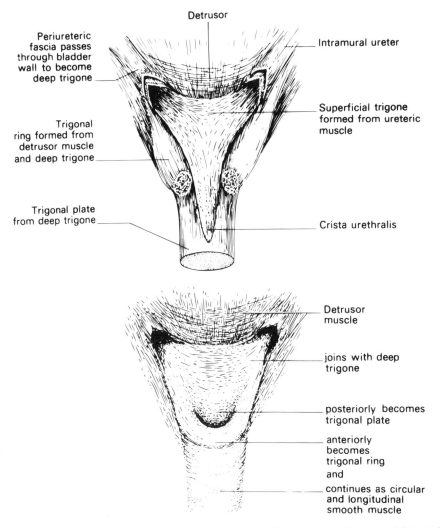

Detrusor

Periureteric fascia passes through bladder wall to become deep trigone

Intramural ureter

Superficial trigone formed from ureteric muscle

Trigonal ring formed from detrusor muscle and deep trigone

Trigonal plate from deep trigone

Crista urethralis

Detrusor muscle

joins with deep trigone

posteriorly becomes trigonal plate

anteriorly becomes trigonal ring and

continues as circular and longitudinal smooth muscle

Figure 2.3   The structure of the urinary trigone and trigonal ring illustrating how the trigonal ring encircles the urethral lumen at the vesical neck. From Asmussen and Miller, Clinical Gynecologic Urology, Oxford: Blackwell Scientific Publications, 1983, with permission.

which surrounds the urethral lumen at the vesical neck. The trigonal plate is a column of trigonal tissue that extends below the level of the trigonal ring, extending along the dorsal aspect of the urethra. The trigonal ring lies between the ends of the striated urogenital sphincter.

α-Adrenergic receptors have been identified in the muscle of the bladder base and the vesical neck, and the trigone/trigonal ring lie within this area. These structures may be important for helping close the vesical neck in response to input from the sympathetic nervous system, although large section histochemistry has not yet been done to localize these receptors in the trigone or trigonal ring. The possibility that the trigonal ring is important in closing the proximal urethra is suggested by the fact that it lies within the area of the vesical neck which is open in patients with myelodysplasia and other forms of denervation injury. The functional association between the trigonal plate and vesical neck closure needs to be confirmed by further study.

Urethra.   The urethra is a complex muscular tube that extends below the lower border of the bladder base (Fig. 2.4). The urethral wall begins about 15%

Figure 2.4 Sagittal section from a 29-year-old cadaver. Cut just lateral to the midline and not quite parallel to it. The section contains tissue nearer the midline in the distal urethra where the lumen can be seen then at the vesical neck. *BM*, bladder mucosa; *CMU*, circular smooth muscle of the urethra; *CU*, compressor urethrae; *D*, detrusor muscle; *LMU*, longitudinal smooth muscles of the urethra; *PB*, perineal body; *PS*, pubic symphysis; *R*, rectum; *T*, trigonal ring; *UL*, urethral lumen; *US*, urethral sphincter; *UVS*, urethrovaginal sphincter; and *V*, vagina. Reprinted with the permission of the American College of Obstetricians and Gynecologists, from Obstet Gynecol 1986; 68:91.

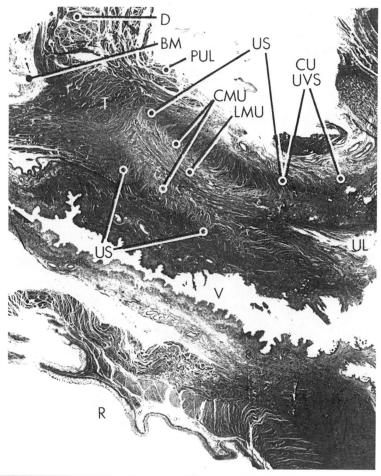

of total urethral length below the beginning of the urethral lumen. The urethra is a multilayered hollow tube, approximately 3 cm–4 cm in length (Fig. 2.5*A*, *B*). The outermost layer of the urethra is the striated urogenital sphincter muscle (sometimes called the striated circular muscle, striated sphincter, or rhabdosphincter). This striated muscle surrounds a thin circular layer of smooth muscle which in turn surrounds a longitudinal layer of smooth muscle. A submucosa with a rich vascular supply lies between this smooth muscle and the urethral mucosa.

Striated Urogenital Sphincter Muscle.   Descriptions of the striated urogenital sphincter muscle in the female have frequently been wrong because the urethra was removed from its surroundings for examination. Studies by Oelrich have corrected many misconceptions about the anatomy of this region and have brought them into line with the functional observations which are made in this area.

The striated urogenital sphincter consists of two different portions: an upper sphincteric portion and a lower arch-like pair of muscular bands (Fig. 2.6). Fibers in the sphincteric portion are oriented circularly and occupy the upper two-thirds of the body of this muscle, surrounding the urethral lumen from approximately 20%–60% of its length. This part is called the sphincter urethrae and corresponds to the rhabdosphincter described by other authors. The fibers in this region do not form a complete circle; rather, the gap between their two ends is bridged by the trigonal plate to complete the circle. This defect in the muscular ring

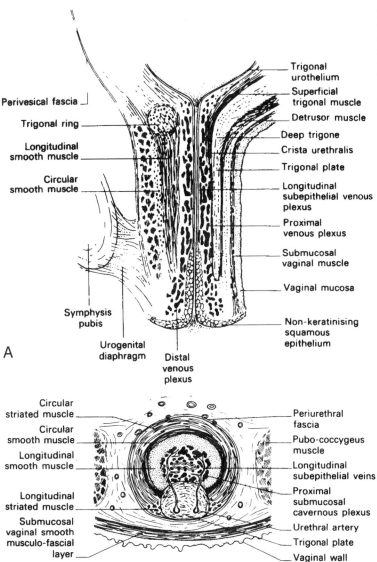

Figure 2.5 Anatomy of the urethra. (*A*) Sagital section. (*B*) Cross-section. From Asmussen and Miller, Clinical Gynecologic Urology, Oxford: Blackwell Scientific Publications, 1983, with permission.

does not impair its contraction since the trigonal plate functions as a tendon and bridges the gap between the ends of the muscles.

The second portion of the striated urogenital sphincter occupies its distal one-third, lying adjacent to the urethral lumen from approximately 60%–80% of its length. This portion consists of two strap-like bands of striated muscle which arch over the ventral surface of the urethra. One of these bands originates in the vaginal wall and is called the urethrovaginal sphincter muscle. The other band of muscle originates near the ischiopubic ramus and is called the compressor urethrae. These muscle bands overlap near the ventral surface of the urethra and are separate structures only in their more lateral projections. This is the muscle which has previously been referred to as the deep transverse perineal muscle. Illustrations of this muscle are often inaccurate and have led to confusion regarding its role in continence.

All three portions of the striated urogenital sphincter muscle are part of the

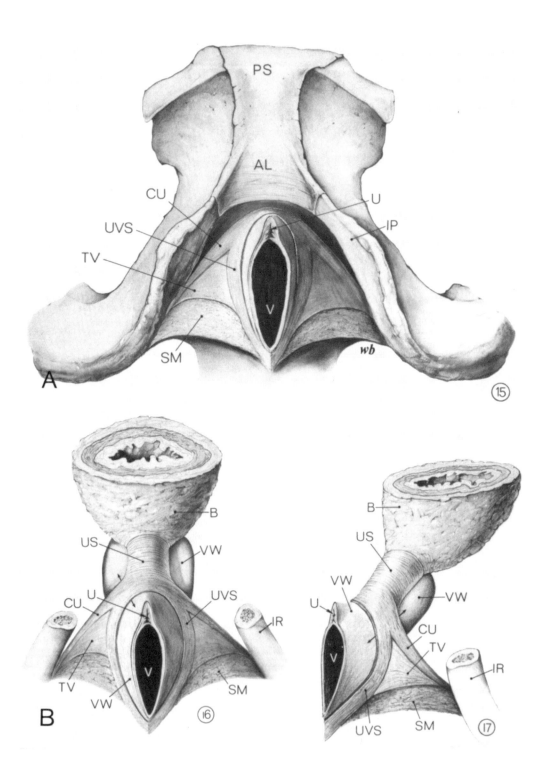

Figure 2.6 Striated urogenital sphincter muscle seen from below after removal of the perineal membrane (*A*) and pubic bones (*B*) including *US*, urethral sphincter; *UVS*, urethrovaginal sphincter; *CU*, compressor urethrae. Bladder (*B*), Ischiopubic ramus (*IR*), transverse vaginae (*TV*) muscle; smooth muscle (*SM*); urethra (*U*); and vagina (*V*), Vaginal Wall (*VW*). From Oelrich, Anat Rec 1983; 205:223–32, with permission of Alan R. Liss Publishers.

same muscle group and function as a single unit. There has been considerable controversy over whether they have somatic or autonomic innervation. There is evidence to suggest that their innervation is complex. The fibers within this muscle are primarily slow-twitch fibers and are therefore well suited to maintaining constant tone over time while still retaining the ability to contract more strongly when additional occlusive force is needed.

Contraction of the striated urogenital sphincter muscle constricts the upper portion of the urethral lumen and compresses the lower one-third of its ventral wall. The striated urogenital sphincter muscle functions primarily as a "back-up" continence mechanism which can maintain urethral closure in spite of vesical neck incompetence or under acute circumstances when the urge to urinate is severe but micturition must be postponed for a few minutes. This striated sphincter is probably the main mechanism by which continent women with an incompetent vesical neck maintain their dryness. However, this muscle is not sufficient to maintain continence by itself when stressed by a cough if the vesical neck is open. This can be demonstrated by the occurrence of stress incontinence in myelodysplastic women who have normal external sphincters but open vesical necks. If the compressor urethrae and urethrovaginal sphincter are excised, as often happens in the performance of a radical vulvectomy, stress incontinence may start abruptly or worsen dramatically. This is powerful testimony to the importance of these structures as an adjunct to the maintenance of urinary continence. Although these women develop no change in resting urethral pressure or urethral support, they become incontinent once this musculature is lost. Sometimes this incontinence is total.

Smooth Muscle. As previously mentioned, the urethral smooth muscle has a separate embryologic origin (Fig. 2.1). Although contiguous with the muscle of the bladder, the urethral smooth muscle is not just a downward extension of the fibers of the detrusor muscle. It has its own special characteristics. There are two distinct smooth muscle layers in the urethra (Fig. 2.4). The circular muscle of the urethra is poorly developed and difficult to identify. It is adjacent to the trigonal ring and extends below it, but the embryologic derivations of these two tissues appear to be different. In contrast to the poorly defined outer circular muscle, the inner longitudinal smooth muscle is well developed and has considerable bulk. This longitudinal smooth muscle is not continuous with the detrusor musculature per se, but does extend to the level of the trigonal ring. It probably functions to shorten the urethra during micturition.

Submucosal Vasculature. The submucosal urethral vasculature is remarkably prominent. Huisman described it as a highly organized arteriovenous complex capable of specific filling and emptying. Although it is technically difficult to study a vascular plexus this small, if the arterial supply to the urethra is clamped, resting urethral pressure will decrease significantly. The submucosal vascular plexus may therefore function as an "inflatable cushion" which helps fill out the urethral wall, aiding mucosal coaptation and helping create a hermetic seal. If urethral pressure studies are carried out using microtip transducer pressure catheters, the vascular pulsations of this submucosal plexus are often recorded during the study and correlate with the patient's pulse as measured in other locations, such as the radial artery.

Glands. A series of submucosal glands is found along the dorsal (vaginal) surface of the urethra (Fig. 2.7). Most of these are concentrated along the lower and middle thirds of the urethra, and the number of glands varies from individual to individual. Most urethral diverticula arise from cystic dilation of these glands and, as a result, urethral diverticula are found most commonly in the distal urethra along its vaginal surface. Since urethral diverticula have submucosal origins, this implies that the urethral fascia has become attenuated over a diverticulum. If a diverticulum is excised surgically, care should be taken to reapproximate this fascia once the lesion has been removed.

Epithelium. The urethral epithelium is hormonally sensitive. Stratified squamous epithelium is found in the distal urethra, while the bladder is lined

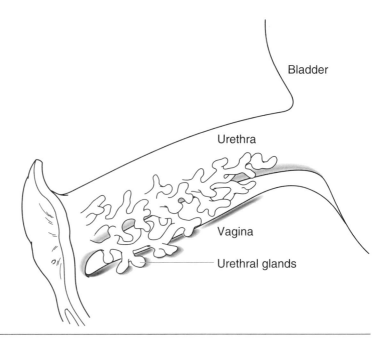

Figure 2.7 Location of the urethral glands between the urethra and the vagina.

by transitional epithelium. The line of demarcation between these two types of epithelia varies depending upon the hormonal status of the individual and other undefined factors. It can occur in the mid-urethra (as it often does after menopause) or it may extend well up into the bladder (as it often does during the reproductive years). So-called "granular trigonitis" is merely squamous metaplasia of the urinary trigone. It is quite common, particularly in women of reproductive age, and should not be regarded as a pathologic finding.

Ureter.

Abdominal Ureter. The course of the pelvic ureter is important to gynecologic surgeons and is given full consideration in the chapter on urologic injury later in this book. However, a few important anatomical landmarks will also be considered here. The ureter is a tubular viscus approximately 25 cm long, divided into abdominal and pelvic portions of equal length. Its small lumen is surrounded by an inner longitudinal and outer circular muscle layer whose coordinated contractions propel urine from the kidney to the bladder. In the abdomen, the ureter lies in the extraperitoneal connective tissue on the posterior abdominal wall and is crossed anteriorly by the left and right colic vessels.

Pelvic Ureter. After passing over the bifurcation of the internal and external iliac arteries just medial to the ovarian vessels, the ureter descends into the pelvis through a special connective tissue sheath (Fig. 2.8A, B). This sheath is attached to the peritoneum of the lateral pelvic sidewall and the medial leaf of the broad ligament. Because of these attachments, the ureter remains adherent to the peritoneum when the retroperitoneal space is entered during surgical dissection, and is not found laterally with the vessels. As it descends further in the pelvis, the ureter crosses under the uterine artery ("water flows under the bridge") as it passes through the cardinal ligament (Fig. 2.8B). A loose areolar plane permits its peristalsis here, creating a "tunnel" through the denser fibrous tissue. At this point the ureter lies along the anterolateral surface of the cervix at a distance of about 1 cm. It then comes to lie on the anterior vaginal wall and proceeds for a distance of about 1.5 cm through the wall of the bladder. During its course through the pelvis the ureter receives blood from the vessels that it passes, specifically the common iliac, internal iliac, uterine, and vesical arteries. A convoluted vessel can be seen running longitudinally along the outer surface of

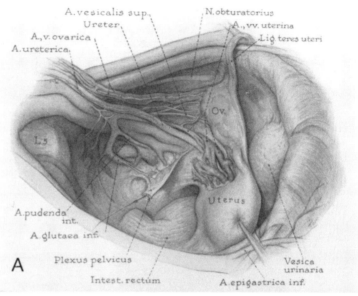

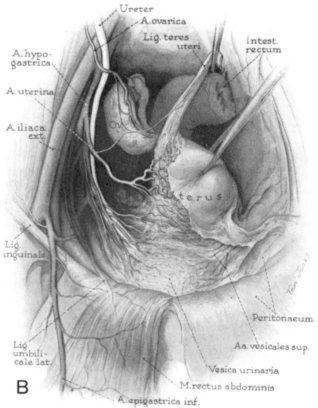

Figure 2.8   The course of the ureter in the pelvis. (*A*) Ureter on pelvic sidewall. (*B*) Ureter on anterior surface of bladder and in relationship to the uterine vessels. From Anson, An Atlas of Human Anatomy, Philadelphia: WB Saunders, 1950; 378–79.

TABLE 2.1. Hypotheses Concerning The Relationship Between Structure And Function In The Urinary Continence Mechanism

Structure	Hypothetical Function
Levator ani (through muscular attachment of urethral supports)	Tonic contraction helps maintain high position of vesical neck and contraction during cough augments vesical neck support; relaxes to change position of vesical neck relative to pubovesical muscles to facilitate micturition.
Connection to arcus tendineus (through fascial attachment of urethral supports)	Assists levators in support and limits the downward excursion of the vesical neck when the levators are relaxed, or overcome during cough
Internal sphincteric mechanism	Maintains vesical neck closure at rest and is necessary in addition to normal support for continence during cough
External sphincteric mechanism	Resting tone contributes to resting urethral pressure, and contraction prevents incontinence when marginally compensated proximal mechanism leaks
Mucosa and submucosal vasculature	Fills the space within the muscular wall of the urethra and forms a hermetic seal

the ureter, providing the blood supply which ultimately derives from these arteries. This intricate blood supply can be damaged by overaggressive ''stripping'' of tissues during attempts to expose the ureter during surgery.

Continence Mechanism   **Subdivisions of the Continence Mechanism.**   Table 2.1 lists the anatomic structures that might influence continence. Clinical observations suggest that these structures can be grouped into two different systems: (*a*) one which has to do with normal support of the lower urinary tract, and (*b*) one which has to do with urethral closure or constriction. Problems with urethral closure can be divided further into: (*1*) those that involve the proximal (internal) sphincter in the vesical neck, and (*2*) those that involve the external sphincter in the urethra.

The internal sphincter lies at the level of the vesical neck and includes the trigonal ring muscle and detrusor loops which have been discussed previously. In patients who have myelodysplasia or who have had previous surgery, the internal sphincter may be open at rest resulting in the development of stress incontinence despite normal anatomic support. The distal (external) urethral sphincter lies below the vesical neck and can be contracted voluntarily. This sphincteric unit includes the striated and smooth muscle of the urethra, its mucosa and submucosa. The distal urethral sphincter has an ancillary role in the maintenance of continence and only functions when urine gets past the vesical neck, as it sometimes does in some continent women. When this occurs, the distal sphincter acts as a ''backup system'' to ensure continence. In men the external urethral sphincter is strong enough to maintain continence by itself, but this is not generally true for women. Although the external sphincter of the female is not strong enough to do this alone, its action may help to minimize incontinence in patients with imperfect support of the urethra and bladder neck.

Location of Structures Involved in Continence.   The spatial relationships of the elements of the sphincteric mechanism are illustrated in Figure 2.9. The internal sphincter mechanism lies in the region where the urethral lumen traverses the bladder wall. This region is often referred to as the vesical neck. It comprises approximately the first 20% of the proximal length of the urethral lumen. The distal sphincteric mechanism is found along the next 20%–80% of the length

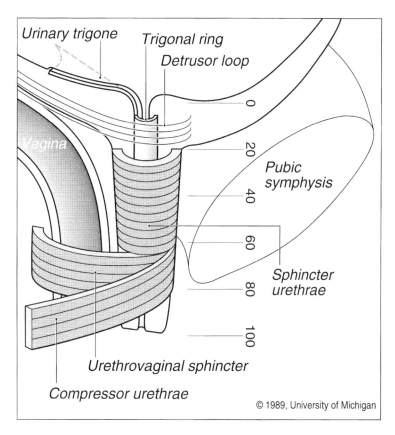

Figure 2.9   Diagrammatic representation showing the component parts of the internal and external sphincteric mechanisms and their locations. The sphincter urethrae, urethrovaginal sphincter and compressor urethrae are all parts of the striated urogenital sphincter muscle.

of the lumen. The bulkiest portion of the distal sphincteric mechanism is the striated urogenital sphincter.

The important structures that support the urethra and vesical neck are attached to the paraurethral tissues in the area from approximately 20%–60% of the urethral length. However, these structures may influence the function of the urethra and vesical neck well beyond this region.

The Nature of Urethral Support.   Poor support of the proximal urethra and vesical neck is by far the most common cause of stress urinary incontinence. Early clinical studies of this region attempted to analyze the relationship between the urethra and the pubic bones using static bead chain cystourethrograms. For some time it was thought that support in this region was provided by bands of connective tissue called the "pubourethral ligaments" which ran from the urethra to the pubic bones. However, it is now apparent that vesical neck support comes from the pubocervical fascia and its attachment to the arcus tendineus fascia pelvis. Extensive dissection in this area does not reveal any direct fibrous connection from the urethra to the pubis that could legitimately be called a "pubourethral ligament."

The urethra is *not* firmly attached to the pubic bones by the "pubourethral ligaments." This is clearly illustrated by the following examples:

- In the normal woman standing erect, the vesical neck lies *above* the attachment of the pubourethral ligaments to the pubic bones (Fig. 2.10).

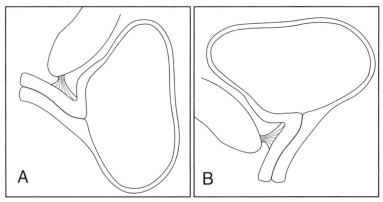

Figure 2.10   Relationship of the pubic bone, vesical neck, and "pubourethral ligaments." (*A*) In the normal woman lying supine, the "ligaments" appear to support the urethra from the pubic symphysis. However, when viewed in the standing woman (*B*) it is apparent that the vesical neck lies above the point of insertion of these "ligaments" so that they cannot be the only structure suspending the urethra.

Figure 2.11   Location and mobility of the normal vesical neck. Note that the vesical neck lies well above the insertion of the pubourethral ligaments into the lower portion of the pubic symphysis.

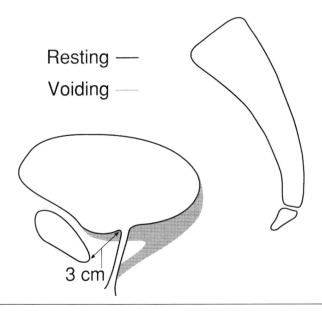

- The positions of the proximal urethra and vesical neck are mobile and are under voluntary control.

     Fluoroscopic studies of the bladder and vesical neck show that contraction of the levator ani muscles can elevate the vesical neck, while relaxation of these same muscles at the time of urination can obliterate the posterior urethrovesical angle (Fig. 2.11). This clearly demonstrates that the levator ani muscles have a role in controlling vesical neck support. The vesical neck normally rests at a level 2–3 cm above the insertion of the pubourethral ligaments, a position which can be explained by the origin and insertion of the levator muscles. The mobile upper portion of the urethra (which is influenced by the levators) joins the lower fixed portion of the urethra at a point 56% along the length of the urethra. This location has been termed the "knee of the urethra" and represents the region where the urethra enters the perineal membrane and is firmly fixed by this structure.

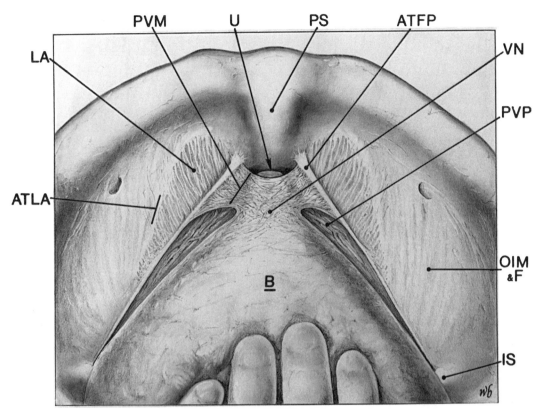

Figure 2.12 Space of Retzius (drawn from cadaver dissection). Pubovesical muscle (*PVM*) can be seen going from vesical neck (*VN*) to arcus tendineus fasciae pelvis (*ATFP*) and running over the paraurethral vascular plexus (*PVP*). *ATLA* = arcus tendineus levator ani; *B* = bladder; *IS* = ischial spine; *LA* = levator ani muscles; *OIM&F* = obturator internus muscle and fascia; *PS* = pubic symphysis; and *U* = urethra. Reprinted from DeLancey, Neurourol Urodynam 1989; 8:53–61, with permission of Alan R. Liss Publishers.

Structure of the Urethral Supportive Mechanism. Observations such as these indicate that urethral support involves both voluntary muscle, and connective tissue. The anterior vaginal wall and urethra arise from the urogenital sinus and are intimately connected. The support of the urethra does not depend on the attachment of the urethra itself to adjacent structures, but rather upon the connection of the vagina and endopelvic fascia to the muscles and fasciae of the pelvic wall.

The tissues that provide urethral support have two lateral attachments, one fascial and one muscular (Figs. 2.12 and 2.13). The paravaginal fascial attachments connect the periurethral tissues and the anterior vaginal wall to the arcus tendineus fasciae pelvis. The muscular attachments connect these same periurethral tissues to the medial border of the levator ani muscle. The position of the vesical neck is maintained by the fascial attachments and the normal resting tone of the levator ani muscles. Relaxation of these muscles at the onset of micturition allows the vesical neck to rotate downward until limited by the elasticity of the fascial attachments, while muscular contraction at the end of urination permits the vesical neck to resume its normal resting position.

The relationship between urethral support and sphincteric function is complex. Miniaturized electronic pressure transducers placed in the urethra demonstrate significant increases in intraurethral pressure during coughing. Many authors attribute these sudden rises in intraurethral pressure to the "transmission" of abdominal pressure to the "intra-abdominal" portion of the urethra. However,

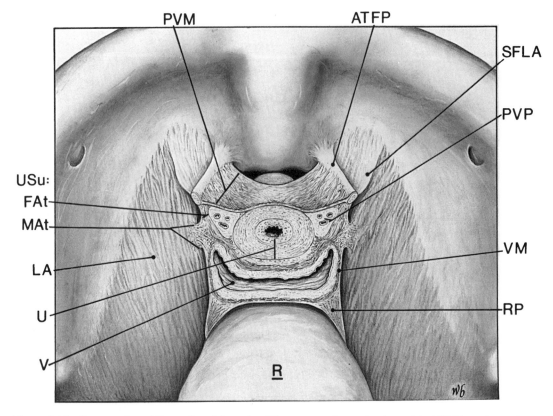

Figure 2.13 Cross-section of the urethra (*U*), vagina (*V*), arcus tendineus fasciae pelvis (*ATFP*), and superior fascia of levator ani (*SFLA*) just below the vesical neck (drawn from cadaver dissection). Pubovesical muscles (*PVM*) lie anterior to urethra and anterior and superior to paraurethral vascular plexus (*PVP*). The urethral supports (*USu*) ("the pubourethral ligaments") attach the vagina and vaginal surface of the urethra to the levator ani muscles (*MAt* = muscular attachment) and to the superior fascia of the levator ani (*FAt* = fascial attachment). Additional abbreviations: *R*, rectum; *RP*, rectal pillar; and *VM*, vaginal wall muscularis. Reprinted from DeLancey, Neurourol Urodynam 1989; 8:53–61, with permission of Alan R. Liss Publishers.

there is no clear anatomic separation between the abdominal and extra-abdominal urethra. There is no single structure which the urethra must pierce in order to exit the abdomen. Furthermore, the urethra is separated from the vaginal lumen throughout its entire length by the vaginal wall and the endopelvic fascia. The urethra is incorporated *into* the pelvic floor rather than piercing some single specific layer between the pelvic floor and the extra-pelvic cavity.

The series of events recorded by microtip transducer pressure catheters during a cough suggests that several pelvic floor structures are involved in maintaining urinary continence. If passive pressure transmission from the intra-abdominal cavity to the extra-abdominal urethra were the only factor involved in continence, then the pressures recorded during a cough would be maximal in the proximal urethra, but clinical measurements reveal that the highest pressure elevations occur in the distal urethra. These pressure elevations occur in a region from 60%–80% of urethral length where the compressor urethrae and urethrovaginal sphincter are located. This suggests that these muscles play an *active* role in augmenting urethral pressure here.

In addition, the pressure rise in the urethra seen during a cough is frequently higher than the pressure rise which is seen in the bladder, resulting in a "pressure transmission ratio" of *over* 100%. This must mean that factors other than passive pressure transmission are at work. Furthermore, the urethral pressure rise *pre-*

cedes the rise in intra-abdominal pressure, suggesting that contraction of the pelvic floor muscles is a natural compensatory reflex that helps maintain continence during periods of increased intra-abdominal pressure. The further fact that some patients have persistent stress incontinence despite adequate urethral suspension suggests that our current theories about the urethra's response to abdominal pressure increases are inadequate. Several recent studies have demonstrated a relationship between denervation injury to the pelvic floor, stress urinary incontinence, and genital prolapse. This new area of investigation may well prove helpful in furthering our understanding of the relationship between structure and function in the maintenance of urinary continence.

Pelvic Floor Anatomy

Since the urethra, bladder, and supporting structures of the pelvis are all part of the pelvic floor, their function cannot be understood without an understanding of the pelvic floor. The pelvic floor is a collection of tissues that spans the opening within the bony pelvis. It lies at the bottom of the abdominopelvic cavity and forms a supporting layer for the abdominal and pelvic viscera (Fig. 2.14). The best way to appreciate the structural role of the pelvic floor is to

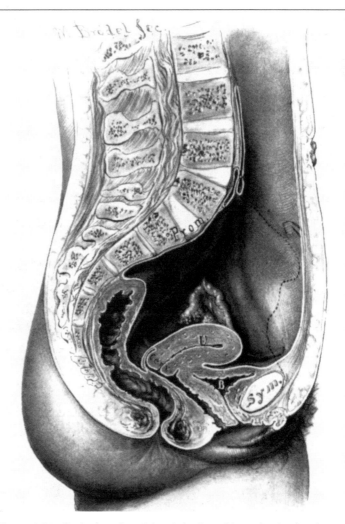

Figure 2.14   Sagittal section of the abdominopelvic cavity showing the position of the pelvic floor at the bottom of this space in the standing woman. From the Max Brödel Collection, Department of Art as Applied to Medicine, Johns Hopkins University.

place a hand on the pelvic contents through an abdominal incision and to press in a caudal direction. The muscles, ligaments, viscera, and fasciae that resist this downward force comprise the pelvic floor. This complex and multifaceted unit includes all of the structures that lie between the pelvic peritoneum and the vulvar skin. In addition to supporting the abdominal and pelvic organs and maintaining continence of urine and feces, the pelvic floor must also permit intercourse, parturition, and the evacuation of excretory products.

The pelvic floor has three supportive layers: the endopelvic fascia, the levator ani muscles, and the perineal membrane/external anal sphincter. The external genital muscles form a fourth layer, but these small muscles are more relevant to sexual function than to pelvic support.

The pelvic viscera are connected to the pelvic sidewalls by the endopelvic fascia (Fig. 2.15). This forms the first layer of the pelvic floor. Neither the fascia alone nor the organs themselves are responsible for the strength of this layer,

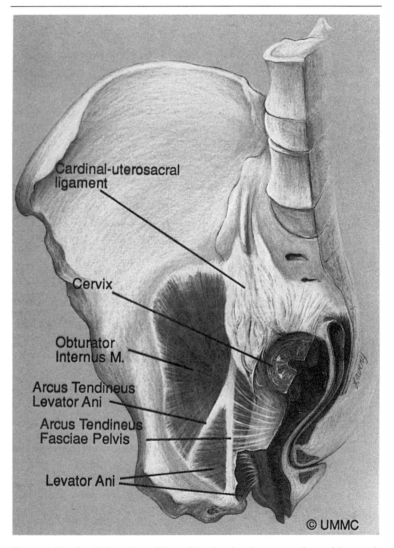

Figure 2.15 Sagittal section of the pelvis showing the connections of the cervix and vagina to the pelvic walls. Fibers going from the vagina to the arcus tendineus fasciae pelvis represent the pubocervical fascia. The corpus of the uterus has been removed, as have the bladder and urethra.

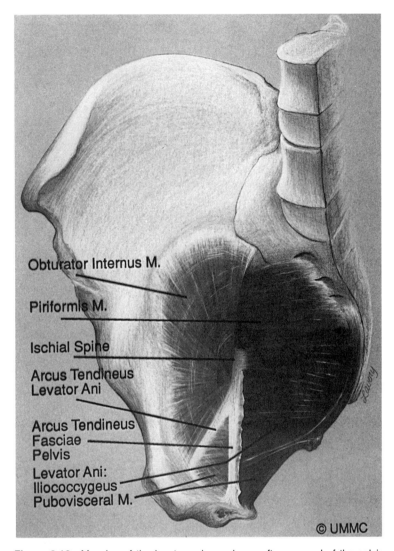

Obturator Internus M.

Piriformis M.

Ischial Spine

Arcus Tendineus
Levator Ani

Arcus Tendineus
Fasciae
Pelvis

Levator Ani:
Iliococcygeus
Pubovisceral M.

© UMMC

Figure 2.16 Muscles of the levator ani are shown after removal of the pelvic organs. Note the relatively horizontal shelf that they form.

which comes from the combination of these two structures. The second layer of the pelvic floor is a sheet-like muscular diaphragm (the pelvic diaphragm) that is formed by the levator ani muscles and their superior and inferior fasciae (Fig. 2.16). This muscle layer spans the opening in the bony pelvis in much the same way that the respiratory diaphragm spans the opening in the bottom of the rib cage. Although anatomy textbooks usually show this muscle in the shape of a deep bowl, in a living woman it is a horizontal sheet with an anterior midline cleft (the urogenital hiatus) through which the urethra, vagina, and rectum pass.

The third layer in the pelvic floor is the perineal membrane (urogenital diaphragm). It lies immediately below the levator ani muscles at the level of the hymenal ring (Fig. 2.17). In the male it forms an uninterrupted sheet that spans the anterior triangle of the pelvic outlet in front of the bituberous diameter. In the female, however, it is incomplete because of the large opening through which the vagina passes. The perineal membrane in the female therefore attaches the edges of the vagina to the ischiopubic ramus rather than forming a supportive

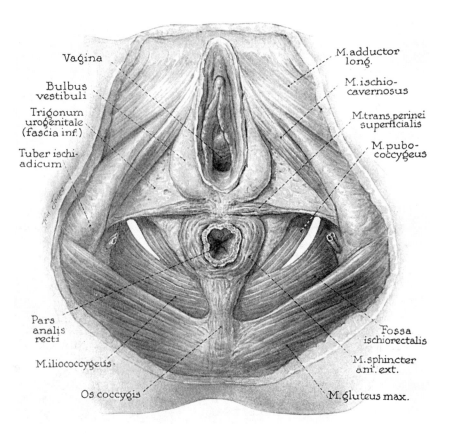

Vagina

Bulbus
vestibuli

Trigonum
urogenitale
(fascia inf.)

Tuber ischi-
adicum

Pars
analis
recti

M.iliococcygeus

Os coccygis

M.adductor
long.

M.ischio-
cavernosus

M.trans.perinei
superficialis

M.pubo-
coccygeus

Fossa
ischiorectalis

M.sphincter
ani.ext.

M.gluteus max.

Figure 2.17   Urogenital diaphragm (trigonum urogenitale) as seen from below. From Anson B. Human Anatomy. Philadelphia: W.B. Saunders, 1950; 361.

sheet as it does in the male. It also provides lateral attachments for the perineal body as well as support for the urethra.

In addition to these major supportive layers, a fourth layer lies below the perineal membrane. This consists of the ischiocavernosus, bulbocavernosus and superficial transverse perineal muscles. Although these muscles are frequently mentioned as being important in closure of the vaginal introitus, they are too small and weak to provide any substantial support. They appear to be related primarily to the vestibular bulb and clitoris, and probably function mainly in sexual responsiveness.

Before considering the details of the structure of the pelvic floor, a brief discussion of its function will be helpful. The primary support for the pelvic organs comes from the levator ani muscles. These muscles close off the pelvic floor so that structures that lie above them rest on their upper surface. This closure is remarkably effective. A small frictionless spherical object placed in the upper vagina would remain in place and would not fall out even though it was not attached to any surrounding structure. The uterus is held in the pelvis by the activity of these muscles in a similar fashion. The levator ani muscles close the pelvis below this level, and this muscular activity represents a major defense against the development of prolapse. The layer of endopelvic fascia and ligaments that attach the uterus and other pelvic organs to the pelvic sidewalls provide important support when the levator ani muscles are relaxed, but are not placed under tension as long as the muscles function normally and keep the pelvic floor closed.

The ligaments and fasciae must also support the pelvic organs when the levator ani muscles have been damaged. In this situation the muscles are no longer able to close the pelvic floor and the fascial attachments of the pelvic organs must prevent their prolapse. The perineal membrane lies below the levator ani muscles and attaches the lateral vaginal wall to the bony pelvis. It also assists in supporting the perineal body. This support is probably not important in the resting state since the perineal body can descend an inch during relaxation of the levator ani muscles. This suggests that the perineal membrane becomes active in support during relaxation of the levator ani, but not when the levators are in their normal state of contraction.

To What is the Pelvic Floor Attached?

The supportive layers described above fill the cylindrical space that lies within the pelvic bones. They attach to the pelvic sidewalls and span the area in between. The term ''pelvic sidewall'' will be used to refer to the vertical walls of the pelvis to which the pelvic floor attaches (Fig. 2.18). The structures that form these walls can be organized conceptually by thinking of a clock face set within the circular space of the pelvis, oriented so that 12 o'clock is located at the pubic symphysis. The region from 11 o'clock to 1 o'clock is formed by

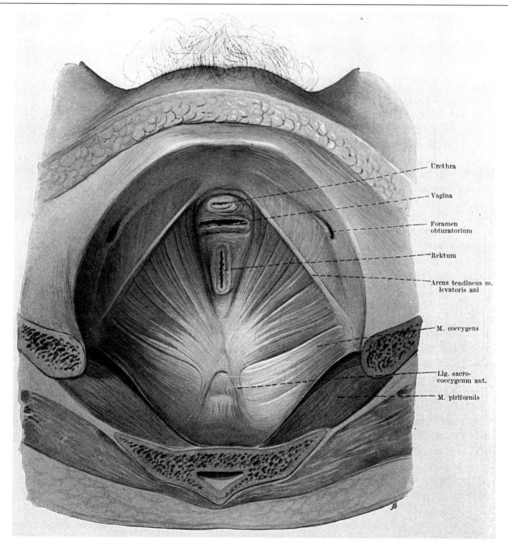

Urethra

Vagina

Foramen obturatorium

Rektum

Arcus tendineus m. levatoris ani

M. coccygeus

Lig. sacro-coccygeum ant.

M. piriformis

Figure 2.18   Pelvic walls and levator ani muscles (shown but not labeled). From Peham and Amreich. Operative Gynecology; 178.

*What Role Does the
Endopelvic Fascia Play in
Supporting the Pelvic
Viscera?*

the pubic bones and pubic symphysis. The region from 1 o'clock to 3 o'clock is the area where the arcus tendineus stretches over the obturator internus muscle, suspended between the pubic bone and the ischial spine. At the 3 o'clock position the bony pelvis is exposed in the region of the ischial spine and from this point to 5 o'clock the piriformis muscle occupies the greater sciatic foramen while the coccygeus muscle delimits its lower border. The posterior aspect of the pelvis from 5 o'clock to 7 o'clock is where the sacrum lies. The remainder of the circle is symmetrical with its opposite side. These walls form the points of origin for the pelvic floor. It is the connection between the pelvic floor and the pelvic walls that provides the structural support of the abdominopelvic cavity.

As previously mentioned, the first layer of the pelvic floor is formed by the endopelvic fascia and the pelvic organs that it connects to the pelvic walls. The endopelvic fascia is a fibromuscular tissue consisting of collagen, elastin, and smooth muscle. The structure of the endopelvic fascia varies considerably in different areas of the pelvis. The cardinal ligaments, for example, consist primarily of perivascular connective tissue while the rectal pillars contain more fibrous tissue but fewer blood vessels. These visceral ligaments and fasciae attach the pelvic organs laterally to the pelvic sidewalls. This combination of viscera and their lateral connections forms a major supportive layer for the pelvic structures (Fig. 2.19).

The upper vagina, cervix, and uterus are attached to the pelvic sidewalls by broad sheets of endopelvic fascia. These sheets of tissue are usually referred to as the cardinal and uterosacral ligaments. They originate over the region of the greater sciatic foramen and lateral sacrum, and insert into the side of the cervix as well as the upper one-third of the vagina. Although the cardinal and uterosacral ligaments have separate names, they are actually a single unit. The endopelvic fascia in this region consists mainly of perivascular collagen and elastin but also

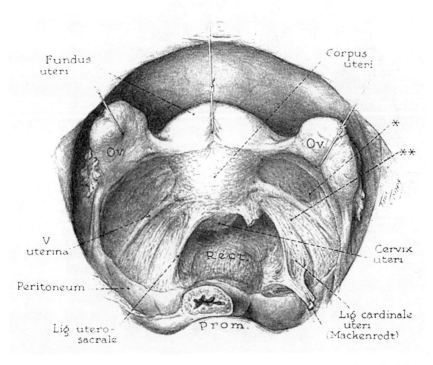

Figure 2.19 Uterus and supportive ligaments. (*, "Clear space" in broad ligament; **, cardinal ligament portion of cardinal/uterosacral ligament complex.) From Anson, An Atlas of Human Anatomy, Philadelphia: W.B. Saunders, 1950; 371.

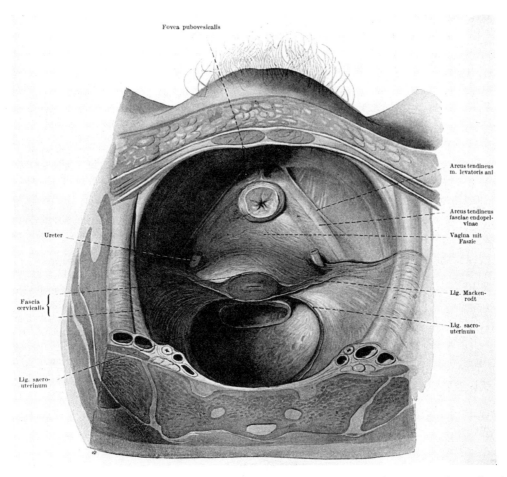

Fovea pubovesicalis

Arcus tendineus m. levatoris ani

Arcus tendineus fasciae endopelvinae

Vagina mit Faszie

Ureter

Lig. Mackenrodt

Fascia cervicalis

Lig. sacrouterinum

Lig. sacrouterinum

Figure 2.20   Upper layer of support showing the cervix after the uterine corpus has been removed as well as the vagina and their lateral attachments to the pelvic walls. From Peham and Amreich, Operative Gynecology; 183.

contains a considerable amount of nonvascular smooth muscle and the autonomic nerves to the uterus and bladder. These ligaments are usually described as running transversely from the pelvic sidewall to the vagina and cervix. Actually, they are oriented vertically and suspend the organs from above. The function of these structures cannot be understood unless they are considered with reference to the *standing* female rather than the anesthetized, supine patient on an operating room table. The vertical orientation of these ligaments in the standing woman will obviously provide better support than a transverse orientation.

Below the level of the uterus, the endopelvic fascia attaches the upper one-third of vagina to the pelvic sidewalls in the same way that the cardinal and uterosacral ligaments provide attachment for the uterine cervix (Fig. 2.20). The middle one-third of the vagina is attached more directly to the lateral pelvic sidewalls by the pubocervical and rectovaginal fasciae, which are nothing more than downward continuations of the cardinal and uterosacral ligaments. These structures attach the lateral margins of the vagina to the pelvic sidewalls on each side, stretching the vagina from one side of the pelvis to the other so that its anterior wall forms a horizontal sheet on which the bladder rests. The posterior attachment of the vagina to the pelvic sidewall creates a similar sheet that prevents the rectum from prolapsing forward. This is the rectovaginal fascia. Although the pubocervical and rectovaginal fasciae are sometimes thought to be separate sheets of tissue, they are actually only combinations of the vagina and its attachments to the pelvic sidewalls.

In the past these ligaments and fasciae were thought to be the most important elements of pelvic support. However, biomechanical analysis suggests that fibrous tissue is poorly suited to support the kind of constant load that gravity and intra-abdominal pressure place on the pelvic floor. The persistent misconception that fibrous ligaments provide the primary support for the pelvis comes from surgical practice, since these are the tissues which are used in operations to repair defective pelvic support. Although these empirical surgical procedures are generally successful, this does not mean that these tissues are normally the ones that hold the uterus, cervix and vagina in place. Neither does it mean, for that matter, that our current reconstructive operations are the best techniques that can be developed to take care of these problems. The levator ani are actually much better suited to supporting a constant load than is the pelvic connective tissue. Muscles are constructed to provide renewable, resilient, and flexible support and are not susceptible to the elongation and breakage that occurs in connective tissue under tension.

Levator Ani Muscles

Few clinicians have seen the levator ani muscles in their entirety and most find them difficult to comprehend. Dickinson observed that ''There is no muscle in the body whose form and function is more difficult to understand than the levator ani.'' Many of our misconceptions about these muscles come from the fact that their shape is greatly distorted by the embalming process. As a result, most of the illustrations in anatomical textbooks bear little resemblance to what clinicians encounter in the examining room.

The levator ani muscle has two different parts (Fig. 2.21). The first part is

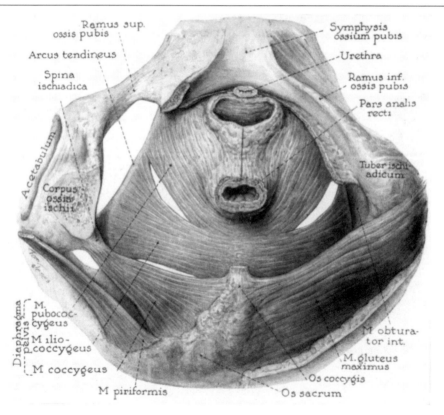

Figure 2.21 Levator ani muscles as seen from below. From Anson B. An Atlas of Human Anatomy. Philadelphia: W.B. Saunders, 1950; 366.

a thick, U-shaped band of muscle that arises from the pubic bones. It attaches to the lateral walls of the vagina and rectum and also sends fibers behind the rectum to act as a sling to pull the rectum toward the pubic bones. This part of the muscle is often called the pubococcygeus but will be referred to here as the pubovisceral muscle (see below). The second component of the levator ani is the iliococcygeus, a thin sheet of muscle that arises from the pelvic sidewall on either side and inserts into a midline raphe behind the rectum.

Several aspects of the structure of the pubovisceral muscle are important to pelvic floor function. Although it is a single continuous body of muscle, it has several portions. Some fibers originate in the pubic bone and attach to the vagina. These are called the pubovaginalis muscle. Other fibers go to the anus and rectum and are called, respectively, the puboanalis and puborectalis muscles. Some of the fibers of the latter also form a thick band that passes behind the rectum to form a sling that pulls the rectum forward towards the pubic bone. A few fibers in this area also go back to attach to the coccyx. This portion is called the pubococcygeus muscle. The overall term ''pubovisceral muscle'' more correctly describes the multifaceted nature of this muscular sling than the term ''pubococcygeus,'' which unfortunately draws attention to its relatively unimportant attachment to two immovable structures: the pubes and coccyx. The pubovisceral muscle has considerable bulk and can easily be palpated during pelvic examination as a distinct ridge just above the hymenal ring running along each lateral wall of the pelvis. This muscle functions to pull the rectum, vagina and urethra anteriorly towards the pubic bones, compressing their lumens closed.

The iliococcygeus muscle arises from the arcus tendineous levator ani which is a fibrous band suspended between the pubic bone and the ischial spine. It is a thin membranous sheet whose muscle fibers join in the midline as a median raphe behind the rectum. The iliococcygeus forms a horizontal sheet which helps support the pelvic viscera. It also has some function in pulling these organs anteriorly towards the pubic bones. The posterior margin of the muscle lies at the sacrospinious ligament where it fuses with the fibers of the coccygeus muscle. This latter muscle runs from the sacrum to the ischial spine and represents a vestigial remnant of the tail-wagging muscle of lower quadrupeds. Because it attaches to immovable structures in the human, it has no function. It is sometimes considered to be part of the pelvic diaphragm, but it is not part of the levator ani since it cannot elevate the anus.

The levator ani muscles exhibit constant resting tone, as does the external anal sphincter. In addition, the levators can be contracted to increase pelvic floor closure during increases in abdominal pressure. The resting tone of these muscles is poorly understood but is critical for pelvic support. The resting tone of these muscles is a phenomenon separate from their voluntary contraction. In many individuals these muscles are flaccid at rest even though they can be contracted forcefully upon command. Because the levator ani muscles maintain closure of the pelvic floor, the viscera that lie above them can rest on this muscular shelf. Constant adjustments in muscular activity maintain closure under many different circumstances and keep the pelvic ligaments from stretching. This muscular factor is critical in pelvic support because fibrous tissues elongate when subjected to constant tension.

Perineal Membrane

The perineal membrane (urogenital diaphragm) is a fibrous layer that spans the anterior triangle of the pelvic outlet (Fig. 2.17). It attaches laterally to the ischiopubic ramus approximately 1–2 cm above its lower (caudal) margin. The perineal membrane fuses medially with the sidewalls of the vagina and with the perineal body. Previous descriptions of the perineal membrane have usually depicted two layers of fascia with a layer of muscle sandwiched in between (the deep transverse perineal muscle). This concept is erroneous and has recently been corrected by Oelrich. Although the perineal membrane does have some smooth muscle and a few striated muscle fibers associated with it that could be termed the ''deep transverse perineal muscle,'' there is no superior diaphragmatic fascia as has previously been supposed. The anterior portion of the perineal membrane is intimately connected with the distal portion of the urethra and with the urethral musculature.

Although the perineal membrane is often thought to be a supportive layer for the pelvic organs, this is not possible in the female. The role of the perineal membrane is to attach the lateral walls of the vagina and the perineal body to the ischiopubic rami. When the levator ani muscles relax, the perineal membrane becomes tight and prevents further downward descent of the perineal body and the lateral vaginal walls beyond its elastic limits. It appears that the smooth and striated muscles of the perineal membrane act to keep it under some kind of resting tone. Since significant descent of the perineal body is possible during voluntary straining, connective tissue cannot be the main supportive layer at rest. The striated muscle in the anterior portion of the perineal membrane has specific functions related to the urethra.

Perineal Body

The mass of fibrous tissue that lies between the vagina and the anus is called the perineal body. This is an ill-defined mass of dense connective tissue without distinct borders. The connective tissue of the perineal body is fused anteriorly with the vaginal wall. Laterally it receives fibers from the bulbocavernous and superficial transverse perineal muscles as well as from the perineal membrane. A significant portion of what is clinically called the perineal body is actually the muscle of the external anal sphincter. The anococcygeal raphe connects the external anal sphincter to the coccyx and forms the dorsal attachment of the perineal membrane. Downward descent of the perineal body is limited by these attachments, especially the connections to the ischiopubic rami.

If the perineal body is incised or torn apart during vaginal birth and is not reapproximated, the support provided by the posterior portions of the perineal membranes is weakened. The interconnections of these two sides in the perineal body provides much of its support. Support of the pelvic outlet is maintained by the normal continuity of the perineal membrane as well as by the strong upward traction exerted by the levator ani muscles. The levator ani muscles are probably more important in maintaining outlet support than are the bulbocavernosus and superficial transverse perineal muscles because the bulk and strength of the levators is much greater than that of these other smaller, superficial muscles.

Although the perineal body is often said to make a substantial contribution to pelvic support, in fact it is relatively unimportant. Patients who have no perineal body at all as the result of a chronic unrepaired fourth degree obstetrical laceration virtually never have prolapse. Similarly, women who have a radical resection of the anus and rectum for cancer have had the entire perineal body removed; these women likewise do not develop significant problems with prolapse. The perineal body can move backwards towards the sacrum 3–4 cm when a weighted speculum is placed in the posterior vagina. This fact indicates that the position of the perineal body is determined by the levator ani muscle rather than by any inherent importance of its own.

How the Continence Mechanism Works

In the normal individual, the urethral lumen is held closed at the level of the vesical neck by the muscle of the trigonal ring and the vesical neck muscle of the detrusor loop. These muscles are controlled by the sympathetic nervous system, acting through α-adrenergic receptors located in this area. Distal to the vesical neck, the striated urogenital sphincter and sparse circular smooth muscle maintain urethral closure at rest. During increases in abdominal pressure—such as those generated by coughing, sneezing, or Valsalva—the urethra must be kept closed, maintaining urethral pressure higher than bladder pressure, or urine loss will occur. This process requires normal function of both the vesical neck and the urethral supports. The urethra can be held closed during elevations of intra-abdominal pressure because the strong connections of the suburethral fascia to the arcus tendineous fascia pelvis and levator ani muscles provide a stable platform against which the lumen can be compressed. However, this closure mechanism will only be effective if the vesical neck keeps the proximal urethra closed.

If the vesical neck is open, urine lying in the proximal urethra will escape before the urethra can be compressed. During a cough, the striated urogenital sphincter muscle contracts to retard urine that may pass beyond the primary continence mechanism at the vesical neck. This mechanism is not, by itself, adequate to maintain perfect continence during rises in abdominal pressure, but helps to minimize stress incontinence. If patients with imperfect urethral support develop damage to the vesical neck, this damage can turn relatively minor problems of support into a major problem with incontinence.

Practical Neurophysiology of the Lower Urinary Tract

Bladder function cannot be understood without reference to neurophysiology. This does not mean that the practicing clinician must master all of the minutiae of neurophysiology and memorize all of the proposed neural pathways involved in bladder control in order to take care of patients with lower urinary tract complaints. It does mean that a basic familiarity with the neurophysiology of the lower urinary tract is necessary for understanding what may be going on in an individual patient. Without this background the physician cannot understand the effect of drugs on the urinary tract. This applies both to the unexpected side effects of seemingly routine medications which may be contributing to a patient's problems, as well as to the desired effects of drugs which are used to achieve a given therapeutic end. The purpose of this section is to lay down a "bare bones" outline of the essentials of lower urinary tract neurophysiology so that the practicing physician will have a frame of reference to use in dealing with patient problems.

The bladder is composed primarily of smooth muscle. It is an involuntary organ which is nonetheless under voluntary control. This makes it unique among the organs of the body. This muscular organ relaxes to permit urine storage and contracts to expel it. During the filling phase of the storage-and-emptying cycle, the bladder receives urine from the ureters and *accommodates* to accept this increasing urine volume without an appreciable rise in bladder pressure. The bladder is normally a *low pressure system*. During normal bladder filling there is also a gradual increase in urethral resistance which helps to prevent urine loss as the bladder fills. This can be shown by electromyography of the urethra and pelvic floor during bladder filling, which demonstrates increased muscle fiber recruitment. As the bladder fills, the detrusor should remain inactive with no involuntary contractions. When the bladder has filled to a specific volume, tension receptors in the bladder sense fullness and, when an appropriate time and place present themselves, a voluntary micturition reflex is initiated. This reflex should lead to complete bladder emptying. This is accomplished by relaxation of the pelvic floor and a resultant decrease in urethral resistance, accompanied by a sustained detrusor contraction which forces urine out of the bladder.

What can go wrong with this seemingly simple system? The bladder can lose its accommodation and become a high pressure system. This can occur due to either a change in the normal visco-elastic properties of the bladder (from such things as tuberculosis or radiation fibrosis) or disrupted neural control, such as is seen in various congenital or neurologic disease states. As the bladder becomes a high-pressure system, back-pressure builds up and is transmitted to the upper tracts, leading to hydronephrosis and kidney damage. If involuntary detrusor contractions develop during bladder filling, due either to a neurologic lesion (detrusor hyperreflexia) or to idiopathic escape of the bladder from cortical suppression (detrusor instability), incontinence will develop. If sensation is increased, patients will develop a small functional bladder capacity which they must empty frequently due to irritation or pain. If sensation is decreased, patients run the risk of bladder overdistension and subsequent deterioration of voiding function. If the bladder and urethra cannot compensate for increases in intraabdominal pressure, urine loss occurs and the patient develops stress incontinence.

Stress incontinence may occur for two reasons. The most common cause is loss of bladder neck and urethral support, leading to displacement of these structures during conditions of increased intra-abdominal pressure (coughing, sneezing, physical activity, etc.). The second, less common, cause is from intrinsic weakness of the sphincteric mechanism itself. Both causes may have a neurologic component since neurologic injury may lead to loss of tone in the supporting muscles as well as in the sphincter itself.

If detrusor contractility is uncoordinated, poor, or absent, the bladder will not empty properly. Similarly, if the pelvic floor does not relax, or worse, if active muscular contraction occurs instead of muscle relaxation, voiding dysfunction may occur. An inability to relax the muscles of the pelvic floor may occur in anxious or nervous patients (particularly during urodynamic studies) or in patients with pelvic floor pain, such as women who have recently had a traumatic vaginal delivery or who have undergone perineal surgery for correction of a rectocele. In some diseases—such as multiple sclerosis—the striated urethral sphincter may actually contract simultaneously with the detrusor during voiding. This condition is called *detrusor-sphincter-dyssynergia* and may result in terrible voiding problems. The pathologic possibilities mentioned in this brief review may occur in many combinations, presenting the clinician with a vast array of potential lower urinary tract problems.

Performance of the seemingly simple processes of urine storage and bladder emptying may thus be seen to require the integration of complex neurologic pathways which are incompletely understood at the present time. The important clinical point is to understand that this seemingly straightforward physiologic process requires an intact *neurourologic axis.* A set of complex pathways runs from the cerebral cortex, down through the mid-brain where the *pontine micturition center* is located, through the spinal cord (particularly the *sacral spinal cord*), to the bladder and urethra. Neurologic lesions anywhere along this axis can affect bladder function. This is why a neurologic screening examination is important in patients with lower urinary tract complaints, particularly in patients with voiding difficulty or incontinence whose problem develops in combination with other neurologic symptoms.

There is little point in presenting a highly complex and detailed discussion of neuroanatomy and the proposed pathways by which these processes are carried out. Most of our detailed knowledge of these areas has come from research on lower animals, particularly cats, which has been extrapolated to human beings. There are many detailed theories as to precisely how the individual parts of this system are interrelated and controlled, but no model has been generally accepted as correct. Rather than forcing the reader to memorize detailed hypothetical pathways which have not been proven in human beings, it seems more logical for our purposes to concentrate on some basic principles of neurophysiology which affect the function of the lower urinary tract.

Practical Neuroanatomy of the Lower Urinary Tract

The lower urinary tract receives innervation from three sources: the *sympathetic* and *parasympathetic* divisions of the *autonomic nervous system,* and the neurons of the *somatic nervous system.* The autonomic nervous system consists of all efferent pathways with ganglionic synapses which lie outside the central nervous system. The autonomic nervous system deals largely with internal visceral control. The sympathetic division of the autonomic nervous system appears to control urine storage, while the parasympathetic division appears to control bladder emptying. The somatic nervous system deals mainly with external bodily neuromuscular control and, as a result, plays only a peripheral role in lower urinary tract function. Somatic innervation is important mainly in regard to the musculature of the pelvic floor and the striated external urethral sphincter.

Neural impulses in both the somatic and autonomic nervous systems move along nerve fibers and affect end organs through the release of *neurotransmitters.* The classic concept of neurotransmission describes a neural impulse which leads to the release of a neurotransmitter at a synapse. This neurotransmitter then binds to a receptor site on the other side of the synapse and triggers a postganglionic effector signal which leads to a discrete activity, such as bladder contraction.

The sympathetic nervous system originates in the thoracolumbar spinal cord. Efferent impulses to the lower urinary tract from the sympathetic nervous system originate in the intermediolateral nuclei of the thoracolumbar spinal cord in segments from T_{11} through L_2 or L_3. They then traverse the lumbar sympathetic ganglia and join the presacral nerve (superior hypogastric plexus). The sympathetic efferents divide into two branches at this point and run in the left and right hypogastric "nerves," which are really elongated nerve plexuses. The hypogastric nerves are joined by the parasympathetic pelvic nerves bilaterally in the inferior hypogastric plexuses of Frankenhauer, from which they spread out to innervate the pelvic organs, including the lower urinary tract, the rectum, and the internal genital organs.

The parasympathetic nervous system originates in the sacral spinal cord. The parasympathetic motor innervation of the lower urinary tract arises in the intermediolateral cell column of the sacral spinal cord in segments S_2–S_4. These fibers exit the ventral nerve roots as the pelvic nerve, running to Frankenhauer's plexus and the pelvic organs. The hypogastric and pelvic nerves also carry afferent autonomic nerve impulses to synapses in the dorsal column of lumbosacral spinal cord.

In addition to its parasympathetic autonomic connections, the sacral spinal cord gives rise to the somatic innervation of the pelvic floor, urethra, and external anal sphincter. The pudendal nerve originates in cord segments S_2–S_4 and innervates the striated urinary sphincter and the striated external anal sphincter. Sensation in the perineum is controlled by sensory fibers which also connect with the sacral spinal cord at this level. This is why examination of perineal sensation, assessment of anal sphincter and pelvic floor tone, and evaluation of the bulbocavernosus and cough reflexes are all relevant to lower urinary tract function. All have intimate relationships to the sacral spinal cord, where the basic sacral micturition reflex is mediated. Figure 2.22 gives a schematic outline of the autonomic and somatic neuroanatomy relevant to bladder control, and shows the sites of action of many common pharmacologic agents (see below).

Classically, the autonomic nervous system has been regarded as a two-neuron system comprised of *preganglionic* neurons arising in the central nervous system and synapsing in autonomic *ganglia* outside the central nervous system. *Postganglionic* neurons then originate in these ganglia and run to the peripheral end organs which they innervate.

The ganglia of the sympathetic nervous system are located adjacent to the spinal cord, between these paravertebral ganglia and the end organ, or adjacent to or within the end organs. Parasympathetic ganglia are all located in or near to the innervated end organ. Some sympathetic ganglia located near parasympathetic ganglia appear to have additional "gatekeeping" functions regulating parasympathetic ganglion transmission. Afferent (sensory) fibers from end organs such as the bladder return to the central nervous system through the peripheral autonomic ganglia.

Recently Elbadawi has reviewed the autonomic innervation of the lower urinary tract. According to him the muscular innervation of the lower urinary tract is derived almost exclusively from postganglionic neurons of the *urogenital short neuron system*. The innervation of the lower urinary tract appears to emanate from peripheral ganglia located only a short distance from their end organs (hence the "short neuron system"). These ganglia appear to be composed of three cell types: cholinergic peripheral neurons, adrenergic peripheral neurons, and small intensely fluorescent cells (SIF) which perform important modulating roles regulating interganglionic vasomotor function and ganglionic neuroimpulse transmission. In addition, there are complex intraganglionic networks of cholinergic and adrenergic fibers. Thus, the efferent autonomic pathways of the lower urinary tract do not necessarily conform to the classic "two neuron" model which has been described. There appears to be a wide variety of modulating synaptic relays. In addition, postganglionic neurons do not necessarily terminate

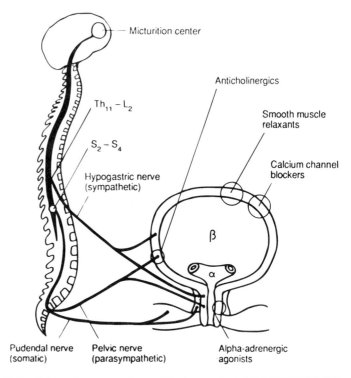

Figure 2.22   Schematic neuroanatomy of the lower urinary tract, with major sites of drug action. From Sourander LB. Gerontology 1990; 3(Suppl 2):19–26, copyright Karger S., with permission.

Neurotransmitters

in the peripheral end organ, but may actually terminate within the ganglia of some systems. Increasing scientific work is revealing that the neural control of the lower urinary tract is more complex than had previously been thought.

The autonomic nervous system affects end organs by the release of neurotransmitters. "Classical" neurotransmission involves a neural impulse which leads to the release of a neurotransmitter at a synapse. The neurotransmitter then binds to a receptor site on the other side of the synapse and triggers a postganglionic effector signal which leads to a discrete activity, such as bladder contraction—a simple, straightforward concept. Traditionally two neurotransmitters have been described in the autonomic nervous system: acetylcholine and norepinephrine. Acetylcholine is also the major neurotransmitter in the somatic nervous system, which is important in contraction of the striated urogenital sphincter and the muscles of the pelvic floor.

Neurotransmitters of the Parasympathetic Nervous System

The autonomic nervous system has preganglionic and postganglionic sites of neurotransmission. In both the sympathetic and parasympathetic systems, the preganglionic neurotransmitter is acetylcholine. In the parasympathetic (bladder motor) system, the postganglionic neurotransmitter is also acetylcholine. The detrusor muscle of the bladder is heavily populated with cholinergic receptors (Fig. 2.23). Acetylcholine is, therefore, the main neurotransmitter involved in bladder contraction which occurs in response to parasympathetic nervous stimulation. This is why nearly all drugs used to reduce unstable or hyperreflexic detrusor activity have anticholinergic properties. Cholinergic receptors are further subdivided into two classes: *muscarinic* receptors and *nicotinic* receptors. Nicotinic receptors do not appear to exist in any significant form in the lower urinary tract. For all practical purposes, therefore, the autonomic cholinergic receptors involved in bladder function can be regarded as muscarinic receptors. These can be blocked by atropine.

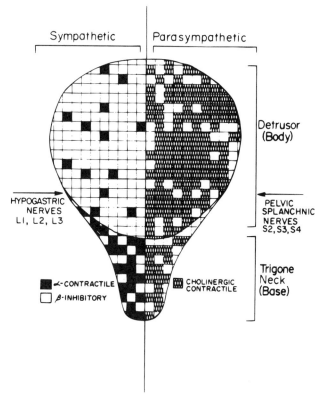

Figure 2.23 Distribution of cholinergic and adrenergic receptors in the bladder and urethra. From Rohner TJ Jr. In Hinman F. (Ed). Benign Prostatic Hypertrophy. New York: Springer-Verlag,1983; 361–72, with permission.

The parasympathetic nervous system appears to control the voiding phase of the micturition cycle. Stimulation of the pelvic nerves produces a strong, sustained bladder contraction which leads to bladder emptying. Drugs with anticholinergic properties such as propantheline, dicyclomine, imipramine, oxybutynin, and others are used in attempts to suppress overactive detrusor contractions by blocking acetylcholine. The use of cholinergic stimulating drugs such as bethanechol chloride does not appear to be clinically useful in promoting bladder emptying even though these drugs will cause bladder muscle strips to contract in a physiology laboratory.

Neurotransmitters of the Sympathetic Nervous System

As in the parasympathetic nervous system, the preganglionic neurotransmitter in the sympathetic nervous system is also acetylcholine. However, postganglionic neurotransmission in the sympathetic nervous system is different. Rather than acetylcholine, the main neurotransmitter here is a catecholamine, norepinephrine, which affects adrenergeric receptors. Adrenergic receptors are further subdivided into *α-receptors* and *β-receptors*. These receptors have different distributions in the lower urinary tract (Fig. 2.23). α-Receptors regulate vasoconstriction and smooth muscle contraction. Within the lower urinary tract they are distributed mainly in the urethra and bladder neck. α-Stimulating drugs such as phenylpropanolamine, ephedrine, and pseudoephedrine will all increase the tone of the urethra and bladder neck by stimulating smooth muscle contraction at these sites. For this reason these drugs have been used in the pharmacologic treatment of stress incontinence in women. Their constricting property at these locations is also the reason why these drugs are contraindicated in men with prostatic hypertrophy, in whom they may cause acute urinary retention. α-Blocking drugs, such as phenoxybenzamine and prazosin (Minipress) will relax the outlet and may cause urinary incontinence. β-Receptors in the urinary tract appear to modulate smooth muscle relaxation, and tend to cluster in the bladder body, as opposed to the bladder base and bladder neck (Fig. 2.23). β-Stimulants tend to cause bladder relaxation. For example, acute urinary retention may occasionally be seen in pregnant women who are given high doses of terbutaline (a β-stimulant) as treatment for premature labor. Unfortunately, β-agonists do not appear to be clinically useful in treating detrusor instability.

The role of the sympathetic nervous system in the control of the lower urinary tract is somewhat controversial and incompletely understood. The parasympathetic system appears to control bladder emptying, and it appears that the sympathetic system helps regulate the storage phase of the micturition cycle. This appears to occur by (*a*) inhibition of bladder contractility through sympathetic blockade of parasympathetic ganglion transmission; (*b*) increasing the accommodation of the bladder through stimulation of β-receptors in the bladder body; and (*c*) increasing outlet resistance through stimulation of α-receptors in the urethra and bladder neck.

Other Neurotransmitters

The phenomenon of atropine resistance—that is, the fact that all bladder contractile activity cannot be blocked by atropine, even with massive doses—has led to the postulation of a *nonadrenergic noncholinergic (NANC)* parasympathetic neurotransmitter system which is responsible for part of the neurotransmission in the bladder. Research work in this area has led to the development of an extensive list of naturally occurring substances in both the peripheral and central nervous systems which affect bladder function, including opioids, vasoactive intestinal polypeptide (VIP), dopamine, serotonin, γ-amino butyric acid (GABA), and a host of others. Some of these substances may well fit the definition of a "classic" neurotransmitter which is released at a synapse in response to a neural stimulus and interacts with a postsynaptic receptor, but many of these substances are probably *neuromodulators* which "fine tune" the effects of neurotransmitters at central and peripheral sites. These developments have significant potential implications for the future development of drugs affecting nervous control mechanisms in the urinary tract and elsewhere.

Central Nervous System Influences and the Micturition Reflex

Micturition is a reflex event which occurs largely in the peripheral autonomic nervous system if permitted to do so by the central nervous system. It is useful to think of this as taking place at a "micturition threshold," a bladder volume at which reflex detrusor contractions occur. The threshold volume which triggers the reflex is variable, not fixed, and can be altered depending upon the balance of the contributions between peripheral sensory afferents coming from the bladder, perineum, and colon, and input from higher centers in the central nervous system. This idea of a floating threshold which can be altered or reset by various influences is key to understanding normal micturition and the effects that neuropathology and other factors can have on it.

There is enormous disagreement among researchers over much of the specific neurophysiology involved in bladder control. The neurophysiology of the bladder in the decerebrate cat is better understood than that of the normal human being. It appears that the most fundamental micturition reflex is a spinal reflex occurring largely in the sacral micturition center at S_2–S_4. This reflex is subject to a variety of influences emanating from higher centers in the nervous system and modulated at several levels as they descend. These influences may permit and enhance the micturition reflex, thereby facilitating complete normal bladder emptying, or they may inhibit the reflex completely until an appropriate time and place for bladder emptying arise. Neuropathology at almost any level of the neurourologic axis may thus have adverse effects on lower urinary tract function.

The spinal cord itself has complex patterns of facilitation and inhibition, many of which are poorly understood. While a detailed description of the ascending afferent and descending efferent pathways is beyond the scope of this chapter, it should be understood that there are multiple complex facilitative and inhibitory interactions which take place among these pathways at the spinal cord level. It is clear that the spinal cord does not function merely as a passive "cable" connecting the lower urinary tract with the higher centers.

Above the level of the cord the most important facilitative motor center for micturition is located in the pontine-mesencephalic gray matter of the brain stem. It is believed that this "pontine micturition center" serves as the final common pathway for all bladder motor neurons. The region known as Barrington's Center in the anterior pons is the main dispatch center for facilitory impulses to the bladder. Transection of the tracts below this level leads to disturbed bladder emptying, while destruction of the regions above this level leads to detrusor hyperreflexia.

The cerebellum modulates both afferent sensory impulses from the bladder and pelvic floor as well as efferent impulses going to the bladder. The cerebellum serves as a major center for coordinating pelvic floor relaxation and the rate, range, and force of detrusor contraction. There are extensive cerebellar interconnections with the brain stem reflex centers. Above this level, the basal ganglia appear to have an inhibitory function on detrusor contractility. This helps explain the detrusor hyperactivity frequently seen in Parkinson's disease, which heavily involves the basal ganglia. The cerebral cortex, particularly the frontal lobes and the genu of the corpus callosum, exert primarily inhibitory influences on the micturition reflex. Thus, facilitative influences which release inhibition occur in the upper cortex and permit the anterior pontine micturition center to send efferent impulses through the spinal cord allowing a sacral reflex micturition reflex to occur with resultant bladder emptying. A schematic representation of the neurophysiology of lower urinary tract control and the disturbances which can arise from lesions at each level is given in Figure 2.24.

Practical Neuropharmacology

The practical neuropharmacology of bladder control is summarized in Figure 2.22. Drugs can exert neurophysiologic effects at all levels of the nervous system, from high CNS effects (such as may occur with the tricyclic antidepressants used in treating nocturnal enuresis) to the end organ effector level in the bladder. However, most of the drugs used in treating disturbances of micturition or urine storage work at the peripheral level of the bladder rather than higher up in the central nervous system. Anticholinergic drugs (such as propantheline) undoubtedly have some ganglionic blocking properties in both the sympathetic and parasympathetic systems, but exert their influences primarily at the bladder synaptic level. These drugs decrease the force of detrusor contractions.

Other drugs which work at the level of the bladder muscle include spasmolytic or direct muscle relaxing drugs such as oxybutynin (Ditropan), and calcium channel blockers such as terodiline (Micturin). Both of these drugs, which are used in the treatment of detrusor overactivity, also have potent anticholinergic effects. Although there are theoretical reasons for thinking that cholinergic agonists like bethanechol chloride (Urecholine) would be useful in stimulating detrusor contractions, these drugs have been very disappointing in clinical practice.

Drugs with α- or β-adrenergic interactions will affect the sympathetic nervous system. α-Agonists such as phenylpropanolamine, ephedrine, and pseudoephedrine, work to stimulate contractility in the urethra and bladder neck and have been used to treat stress incontinence pharmacologically. α-Antagonists, such as phenoxybenzamine or prazosin (Minipress) will lower tone in this region and may cause incontinence. Because they lower outlet resistance, these drugs may have some utility in the management of voiding disorders and in treating those patients with "urethral syndrome" whose condition is due to urethral spasm. The role of β-mimetic or β-blocking drugs is less sure. Although β-agonists like terbutaline should have a relaxant effect on the detrusor muscle, use of these drugs in treating detrusor overactivity has not been successful.

Since prostaglandins cause smooth muscle contractions, attempts have been made to utilize these drugs to enhance bladder emptying after surgery. These attempts have not been very successful. Anecdotal success has been reported in treating women with urge-symptoms occurring around the time of menstruation using prostaglandin synthetase inhibitors, but these drugs would appear to be

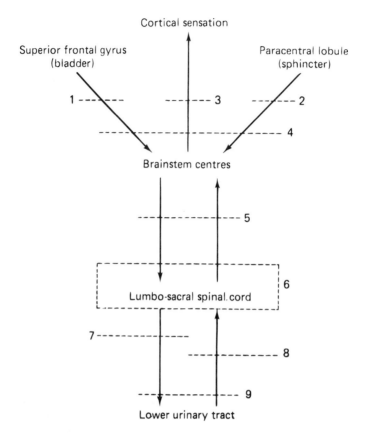

Figure 2.24 Simplified scheme of the interaction of various levels of the nervous system in micturition. From Torrens M.. In Torrens M. and Morrison JFB (Eds). The Physiology of the Lower Urinary Tract. New York: Springer-Verlag, 1987; 333–50, with permission.

The locations of certain possible nervous lesions are denoted by numbers and explained as follows:

1. Lesions which isolate the superior frontal gyrus prevent voluntary postponement of voiding. If sensation remains intact this produces urge incontinence. If the lesion is larger there will be additional loss of social concern about incontinence.

2. Lesions isolating the paracentral lobule, sometimes associated with a hemiparesis, will cause spasticity of the urethral sphincter and urinary retention. This will be painless if sensation is abolished. Minor degrees of this syndrome may cause difficulty in initiating micturition.

3. Pathways of sensation are not known accurately. In theory, an isolated lesion of sensation above the brain stem would lead to unconscious incontinence. Defective central conduction of sensory information would explain nocturnal enuresis.

4. Lesions above the brain stem centers lead to involuntary voiding that is coordinated with sphincter relaxation.

5. Lesions below the brain stem centers but above the lumbosacral spinal cord lead, after a period of bladder paralysis associated with spinal shock, to involuntary reflex voiding that is not coordinated with sphincter relaxation (detrusor-sphincter-dyssynergia).

6. Lesions that destroy the lumbosacral spinal cord or completely destroy the nervous connections between the central and peripheral nervous system result in a paralyzed bladder which contracts only weakly in an autonomous fashion because of its remaining ganglionic innervation. However, if the lumbar sympathetic outflow is preserved in the presence of destruction of the conus medullaris and/or of the cauda equina, then there may be some residual sympathetic tone in the bladder neck which may be sufficient to be obstructive.

7. A lesion of the efferent fibers alone leads to a bladder of decreased capacity and decreased compliance associated experimentally with an increased number of adrenergic nerves.

8. A lesion confined to the afferent fibers produces a bladder with increased compliance and capacity.

9. As there are ganglion cells in the bladder wall it is technically impossible to decentralize the bladder completely, but congenital absence of the bladder ganglia may exist producing megacystis.

useful only on a case-by-case basis. Prostaglandins may play a local neuromodulating role in bladder function.

Occasionally patients with detrusor-sphincter dyssynergia who have striated urethral sphincter contractions occurring simultaneously with a detrusor contraction will benefit from muscle relaxants such as diazepam. However, many patients with this condition will have complex neurologic problems which require multi-agent pharmacotherapy to control their other neurologic symptoms. These patients will often find it necessary to use clean intermittent self-catheterization to empty their bladders.

The neurophysiology and neuropharmacology of the lower urinary tract is quite complicated and poorly understood at the present time. However, a solid understanding of the basic principles of neural activity and bladder physiology will give practicing clinicians a firm foundation on which to pursue the clinical management of their patients, and will help them realize when specialist neurologic or neurourologic consultation is needed.

SUGGESTED READING

Anatomy and Development of the Urethra and Bladder

Berkow SG. The corpus spongiosum of the urethra: Its possible role in urinary control and stress incontinence in women. Am J Obstet Gynecol 1953; 65:346–51.

DeLancey JOL. Correlative study of paraurethral anatomy. Obstet Gynecol 1986; 68:91–97.

DeLancey JOL. Structural aspects of the extrinsic continence mechanism. Obstet Gynecol 1988; 72:296–301.

DeLancey JOL. The pubovesical ligament, a separate structure from the urethral supports ("Pubo-Urethral Ligaments"). Neurourol Urodynam 1989; 8:53–61.

Droes JThPM. Observations on the musculature of the urinary bladder and urethra in the human foetus. Br J Urol 1974; 46:179.

Gosling JA, Dixon JS, Critchley HOD, Thompson SA. A comparative study of the human external sphincter and periurethral levator ani muscles. Br J Urol 1981; 53: 35–41.

Gosling JA. The structure of the female lower urinary tract and pelvic floor. Urol Clin N Am 1985; 12:207.

Huffman J. Detailed anatomy of the paraurethral ducts in the adult human female. Am J Obstet Gynecol 1948; 55: 86–101.

Huisman AB. Aspects on the anatomy of the female urethra with special relation to urinary continence. Contrib Gynecol Obstet 1983; 10:1–31.

Krantz KE. The anatomy of the urethra and anterior vaginal wall. Am J Obstet Gynecol 1951; 62:374–86.

Oelrich TM. The striated urogenital sphincter muscle in the female. Anat Rec 1983; 205:223–32.

Ricci J, Lisa JR, Thom CH. The female urethra: A histologic study as an aid in urethral surgery. Am J Surg 1950; 79: 499–05.

Clinical and Physiologic Observations about the Lower Urinary Tract

Constantinou CE. Resting and stress urethral pressures as a clinical guide to the mechanism of continence in the female patient. Urol Clin N Am 1985; 12:247.

Elbadawi A. Neuromuscular mechanisms of continence. In Yalla SV, McGuire EJ, Elbadawi A, Blaivas JG (Eds). Neurourology and Urodynamics. 3–35. New York: Macmillan Publishing Company, 1989.

Enhorning G. Simultaneous recording of the intravesical and intra-urethral pressures. Acta Obstet Gynecol Obstet Suppl 1961; 276:1–68.

Hilton P, Stanton SL. Urethral pressure measurement by microtransducer: The results in symptom-free women and in those with genuine stress incontinence. Br J Obstet Gynecol 1983; 90:919.

Hodgkinson CP. Relationships of the female urethra in urinary incontinence. Am J Obstet Gynecol 1953; 65:560.

Jeffcoate TNA, Roberts H. Observations on stress incontinence of urine. Am J Obstet Gynecol 1952; 64:721–38.

McGuire EJ. Urodynamic findings in patients after failure of stress incontinence operations. Prog Clin Biol Res 1981; 78:351.

Muellner SR. Physiology of micturition. J Urol 1951; 65: 805–10.

Noll LE, Hutch JA. The SCIPP line—An aid in interpreting the voiding lateral cystourethrogram. Obstet Gynecol 1969; 33:680–89.

Reid GC, DeLancey JOL, Hopkins MP, Roberts JA, Morley GW. Urinary incontinence following radical vulvectomy. Obstet Gynecol 1990; 75:852–58.

Richardson AC, Edmonds PB, Williams NL. Treatment of stress urinary incontinence due to paravaginal fascial defect. Obstet Gynecol 1981; 57:357–62.

Rud T, Anderson KE, Asmussen M, Hunting A, Ulmsten U. Factors maintaining the intraurethral pressure in women. Invest Urol 1980; 17:343–47.

Smith P. Age changes in the female urethra. Br J Urol 1972; 44:667–76.

Versi E, Cardozo LD, Studd JWW, Brincat M, O'Dowd TM, Cooper DJ. Internal urinary sphincter in maintenance of female continence. Br Med J 1986; 292:166–67.

Westby M, Asmussen M, Ulmsten U. Location of maximum intraurethral pressure related to urogenital diaphragm in the female subject as studied by simultaneous urethrocystometry and voiding urethrocystography. Am J Obstet Gynecol 1982; 144:408–12.

Anatomy of Pelvic Supportive Structures

Campbell RM. The anatomy and histology of the sacrouterine ligaments. Am J Obstet Gynecol 1950; 59:1–12.

DeLancey JOL. Anatomic causes of vaginal prolapse after hysterectomy. Am J Obstet Gynecol 1992; 166:1717–28.

Dickinson, RL. Studies of the levator ani muscle. Am J Dis Wom 1889; 22:897–917.

Lawson JO. Pelvic anatomy. I. Pelvic floor muscles Ann R Coll Surg Engl 1974; 54:244–52.

Lawson JO. Pelvic anatomy. II. Anal canal and associated sphincters. Ann R Coll Surg Engl 1974; 54:288–300.

Range RL, Woodburne RT. The gross and microscopic anatomy of the transverse cervical ligaments. Am J Obstet Gynecol 1964; 90:460–67.

Richter K. Lebendige anatomie der vagina. Geburtshilfe Frauenheilkd 1966; 26(9):1213–23.

Physiologic Study of the Pelvic Floor

Snooks SJ, Badenoch DF, Tiptaft RC, et al. Perineal nerve damage in genuine stress urinary incontinence: An electrophysiological study. Br J Urol 1985; 57:422.

Smith ARB, Hosker GL, Warrell DW. The role of partial denervation of the pelvic floor in the etiology of genitourinary prolapse and stress incontinence of urine: A neurophysiological study. Br J Obstet Gynecol, 1989; 96:24–28.

Parks AG, Porter NH, Melzak J. Experimental study of the reflex mechanism controlling muscles of the pelvic floor. Dis Colon Rectum 1962; 5:407–14.

Neurophysiology

Bock G, Whelan J (Eds). Neurobiology of Incontinence. New York: John Wiley, 1990 (Ciba Foundation Symposium 151).

Burnstock G. Nervous control of smooth muscle by transmitters, co-transmitters, and modulators. Experientia 1985; 41:869–74.

Burnstock G. The changing face of autonomic neurotransmission. Acta Physiol Scand 1986; 126:67–91.

Caine M (Ed). The Pharmacology of the Urinary Tract. New York: Springer-Verlag, 1984.

Daniel EE, Cowan W, Daniel VP. Structural bases of neural and myogenic control of human detrusor muscle. Can J Physiol Pharmacol 1983; 61:1247–73.

DeGroat WC. Nervous control of the urinary bladder of the cat. Brain Res 1975; 87:201–11.

Elbadawi A. Neuromuscular mechanisms of micturition. In Yalla SV, McGuire EJ, Elbadawi A, Blaivas JG (Eds).

Neurourology and Urodynamics: Principles and Practice. New York: Macmillan 1988; 3–35.

Elbadawi A. Neuromorphologic basis of vesicourethral function I. Histochemistry, ultrastructure, and function of the intrinsic nerves of the bladder and urethra. Neurourol Urodynam 1982; 1:3–50.

Fletcher TF, Bradley WE. Neuroanatomy of the bladder urethra. J Urol 1978; 119:153–60.

Kirby RS, Milroy EJ, Mitchell MI (Eds). Role of the sympathetic nervous system in the lower urinary tract. Clinical Science 1986; 70(Suppl 14):1s–81s.

Kluck P. The autonomic innervation of the human urinary bladder, bladder neck and urethra: A histochemical study. Anat Rec 1980; 198:439–47.

Morrison JFB. Bladder control: Role of higher levels of the central nervous system. In Torrens M, Morrison JFB (Eds). Physiology of the Lower Urinary Tract. New York: Springer-Verlag 1987; 237–74.

Nathan PW. The central nervous connections of the bladder. In Williams DI, Chishold GD (Eds). Scientific Foundations of Urology, Vol. 2. Chicago: Year Book Medical Publishers 1976; 51–58.

Rohner TJ Jr. Changes in adrenergic receptors in bladder outlet obstruction. In Himan F Jr (Ed). Benign Prostatic Hypertrophy. New York: Springer-Verlag 1983; 410–13.

Schmidt RA. Urethrovesical reflexes and their inhibition. In Hinman F Jr (Ed). Benign Prostatic Hypertrophy. New York: Springer-Verlag 1983; 361–72.

Sourander LB. Treatment of urinary incontinence: The place of drugs. Gerontology 1990; 3(Suppl. 2):19–26.

Torrens M. Human physiology. In Torrens M, Morrison JFB (Eds). The Physiology of the Lower Urinary Tract. New York: Springer-Verlag, 1987; 333–50.

Torrens M, Morrison JFB (Eds). The Physiology of the Lower Urinary Tract. New York: Springer-Verlag, 1987.

Van Arsdalen K, Wein AJ. Physiology of micturition and continence. In Krane RJ, Siroky MB (Eds). Clinical Neuro-Urology, 2nd ed. Boston: Little, Brown 1991; 25–82.

3   Evaluating Symptoms

Patients seek medical care because of *symptoms*. A symptom is a subjective complaint which bothers the patient and from which she wants relief, either because the symptom itself is troublesome or because she is worried that the symptom may be related to some other hidden disease process, such as cancer. The physician's responsibility is to evaluate symptoms and to explain their underlying pathophysiology so that they may be eliminated or alleviated.

Like symptoms in any other organ system, those arising in the lower urinary tract have their origins in some alteration of the normal physiology or anatomy of the bladder and urethra. In its healthy state the bladder is a simple organ with a simple function. Its job is to receive urine from the kidneys through the ureters and to store that urine effortlessly and without discomfort until it can be voluntarily expelled without effort or discomfort at a socially acceptable time and place. As a result, the authors believe that urinary tract complaints can be grouped into four major categories: abnormal storage (incontinence); abnormal emptying (voiding difficulty); sensory disorders; and abnormal bladder contents (Table 3.1). Grouping symptoms in this fashion helps focus our attention on the potential pathophysiologic processes which may be responsible for them and contributes to developing a logical plan for evaluating patient complaints.

Because patients present with *symptoms* and not with ready-made diagnostic labels, this book has been organized around major symptom complexes: incontinence, voiding difficulty, sensory disorders, prolapse, etc. By organizing the text in this way the authors hope to anchor it firmly in the "real world," and thereby provide a guide by which patients may be moved more swiftly and confidently along the path to diagnosis and treatment. This chapter introduces symptoms and their significance, highlights the features of routine physical diagnosis which are of particular importance in evaluating patients with lower urinary tract complaints, and surveys the main laboratory tests which are useful in the initial evaluation of these patients. Details of specific symptom complexes and diagnostic categories are elaborated in individual chapters or sections throughout this book, but they assume a basic familiarity with the material presented here.

Symptoms and Their Significance

The initial approach to a patient with lower urinary tract complaints does not differ from the initial evaluation of any other clinical problem. The patient's chief complaint must be elucidated and set within the context of a thorough history of the present illness. The character, onset, and duration of the complaint should be recorded, along with factors which make it worse or better. Previous attempts at therapy—particularly previous surgical operations—and their results must be recorded. This material must be supplemented by a thorough investigation of other potentially relevant urinary tract symptoms, the patient's general medical, surgical, and gynecologic history, and appropriate laboratory investigations. This process is accomplished best if it is done in a systematic and orderly fashion. Many clinicians have organized their practice so that a standard questionnaire is either filled out by the patient, or a standard urogynecology database is completed by the physician during the initial patient interview. We believe that one of the major ways in which clinicians go wrong in dealing with lower

TABLE 3.1.   Categories of Bladder Symptoms

Abnormal storage	Abnormal sensation
Stress incontinence	Urgency
Urge incontinence	Dysuria
Mixed incontinence	Pain
Frequency	Pressure
Nocturia	Decreased sensation
Nocturnal enuresis	Abnormal contents
Abnormal emptying	Abnormal color
Hesitancy	Abnormal smell
Straining to void	Hematuria
Poor stream	Pneumaturia
Intermittent stream	Stones
Incomplete emptying	Foreign bodies
Postmicturition dribble	Miscellaneous complaints
Acute urinary retention	

urinary tract problems is by taking an inadequate history. It is absolutely essential that this is done in an orderly and systematic way. This chapter attempts to bring some order to the evaluation of lower urinary tract symptoms in women and provides a general framework for understanding symptoms and their significance which can be expanded throughout the course of this book as the various symptom complexes are discussed.

The following questions should be asked of all patients:

- **What bothers you about your bladder?** Write down the patient's complaint *in her own words*. Looking at what the patient *actually says* may be invaluable in sorting out *exactly* what bothers her. Pay precise attention to what she says and do not "interpret" her chief complaint and force it into a preconceived medical diagnosis, or this may put you on the wrong track from the beginning. For example, one of the authors recently saw a patient whose chief complaint had been recorded by the resident as "stress incontinence with coughing, laughing, or sneezing." When the patient was questioned in more detail, her chief complaint was "Whenever I get really tickled and laugh real hard, I wet all over myself—I just can't control my bladder when I laugh like that." Furthermore, she did *not* leak urine with coughing or sneezing at all: The *only* time she leaked urine was during bouts of semi-hysterical laughter, when she was really "tickled." This had started about the age of 14 (the patient remembered her first episode specifically: It had begun while watching a very funny movie in a theater with some friends). The patient was ultimately found to have "giggle micturition," a specific condition in which uncontrolled laughter triggers a micturition reflex and results in nearly complete bladder emptying (see Chapter 11, "Atypical Causes of Incontinence"). The resident had "interpreted" what the patient had said and embellished it to fit into a preconceived diagnostic pattern. He had, as a result, missed the diagnosis completely.

  Patients will sometimes do this themselves, going through a process of self-diagnosis and then presenting their conclusions to the clinician as their "symptoms." Beware the patient who says "I have stress incontinence" without finding out what she means by this! She may think that "stress incontinence" means losing urine because she is "stressed out" by the pressures of family, job, and daily life, when her complaint is really urge incontinence due to detrusor instability, made worse by her pressured lifestyle. Or she may think (as do many physicians) that *all* female urinary incontinence is "stress incontinence." Patients sometimes know too much for their own good. This frequently gets in the way of a proper diagnostic evaluation.

- **When did your problem *first* begin?**
- **Has it been getting better or worse, or has it stayed the same since it started?**
- **What makes it worse or better?** Find out the exact circumstances in which

the patient first started noticing her problem. Some conditions may have been present for some time, but have become clinically bothersome only recently. Others may have an acute onset which can be linked to an obvious precipitating cause such as a change of medication, the development of diabetes, or undergoing a surgical procedure. If the problem has been around for some time, find out if anything makes it better or worse. For example, some women give up doing aerobic exercises because it precipitates stress incontinence or makes it much worse. Others find that irritative bladder symptoms are made worse by drinking coffee or sodas with artificial sweeteners in them.

- **How much does this bother you?** Urinary tract symptoms are difficult to quantify and may have a markedly different impact on the quality of life depending upon the patient. Slight stress incontinence is often noticed during a routine pelvic examination, but many women are not bothered by it. It is an occasional annoyance rather than a clinical problem. Just because stress incontinence can be demonstrated does not mean it needs surgical repair! On the other hand, there are many women who have only slight clinical leakage but who are absolutely devastated by this loss of urine. Some women may have become house bound by their bladder problems and cut themselves off from all social activity. Some women are sexually incapacitated by incontinence, recurrent bladder infections, or urethral pain. All of these women merit sympathetic understanding, but the nature and scope of both their workup and their treatment needs to be altered to fit individual circumstances.

- **Have you had any treatment for this problem before, and if so, did it help?** Knowing what has been done for the patient previously will help the clinician avoid repeating a previous failed therapy. If a previous treatment has "failed," find out if the patient had an adequate trial of therapy. Some treatments are abandoned prematurely without a fair chance to work. Drugs are sometimes given in inadequate dosages for an inadequate period of time. If previous surgery has failed, find out if it was done for the right reasons and whether or not it was done correctly. A retropubic urethropexy for stress incontinence may be precisely the right operation for some patients, but if done with chromic catgut suture it may fail a few weeks after the operation because the suture dissolved before adequate scar tissue formation had occurred. In all cases of "failed" therapy, try to find out what kind of diagnostic evaluation the patient had before the therapy was undertaken in the first place. Many patients have been treated without an adequate evaluation.

After the initial complaint has been fleshed out, be sure to ask about *other* urinary tract symptoms that may also be present. Obtaining pertinent negative answers is as important as finding out the chief complaint. Unexpected positive findings may change the initial diagnostic plan. The patient who complains of stress incontinence but who also mentions that she has been passing blood in her urine for the last four months has just changed both the nature and the order of her diagnostic evaluation.

The initial interview with the patient, and the subsequent physical examination, should allow the physician to formulate a diagnostic plan, which can be modified to fit the circumstances of individual patients. The authors believe that the initial diagnostic evaluation should consist of:

- A thorough history, including a general medical history
- A good physical examination, including a neurologic screening exam and a "stress test" with a full bladder
- Estimation of residual urine after voiding
- Urinalysis, with culture and cytology in selected cases

When this has been done, the clinician will have the basic information necessary to proceed with further testing and to formulate an acceptable plan of

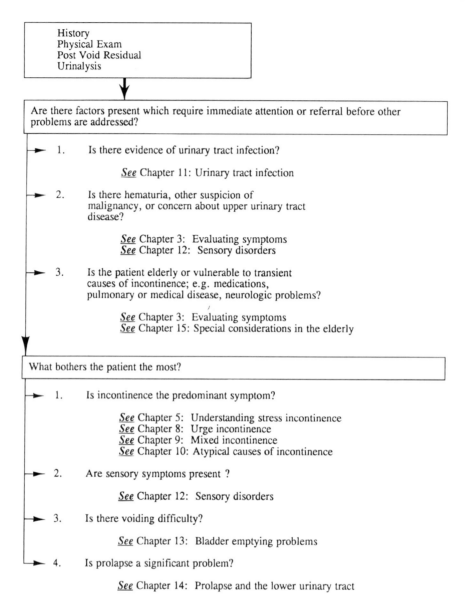

History
Physical Exam
Post Void Residual
Urinalysis

Are there factors present which require immediate attention or referral before other problems are addressed?

1.   Is there evidence of urinary tract infection?

     See Chapter 11: Urinary tract infection

2.   Is there hematuria, other suspicion of malignancy, or concern about upper urinary tract disease?

     See Chapter 3: Evaluating symptoms
     See Chapter 12: Sensory disorders

3.   Is the patient elderly or vulnerable to transient causes of incontinence; e.g. medications, pulmonary or medical disease, neurologic problems?

     See Chapter 3: Evaluating symptoms
     See Chapter 15: Special considerations in the elderly

What bothers the patient the most?

1.   Is incontinence the predominant symptom?

     See Chapter 5: Understanding stress incontinence
     See Chapter 8: Urge incontinence
     See Chapter 9: Mixed incontinence
     See Chapter 10: Atypical causes of incontinence

2.   Are sensory symptoms present ?

     See Chapter 12: Sensory disorders

3.   Is there voiding difficulty?

     See Chapter 13: Bladder emptying problems

4.   Is prolapse a significant problem?

     See Chapter 14: Prolapse and the lower urinary tract

Figure 3.1   Initial evaluation of the patient with lower urinary tract complaints.

treatment. Figure 3.1 outlines the initial basic diagnostic workup, and shows how it relates to the organization of this book.

Abnormal Storage

Urine should be stored without effort and without leakage. The bladder should hold urine comfortably until it can be released voluntarily at a socially acceptable time and place. Failure to store urine in this fashion results in urinary incontinence. The common symptoms associated with abnormal urine storage are given in Table 3.2.

Involuntary urine loss which is clinically troublesome is _urinary incontinence._ This is only a _symptom_ with many possible causes and is not, in itself, a diagnosis. Many medical practitioners have the mistaken impression that _all_ female urinary incontinence is stress incontinence. This is not true. Urinary incontinence in women has many potential causes. Although stress incontinence

TABLE 3.2. Symptoms of Abnormal Urine Storage

Incontinence—Involuntary loss of urine, which is a social or hygienic problem and which is objectively demonstrable

Stress incontinence—Loss of urine coincident with increased intra-abdominal pressure, as with sneezing, coughing, or jumping

Urge incontinence—Loss of urine accompanied by a strong desire to void

Mixed incontinence—Symptoms of both stress and urge incontinence

Unconscious incontinence—Loss of urine occurring without urgency and without conscious recognition of leakage

Frequency—The number of voids per day, from waking in the morning until falling asleep at night

Nocturia—The number of times the patient is awakened from sleep to void at night

Nocturnal enuresis—Urinary incontinence occurring during sleep

TABLE 3.3. Etiology of Female Urinary Incontinence

I. Extraurethral incontinence
  A. Congenital
    1. Ectopic ureter
    2. Bladder exstrophy
    3. Other
  B. Acquired (fistulae)
    1. Ureteric
    2. Vesical
    3. Urethral
    4. Complex combinations
II. Transurethral incontinence
  A. Genuine stress incontinence
    1. Bladder neck displacement
    2. Intrinsic sphincter dysfunction
    3. Combined
  B. Detrusor overactivity
    1. Idiotrophic detrusor instability
    2. Neuropathic detrusor hyperreflexia or reflex neurogenic incontinence
  C. Mixed incontinence (genuine stress incontinence and detrusor overactivity)
  D. Urinary retention with bladder distension and overflow incontinence
    1. Genuine stress incontinence
    2. Detrusor hyperactivity with impaired contractility ("DHIC")
    3. Combinations
  E. Urethral diverticulum
  F. Congenital urethral abnormalities, e.g., episadias
  G. Uninhibited urethral relaxation or "urethral instability" (rare)
  H. Functional and transient incontinence (common, especially in the elderly)
    1. Delirium
    2. Infection
    3. Atrophic urethritis and vaginitis
    4. Pharmacological causes
    5. Psychological causes
    6. Excessive urine production, e.g., diabetes mellitus, diabetes insipidus, hypercalcemia, resorption of lower extremity edema fluid, etc.
    7. Restricted mobility
    8. Stool impaction

is the most common reason for women to lose urine, all incontinence in women is *not* stress incontinence. A classification of female urinary incontinence and its causes is given in Table 3.3. The first task of a clinician faced with an incontinent female patient is to place her problem in the appropriate diagnostic category so that effective treatment can be started. This section provides an overview of female urinary incontinence and suggestions for beginning the basic workup. Details of particular clinical problems will be dealt with separately in the chapters which follow.

Our guiding principle in approaching incontinent patients is an ancient rule of medical practice: *Primum non nocere*, "First of all do no harm." Harm can be done to an incontinent patient in two ways: First, by failing to do something that should have been done; and second, by doing something that should not have been done. The "sins of omission" lie in failing to diagnose an underlying condition which manifests itself as urinary incontinence, such as diabetes, congestive heart failure, a stroke or some other neurologic problem. The "sins of commission" involve doing something actively harmful to the patient, such as thoughtlessly placing an indwelling urinary catheter which leads to urosepsis, or operating on a patient in whom surgery was not indicated or (worse yet) was contraindicated.

The initial evaluation of a patient with urinary incontinence should consist of a careful and detailed history, a thorough physical examination, a urinalysis (with urine culture as appropriate), estimation of residual urine, and a frequency/volume bladder chart. Based on this information, a conservative plan of treatment can be initiated or more extensive investigations can be planned, particularly if potentially harmful or dangerous intervention—such as surgery—is contemplated, or if the initial evaluation has led to the suspicion of a more complex pathophysiology (see Chapter 4, "Practical Urodynamics").

The most important starting place in evaluating urinary incontinence is the patient's history. The International Continence Society has defined urinary incontinence as "involuntary urine loss which is a social or hygienic problem and which is objectively demonstrable." *Occasional* urine loss, such as when exercising vigorously with a full bladder, is quite common in women, but this is usually nothing more than a transient annoyance. This becomes *clinical incontinence* when it begins to trouble the patient or her caregivers. Unfortunately, many women have assumed that since occasional stress incontinence is so common, any degree of urine loss is "woman's lot," no matter how severe. Regular troublesome urine loss is *not* normal and should be evaluated. The criterion that it be "objectively demonstrable" merely means that it must be proven that urine loss is occurring and that the patient's "wetness" is not due to something else, such as perspiration, a vaginal discharge, or unusual circumstances such as a leaking waterbed. Although this may seem to be an overly basic point, neglect of this principle has sometimes had unfortunate consequences for patients.

There may be a considerable time lag between the development of clinical urinary incontinence and the patient's presentation to a physician for evaluation and treatment, because of embarrassment, fear (particularly of surgery), or the feeling that urine loss is "normal" in women as they age. The history should document when the incontinence began, the factors associated with it, and its course since it started. Has it stayed the same and the patient is just tired of it? Or has it suddenly worsened? Precipitating or exacerbating factors must be elucidated. Interval treatments should be described and whether or not they improved the situation. This is particularly important when patients have had previous surgery or have undergone complex pharmacologic treatment. Previous medical records must often be reviewed, as many patients (we are sorry to say) have no idea what was done to them or why. A history of urinary incontinence which began abruptly mandates a careful exploration for possible etiologic factors, such as trauma, abrupt change in social circumstances, treatment with a new drug, etc. Incontinence beginning in association with neurologic symptoms should prompt a careful neurologic evaluation.

Urine loss may be *continuous* or *intermittent, conscious* or *unconscious.* Most urine loss is *intermittent;* that is, the patient has periods of dryness broken by episodes of incontinence. The patient must be questioned as to the nature of her incontinent episodes to see if any pattern is present. *Continuous urinary incontinence* is rare. It is most often seen either with a congenital anomaly such as an ectopic ureter or with a fistula. Most congenital anomalies are picked up by pediatricians before the patient begins seeking gynecologic care, but occasionally a subtle anomaly is missed. In industrialized countries like the United States, fistulae are most commonly seen in association with malignancy, and following surgery or radiation therapy. Obstetric fistulae are still very common in nonindustrialized countries where access to health care is poor. Patients with fistulae are uncommon. More commonly women say that they "are never dry" to emphasize the severity of their incontinence. Careful questioning soon makes it obvious that these women have severe intermittent incontinence rather than continuous urine loss. Some women, particularly those who have had multiple unsuccessful surgical operations for stress incontinence, may develop continuous incontinence from fibrosis, scarring, and virtual destruction of the urethra which then becomes an open conduit for urine from the bladder to the outside world.

Conscious urine loss means that the patient is immediately aware that she has leaked and knows that she is wet. Some women complain of continually being "damp" and may suffer from excessive vulvar sweating or a vaginal discharge rather than urinary incontinence. Others may leak a drop or two of urine from time to time and not be aware that they have leaked only because the volume of loss is so small. This is different from the patient who has a large volume leak to which she remains oblivious until it is brought to her attention. This usually implies serious accompanying neurologic or psychiatric pathology.

The difference between *established incontinence* and *transient incontinence* is also important, particularly in the elderly. Many medical conditions and environmental factors can contribute to the development of urinary incontinence in patients, including delirium, infection, urogenital atrophy, drug interactions, psychiatric illness, endocrine disorders, excessive urine production, restricted mobility, and problems such as stool impaction. These factors must all be evaluated, particularly in patients with incontinence of recent onset. Since many of these factors are reversible, a little careful thought and good basic medical care may solve a patient's incontinence problem quickly and simply.

Incontinence should be evaluated as to its pattern and severity. Ask how often the patient loses urine and under what circumstances: multiple times each day, once or twice a week, once a month under conditions of extreme stress, etc. It is useful to have the patient describe a typical example of urine loss and to write it down in her own words: "I wet my pants every time I cough or sneeze," or "When I have to go I can't get to the bathroom in time." How much the problem bothers the patient may be estimated by having her complete a visual analog scale, where she rates the distress caused by her urine loss from 1–10 or by marking a point on a line of standard length.

The patient should be asked if she wears protective pads because of her leakage, and if so, what kind: a small amount of tissue paper stuffed into her underwear, a "mini pad," a tampon or regular menstrual pad, or a heavy-duty incontinence pad such as Serenity, Depends, Attends, etc. How often does she change them? When she changes them are they damp, wet, or soaked? It must be remembered that the amount of urine she loses has no necessary relationship to how much she is troubled by it. Similarly, some women will change their pad each time they void simply as a matter of personal hygiene, irrespective of whether or not it is wet. Others will wear a pad until it is completely soaked, dry it out, and attempt to reuse it because of the expense involved in buying pads. It is also worthwhile to ask patients if they have limited their social activities due to their incontinence; if so, get them to tell you what they have stopped doing and why. This gives a clearer picture of the changes incontinence is making in a woman's life. Some women have given up active sports and regret this but are able to function otherwise. Other women, however, have become house bound recluses, cut off from formerly pleasurable social interactions such as visiting friends, going shopping, attending church services, etc. One of the authors has recently seen a former Olympic athlete who has had to give up competing in her sport because of stress incontinence. For most women the elimination of violent physical exercise from their lives would not be too troublesome, but for this patient it has been devastating.

The impact of urinary incontinence on sexual activity may be profound.

Patients seldom volunteer this information, even though it may be the real reason they have sought medical help. Physicians should be sensitive to this fact and should make an effort to explore this area of sexuality with their patients. Just learning that other women also have this problem may bring significant emotional relief to some patients.

Intermittent urinary incontinence usually falls into one of four basic presentations: stress incontinence, urge incontinence, mixed incontinence, and overflow incontinence. Sorting patients out according to their predominant symptoms helps facilitate the rest of the evaluation and to develop an initial plan of action.

Stress Incontinence.   Stress incontinence is involuntary urine loss occurring during periods of increased intra-abdominal pressure, such as with sneezing, coughing, lifting, running, or vigorous exercise, particularly exercise which involves repetitive bouncing movements, such as high-impact aerobics. Urine is typically lost in spurts occurring with each rise in intra-abdominal pressure. Most commonly, this is due to downward displacement of the bladder neck with physical exertion so that the closure mechanism is inefficient. Less often this occurs due to intrinsic urethral weakness or dysfunction (see Chapter 5, "Understanding Stress Incontinence"). In some cases, however, physical activity may precipitate an uncontrolled detrusor contraction which is interpreted by the patient as "stress incontinence" and described to the physician as such. Demonstration of *repetitive* urine loss in spurts with each cough during physical examination establishes stress incontinence as a clinical condition. Care must be taken, however, to ensure that this finding represents the patient's complaint and the reason she has sought help.

Urge Incontinence.   Urge incontinence is urine loss accompanied by a strong desire to void (urgency). The patient with this problem typically experiences a sudden need to void and begins to lose urine involuntarily before she can make it to the toilet. This may occur just as she reaches the toilet while she is lowering her undergarments and may involve only a few drops of urine, or it may involve complete bladder emptying. Most of these patients suffer from detrusor overactivity, which may lead to associated symptoms of frequency, urgency, nocturia and nocturnal enuresis. Unstable detrusor activity may also present as sudden loss of urine without forewarning symptoms. Patients who experience complete bladder emptying for no apparent reason may be assumed to suffer from detrusor overactivity.

Urge incontinence may be associated with specific "triggers," such as leaving a warm house and walking into a cold winter wind, or rushing home from shopping with a full bladder and jangling keys to open a door only to have the bladder empty uncontrollably. Many times the presence of water serves as a trigger for urge incontinence—turning on a tap to wash dishes, climbing into a running shower, or getting into or out of a swimming pool. Occasionally women will report (and often they must be asked) that complete bladder emptying occurs during sexual intercourse at the time of orgasm.

In evaluating urge incontinence it is important to differentiate between patients whose urgency is due to the fear of leaking and those whose urgency is due to increasing bladder pain or fear of pain. Some patients may lose urine because their bladder hurts so much that they must empty it in order to obtain relief from the pain even though toilet facilities are not available. "Painful" urge incontinence is usually associated with a sensory bladder disorder, which may also cause frequency and urgency (see Chapter 8, "Urge Incontinence and the Unstable Bladder," and Chapter 12, "Sensory Disorders of the Bladder and Urethra").

Mixed Incontinence.   Mixed incontinence refers to the presence of both stress and urge incontinence. If patients are evaluated with a standardized questionnaire, most of them will have multiple symptoms. It is quite common to see patients who have both stress and urge incontinence. This makes it extremely important to take a good history to find out exactly which symptoms bother the patient the most and which symptoms are "incidental findings" as far as the patient is concerned. Care should be taken to address the problem that bothers the patient the most. Not infrequently, definitive diagnosis of a patient's complaint is difficult on the basis of her history alone. Patients with mixed symptoms often require further evaluation in order to understand the pathophysiology of their complaints (see Chapter 9, "Mixed Incontinence").

Overflow Incontinence. Overflow incontinence occurs when urine leaks from an overdistended bladder which does not empty properly. This may present as "stress incontinence" because the pressure in the overdistended bladder overcomes the resistance of the bladder outlet. It may also present as urge incontinence. In this case bladder overdistension triggers an unstable detrusor contraction that causes leakage, but because the detrusor is weak and inefficient (in addition to being overactive) the abnormal contraction does not empty the bladder completely. This means that a large chronic residual urine remains, and the process is set up to occur again. This is one reason why measurement of the postvoid residual urine is an important part of the incontinence evaluation. A large residual urine also creates significant "dead space" in the bladder creating a low functional bladder capacity. This often results in urinary frequency, urgency, and nocturia. Removal of the residual urine by a program of clean intermittent self-catheterization may eliminate all of these symptoms without recourse to any other therapy (see Chapter 10, "Atypical Causes of Incontinence").

Frequency refers to the number of times a patient empties her bladder during her waking hours. Normal, healthy women without urinary tract complaints void about 6 times per day, with an average voided volume of 250 ml, and an average maximum voided volume of around 500 ml. The maximum voided volume is referred to as the *functional bladder capacity,* because it is the largest volume held by the bladder under normal circumstances. This is often the first volume voided in the morning after a night's sleep. The *cystometric bladder capacity* is the largest infused volume tolerated by the patient during a urodynamic study. The *structural bladder capacity* is the capacity of the bladder measured during deep anesthesia after sensory input has been abolished. The functional capacity may be reduced by processes such as inflammation which increase bladder sensitivity, by uninhibited bladder contractions which reduce the degree to which the bladder can be filled, by habit, by fear of leakage, by large residual urines which result in unusable "dead space" in the bladder, or by true structural limitations of bladder capacity. The structural capacity is reduced only by anatomic changes, such as fibrosis from radiation injury, tuberculosis, surgery, etc. The average daily urine output for most women is around 1500 ml, and is almost always less than 2500 ml. The actual volume voided for any individual depends upon her fluid intake and her bladder habits; therefore, complaints regarding changes in urinary frequency must be assessed in light of the patient's normal habits and fluid intake. Patients are notoriously unreliable in reporting their frequency of urination. The only way to assess this accurately is by having the patient keep a frequency/volume bladder chart.

A frequency/volume chart is simply a modified fluid balance sheet which the patient keeps herself. To do this she must measure her voided urine volumes and record both the amount and the time on a chart. A separate column can be used to keep an account of fluid intake, which can be estimated in "cups," or the intake can be estimated by looking at the recorded urine output. An additional column can be used to have the patient record associated symptoms or note relevant clinical details (Fig. 3.2). The longer the patient keeps a record of this kind, the more accurate is the information collected. Preferably this information should be recorded for several days. The process is facilitated by providing the patient with a graduated plastic "hat" which fits over the toilet rim and under the seat to collect the voided urine (Fig. 3.3). The bladder chart provides an objective record of minimum and maximum voided volumes, average voided volumes, daily urine output, and the time intervals between voids. This record provides invaluable information in assessing patient urinary tract function and should be part of the routine work-up of virtually all patients.

NAME_____PHONE(H)_____(W)_____

	DAY ONE				DAY TWO		
TIME	INTAKE	OUTPUT	SYMPTOMS	TIME	INTAKE	OUTPUT	SYMPTOM
TOTAL							

Figure 3.2   Frequency/volume bladder chart.

An example of a normal bladder chart is given in Figure 3.4. Examination of this chart, which was kept for two days, shows normal fluid intake and output, normal urinary frequency, and one episode of nocturia which was probably related to a drink just before bedtime.

In contrast, a series of abnormal bladder charts are shown in Figures 3.5–3.11. The patient in Figure 3.5 has complaints of frequency, urgency, and urge incontinence. Examination of this chart shows a grossly elevated urine output which is clearly related to excessive fluid intake, even though the patient thought that her drinking habits were ''normal.'' Figure 3.6 shows a patient with a slightly

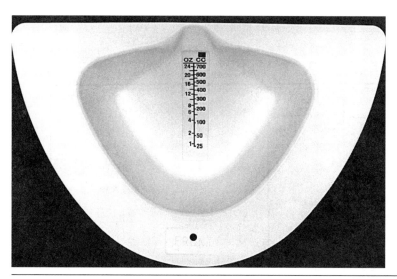

Figure 3.3 Plastic collecting hat to help patients measure their voided volumes.

different problem: early morning urinary frequency associated with taking a diuretic. Once the effects of her medication have worn off, the patient appears to have normal bladder function. Figure 3.7 shows a patient with relatively low fluid intake associated with frequency, urgency, and urge incontinence. Her average bladder capacity is around 120 ml (4 oz.), and her functional bladder capacity does not appear to exceed 360 ml (12 oz.). This patient probably has an unstable bladder and has limited her fluid intake in order to minimize her bladder symptoms. Figure 3.8 shows a patient with normal fluid intake and a normal functional bladder capacity, but symptoms of mixed stress and urge incontinence. Her incontinent episodes are clearly documented and several are directly related to physical activity.

It should be obvious from these examples that a frequency/volume bladder chart provides extremely important information regarding bladder function in patients with lower urinary tract complaints. Better still, this information costs nothing to obtain, involves the patient in her own care, and provides objective baseline data on bladder function against which future therapy can be assessed.

Nocturia refers to *awakening from sleep* with the need to void. Many patients are up late at night because of jobs or habit or because they cannot sleep. Urinating at night because you are up late watching a movie on television and drinking coffee is *not* nocturia! Most patients sleep through the night without awakening to urinate. Other women often get up once per night to void. This is entirely normal. It is also important to realize that nocturia normally increases with age. It is not abnormal for an 80-year old woman to be awakened from sleep twice per night to void. Four or five or six trips to the toilet per night is abnormal at any age. Nocturia may be associated with excessive fluid intake before bedtime, taking diuretic medications at inappropriate times, resorption of edema fluid from the lower extremities, or inadequate secretion of ADH (Anti-Diuretic Hormone) at night.

Bladder charts demonstrating various causes of nocturia are shown in Figures 3.9–3.11. The bladder chart in Figure 3.9 shows a patient with nocturia and a normal fluid intake which stopped well before bedtime. The pattern on this chart suggests that the patient has a nighttime diuresis due to mobilization of fluid which has accumulated during the day. In contrast, the patient in Figure 3.10 is an alcoholic with nocturia. All of her fluid intake after 4:00 PM consisted of bourbon-and-soda, which resulted in a significant diuresis and frequent trips to the toilet throughout the night. Finally, Figure 3.11 shows a patient with multiple recurrent episodes of nocturia. In this case, however, the nocturia occurred in

NAME_____PHONE(H)_____(W)_____

	DAY ONE				DAY TWO		
TIME	INTAKE	OUTPUT	SYMPTOMS	TIME	INTAKE	OUTPUT	SYMPTOM
7AM		400 cc	slight trouble starting stream	7AM	200 cc	450 cc	
7:30	240 cc			8AM	200 cc		
8:30	200 cc			9:30		200 cc	at same time as bowel mvmt.
9:30		250 cc	at same time as bowel mvmt	11:30	240 cc		
				12:00	333 cc		
12 noon	300 cc			12:30		300 cc	
1 pm		300 cc		3 pm		250 cc	
3 pm	240 cc						
4:30		250 cc	before leaving work	4:30	200 cc		
				5 pm	150 cc		
				6:30		275 cc	
6 pm	250 cc			7 pm	350 cc		
7 pm	500 cc						
8 pm		200 cc		9 pm	300 cc		Irish coffee
9 pm	150 cc			10 pm Bedtime	200 cc	300 cc	
10:30 Bedtime		300 cc		2 AM		400 cc	
TOTAL	1880 cc	1700 cc			2173 cc	2175 cc	

Figure 3.4   Frequency/volume chart from a normal patient.

association with daytime urinary frequency, urgency, and urge incontinence. The cause of this patient's nighttime problem is probably the same as her problem during the day: uncontrolled bladder contractions.

Enuresis is often used as a synonym for *"nocturnal enuresis,"* or bedwetting. Properly speaking, however, enuresis actually refers to urine loss at any time, not just at night. *Nocturnal enuresis* refers to urine loss during sleep. Many patients with urge incontinence report awakening from sleep with an urge to urinate and leaking urine before they can get to the toilet. This is urge incontinence occurring at night, not nocturnal enuresis.

NAME______________________________PHONE(H)______________(W)______________

DAY ONE

TIME	INTAKE	OUTPUT	SYMPTOMS
6:50		880 cc	urge-woke me up
7 Am	500 cc	100 cc	
8:20		350 cc	
9:20	360 cc	350 cc	urge + leak
10:30	240 cc		
11:30–12 N	1750 cc	600 cc	+ urge leak (coming in door + trying to get coat off)
12:30		400 cc	
2 pm	400 cc	950 cc	urge
2:45	800 cc		
3:40	100 cc	700 cc	
4 pm	1100 cc		Big gulp
4:45	500 cc	500 cc	urge, leak+
5:10		300 cc	
6 pm		400 cc	urge, leak+ while getting dinner
6:30	400 cc		
7:35	250 cc	550 cc	urge
8:10	1050 cc		
8:40		650 cc	
9:30	700 cc	500 cc	
10 pm	500 cc		
10:50	300 cc	800 cc	severe urge
— Bedtime —			
12:50	200 cc	950 cc	urge
3 am	300 cc	750 cc	urge
4:45	200 cc	700 cc	urge
6:30	300 cc	700 cc	urge, leak ++
TOTAL	> 8,000	> 9,000	

DAY TWO

TIME	INTAKE	OUTPUT	SYMPTOM
6:20		550 cc	
6:35	100 cc	150 cc	
8:10	500 cc	500 cc	urge ++ leak
8:30	500 cc		
9:30	500 cc	700 cc	urge
10:30		600 cc	
11:30	300 cc	200 cc	
12:45	800 cc		
2:10		400 cc	
3:45	300 cc	275 cc	urge, ++ leak before getting pants down
5:10	950 cc	300 cc	urge, leak + unlocking door
6:15	400 cc	300 cc	
6:45	400 cc		
7:50	550 cc	300 cc	
8:20	500 cc		
8:50	200 cc	200 cc	
— Bedtime —			
11:10	200 cc	950 cc	urge, leak+
1:50	800 cc	700 cc	
4:10	550 cc	900 cc	urge
5:40		900 cc	urge
TOTAL	> 7,500	> 7,500	

Figure 3.5 Frequency/volume chart from a patient with excessive fluid intake resulting in excessive urine output.

Nocturnal enuresis may be further subdivided into *primary* and *secondary* nocturnal enuresis. Primary nocturnal enuresis begins in childhood and persists into adulthood, whereas secondary nocturnal enuresis refers to the onset of this symptom as an adult, either with no prior history of childhood bedwetting or after a prolonged period of dryness. These are different problems. Primary nocturnal enuresis is usually the result of delayed maturation of the mechanisms of normal bladder control which then allows a normal micturition reflex to occur at an abnormal time (during sleep), whereas secondary nocturnal enuresis is more commonly associated with unstable bladder contractions. Some patients with

NAME_____ PHONE(H)_____ (W)_____

DAY ONE   **DAY TWO**

TIME	INTAKE	OUTPUT	SYMPTOMS	TIME	INTAKE	OUTPUT	SYMPTOM
7AM		300cc		7AM		400cc	had to hurry
7:30	200cc		this is when I take my water pill	7:30	250cc		
8:30	100cc			8 AM	250cc		water pill
9:30		150cc		9:30		200cc	
10:30		200cc		10:15		200cc	
11:30		150cc	I'm living in the bathroom	10:50		150cc	
12 noon	300cc			11 am	150cc		
12:30		150cc		11:15		200cc	
12:45		50cc	felt like I needed to go again	12 noon	300cc	200cc	
2pm	150cc	300cc		1 pm		150cc	
2:45		150cc		2 pm		100cc	
4pm	150cc	150cc		3 pm	240cc		
5:30	200cc			4:30		250cc	
6:30	500cc		dinner	5:00	240cc		
7pm	150cc	200cc		6 pm	500cc		
9 pm	300cc			6:30	300cc	200cc	
10:30		150	Bedtime	8 pm	150cc		
				9:30	200cc	300cc	Bedtime
TOTAL	2050cc	1950cc			2580cc	2350cc	

Figure 3.6   Frequency/volume chart demonstrating urinary frequency associated with diuretic use.

nocturia and nocturnal enuresis suffer from inadequate secretion of ADH at night and thus produce abnormally large amounts of urine while they are asleep. These patients may be helped by the use of synthetic ADH (desmopressin) at bedtime.

Abnormal Emptying

Symptoms related to abnormal emptying can be due either to voiding dysfunction or outflow obstruction (Table 3.4). Abnormal emptying is more common in men than in women due to the problem of prostatic hypertrophy in males. As a result, less attention has been devoted to the study of female voiding problems and they are not understood as well as those occurring in men.

NAME_____PHONE(H)_____(W)_____

DAY ONE   DAY TWO

TIME	INTAKE	OUTPUT	SYMPTOMS	TIME	INTAKE	OUTPUT	SYMPTOM
7am		200	urge, leak ++				
7:30	150						
8am		50					
10am		75	urge				
12:30	150	100	urge				
2pm		75	urge w/ leak ++				
4pm		75					
5pm	200	50					
6pm	150	100	urge, leak while washing up.				
7:30	200	50					
9:30		125					
10pm		50					
2am		125	urge, leak ++				
TOTAL	850	975					

Figure 3.7 Frequency/volume chart from a patient with frequency, urgency, and urge incontinence in association with low fluid intake.

"Normal" voiding occurs when relaxation of the pelvic floor and urethra is followed by voluntary initiation of a sustained detrusor contraction which empties the bladder completely, effortlessly and painlessly. Women have less appreciation of their voiding patterns than do men, largely because urination is not the same sort of "social event" for females as it is for males. Force of stream, cast distance of the urinary stream, and accuracy of placement of the urinary stream are all things that men can describe with some certainty. Indeed, many males have even competed with each other in these areas during childhood

NAME_____ PHONE(H)_____ (W)_____

DAY ONE   DAY TWO

TIME	INTAKE	OUTPUT	SYMPTOMS	TIME	INTAKE	OUTPUT	SYMPTOM
8:30		450 cc	had to hurry no leak	7 AM		400cc	+ leak while hurrying
9 AM	250 cc			7:30	250 cc	100 cc	just before leaving house
11 AM			+ sneeze	8 Am			
11:30		200 cc		10 Am	200 cc		
12 noon	500 cc			11 Am		200 cc	coughed + leaked ++
				11:30			
2:30	150 cc	250 cc	some urge	12:30	450 cc	150 cc	
3 pm		50 cc	went just before aerobics	1 pm			
			++ leak with jumping jacks	3 pm		300 cc	leaked ++ on way to toilet
				3:30	250 cc		
4 pm	300 cc			5 pm		250 cc	leaked at the front door
5 pm	250 cc			5:30	300 cc		
5:30		250 cc	++ leak when trying to put key in lock	6:30	500 cc	200 cc	coughed with full bladder, ++ leak
6 pm	150 cc		urge while washing lettuce	8:30	150 cc		
6:30	500 cc						
7 pm			+ leak while laughing.	10:30		200 cc	had to hurry
7:30		150 cc		Bedtime —			
8:30	150 cc	200 cc					
10:30		150 cc					
— Bedtime —							
TOTAL	2250 cc	1700 cc			2100 cc	1800 cc	

Figure 3.8 Frequency/volume chart from a patient with normal fluid intake and normal urinary output, but with symptoms of stress and urge incontinence.

contests. Voiding function for women is a much more private event, usually gauged only by the sounds coming from the next toilet stall in a public restroom. As a result, women tend to judge their voiding habits as ''normal'' because they have limited experience in comparing their voiding patterns with others. This makes it more difficult to evaluate voiding disorders—particularly subtle ones—in a female patient population. In addition, there are variations in the way women void, particularly as compared to men. Many women relax the pelvic floor and then contract the detrusor muscle to urinate, but some women do not void in this manner. Some women void by relaxing the outlet and then

NAME_____PHONE(H)_____(W)_____

	DAY ONE				DAY TWO		
TIME	INTAKE	OUTPUT	SYMPTOMS	TIME	INTAKE	OUTPUT	SYMPTOM
7 AM		400 cc	Some urge	7:30		250 cc	
7:30	200 cc		Coffee	8 AM	200 cc		
8:30	200 cc	100 cc	Coffee	10 AM	150 cc		
10 AM	150 cc			11 AM		100 cc	
12 NOON	300 cc	100 cc	lunchtime	12 NOON	200 cc		
1 PM	200 cc						
3:30	150 cc			3 PM		150 cc	
4 PM		150 cc		3:30	150 cc		Coffee
5 PM	200 cc						
6:30	150 cc			5 PM	240 cc		Coke
7 PM	150 cc	100 cc					
9 PM	250 cc		stopped drinking for the night	6:30	200 cc		
				7 PM	240 cc	200 cc	
				8:30	150 cc		
11 PM		150 cc					
Bedtime				11 PM		100 cc	tried to drink less this day
				Bedtime			
2 AM		250 cc	woke me up	1 AM		200 cc	woke me
3:30		200 cc	woke me up	3:30		200 cc	woke me
4:30		250 cc		5 AM		100 cc	
5 AM		100 cc	still awake				
TOTAL	1950 cc	1800 cc			1530 cc	1300 cc	

Figure 3.9 Frequency/volume chart demonstrating increased diuresis at night from mobilization of edema fluid which has accumulated during the day.

strain to empty the bladder by an unconscious but sustained Valsalva maneuver. Other women may void entirely by pelvic floor relaxation, letting the urine drain out of the bladder like oil running out of an automobile engine when the plug is pulled from the oil pan. In spite of these differences, women void more rapidly and with higher peak flow and mean flow rates than do men, due to the shorter female urethra and the absence of a potentially obstructing prostate. Voiding symptoms in women are usually due to urethral spasm, infection, inadequate relaxation of the pelvic floor, poor detrusor activity, functional obstruction by a prolapse which kinks the urethra, or the development of outflow obstruction

NAME_____PHONE(H)_____(W)_____

	DAY ONE				DAY TWO		
TIME	INTAKE	OUTPUT	SYMPTOMS	TIME	INTAKE	OUTPUT	SYMPTOM
6 AM		100 cc		6AM		100 cc	
7 AM	8 oz	100 cc		7 AM	8 oz		
7:30	8 oz			7:30	4 oz		
				10:30		150 cc	
11 AM		200 cc		1 PM	6 oz		
				4:30	8 oz		
				5 PM	8 oz		
5:30	16 oz			6 PM	8 oz	200 cc	
6 PM	8 oz			7 pm		150 cc	
6:30		200 cc	Some urge				
8pm		200 cc		8 PM		200 cc	
9 pm		200 cc		8:30		100 cc	
Bedtime				Bedtime			
10 pm		100 cc	got back out of bed	9 PM		200 cc	
12 pm		100 cc	had to go	11 PM		100 cc	woke up and needed to go
2 am		60 cc	had to go	2 AM		100 cc	needed to hurry
4 AM		100 cc		4 AM		60 cc	woke me up
5 AM		60 cc		5 AM		60 cc	
TOTAL	40 oz	1420 cc			42 oz	1420 cc	

Figure 3.10   Frequency/volume chart demonstrating nocturia as the result of heavy alcohol intake in the afternoon and evening. All fluid intake after 4:30 PM consists of bourbon-and-soda.

following bladder neck surgery for stress incontinence. Neurologic disease may also cause voiding difficulty in women.

Hesitancy refers to difficulty initiating the urine stream. Relaxation of the pelvic floor precedes the initiation of a voluntary detrusor contraction during normal voiding. Hesitancy may result if relaxation of the pelvic floor muscles is inadequate, or if active contraction of these muscles takes place when the patient attempts to urinate (detrusor-sphincter dyssynergia). Poor muscular relaxation may often be corrected using biofeedback techniques. Neuropathology is often responsible for active detrusor-sphincter dyssynergia. Overdistension of

NAME_____PHONE(H)_____(W)_____

	DAY ONE				DAY TWO		
TIME	INTAKE	OUTPUT	SYMPTOMS	TIME	INTAKE	OUTPUT	SYMPTOM
8:25AM		2½ oz	running in and clutching myself	7:05	4½ oz	2½ oz	really ran
8:35		2½ oz		9:20		5 oz	+++ leak + urge
9:20	8 oz			10:35		2½ oz	just to be safe
11:25		2½ oz	awakened from a nap	12 NOON	3 oz		
11:40	4½ oz	1 oz	washing hands. thought I was through	12:30		1 oz	not much out
12:20		1½ oz		1:30	4½ oz		
12:40		1 oz	+ leak getting ready to bathe	1:45	11 oz	1 oz	+++ leaked most of it before I could get there
1:10 PM	4½ oz			2 PM			
1:25	11 oz			4:50		2½ oz	
2:30		1½ oz		5:55pm		1½ oz	almost didn't make it
2:45		1½ oz	+++ leak at bank machine	6 pm	4½ oz		
3:35	4½ oz			7 pm		1 oz	just needed to go
3:40		1½ oz	changed pad	7:30		2½ oz	needed to go when I stood up
5:50		2 oz	almost didn't make it.	7:40	4½ oz		
6:05		1 oz	Had to run back in.	10PM	6 oz	2½ oz	
6:45	11 oz			10:50		3½ oz	before Perry Mason
7:15	4½ oz			11:20	2 oz	2¾ oz	
7:30		2½ oz	had to go	12:35		2 oz	Bedtime
9:25		3 oz	+ leak while hurrying	2:05AM		3 oz	awakened and clutched myself washing hands + had to do more
10:15	7 oz		cross-legged to toilet	2:10		1 oz	
10:20		1 oz		2:12	3 oz		
11 PM		1 oz		3:40		4 oz.	+++ leak on way to toilet
11:30		2½ oz	Bedtime				
12:15		1½ oz		5:50AM		2¾ oz / 2 oz	just leaving and had to do more
1:15	1 oz	2½ oz		7AM		5 oz	+ leak
3:05AM		3½ oz	+ leak on way				
4:20AM		3 oz	clutching and				
5 AM		2½ oz	cross-legged				
TOTAL	56 oz	41½ oz			45½ oz	46½ oz	

Figure 3.11 Frequency/volume bladder chart demonstrating multiple episodes of nocturia associated with daytime urgency, frequency and urge incontinence.

the bladder may cause hesitancy by overstretching the detrusor muscle. This is sometimes seen in normal women who accumulate large urine volumes during sleep and experience some hesitancy with their first void the following morning. An underactive detrusor contraction may also cause hesitancy since it may be unable to produce enough force to empty the bladder promptly and efficiently.

Straining to void is the need to engage the abdominal musculature in order to empty the bladder. Many women normally void by abdominal straining but do not realize it. This is often the case in women with severe stress incontinence and an incompetent urethral sphincter, where relaxation of the pelvic floor and

TABLE 3.4. Symptoms of Abnormal Bladder Emptying

Hesitancy—Trouble initiating voiding
Straining to void—Voiding by conscious abdominal straining
Poor stream—Decreased force of flow of the urinary stream
Intermittent stream—A "stop-and-start" pattern of urination
Incomplete emptying—a persistent feeling of bladder fullness after voiding
Postmicturition dribble—Urine loss occurring just after normal voiding has been
  completed
Acute urinary retention—Sudden inability to void resulting in painful bladder over-
  distension and the need to catheterization to obtain relief

abdominal straining suffice to empty the bladder rapidly without the need to contract the detrusor muscle. Conscious straining to empty the bladder is a good clue that voiding function is not optimal.

Poor stream refers to decreased force of flow. Since women void with much higher peak and average flow rates than men, a woman who has a noticeable change in her urine flow merits investigation.

Intermittent stream refers to a "start and stop" pattern of urination, which may reflect outflow obstruction, inefficient detrusor contraction, poor pelvic floor relaxation, or active urethral contraction while the patient is attempting to void (detrusor-sphincter dyssynergia).

Incomplete emptying refers to the feeling that urine is present after voiding and cannot be expelled. However, this feeling may or may not be related to increased residual urine. This symptom is often present in patients with significant urogenital prolapse, such as a large cystocele, rectocele, or enterocele, and in patients with unstable detrusor contractions which cause postvoid urgency, as well as patients with increased residual urine volumes.

Postmicturition dribble refers to urine loss occurring as the patient stands up after normal voiding has been completed. This symptom may be related to a urethral diverticulum in some patients, to an after-contraction of the bladder muscle, or to a cystocele.

Acute urinary retention may be defined as a sudden inability to void over a 24-hour period which requires catheterization and results in a bladder emptying of at least 50% of the maximum cystometric bladder capacity. It is usually painful. Acute retention may have many precipitating factors, such as trauma, surgery (especially vaginal surgery or surgery on the bladder neck), obstetrical manipulation or vaginal delivery, neurologic disease, acute pelvic pathology such as a tumor, or psychologic conditions. A past history of acute urinary retention should be noted, with particular attention to the details surrounding the episode. Voiding difficulty of any kind—and acute urinary retention in particular—which presents in association with neurologic symptoms requires an especially careful workup to detect potentially serious, life threatening pathology. Occult neurologic conditions such as multiple sclerosis may present initially in this way, without other symptoms developing for a long time after the initial episode of bladder dysfunction.

Abnormal Sensation   Bladder and urethral sensation are among the most poorly understood areas of lower urinary tract physiology. Objective measurement of bladder sensation is difficult and is highly dependent upon patient cooperation. Patient symptoms may correlate poorly with cystometric findings. Abnormal bladder sensation may be divided into two categories: *hypersensitive* states where patients complain of irritative symptoms, or *hyposensitive* states where bladder sensation is diminished or absent (Table 3.5).

Urgency is defined as "a strong desire to void." This is probably the most common bladder symptom since it occurs in normal individuals when their bladders approach capacity. This feeling becomes abnormal when it is present most of the time, causing the patient to rush to the toilet continually. It is useful

TABLE 3.5.   Symptoms of Abnormal Bladder Sensation

Urgency—A strong desire to void
Dysuria—Burning or pain with urination
Bladder pain—Conscious, hurting, subrapubic pain in the bladder
Flank pain—Pain between the lower rib cage and the ilial crest
Pressure—A feeling of heaviness or constant force being exerted on the bladder
   or lower pelvis
Loss of bladder sensation—Decreased sensation in the bladder or urethra

clinically to separate urgency into (*a*) urgency experienced because the patient is afraid of leaking urine, and (*b*) urgency due to increasing pain or fear of pain. Urgency is often associated with frequency, and may be associated with urge incontinence. Urgency and frequency without incontinence are more commonly due to abnormal sensation. At urodynamic investigation patients with urgency and frequency, but not incontinence, tend to have an early first sensation of fullness, an early first desire to void, and a low cystometric capacity. The cystometrogram is usually stable, although some patients present with low level detrusor contractions (below 15 cm H_2O). Frequency-volume bladder charts often reveal frequent small voids but a normal first morning voided volume, indicating that the problem goes away when they are asleep. Urgency and frequency associated with urge incontinence are more likely to be caused by unstable bladder contractions, particularly if nocturia and nocturnal enuresis are also present. However, these symptoms may also be caused by urinary tract infection, bladder stones, bladder tumors, and a host of other conditions. Many women who are seen for ''recurrent urinary tract infections'' often have frequency and urgency from another cause. This should be suspected in women with persistently negative urine cultures or women whose infections are poorly documented despite multiple courses of antibiotics.

Dysuria is burning on urination and should be differentiated from *bladder pain.* The symptom of bladder pain refers to a bladder that *hurts,* and this must be distinguished from ''fullness,'' ''discomfort,'' ''aching,'' or other vague symptoms. Dysuria is usually experienced in the urethra, whereas bladder pain is generally suprapubic in location. Many patients experience urinary urgency but report this as ''pain'' when they give their histories. The distinction between bladder discomfort and bladder pain is important and must be clearly delineated. The patient with a painful bladder falls into an entirely different category and is not easy to treat. Often these women have pain related to the degree of bladder filling and will relate that their pain is relieved by voiding, setting up a cycle of pain, frequency and urgency due to pain or fear of pain, and increasing debilitation which is truly tormenting. Burning on urination, or dysuria, may be associated with this as part of a painful symptom complex, but isolated dysuria is more commonly linked to acute urinary tract infection. Both symptoms—dysuria and bladder or urethral pain—may be linked to other painful conditions in the pelvis, aggravated by sexual intercourse, and develop into a chronic, generalized, debilitating pelvic pain syndrome which is daunting to deal with from a clinical perspective and even worse to live with for the patient.

The first step in evaluating such patients is to rule out a local cause for the problem, such as a bladder stone, intercurrent infection, bladder tumor, or other local pathology. Older women frequently have some of these symptoms as a result of estrogen deprivation after menopause. Urogenital atrophy presenting in combination with any of these symptoms should be treated by aggressive hormone replacement therapy, unless contraindicated for other reasons. Evaluation of patients with painful bladder symptoms often requires tact, time, and referral to a specialized chronic pain treatment center. Urinalysis, urine culture and sensitivity, and urinary cytology, should all be obtained during the initial evaluation of these patients. Urethrocystoscopy, often under general anesthesia so that biopsies may be obtained and the structural bladder capacity may be

TABLE 3.6. Causes of Flank Pain[a]

Urinary tract causes	Renal tumor
Acute ureteral obstruction	Renal cell carcinoma
Stone	Transitional cell carcinoma
Blood clot	Wilms' tumor
Papillary necrosis	Trauma to the kidney
Chronic ureteral obstruction	Renal infarction
Congenital anomaly	Vesicoureteral reflux
Tumor	Nonurinary tract causes
Stricture of ureter	Gallbladder disease
Previous surgery	Appendicitis
Radiation therapy	Pancreatitis
Retroperitoneal fibrosis	Diverticulitis
Stone	Other gastrointestinal disease
Renal inflammation	Chest disease
Acute pyelonephritis	Salpingitis
Perinephric abscess	

[a] From AJ Bueschen, In: Walker, Hall, and Hurst (Eds), Clinical Methods, 3rd ed.; Boston: Butterworths 1990:845–46, with permission

evaluated, should be considered early in the investigation of these patients. Simultaneous laparoscopy is also sometimes useful in evaluating patients with complex symptoms of lower urinary tract pain and may reveal endometriosis on the bladder serosa. Cystometry in patients with these symptoms typically shows a hypersensitive, low capacity bladder, sometimes with decreased compliance.

Flank pain refers to pain in the body between the lower rib cage and the iliac crest, usually in the midaxillary line or slightly posterior. It is generally due to stimulation of sensory nerve endings in the ureter or renal capsule, but may also have a nonurinary cause. When flank pain is due to distension of the urinary tract, the degree of pain is related to the rapidity of the distension and not the degree of distension. A patient with acute obstruction of a ureter due to an impacted kidney stone will have excruciating pain, whereas a patient with long-standing chronic obstruction and severe upper tract dilatation may have almost no pain at all. The differential diagnosis of flank pain is outlined in Table 3.6.

Feelings of "fullness" or "pressure" in the lower abdomen or bladder region are common, but often there are no significant findings on physical examination to account for these symptoms. On the other hand, women with large cystoceles, enteroceles, or complete vaginal vault prolapse often have multiple urinary tract complaints associated with their anatomic defect. Acute urinary retention is often extremely painful, and chronic urinary retention may present with uncomfortable fullness. The bladder can usually be palpated abdominally when it contains 150 ml of urine or more, and often will be seen as a low, suprapubic distension on abdominal examination. Pelvic examination should almost always pick up a distended bladder.

Decreased sensation is less common than bladder hypersensitivity and generally represents some form of denervation injury. Injury of this kind can result from dysfunctional voiding and the development of a "holding" pattern of urination in which the patient voids infrequently and gradually overdistends her bladder. The end result is a large capacity bladder with a diminished first desire to void. Women in jobs where timely access to toilet facilities is limited seem to be at risk for this kind of problem. These habits may develop in childhood out of fear of embarrassment at using school toilets or displeasure at the state of public restrooms. Radical pelvic surgery often causes severe denervation injury. Diminished or absent bladder sensation and voiding dysfunction are quite common following radical hysterectomy, abdominoperineal resection for rectal cancer, and similar procedures. The sudden onset of decreased bladder sensation

TABLE 3.7. Abnormal Bladder Contents

Abnormal color	Stones
Abnormal smell	Foreign bodies
Hematuria	Miscellaneous
Pneumaturia	

or acute urinary retention should prompt a thorough neurologic investigation to look for a precipitating cause.

Diminished perineal sensation in the sacral dermatomes may be a clue to previously unexpected neuropathy. *Unconscious urine loss* occurs when the patient is not aware of having lost urine. Sometimes the amount of urine lost is so small that the patient does not know it has happened until she checks her pad. This is different from a patient who is discovered sitting in a pool of urine, oblivious to this fact. These patients are more likely to have some degree of dementia or a significant neurologic disease. In a previously normal patient, onset of urine loss of this type is worrisome and must be investigated promptly to find the underlying medical factors.

Abnormal Bladder Contents

Patients frequently complain that there is something "abnormal" about their urine; either it "looks funny" or "smells funny." Some patients are simply unaware that the concentration of urine differs with fluid intake and that ingestion of certain foods may impart unusual odors to their urine. Other patients may have potentially significant problems with infection, stones, foreign bodies, or urinary tract malignancy (Table 3.7). Occult problems with the urine which may mirror pathologic processes in other organ systems will be dealt with later, when urinalysis is considered in more detail.

Urine normally has a color which ranges from clear to dark amber depending upon its concentration; however, upon occasion the patient may note an abnormal urine color. This may be due to a wide variety of causes, some of which are quite unusual. These are detailed in Table 3.8.

Pneumaturia refers to passage of gas in the urine. In women this is seen most commonly after sexual intercourse. However, it may also be seen in cases where a fistula between the urinary and gastrointestinal tracts exists, in the presence of an infection with gas forming organisms (seen more frequently in diabetics), or after the introduction of air into the urinary tract by instrumentation (such as cystoscopy).

Hematuria is passage of blood in the urine. It may either be gross or microscopic. Gross hematuria is usually observed by the patient and causes her to seek medical care promptly. Microscopic hematuria is usually detected only on urinalysis where greater than 2 red blood cells per high-power field are present on microscopic examination. Bright red urine suggests a source in the bladder or urethra. Dark brown urine suggests a source higher up in the urinary tract. "Wormlike" clots may indicate bleeding within a ureter. Vaginal or rectal bleeding is often mistaken for "blood in the urine" if the patient only notices the symptom by observing the color of the water in the toilet after urination or looking at the toilet paper after she has wiped herself.

Hematuria must be evaluated promptly, as 22% of patients will have a significant urologic problem irrespective of whether the hematuria is gross or microscopic. Most bladder cancers present with hematuria as an initial symptom.

The differential diagnosis of hematuria is given in Table 3.9. The patient's history should be reviewed thoroughly, paying special attention to the pattern of bleeding and associated symptoms such as pain, fever, renal colic, weight loss, smoking, exposure to chemicals or industrial dyes, trauma, bleeding from other sites, family history, recent dental or genitourinary manipulation which may indicate endocarditis, travel history (tuberculosis or schistosomiasis), and a careful drug history. Many drugs are associated with acute interstitial nephritis, which is a common cause of hematuria (Table 3.10).

TABLE 3.8. Causes of Colored Urine[a]

Color of Urine	Associated Conditions
Watery	Dilute urine
Yellow-orange	Normal urochrome pigments
	Phenazopyridine (HCl) (Pyridium)
Green	Pseudomonas infection
	Methylene blue or other blue dyes
	Elevated urinary copper level
	Phenol
	Iodochlorhydroxyguin
	Amitriptyline hydrochloride
	"Chlorophyll" breath fresheners
Brown	Bile
	Feces
Black	Melanoma
	Alkaptonuria
	Phenol (as a vehicle for iv drugs)
	Malaria ("Blackwater Fever")
	α-Methyldopa
Purplish	Porphobilin
Red	Hemoglobin
	Laxatives containing phenolphthalein
	Myoglobin
	Senna
	Beets
	Rifampin
Milky white	Pus
	Chyle
	Phosphates

[a] From DM Roxe, In: Walker, Hall, and Hurst (Eds), Clinical Methods, 3rd ed. Boston: Butterworths 1990:868–871.

TABLE 3.9. Differential Diagnosis of Hematuria[a]

Acquired glomerular and tubulointerstitial renal disease
  Primary
  Secondary to systemic disease
Hereditary renal disease
  Alport's syndrome
  Polycystic kidney disease
Infection
  Ordinary
  Exotic (including tuberculosis and schistosomiasis)
Papillary necrosis
  Sickle hemoglobin
  Analgesic abuse
  Diabetes mellitus
Trauma
Calculi
Neoplasia
  Primary
  Metastatic
Coagulopathy
  Congenital
  Acquired

[a] From WG Kirkpatrick, In: Walker, Hall, and Hurst (Eds); Clinical Methods, 3rd ed., Boston: Butterworths 1990:849–850, with permission.

TABLE 3.10. Drugs Associated With Acute Interstitial Nephritis

Antibiotics
Penicillins (especially Methicillin, Ampicillin)
Cephalosporins
Sulfonamides
Rifampin
Isoniazid
Nonsteroidal Anti-Inflammatory Drugs
Indomethacin
Phenylbutazone
Fenoprofen
Naproxen
Tometin
Mefenamic acid
Diuretics
Thiazides
Furosemide
Triamterene
Miscellaneous
Phenytoin
Cimetidine
Allopurinol
Azathioprine

[a] From WG Kirkpatrick, In: Walker, Hall, and Hurst (Eds); Clinical Methods, 3rd ed., Boston: Butterworths 1990:849–850, with permission.

Patients who complain of hematuria should have a complete urinalysis, including microscopic and chemical analysis, to confirm the presence of blood, since other substances can also color the urine red. Proteinuria associated with hematuria is suggestive of a renal parenchymal problem, and should be followed up by a 24-hour urine collection for protein and creatinine. A 24-hour protein excretion of greater than 1000 mg is highly diagnostic of renal disease.

In addition to urinalysis, a urine culture should be performed, along with serum electrolytes, blood urea nitrogen, creatinine, and a complete blood count. Coagulation studies are appropriate in selected patients, and black patients should be screened for sickle cell trait and sickle cell disease.

Finally, all patients with persistent hematuria should undergo cystoscopy and intravenous urography to rule out malignancy. Some urologists feel that computerized axial tomography of the abdomen and pelvis is mandatory if gross hematuria is present and no etiology has been identified.

It should not be the place of the general gynecologist to perform a comprehensive evaluation of patients with hematuria. These patients will usually require referral to a urologist or nephrologist for a complete work-up, but much of the preliminary evaluation can be completed at an initial clinic visit. As many as 15% of patients will have no etiology discovered for their hematuria after a careful diagnostic evaluation. These patients have an excellent prognosis, but should be followed regularly with urinalysis and urinary cytology at a minimum.

Urine with an abnormal smell is often infected, but the odor may be due to ingestion of unusual foods. Asparagus is notorious for producing this symptom.

Urinary tract stones and foreign bodies can be detected by intravenous urography and cystoscopy, usually in patients who present with pain or passage of unusual substances. These patients generally require urologic referral. Patients with psychiatric problems not infrequently insert foreign objects into the bladder and urethra, and the urologic literature is replete with unusual anecdotes of such instances.

Past Medical and Surgical History

Once the nature of the basic urologic complaint has been defined, and its course, duration, and previous treatment outlined, it must be set within the context of the patient's past medical and surgical history. Many systemic disease

TABLE 3.11. Causes of Fecal Incontinence[a]

Normal Pelvic Floor
    Diarrheal states
        Infectious diarrhea
        Inflammatory bowel disease
        Short-gut syndrome
        Laxative abuse
        Radiation enteritis
    Overflow
        Impaction
        Encopresis
        Rectal neoplasms
    Neurological conditions
        Congenital anomalies (e.g., myelomeningocele)
        Multiple sclerosis
        Dementia, strokes, tabes dorsalis
        Neuropathy (e.g., diabetes)
        Neoplasms of brain, spinal cord, cauda equina
        Injuries of brain, spinal cord, cauda equina
Abnormal pelvic floor
    Congenital anorectal malformation
    Trauma
        Accidental injury (e.g., impalement, pelvic fracture)
        Anorectal surgery
        Obstetrical injury
    Aging
    Pelvic floor denervation (idiopathic neurogenic incontinence)
        Vaginal delivery
        Chronic straining at stool
        Rectal prolapse
        Descending perineum syndrome

[a] From Madoff, Williams, Caushaj; N Engl Med J 1992; 326:1002–1007.

processes may produce local urinary tract symptoms, including congenital defects (particularly of the lower spine and cauda equina, as well as of the genitourinary tract), diabetes mellitus, thyroid disorders, and neurologic disease. Cardiovascular, pulmonary, and renal diseases are all relevant to the patient's current condition and urinary tract function.

A gastrointestinal history is particularly important, as many women with urinary tract complaints have concurrent bowel complaints. A surprising number of women with urinary incontinence also have problems with incontinence of flatus or stool. This may, in fact, be the real reason they have sought clinical help and yet they may be too embarrassed to admit it. Possible causes of fecal incontinence are given in Table 3.11. The frequency of bowel movements, their character and consistency, and the presence of incontinence of gas, liquid stool or solid stool are important questions. Alternating constipation and diarrhea is a frequent sign of irritable bowel syndrome, and this has a significant association with unstable bladder activity in women. The presence of fecal incontinence in association with urinary incontinence should prompt a more thorough gastrointestinal referral for consideration of specialized studies of colorectal function, such as anorectal manometry and defecography.

The patient's surgical history is important, particularly surgery relating to the genitourinary tract and the lumbosacral spine. It is surprising how many patients have had major surgery and yet have no idea as to what operation was performed or why it was done. Review of the patient's previous medical records may be necessary, particularly if further surgery is contemplated. This is particularly important in cases where the patient has had previous incontinence surgery which failed.

Among the most important—and frequently neglected—aspects of the patient's medical history is a thorough appreciation of the effects of drugs on the

TABLE 3.12.   Common Drugs Affecting Lower Urinary Tract Function[a]

Drug Class	Effects
Sedative hypnotics	
Benzodiazepines	Long-acting drugs such as diazepam and flurazepam may accumulate and cause confusion and secondary incontinence, particularly in elderly patients
Alcohol	Alcohol impairs mobility, causes diuresis, and can impair the sensorium
Diuretics	Loop diuretics such as furosemide, ethacrynic acid, and bumetamide can overwhelm bladder capacity and cause urgency, frequency, and incontinence
Anticholingeric agents	Anticholinergic drugs typically impair
Antihistamines	detrusor contractility and may cause
Antidepressants	urinary retention with secondary
Antipsychotics	overflow incontinence; they are
Disopnamide	common in over-the-counter cold
Opiates	remedies; in addition, many
Antispasmodics	prescription drugs have anticholinergic
Dicyclomine	properties; antipsychotic drugs may
Donnatol	cause sedation, immobility, and rigidity
Anti-Parkinsonian agents	in addition to their anticholinergic
Trihexyphenidyl	effects
Benztropine mesylate	
α-Adrenergic agents	Sympathomimetic drugs, often found in
Sympathomimetics (decongestants)	over-the-counter cold remedies, can increase urethral sphincter resistance
Sympatholytics (Prazosin, Terazosin, Doxazosin)	and lead to voiding difficulty; sympatholytic drugs such as prazosin, may lower urethral tone and cause incontinence
Calcium channel blockers	Calcium antagonists may occasionally cause urinary retention and overflow incontinence by reducing bladder smooth muscle contractility

[a] From AHCPR Clinical Practice Guidelines on Urinary Incontinence in Adults, 1992.

lower urinary tract. Diuretics, anticholinergics, muscle relaxants, antipsychotics, antihypertensive and cardiac drugs all may have surprising effects on lower urinary tract function. All medications—including over-the-counter preparations—should be reviewed with the patient. If the physician is unfamiliar with a particular drug he should make the effort to familiarize himself with it and its side effects. Many lower urinary tract disorders can be solved by a simple change of drug therapy. Common drugs affecting the lower urinary tract are listed in Table 3.12.

Physical Examination   The physical examination of the patient is crucial in the evaluation of urogynecologic complaints. The general physical examination differs little from that of any other patient in whom systemic or general medical problems are relevant to her overall care. The patient's general medical condition obviously forms the background against which all treatment decisions must be made once a diagnosis is reached. This is especially important if surgery is contemplated.

Any initial clinical encounter begins with a process which may be loosely called "sizing up the patient." A cursory visual examination as the patient comes into the room will tell you if she is mobile or in a wheelchair, whether she is crippled by arthritis or stands erect, whether she is enormously obese or has a normal body build. Body movements, gait and speech all help determine whether she has had a devastating neurologic illness such as a stroke or progressive multiple sclerosis. Does she understand your questions? Can she follow simple directions? Can she follow complex instructions? Mental status is important in dealing with incontinence, particularly in the elderly. When the patient's mental acuity is in doubt, it may be useful to perform a brief mental status examination, such as the Folstein mini-mental status exam. Mobility and dexterity are also important. Incontinence in otherwise functional but poorly mobile patients may be solved by providing them with improved access to toilet facilities, such as a bedside commode. Poor manual dexterity may mean that the patient can get to the toilet in time but has trouble undressing fast enough to maintain continence. Improvements in clothing such as eliminating buttons and replacing them with Velcro fasteners may solve this type of problem.

General medical problems are likewise important. Conditions which chronically increase intra-abdominal pressure, such as obesity, ascites, or obstructive pulmonary disease are relevant to patients with prolapse or stress incontinence. Cardiac status is important in patients with complaints of nocturia and edema. A neurologic screening exam is always important, particularly in patients whose lower urinary tract complaints present against a background of neurologic symptoms.

Attention to neurologic signs and symptoms is important for two reasons. First of all, an intact neurourologic axis is necessary for the proper functioning of the lower urinary tract and disorders at any level of the nervous system may affect bladder function (Table 3.13). Not all of these disorders are bizarre rarities: The incidence of bladder dysfunction is quite high in a number of common neurologic conditions (Table 3.14). Secondly, neurologic lesions are more common in patients who present with lower urinary tract complaints than they are in the general population. If the patient presents without any gross neurologic deficit, the chances of finding a neurologic lesion are small; nonetheless, there is a significant cohort of patients who present with urinary tract complaints and who have a significant neurologic component to their problem. It is tragic to miss a correctable condition such as a benign tumor compressing the spinal cord when failure to do so could have devastating consequences. If the history is suspicious for a possible neurologic lesion, obtain a neurologic consult, and build a close relationship with an interested neurologic practitioner.

A screening neurologic examination need not take long to perform. The importance of a mental status examination has been emphasized above. The cranial nerves can be examined rapidly, along with gait, balance and cerebellar function. Deep tendon reflexes and muscle strength of the extremities can also be assessed easily. The lumbosacral spine should be palpated and examined in all patients. The presence of a sacral dimple may indicate significant spinal dysraphism, for example.

The major emphasis in the screening examination should be on the lumbosacral and pelvic areas, since the motor innervation of the bladder and urethra comes from this area. Tone, strength, and movement of the lower extremities help evaluate the integrity of the cauda equina. It is particularly useful to have the patient attempt to abduct and spread her toes laterally because the innervation of these lateral abductors comes directly from the lower sacral segments of the spinal cord, especially S3. An inability to do this, particularly when associated with dysmorphic feet (Fig. 3.12), may be a clue to a subtle congenital abnormality of the spine which may warrant further radiographic evaluation. A plain upright KUB film will often show an occult spina bifida; however, radiologists may overlook subtle findings unless they are specifically asked to look for the presence of these abnormalities. Magnetic resonance imaging is an extremely accurate way of looking for spinal anomalies, and should be considered in cases where the suspicion of a neurologic lesion is high.

Examination of perineal sensation and the integrity of the sacral reflexes is important. This is usually done best with the patient in the dorsal lithotomy or lateral Sims position. The perineal region is supplied with sensory afferent nerve fibers from the posterior spinal roots of S2–S4 (Fig. 3.13). The exact distribution of the dermatomes is variable in this region but sensation should still be normal

TABLE 3.13.   Neurological Causes of Bladder Dysfunction[a]

Diffuse cerebral causes
  Alzheimer's disease
  Pick's disease
  Huntington's disease
  Myxedema
Focal or multifocal cerebral causes
  Parkinson's disease
  Head injury
  Multiple sclerosis
  Cerebrovascular disease
  Frontal tumor
  Hydrocephalus
Spinal cord causes
  Trauma
  Multiple sclerosis
  Transverse myelitis
  Vitamin B_{12} deficiency
  Cervical spondylotic myelopathy
Cauda equina causes
  Central lumbar disc prolapse
  Trauma
  Spina bifida
  Herpes zoster
  Sacral agenesis
Peripheral nerve causes
  Diabetes mellitus neuropathy
  Pelvic surgery or irradiation
  Autonomic degenerations
  Familial amyloid neuropathy
  Alcoholic neuropathy
  Guillain-Barré syndrome
  Drug and heavy metal toxic neuropathy
  Familial dysautonomia (Riley-Day syndrome)
  Other congenital disorders
    Prophyric neuropathy, peroneal muscular atrophy, Friedrich's ataxia, heredi-
    tary sensory-motor and autonomic neuropathies
  Other diseases:
    Uremic neuropathy, vasculitic neuropathy, Chagas disease, leprous neuritis

[a] From DN Rushton, In: Bradley, Daroff, Fenichel, and Marsden (Eds); Neurology in Clinical Practice; Boston: Butterworth-Heinemann 1991:665–676, with permission.

TABLE 3.14.   Incidence of Neuropathic Bladder in Neurological Disease[a]

Condition	Incidence
Abdominoperineal resection	10%–44%
Radical hysterectomy	7%–80%
Polio (almost always recovers)	4%–42%
Diabetic neuropathy	2%–83%
Lumbar disc disease	6%–18%
Multiple sclerosis	
Presenting symptom	2%–12%
Overall incidence	33%–78%
Parkinsonism	37%–70%
Stroke	34%–53%
Meningomyelocele	97%

[a] From MJ Torrens, In: Jordan and Stanton (Eds); The Incontinent Woman; London: Royal College of Obstetrics and Gynaecologists, 1982, with permission.

Figure 3.12 Dysmorphic feet in a 56-year-old woman with recurrent urinary tract infections, mixed stress-urge incontinence, and voiding dysfunction. Evaluation revealed a tethered spinal cord and significant spinal dysraphism. Physical examination also revealed a sacral dimple and large sacral lipoma (courtesy Dr. N.T.M. Galloway).

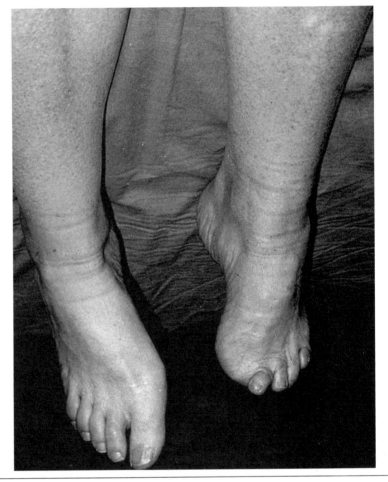

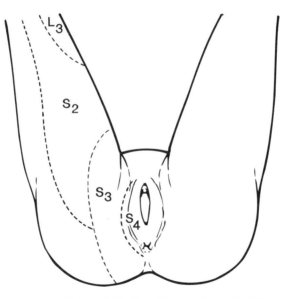

Figure 3.13 Distribution of the sacral sensory dermatomes.

and symmetrical. Gross abnormalities of perineal sensation merit further neurologic investigation. Lightly stroking the skin lateral to the anus should cause the sphincter to "wink" by reflex contraction. This is sometimes rapid and difficult to see. Lightly tapping the clitoris with a gloved finger should elicit the same response in the anal sphincter (bulbocavernosus reflex). To avoid startling or worrying patients it is important to let them know that you are going to tap them in this region before doing so. A voluntary cough should normally produce a reflex contraction of the pelvic floor ("cough reflex"). Absence of these three reflexes helps confirm the suspicion of a neurologic lesion affecting S2–S4 when this occurs within the context of other neurologic signs or symptoms; however, the absence of one of these reflexes alone is not sufficient to establish a neurologic diagnosis as these reflexes may be difficult to elicit in some otherwise normal women.

The pelvic examination is a crucial part of the evaluation of the patient with lower urinary tract complaints. The vulva should be examined for lesions, excoriations from scratching, and skin breakdown from the effects of constant urinary leakage. The presence of urogenital atrophy should be noted and treated in all symptomatic patients unless there is a direct contraindication to the use of estrogen.

It is important to evaluate pelvic support and muscle tone, since the presence of prolapse and weakness of the levator ani muscles both influence urinary continence. A gloved examining finger should be inserted into the vagina. The patient should then be asked to tighten the muscle and elevate the examining finger while it rests over the levator plate, slightly lateral to the midline of the posterior vagina (at roughly the 5 o'clock and 7 o'clock positions). This allows the examiner to assess the tone of the muscle, which can be rated on a scale of 0–5 (see Chapter 6, "Conservative Management of Stress Incontinence"). This procedure should become part of every practitioner's routine pelvic examination. This will allow the examiner to become familiar with the assessment of pelvic floor strength in asymptomatic women and to compare them with patients who have incontinence or prolapse. Many women do not realize that they can contract these muscles until they are instructed how to do so, and proper instruction in the performance of pelvic muscle exercises is a mandatory part of any successful program to improve pelvic muscle tone and strength. If the pubococcygeus and puborectalis muscles are identified routinely for patients during pelvic examinations and if patients are instructed to exercise these muscles regularly, it may be possible to prevent or delay some of the problems associated with pelvic relaxation.

The examining finger can next be used to assess the tenderness of the circumvaginal structures, particularly the posterior urethra and the bladder neck. Massaging the urethra may produce a dribble of urine or pus from the external urethral meatus, suggesting that the patient might have a urethral diverticulum or urethritis.

All patients with urinary incontinence should be examined with a full bladder and undergo some form of "stress test." The patient should be asked to cough and bear down while the mobility of the urethra is observed. Downward and outward mobility of the urethra and bladder neck accompanied by urine loss is strongly suggestive of stress incontinence. Urine is usually lost in small spurts, with each cough (Fig. 3.14). Repetitive attempts should be made to reproduce the finding of stress incontinence and to have the patient confirm that what has just been demonstrated reproduces her complaint. Delayed urine loss, particularly large volume loss or complete bladder emptying occurring after coughing, is suggestive of unstable bladder activity. If stress incontinence is demonstrated but the patient says her problem is something else, pay attention to her. Not all stress incontinence needs treatment and sometimes surgical suspension of the bladder neck makes other problems worse. Listen to the patient and correlate her symptoms with the findings on physical examination. If stress incontinence is not demonstrated in the standard lithotomy position, the stress test should be

Figure 3.14 Demonstrable stress incontinence associated with bladder neck hypermobility and a cystourethrocele.

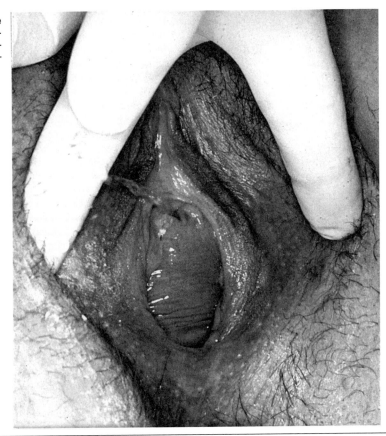

repeated in the standing position with the patient's feet comfortably separated at shoulder width. Placing an absorbent plastic-backed pad on the floor under the patient's feet is a good idea during this test.

Evaluation of the mobility of the urethra and bladder neck can be aided by placing a sterile lubricated Q-tip into the urethra to the level of the bladder neck and having the patient strain. Downward movement of the bladder neck then causes the Q-tip to rise upwards. Some clinicians find observation of the exaggerated arc created by this maneuver to be useful in assessing bladder neck displacement. An alternate method of performing this test is to use a 14 Fr plastic female self-catheterization catheter instead of a Q-tip. If the test is done after the patient has voided, the sterile catheter can be used to measure the postvoid residual urine and to collect a sterile specimen for analysis (Fig. 3.15).

Many attempts have been made to quantify bladder neck mobility using the "Q-tip test." The angle of the Q-tip in relationship to the horizontal can be measured using an orthopedic goniometer. The resting and straining angles can be measured and the difference between them calculated. Many authors consider an upward movement of more than 30 degrees to be "hypermobile." It should be emphasized, however, that this test is *only* a test for increased mobility of the bladder neck and urethra. By itself it does *not* establish the diagnosis of stress incontinence. Many women have hypermobility of the bladder base and urethra but remain continent. Many other women with different causes of incontinence and many women with terrible stress incontinence due to intrinsic urethral weakness ("Type III" incontinence) will have a normal "Q-tip test." Bladder neck displacement in women with stress incontinence is important because it has implications for the choice of surgical operation for this problem, but the

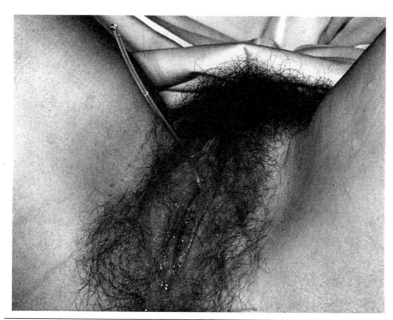

Figure 3.15 Demonstration of bladder neck hypermobility using a 14 Fr plastic female self-catheter after collection of a sterile urine specimen.

importance of the "Q-tip test" per se has been stressed too dogmatically in the past by many writers.

Examining patients with a ring forceps adds additional information about the role that loss of urethral support may play in causing stress incontinence in any individual patient (Fig. 3.16 *A–C*). Once stress incontinence has been demonstrated consistently, the end of a pair of ring forceps may be inserted into the vagina, separated by 2 or 3 cm, and placed on either side of the urethra in the paraurethral sulci. Most of the time only the ring itself needs to be inserted beyond the hymenal ring to do this. Proper position of the instrument may be checked by palpation. The patient should then be asked to cough, but no attempt should be made to elevate the vesical neck. Stress incontinence should still be demonstrable at this time. Next, the handles of the ring forceps should be elevated, keeping them parallel to the floor, until they come up to the bottom of the pubic arch. This should not *elevate* the anterior vaginal wall as much as prevent it from *descending*. If stress incontinence still persists when this is done, the patient may have a form of incontinence that will not be cured by a simple bladder neck suspension operation.

Performing this maneuver properly requires some skill and practice, since overzealous elevation of the vesical neck will simply obstruct the urethra and will not be a reliable test of vesical neck stabilization. Several urodynamic studies have confirmed this fact. The important information derived from this test comes not from seeing that improved support stops stress incontinence, but rather from seeing persistent leakage in some patients after this support has been provided. This finding suggests that an element of intrinsic weakness of the vesical neck and proximal urethra is present in such women, rather than simple displacement of these structures. These patients should be evaluated thoroughly to determine whether or not this is true. If "Type III" incontinence is confirmed, more extensive surgery (such as a suburethral sling operation) will need to be performed.

Evaluation of patients for the presence of prolapse is mandatory, especially if incontinence surgery is contemplated. Although hysterectomy is *not* always necessary in the treatment of stress incontinence, performance of a bladder neck suspension operation without treatment of concomitant prolapse is foolish and may lead to significant complications. If the posterior vagina is pulled anteriorly as the bladder neck is elevated, the cul-de-sac of Douglas can be widened. This

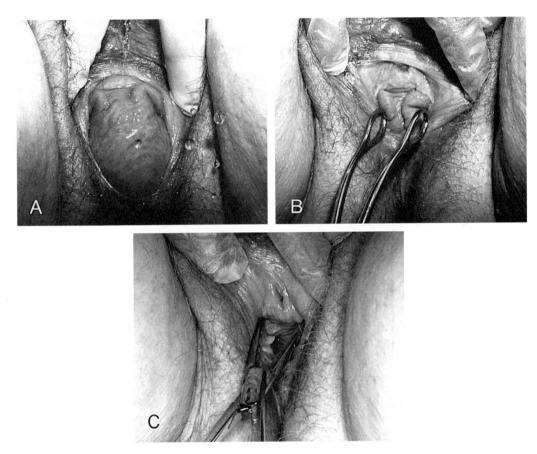

Figure 3.16 Examination of the stress-incontinent patient using ring forceps. *A.* Stress incontinence is demonstrated in association with bladder neck hypermobility and a cysto-urethrocele. *B.* The ring forceps is inserted just beyond the hymeneal ring. *C.* Support (not elevation or obstruction) of the vesical neck and urethra stops the stress incontinence. This suggests that the patient's stress incontinence is due to poor urethral support. If stress incontinence persists when proper support is provided, this suggests a more complex problem which may involve intrinsic sphincteric weakness.

may result in the worsening of a rectocele, the rapid development of an enterocele, vaginal vault eversion, or uterine procidentia.

The assessment of prolapse is greatly assisted by the routine use of a Sims vaginal speculum or by the posterior blade of an ordinary Graves speculum. This can be used to retract either the anterior or posterior vaginal wall while the other wall is inspected. This is very useful in the assessment of vaginal relaxation, particularly when a large prolapse is present. Having the patient cough or bear down while the speculum is positioned in the posterior vagina aids in the observation of bladder neck mobility and may facilitate the demonstration of stress incontinence. However, care should be taken not to pull the bladder neck down by depressing the posterior vagina too much or a "false positive" exam for stress incontinence may be created. If a large prolapse—such as a complete posthysterectomy vaginal vault prolapse—is present, the speculum blade may be used to reposition the prolapse into its normal position while the patient coughs. Because massive prolapse can kink and compress the urethra and thereby mask an otherwise incompetent continence mechanism, replacing the prolapse and holding it in place while the patient coughs is a useful test for detecting unsuspected stress incontinence. A cube pessary can also be used for this purpose.

The importance of examining patients in the upright as well as the dorsal lithotomy position should also be emphasized. Most incontinent women have more problems with incontinence while they are erect and active than when they are recumbent. The importance of performing a "cough stress test" in the standing position has already been mentioned, particularly if the patient's complaint of stress incontinence has not been confirmed during examination in the dorsal lithotomy position. The patient with prolapse should also be examined in the upright position. Her right foot should be placed on a small stool or the footstep of the examining table and a vaginal examination carried out with her standing. A cystocele, rectocele, or uterine descent is often much more pronounced in this position than when the patient is lying down. The use of a thumb in the vagina with a forefinger in the rectum also allows a much better examination for the presence of an enterocele. Small bowel descending into the cul-de-sac is easily trapped between the two examining fingers if an enterocele is present. The examination and management of patients with prolapse is discussed in more detail in Chapter 14, "Prolapse and the Lower Urinary Tract."

Incontinent patients should be examined with a *full* bladder, particularly patients complaining of stress incontinence. A primary goal of the examination is to demonstrate repetitive urine loss, and this may not be possible in patients with an empty or only partially full bladder. Although it may be difficult to break old habits, patients should be encouraged to come for their urogynecologic evaluation with a full bladder and they should *not* empty it prior to being examined. The patient may be allowed to void after the cough stress test. A routine pelvic examination may then be performed. If a urine flowmeter is available, this provides an opportunity to obtain further information on voiding function. Immediately after voiding, the volume voided should be recorded and the patient should be checked for the presence of residual urine. This can be estimated crudely by palpation, or it can be calculated by ultrasound measurements. Most clinicians will prefer simply to catheterize the bladder since this is more accurate than palpation and much cheaper than ultrasound, and also allows a sterile urine specimen to be collected for urinalysis and culture. If a small plastic female self-catheter is used to collect the residual urine, it can serve as a "surrogate Q-tip" for evaluating urethral mobility (see above). If the voided volume is small and incontinence has not been demonstrated in a patient who complains of this problem, her bladder should be filled to capacity with sterile water or saline. This can be done simply by filling the bladder, or a simple cystometrogram can be performed if the filling line is connected to a simple manometer (see Chapter 4, "Practical Urodynamics"). Alternatively, a urethroscope or cystoscope can be used to fill the bladder. Information on bladder capacity and sensation can be obtained in this way, and the presence of stress incontinence can be determined reliably by having the patient cough with a full bladder. If a urethroscope is used for bladder filling, the inside of the bladder and urethra can also be examined.

Urinalysis, Culture, and Cytology

Examination of the urine is a mandatory part of the evaluation of any patient with lower urinary tract complaints and is one of the most cost-effective parts of patient evaluation. A "clean-catch" voided specimen is suitable for routine urinalysis, provided it is truly a "clean" specimen. Obtaining such a specimen is more difficult in women (especially pregnant women) than in men. The cleanest way for women to obtain a voided specimen is to have them use a private toilet, remove all of their lower garments, straddle or sit on the toilet while facing the back, spread the labia with one hand and cleanse themselves thoroughly with a moist "towelette" from front to back, void the initial portion of the urine stream into the toilet while keeping the labia apart and collect the midstream portion of the voided urine as the specimen. Attempting to base a clinical plan upon voided urine contaminated with menstrual blood, large clumps of squamous epithelial cells, or vulvar and vaginal bacteria is hopeless, and culturing such urine is equally unhelpful in caring for a symptomatic patient. It is, therefore,

TABLE 3.15. Criteria for Classification of Positive Microscopic Urinary Sediment Exam Using Brightfield Microscopy on Spun Urine Specimens[a]

1. More than five erythrocytes, leukocytes, or renal tubular cells per high-power field (430×)
2. More than 3 hyaline casts, more than one granular cast, or the presence of any other type of cast per low-power field (100×)
3. More than one (three to five) bacteria per high-power field (430×)
4. The presence of fungi, parasites, or viral inclusions
5. The presence of significant crystals (e.g., cystine) or a large number of crystals (e.g., uric acid)

Note: The presence of these findings proves an abnormality. Absence of these findings does *not* prove the absence of an abnormality, particularly if the urine is dilute.

[a] Based on Schuman and Greenberg. Am J Clin Pathol 1979; 71:452–456; and Szwed and Schaust. Am J Med Technol 1982; 48:141–143

more useful in many cases to obtain a urine sample for urinalysis and culture by sterile in-and-out catheterization. This can usually be done at the same time that residual urine is measured after voiding.

Urine should be examined while it is still fresh, because particulate matter settles out with standing, casts may dissolve, bacteria grow, and the pH change. Approximately 10 ml of urine is needed for a microscopic examination. Uncentrifuged urine should be examined routinely with the use of a "dipstick" for chemical abnormalities. A variety of dipsticks are available which will test for urine specific gravity, pH, protein, glucose, ketones, blood, bilirubin, nitrites, leukocyte esterase, etc. Urine should be evaluated while fresh and the instructions for a particular test strip should be followed carefully to avoid misleading results. Microscopic examination of unspun urine can detect the probable presence of urinary tract infection if one or more bacteria are present per high-power field. The presence of white blood cells is suggestive, but less indicative, of acute infection than the presence of bacteria.

Examination of the urinary sediment is particularly useful in looking for renal disease. For a proper examination, the urine should be centrifuged for five minutes at 2,000 rpm, the supernatant fluid discarded, and the sediment examined after resuspending it on a microscope slide in a small amount of the remaining urine. The traditional criteria for classifying a urinary sediment examination as "positive" are given in Table 3.15.

Urine specific gravity will depend upon a patient's state of hydration, normal production of ADH from the posterior pituitary, and renal function. Specific gravity is measured relative to water according to the formula:

$$\text{Specific Gravity} = \text{Weight of urine/weight of water.}$$

Normal urine specific gravity ranges from 1.003–1.040. Values above 1.032 are quite concentrated and may reflect the presence of extraneous solutes such as IVP dye, mannitol, etc. Low values will be found in patients with hyocalcemia, hypokalemia, protein malnutrition, and polydipsia who are not able to concentrate urine effectively. Diuretic use may also produce urine with a low specific gravity.

Urinary pH is an expression of urinary acid excretion. Normal urine has a pH between 5 and 9. Highly alkaline urine may reflect the presence of an infection with a urea splitting bacteria such as *Proteus* species. If the patient suffers from systemic acidosis but is excreting an alkaline urine, this may indicate renal tubular acidosis.

Protein is not normally present in urine and enters the urinary tract either through tubular damage or altered glomerular permeability to protein. Most reagent test strips measure albumin, which enters the urine through the glomerulus. As a result, dipstick testing for protein is only useful for detecting albumin and may miss other proteins which may be present in the urine, such as globulins or light chains.

Glucose is found in normal urine in small amounts (<100 mg/dl) but is usually masked on dipsticks by the presence of ketones, ascorbic acid and other substances. Large amounts of glucose in the urine are usually associated with diabetes mellitus. Pregnancy alters glucose reabsorption in the kidney and therefore often produces a physiologic renal glycosuria which resolves in the postpartum period.

Ketones appear in urine as a by-product of fat metabolism. They are most likely to be found in fasting patients or diabetics in ketoacidosis.

Bilirubin and urobilinogen are found in the urine of patients with abnormal liver function or abnormal bilirubin metabolism. Indirect bilirubin is bound to albumin and does not appear in the urine, but conjugated bilirubin is water soluble and therefore appears in the urine in amounts which correlate roughly with the level of "direct" serum bilirubin. Conjugated bilirubin is usually detected in the urine when it is present in amounts greater than 0.2 mg/dl. False negative tests for urinary bilirubin may be caused by ascorbic acid. Phenothiazines may cause false positive tests.

Urobilinogen is produced as a by-product of bowel flora acting upon conjugated bilirubin. Urobilinogen is then reabsorbed into the portal circulation. The amount of urobilinogen presented to the kidney for excretion can therefore be raised by increased bilirubin production or decreased hepatic clearance of bilirubin. Hemolysis or liver dysfunction will increase the amount of urobilinogen in the urine by increasing the load which is presented to the kidney. Biliary obstruction can lower urobilinogen production by reducing the amount of bilirubin which reaches the bowel. Antibiotics acting upon bowel flora can reduce urobilinogen production by decreasing the bacterial population of the gut. When bilirubin and urobilinogen are analyzed together they can help to distinguish between biliary obstruction, hemolysis, or liver disease.

Hemoglobin should not be present in the urine. It appears either as the result of direct bleeding into the urinary tract, or as the result of intravascular hemolysis with subsequent hemoglobin clearance by the kidney. Myoglobin from injured muscle will also react with the reagent strip for hemoglobin. Ascorbic acid may cause a false negative reaction for hemoglobin on dipstick analysis. Povidone-iodine solutions may cause false positive reactions.

Nitrites appear in the urine from the reduction of nitrates by bacteria. This causes a color change on the nitrite reaction strip on a dipstick and is a useful indicator of bacteriuria. Its usefulness goes up when it is found in association with *leukocyte esterase*, an enzyme associated with pyuria. A negative test for nitrite does not rule out urinary tract infection, as some bacteria do not reduce nitrates. Also, the infected urine may be evacuated from the bladder before the reaction can take place, particularly in patients with urgency and frequency. Although leukocyte esterase is quite a sensitive test for pyuria, phenazopyridine (Pyridium), vitamin C, and high protein levels may interfere with the test results. Urine culture should be obtained when there is any question of infection in a symptomatic patient.

Urinary sediment may contain a variety of cells and casts and is usually evaluated after centrifugation (Table 3.15). Hematuria is manifested by the presence of red blood cells and has an extensive differential diagnosis (Table 3.9). The presence of white blood cells usually indicates an infection, but this may also be found in collagen-vascular disease or allergic interstitial nephritis, particularly if red blood cells are also present. Epithelial cells from any part of the urinary tract may be sloughed into the urine. Squamous epithelial cells from the vulva and vagina are frequently present—particularly if the "clean catch" urine is not so clean. Vulvar and vaginal contamination can also result in increased numbers of bacteria, leukocytes, and other foreign cells, such as spermatozoa or trichomonads. Casts are formed in the renal tubules by hyalinized protein and may incorporate red cells or white cells. The presence of such cells in renal

TABLE 3.16.   Risk Factors for Bladder Cancer

Gross hematuria
Microhematuria
Male:female 3:1
Heavy smoker
Occupational exposure to industrial chemicals
Persistent irritative voiding symptoms
Age over 50 years
Analgesic abuse (phenacetin)
Chronic urinary tract infection
Treatment with cyclophosphamide

casts suggests that they have originated in the kidney and raise the important possibility of renal disease.

Urine can also be examined for the presence of abnormal or malignant cells by *urinary cytology.* The usefulness of this test depends upon the quality of the cytology laboratory performing the work and on the nature of the population being screened. There is little evidence which justifies the use of routine urine cytology in the general population; however, patients at risk for bladder malignancy should be screened. A list of risk factors is given in Table 3.16. By itself, urinary incontinence probably does not justify the routine use of cytology, but patients with persistent irritative voiding symptoms should be screened, particularly if another risk factor is present. Carcinoma-in situ of the bladder often cannot be localized even by cystoscopy and biopsy. Therefore, urinary cytology has an important role to play in the diagnosis and management of this condition. Specimens for cytology should be fresh and the yield may be improved by washing the bladder with normal saline. The first voided urine specimen in the morning should *not* be used for cytology, because concentrated urine will lyse free urothelial cells and render cytologic examination less useful.

Next Step

At this point in the evaluation process, the clinician should be able to answer the following questions:

- **What is the patient's main complaint?**
- **How has this complaint developed or progressed?**
- **Is urinary incontinence a problem?**
- **Has stress incontinence been demonstrated and is it relevant to the patient's main complaint?**
- **Does she have symptoms related to voiding difficulty?**
- **Does she have an elevated postvoid residual urine?**
- **Does she have a problem with bladder sensitivity?**
- **Is there evidence of genital prolapse?**
- **Is there evidence of estrogen deficiency?**
- **Is the urine normal?**
- **Are there acute medical problems which need immediate attention?**

By now the nature of the patient's complaint should be fairly clear, even if the precise etiology of her symptoms is not. These symptoms will fall into four main categories:

1. Abnormal Storage (Incontinence).   It should be clear at this point if the patient has stress incontinence, urge incontinence, or mixed incontinence. If she complains of stress incontinence, and this has been demonstrated, it is acceptable to proceed with conservative management immediately. If urge incontinence is her main complaint, a frequency/volume chart will provide additional information useful in planning a course of treatment. Conservative therapy may also be initiated, and the patient reevaluated in a few weeks. If a large residual urine is present, if the patient has unusual or atypical symptoms, or if surgery is contemplated, further evaluation is usually necessary.

2. Abnormal Emptying (Voiding Problems). Symptoms of voiding dysfunction or the presence of a large postvoid residual urine need further evaluation, generally with more sophisticated urodynamic testing. This is especially true in the presence of neurologic findings (see Chapter 13, "Bladder Emptying Problems").

3. Abnormal Sensation. A hypersensitive bladder requires a more thorough investigation, including careful urinalysis and culture. Cytology, cystoscopy, and radiographic imaging studies may all be necessary. An individual approach is needed based upon the symptoms and physical findings in each patient (see Chapter 11, "Sensory Disorders of the Bladder and Urethra").

4. Abnormal Bladder Contents. Further evaluation of abnormal urine will depend upon the nature of the abnormality. This may range from simple urine culture to a full-scale oncologic work-up or admission to a nephrology service.

Succeeding chapters in this book provide additional information about the etiology and treatment of these symptom complexes. Arriving at the patient's final diagnosis can be aided greatly by the selective use of appropriate urodynamic studies, which are discussed in Chapter 4. Not all of these studies are complex or expensive (e.g., frequency/volume bladder charts). However, it is important to remember that all urodynamic studies are an adjunct to the basic history and physical examination, not a substitute for careful initial patient evaluation. Urodynamic studies which do not reproduce the patient's complaint are of limited usefulness.

REFERENCES

General Evaluation

Abrams P, Blaivas JG, Stanton SL, Anderson JT. The standardisation of terminology of lower urinary tract function. Scand J Urol Nephrol Suppl 1988; 114:5–18.

Barker JC, Mitteness LS. Nocturia in the elderly. Gerontologist 1988: 28:99–104.

Bhatia NN, Bergman A. The pessary test in women with urinary incontinence. Obstet Gynecol 1985; 65:220–226.

Bissada NK, Finkbeiner, AE. Urologic manifestations of drug therapy. Urol Clin NA 1988; 15:725–36.

Bueschen, AJ. Flank pain. In Walker HK, Hall, WD, Hurst, JW (Eds), Clinical Methods: The History, Physical, and Laboratory Examinations. Boston: Butterworths, 1990; 845–46, 3rd ed.

Bump, RC, Sugerman, HJ, Fantl, JA, McClish, DK. Obesity and lower urinary tract function in women: Effect of surgically induced weight loss. Am J Obstet Gynecol 1992; 167:392–99.

Carlton, CE, Scardino, PT. Initial evaluation, including history, physical examination, and urinalysis. In Walsh, PC, Gittes, RF, Perlmutter, AD, Stamey, TA (Eds.), Campbell's Urology 5th ed.; Philadelphia: W.B. Saunders, 1986; 276–85.

Carenza L, Nobili F, Siacobini S, et al. Voiding disorders after radical hysterectomy. Gynecol Oncol 1982; 13: 213–19.

Coolsaet BLRA, Blok C, van Venrouji GEFM, et al. Subthreshold detrusor instability. Neurourol Urodynam 1985; 4:309–11.

Cardozo LD, Stanton SL, Bennett AE. Design of a urodynamic questionnaire. Br J Urol 1978; 50:269–74.

Dwyer PL, Lee ETC, Hay DM. Obesity and urinary incontinence in women. Br J Obstet Gynaecol 1988;95:91–96.

Eckford SD, Persad RA, Brewster SF, Gingell JC. Intravesical foreign bodies: Five-year review. Br J Urol 1992; 69: 41–45.

Farrar DJ, Whiteside CG, Osborne JL, Turner-Warwick RT.

A urodynamic analysis of micturition symptoms in the female. Surg Gynecol Obstet 1975; 141:875–81.

Folstein MF, Folstein SE, McHugh PR. "Mini-mental state: " A practical method for grading the cognitive state of patients for the clinician. J Psychiat Res 1975; 12:189–98.

Fraser A. The late effects of Wertheim's hysterectomy on the urinary tract. J Obstet Gynaecol Br Commw 1966; 73: 1002–2007.

Gardy M, Kozminski M, DeLancey J, et al. Stress incontinence and cystoceles. J Urol 1991; 145:1211–13.

Glen ES, Small DR, Morrison LM, et al. Urological history-taking and management recommendations by microcomputer. Br J Urol 1989; 63:117–21.

Hodgkinson CP. Urinary stress incontinence in the female: A programme of preoperative investigation. Clin Obstet Gynecol 1963; 6:154–77.

Jarvis GJ, et al. An assessment of urodynamic examination in the incontinent woman. Br J Obstet Gynaecol 1980; 87:893–96.

Jordan JA, Stanton SL (Eds). The Incontinent Woman. London: Royal College of Obstetricians and Gynaecologists, 1982.

Kadar N. The value of bladder filling in the clinical detection of urine loss and selection of patients for urodynamic testing. Br J Obstet Gynaecol 1988; 95:698–704.

Koefoot RB, Webster GD. Urodynamic evaluation in women with frequency, urgency symptoms. Urology 1983; 6: 648–51.

Kolbl H, Riss P. Obesity and stress urinary incontinence: Significance of indices of relative weight. Urol Int 1988; 43:7–10.

Madoff RD, Williams JG, Caushag PF. Fecal incontinence. New Eng J Med 1992; 326:1002–07.

Ostergard DR. The effect of drugs on the lower urinary tract. Obstet Gynecol Surv 1979; 34:424–32.

Rees DLP, Whitfield HN, Islam AKM, et al. Urodynamic findings in adult females with frequency and dysuria. Br J Urol 1975; 47:853–60.

Richer C, Decker N, Belin J, Imbs, JL, Montastruc JL, Giudicelli JF. Odorous urine in man after asparagus. Br J Clin Pharmacol 1989; 27:640–41.

Robertson JR. Ambulatory gynecologic urology. Clin Obstet Gynecol 1974; 17:255–75.

Susset J, et al. Urodynamic assessment of stress incontinence and its therapeutic implications. Surg Gynecol Obstet 1976; 142:343–52.

Vertuno LL, Kozeny GA. Nocturia. In Walker HK, Hall WD, Hurst JW (Eds) Clinical Methods: The History, Physical, and Laboratory Examinations. 3rd ed. Boston: Butterworths 1990; 847–48.

Urinary Incontinence Guideline Panel. Urinary Incontinence in Adults: Clinical Practice Guidelines. AHCPR Pub. No. 92-0038. Rockville, MD: Agency for Health Care Policy and Research, Public Health Service, U.S. Department of Health and Human Services, 1992.

Wall LL, Hewitt JK. Urodynamic characteristics of women with complete post-hysterectomy vaginal vault prolapse. Urology; In Press.

Walter S, Olesen KP. Urinary incontinence and genital prolapse in the female: Clinical, urodynamic and radiological examinations. Br J Obstet Gynaecol 1982; 89:393–401.

Walters MD, Shields LE. The diagnostic value of history, physical examination, and the Q-tip cotton swab test in women with urinary incontinence. Am J Obstet Gynecol 1988; 159:145–49.

Warrell DW. Investigation and treatment of incontinence of urine in the female who has had a prolapse repair operation. Br J Urol 1965; 37:233–39.

Wein AJ. Practical uropharmacology. Urol Clin NA 1991; 18:269–81.

Whorwell PJ, McCallum M, Creed Fh. et al. Non-colonic features of irritable bowel syndrome. Gut 1986; 27:37–40.

Whorwell PJ, Lupton EW, Erduran D, et al. Bladder smooth muscle dysfunction in patients with irritable bowel syndrome. Gut 1986; 27:1014–17.

Yarnell JWG, Voyle GJ, Sweetnam PM, Milbank J, Richards CJ, Stephenson TP. Factors associated with urinary incontinence in women; J. Epidemiol Comm Heal 1982; 36: 58–63.

Frequency/Volume Bladder Charts

Boedker A, Lendorf A, H-Nielsen A, Glahn B. Micturition pattern assessed by the frequency volume chart in a healthy population of men and women. Neurourol Urodynam 1989; 8:421–22.

Diokno AC, Wells TJ, Brink CA. Comparison of self reported voided volume with cystometric bladder capacity. J Urol 1987; 137:698–700.

Larrson G, Victor A. Micturition patterns in a healthy female population, studied with a frequency/volume chart. Scand J Urol Nephrol Suppl 1988; 114:53–57

Larrson G, Abrams P, Victor A. The frequency/volume chart in detrusor instability. Neurourol Urodynam 1991; 10: 533–43.

Larsson G, Victor A. The frequency/volume chart in genuine stress incontinent women. Neurourol Urodynam 1992; 11: 23–31.

McCormack M, Infante-Rivard C, Schick E. Agreement between clinical methods of measurement of urinary frequency and functional bladder capacity. Br J Urol 1991; 69:17–21.

Wyman JF, Choi SC, Harkins SW, Wilson MS, Fantl JA. The urinary diary in the evaluation of incontinent women: a test-retest analysis. Obstet Gynecol 1988; 71:812–17.

Clinical NeuroUrology

Andersen JT, Bradley WE. Neurogenic bladder dysfunction in protruded lumbar disk and after laminectomy. Urology 1976; 8:94–96.

Andersen JT, Bradley WE. Abnormalities of detrusor and sphincter function in multiple sclerosis. Br J Urol 1976; 48:193–98.

Andersen JT, Hebjorn S, Frimodt-Moller C, et al. Disturbances of micturition in Parkinson's disease. Acta Neurol Scand 1976; 53:161–70.

Andersen JT, Bradley WE. Bladder and urethral innervation in multiple sclerosis. Br J Urol 1976; 48:239–43.

Awad S, Gajewski JB, Sogbein SK, et al. Relationship between neurological and urological status in patients with multiple sclerosis. J Urol 1984; 132:499–502.

Beck RP, Warren KG, Whitman P. Urodynamic studies in female patients with multiple sclerosis. Am J Obstet Gynecol 1981; 139:273–76.

Bemelmans BLH, Hommes OR, Van Kerrebroeck PEV, Lemmens WAJG, Doesburg WH, Debruyne FMJ. Evidence for early lower urinary tract dysfunction in clinically silent multiple sclerosis. J Urol 1991; 145:1219–24.

Blaivas JG, Labib KB. Acute urinary retention in women: Complete urodynamic evaluation. Urology 1977; 10: 383–89.

Bors E, Turner RD. History and physical examination in neurological urology. J Urol 1960; 83:759–67.

Bradley WE. Diagnosis of urinary bladder dysfunction in diabetes mellitus. Ann Int Med 1980; 92:323–26.

Brocklehurst JC, Andrews K, Richards B, et al. Incidence and correlates of incontinence in stroke patients. J Am Geriatr Soc 1985; 33:540–42.

Brooks ME, Moreno M, Sidi A, Braf ZF. Urologic complications after surgery on lumbosacral spine. Urology 1985; 26:202–04.

Caplan LR, Kleeman FJ, Berg S. Urinary retention probably secondary to herpes genitalis. NEJM 1977; 297:920–21.

Doran J, Roberts M. Acute urinary retention in the female. Br J Urol 1976; 47:793–96.

Ellenberg M, Weber H. The incipient asymptomatic diabetic bladder. Diabetes 1967; 16:331–35.

Ellenberg M. Development of urinary bladder dysfunction in diabetes mellitus. Ann Int Med 1980; 92:321–23.

Emmett JL, Love JG. Urinary retention in women caused by asymptomatic protruded lumbar disk: Report of 5 cases. J Urol 1968; 99:597–606.

Emmett JL, Love JG. Vesical dysfunction caused by protruded lumbar disk. J Urol 1971; 105:86–91.

Fidas A, MacDonald HL, Elton RA, McInnes A, Wild SR, Chisholm GD. Prevalence of spina bifida occulta in patients with functional disorders of the lower urinary tract and its relation to urodynamic and neurophysiological measurements. BMJ 1989; 298:357–59.

Frimodt-Moller C. Diabetic cystopathy: Epidemiology and related disorders. Ann Int Med 1980; 92:318–21.

Frimodt-Moller C, Mortensen S. Treatment of diabetic cystopathy. Ann Int Med 1980; 92:327–28.

Goldstein I, Siroky MB, Sax DS, et al. Neurourologic abnormalities in multiple sclerosis. J Urol 1982; 128:541–45.

Galloway NTM, Tainsh J. Minor defects of the sacrum and neurogenic bladder dysfunction. Br J Urol 1985; 57: 154–55.

Galloway NTM. Classification and diagnosis of neurogenic bladder dysfunction. Prob Urol 1989; 3:1–39.

Garfield J, Lytle SN. Urinary presentation of cauda equina lesions without neurological symptoms. Br J Urol 1970; 42:551–54.

Kham Z, Hertanu J, Yang WC, et al. Predictive correlation of urodynamic dysfunction and brain injury after cerebrovascular accident. J Urol 1981; 126:86–88.

Kogan BA, Solomon MH, Diokno AC. Urinary retention secondary to Landry-Guillain-Barre syndrome. J Urol 1981; 126; 643–44.

McGuire EJ, Wagner FC Jr. The effects of sacral denervation on bladder and urethral function. Surg Gynecol Obstet 1977; 144:343–46.

McGuire EJ, Savastano JA. Urodynamic findings and long term outcome management of patients with multiple sclerosis induced lower urinary tract dysfunction. J Urol 1984; 132:713–15.

Mastri AR. Neuropathology of diabetic neurogenic bladder. Ann Int Med 1980; 92:316–18.

Mayo M, Chetner MP. Lower urinary tract dysfunction in multiple sclerosis. Urology 1992; 39:67–70.

O'Flynn KJ, Murphy R, Thomas DG. Neurogenic bladder dysfunction in lumber intervertebral disc prolapse. Br J Urol 1992; 69:38–40.

Pavlakis AJ, Siroky MB, Goldstein I, et al. Neurourologic findings in Parkinson's disease. J Urol 1983; 129:80–83.

Peterson T, Pedersen E. Neurourodynamic evaluation of voiding dysfunction in multiple sclerosis. Acta Neurol Scand 1984; 69:402–11.

Philp T, Read DJ, Higson RH. The urodynamic characteristics of multiple sclerosis. Br J Urol 1981; 53:672–75.

Rushton DN. Neurourology. In Bradley WG, Daroff RB, Fenichel GM, Marsden CD (Eds) Neurology in Clinical Practice; Boston: Butterworth Heinemann 1991:665–76.

Schiff HI. The neurogenic bladder in diabetes. NY St J Med 1982; 82:922–26.

Scot PJ. Bladder paralysis in cauda equina lesions from disc prolapse. J Bone Joint Surg 1965; 47B:224–35.

Susset JG, Peters ND, Cohen SI, et al. Early detection of neurogenic bladder dysfunction caused by protruded lumbar disk. Urology 1982; 20:461–63.

Tsuchida S, Noto H, Yamaguchi O, et al. Urodynamic studies on hemiplegic patients after cerebrovascular accident. Urology 1983; 21:315–18.

Wheeler JS Jr., Siroky MB, Pavlakis AJ, et al. The changing neurourologic pattern of multiple sclerosis. J Urol 1983; 130:1123–26.

Wheeler JS Jr., Sax DS, Krane RJ, et al. Vesico urethral function in Huntington's chorea. Br J Urol 1985; 57: 63–66.

Wheeler JS Jr., Culkin DJ, O'Hara RJ, et al. Bladder dysfunction and neurosyphilis. J Urol 1986; 136:903–05.

Yalla SV, Andriole GL. Vesicourethral dysfunction following pelvic visceral ablative surgery. J Urol 1984; 132: 503–09.

Assessment of Residual Urine

Haylen BT. Residual urine volumes in a normal female population: Application of transvaginal ultrasound. Br J Urol 1989; 64:347–49.

Haylen BT. Verification of the accuracy and range of transvaginal ultrasound in measuring bladder volumes in women. Br J Urol 1989; 64:350–52.

Haylen BT, Frazer MI, MacDonald JH. Assessing the effectiveness of different urinary catheters in emptying the bladder: an application of transvaginal ultrasound. Br J Urol 1989; 64:353–56.

Hendrikx AJM, Doesburg WH, Stappen W, et al. Ultrasonic determination of the residual urine volume. Urol Int 1989; 44:96–102.

Ireton RC, Krieger JH, Cardenas DD, et al. Bladder volume determination using a dedicated, portable ultrasound scanner. J Urol 1990; 143; 909–11.

Mainprize TC, Drutz HP. Accuracy of total bladder volume and residual urine measurements: Comparison between real-time ultrasonography and catheterization. Am J Obstet Gynecol 1989; 160:1013–16.

Williot P, McLorie GA, Gilmour RF, et al. Accuracy of bladder volume determinations in children using a suprapubic ultrasonic bi-planar technique. J Urol 1989; 141: 900–02.

Wise BG, Burton G, Cutner A, Cardozo LD. Effect of vaginal ultrasound probe on lower urinary tract function. Br J Urol 1992; 70:12–16.

Hematuria

Abuelo JG. Evaluation of hematuria. Urology 1983; 21: 215–25.

Birch DF, Fairley KF, Whitworth JA, Forbes IK, Fairley JK, Cheshire GR, Ryan GB. Urinary erythrocyte morphology in the diagnosis of glomerular hematuria. Clin Nephrol 1983; 20:78–84.

Burkholder GV, Dotin LN, Thomason WB, Beach PD. Unexplained hematuria: How extensive should the evaluation be? J Am Med Assoc 1969; 210:1729–33.

Carson CC III, Segura JW, Greene LF. Clinical importance of microhematuria. J Am Med Assoc 1979; 241:149–50.

Golin AL, Howard RS. Asymptomatic microscopic hematuria. J Urol 1980; 124:389–91.

Kirkpatrick WG. Hematuria. In Walker HK, Hall WD, Hurst JW (Eds); Clinical Methods: The History, Physical, and Laboratory Examinations. 3rd ed. Boston: Butterworths 1990:849–50.

Mariani AJ, Mariani MC, Macchioni C, Stams UK, Hariharan A, Moriera A. The significance of adult hematuria: 1,000 hematuria evaluations including a risk-benefit and cost-effectiveness analysis. J Urol 1989; 141:350–55.

Turner AG, Hendry WF, Williams GB, Wallace DM. A haematuria diagnostic service. Br Med J 1977; 2:29–31.

Urinalysis

Bolann BJ, Sandberg S, Digranes A. Implications of probability analysis for interpreting results of leukocyte esterase and nitrite test strips. Clin Chem 1989; 35:1663–68.

Carel RS, Silverberg DS, Kaminsky R, Aviram A. Routine urinalysis (dipstick) findings in mass screening of healthy adults. Clin Chem 1987; 33:2106–08.

Hindman R, Troic B, Bartlett R. Effect of delay on culture of urine. J Clin Microbiol 1976; 4:102–03.

Kellogg JA, Manzella JP, Shaffer SN, Schwartz BB. Clinical relevance of culture versus screens for the detection of microbial pathogens in urine specimens. Am J Med 1987; 83:739–45.

Kunin CM, DeGroot JE. Self-screening for significant bacteriuria: Evaluation of dip-strip combination nitrite/culture test. J Am Med Assoc 1975; 231:1349–53.

Pezzlo M, Wetkowski MA, Peterson EM, De la Maza LM. Detection of bacteriuria and pyuria within two minutes. J Clin Microbiol 1985; 21:578–81.

Pezzlo M. Detection of urinary tract infections by rapid methods. Clin Microbiol Rev 1988; 1:268–80.

Pouchot J, Launay I, Cahen P, Boussougant Y, Vinceneux P. Significance of crystal clear urine. Lancet 1990; 336: 320–21.

Raymond JR, Yarger WE. Abnormal urine color: Differential diagnosis. South. Med. J. 1988; 81:837–41.

Roxe DM. Urinalysis. In Walker HK, Hall WD, Hurst JW (Eds); Clinical Methods: The History, Physical, and Laboratory Examinations. 3rd ed. Boston: Butterworths 1990: 868–71.

Schumann GB, Greenberg NF. Usefulness of macroscopic

urinalysis as a screening procedure: A preliminary report. Am J Clin Path 1979; 71:452–56.

Shaw ST, Poon SY, Wong ET. "Routine urinalysis:" Is the dipstick enough? J Am Med Assoc 1985; 253:1596–1600.

Szwed JJ, Schaust C. The importance of microscopic examination of the urinary sediment. Am J Med Technol 1982; 48:141–43.

Wenk RE, Dutta D, Ruderst J, Kim Y, Steinhagen C. Sediment microscopy, nitrituria, and leukocyte esterasuria as predictors of significant bacteriuria. J Clin Lab Automat 1982; 2:117–21.

Wenz B, Lampasso JA. Eliminating unnecessary urine microscopy: Results and performance characteristics of an algorithm based on chemical reagent strip testing. Am J Clin Path 1989; 92:78–81.

Wilson DM. Urinalysis and other tests of renal function. Minn Med 1975; 58:9–17.

Urinary Cytology

Farrow GM, Ultz DC, Rife CC, Greene LF. Clinical observations on sixty-nine cases of in situ carcinoma of the urinary bladder. Cancer Res 1977; 37:2794–96.

Heney NM, Szyfelbein WM, Daly JJ, Prout GR, Bredin HC. Positive urinary cytology in patients without evident tumor. J Urol 1977; 117:223–24.

Morrison AS. Public health value of using epidemiologic information to identify high-risk groups for bladder cancer screening. Semin Oncol 1979; 6:184–88.

Murphy WM. Current status of urinary cytology in the evaluation of bladder neoplasms. Hum Pathol 1990:21:886–96.

4   Practical Urodynamics

Even the most searching history and thorough physical examination may fail to uncover the true nature of bladder dysfunction in some women. Some patients are simply unable to separate their symptoms as precisely as a trained urogynecologist would like. Others have already made their "own diagnosis" and view their symptoms through this artificial filter. Some clinicians do not question their patients closely enough to find out *exactly* what is troubling them, and thereby run the risk of basing therapy on a superficial understanding of the patient's complaint. There are pitfalls present in taking a history during every clinical encounter and these will vary with the patient population involved. There are obvious differences in taking histories from patients in a small midwestern university town as opposed to those presenting for care at an inner city charity hospital in the deep south.

A "urodynamic study" is any test which provides objective information about lower urinary tract function. These studies vary in complexity from the simple frequency/volume bladder chart to complex fluoroscopic video urodynamics with simultaneous pelvic floor electromyography. Urodynamic testing is an *adjunct to,* not a *substitute for,* a thorough history and physical examination. Used together with the patient's clinical presentation and medical background, urodynamic testing can reveal a wealth of information about urethral function, bladder storage, and the process of voiding. If the pieces do not mesh together, however, the clinician should step back and rethink the diagnosis.

Object of All Urodynamic Testing is to Reproduce the Patient's Symptoms Under Controlled Conditions

Simple urodynamic tests are widely available and performing them should be within the scope of practice of all physicians who provide primary care. Training programs in gynecology, medicine, family practice, and geriatrics—not to mention many urology residencies—do not always do a good job of familiarizing physicians with the use and interpretation of these tests. Combined with a good history and physical examination, simple urodynamic tests can lead to a preliminary diagnosis and the formulation of an initial, conservative treatment plan for most patients. The most difficult part of these tests is developing the clinical skills necessary to select the proper test and to interpret its meaning in the case of any individual patient. If residents had more training in the evaluation and management of the incontinent patient, these obstacles would be more easily overcome.

Complex urodynamic testing, on the other hand, requires special equipment and training. Testing of this kind is not normally part of primary health care for women and it is usually necessary to refer patients who need these studies to a tertiary care medical center. Complex urodynamic testing greatly increases diagnostic accuracy and often explains why previous therapies have failed. Such testing is particularly helpful in difficult or complex cases. The primary care physician should understand when such testing is indicated and what it can tell him. He should be able to identify an appropriate referral center and should be able to work with that center to develop further care plans for his patients. Much of the controversy regarding the use of urodynamic testing arises from the misuse and misreading of complex urodynamic studies. The practice of immediately referring a patient with lower urinary tract symptoms for urodynamic studies without any prior evaluation should be condemned. Not only can many problems be solved without the use of complex studies, but patients who are referred for testing without proper preparation often have studies which provide erroneous or useless information. It is particularly important for patients to keep a frequency/volume bladder chart before urodynamic studies are done, to have acute urinary tract infections treated, and to have long-term indwelling catheters removed and to be started on intermittent catheterization before comprehensive studies are undertaken. Unfortunately, some urodynamic laboratories consist only of a machine and the technician who switches it on. The referring physician often then receives a computerized printout of various urodynamic parameters without any indication of its clinical meaning or potential applicability to the patient in question. This approach is not helpful.

Physicians often ask "Can I operate on this patient without urodynamic studies?" The *real* question which should be asked is "What can I do to understand this patient's problem and formulate a reasonable treatment plan?" The result of all urodynamic evaluation should be to help solve the patient's problem, not generate a surgical case list! The following suggestions should be useful in evaluating a patient's complaint:

Use the simplest, least expensive tests first. These include urinalysis, urine culture, frequency/volume bladder charts, cough stress-testing, and measurement of postvoid residual urine.

Only employ tests with which you are familiar. Although simple cystometry is easy to perform, the results may be difficult to interpret if the clinician does not have extensive experience with lower urinary tract dysfunction. Although the procedure for performing simple cystometry is outlined in this text, the help and advice of a more experienced practitioner is particularly useful in getting started with the performance and interpretation of these tests.

Employ more complex testing only if it will affect patient management. Complex urodynamic studies should only be performed by trained practitioners who do these studies often. If it is necessary to refer several patients for complex studies each week, it may be worthwhile to obtain additional training in this area, but the practice of purchasing expensive urodynamic testing equipment and then using it on everybody who walks through the door in order to pay for it should not be encouraged. Patients for whom complex studies are appropriate include those with an unclear history, failed conservative therapy, increasingly complex pharmacotherapy, and patients for whom the risks are high, such as those who are contemplating surgery to correct their problem. More precise diagnosis is needed as the risks of therapy increase.

This chapter is organized into three sections. The first deals with the simple urodynamic tests that should be part of the evaluation of most patients with urinary incontinence (Table 4.1). The second section deals with cystometry in both its simple and complex forms. The technique of simple cystometry is described, along with the interpretation of normal and abnormal cystometrograms. Complex subtracted cystometry is reviewed, with an emphasis on the indications for its use, the additional information that it can provide, and the variations that exist in terms of urodynamic techniques. Complex uroflowmetry and pressure flow voiding studies are also discussed. The reader should become familiar with

TABLE 4.1. Simple Urodynamic Tests

Frequency/volume bladder chart	Simple uroflowmetry
Cough stress test with a full bladder	Urinalysis
Simple bladder filling	Urine culture
Perineal pad testing	Urine cytology
Measurement of postvoid residual urine	

the interpretation of simple and complex cystometry and voiding studies in this section. The third section deals with other urodynamic tests, some of which are widely available and others which require referral to specialized centers. Some other tests have very specific uses (such as the diagnosis of a vesico-vaginal fistula) and will be discussed in later chapters in relation to specific disorders.

Simple Urodynamic Testing
Demonstration and Quantification of Urine Loss

Common sense dictates that urinary incontinence ought to be demonstrated objectively before performing major surgery for this complaint. This is not to suggest that patients would lie about urine loss in hopes of having an operation; rather, failure to demonstrate incontinence may suggest a milder problem more amenable to conservative therapy or even the possibility of misdiagnosis. It is still striking how many women undergo surgery each year for incontinence based upon their histories alone. Terrible tragedies result from this practice, both for the patient and for the surgeon. Remember that the clinical diagnosis of incontinence does not exist until it has been seen to occur!

Standing Cough Stress Test. This is a simple way of confirming stress incontinence. To perform this test, the patient is asked to come to the clinic with a comfortably full bladder. She stands with her legs shoulder-distance apart, turns her head to the side, and is asked to cough vigorously. An *immediate* loss of urine confirms a clinical diagnosis of stress incontinence. If no leakage is demonstrated, the patient may be asked to cough forcefully six to eight more times in an attempt to demonstrate stress leakage. Some clinicians perform this test with the patient in the dorsal lithotomy position, but if the test is negative it must be repeated in the standing position. It therefore seems best to do this test with the patient standing (over an absorbent plastic-backed pad!). This also allows patients to be examined in the erect position for concurrent genital prolapse. Delayed leakage after coughing or prolonged leakage of urine suggests cough-induced detrusor instability and should warrant further, more extensive, testing in order to make a more precise diagnosis.

Attempts have been made to check for the presence of surgically correctable stress incontinence by elevating the bladder neck while the patient coughs and seeing if her leakage stops. This is generally done by elevating the bladder neck with two fingers ("Bonney test") or the two sides of a rubber-shod clamp ("Marshall test"). If previously demonstrated stress incontinence disappears when this is done, the theory states that a bladder neck suspension operation will be successful. However, it is easy to occlude and compress the urethra while doing these tests, giving falsely reassuring results. Even patients with high pressure detrusor instability can be made dry if the urethra is held closed by the examiner's finger! The proper technique for evaluating urethral support has been discussed in Chapter 3. The urethra should not be *elevated,* but only *supported.* The most important information which can be obtained from doing this is *not* who has a "positive" test, but rather who has a "negative" test. Women who continue to leak after the urethra has been repositioned should undergo further examination to see if they leak because of intrinsic urethral weakness ("Type III" stress incontinence).

Simple Bladder Filling. If incontinence cannot be demonstrated during the cough stress test in a patient for whom this is a major complaint, the reason may be that her bladder is not full enough to reproduce her symptoms. Simple retrograde bladder filling can be used to overcome this problem. The easiest way to accomplish this is by using a 12 Fr red rubber catheter connected to a bag of sterile water or saline. The catheter is inserted into the bladder, taped to the thigh, and then opened at a moderate flow. By reading the markings on the side of the bag and having the patient note her sensations, the bladder volumes at first sensation, first desire to void, strong desire to void, urgency, and bladder capacity can be noted. The catheter is then removed and the patient is asked to cough vigorously. Urine loss *immediately* upon coughing confirms her complaint of stress incontinence. If the patient experiences urgency and has a large volume leak, it is likely that she has detrusor instability. Some clinicians measure urine flow after retrograde bladder filling, but it should be remembered that urethral instrumentation decreases urine flow and that uroflowmetry performed under these circumstances may be unreliable.

Perineal Pad Testing.   Should the cough stress test or simple bladder filling fail to demonstrate stress incontinence in the patient with this complaint, many clinicians proceed with a perineal pad test. This test is based on the premise that laboratory urodynamic studies fail to reproduce the conditions of daily life under which patients lose urine. An attempt is therefore made to identify urine loss by having the patient wear a preweighed perineal pad which is reweighed after she goes through a standardized series of exercises over time (Table 4.2).

Many variations on this technique exist, including the length of time the test is carried out, the volume of urine in the bladder, and the amount of exercise the patient is required to perform. While useful for documenting the presence of incontinence in selected patients, these tests are difficult to use as objective measurements of incontinence because there is significant test-retest variability and little correlation between the amount of urine loss demonstrated and the degree to which the incontinence bothers the patient. Attempts to use dyes such as Pyridium to color the urine and confirm incontinence in these patients may lead to false positive tests because the periurethral tissues are stained with the dye during normal urination which may rub off on the pad. Patients with a small pad-weight gain (less than 2 grams) during the course of a 1-hour test should be viewed with special caution, as weight gain of this degree may be caused by vaginal discharge, perspiration, or other factors. At the completion of the test, the cough stress test should be performed again after which the patient should empty her bladder. The volume voided should be recorded. A negative test with

TABLE 4.2.   Instructions For Preparing A Perineal Pad Test (International Continence Society 1-Hour Pad Test)

The total amount of urine lost during the test period is determined by weighing a collecting device such as a diaper or absorbent pad, usually a preweighed sanitary napkin. The pad should be worn inside waterproof underpants or should have a waterproof backing. Care should be taken to use a collecting device of adequate capacity.

Immediately before the test begins the collecting device should be weighed accurately, at least to the nearest gram.

1. Test is started without the patient voiding.
2. Preweighed collecting device is put on and the first 1-hour test period begins.
3. Subject drinks 500 ml of sodium-free liquid within a short period (maximum 15 minutes), then sits or rests.
4. Half-hour period: Subject walks, including stair climbing equivalent to one flight up and down.
5. During the remaining period the subject performs the following activities:
   a. Standing up from sitting, 10 times
   b. Coughing vigorously, 10 times
   c. Running in place for 1 minute
   d. Bending to pick up a small object from the floor, 5 times
   e. Washing hands in running water for 1 minute
6. At the end of the 1-hour test, the collecting device is removed and weighed.
7. If the test is regarded as representative of the patient's urine loss, she voids and the voided volume is recorded.
8. If the test is not representative, it should be repeated, preferably without voiding.

If the collecting device becomes saturated or filled during the test, it should be removed and weighed, and replaced by a fresh device. The total weight of urine lost during the test period is taken to be equal to the gain in weight of the collecting device(s). In interpreting the results of the test, it should be borne in mind that a weight gain of up to 2 g in 1 hour may result from weighing errors, sweating, or vaginal discharge. The activity program may be modified according to the subject's physical ability.

Based on Abrams, et al. Scand J Urol Nephrol Suppl 1988; 114:5–18, with permission.

less than 250 ml in the bladder is unreliable and should be repeated. If the patient's bladder cannot hold this amount in order to perform a test, this is also abnormal and is an indication for further testing.

Some clinicians advocate an extended pad test which can be performed during specific activities which cause incontinence in selected patients (such as running or aerobics), or tests which are done for prolonged periods of time using multiple pads. The patient is given preweighed pads which must be kept in self-sealing bags and returned to the clinic for weighing. Although tests of this type are useful in research, pad tests which extend for more than a few hours are cumbersome and are unlikely to be popular with busy practicing clinicians. Patients who require testing of this kind might actually benefit more from ambulatory urodynamic studies as these become more widely available.

It must also be pointed out that perineal pad testing, by itself, is only useful for documenting that incontinence *exists*. It does not determine the etiology of the problem, nor determine what needs to be done about it. Patients may have incontinence for a variety of reasons, including detrusor muscle overactivity, overflow incontinence from a large residual urine, stress incontinence, or other causes, and these etiologies must be excluded by a thorough evaluation.

Documentation of Voiding Dysfunction

Measurement of Postvoid Residual Urine. Measurement of postvoid residual urine should be part of every patient evaluation. The most common techniques used for measuring residual urine include bimanual palpation, catheterization, and ultrasound.

Bimanual palpation is available to every clinician, is inexpensive, and carries no additional risk of infection. Estimation of residual urine by palpation of the bladder has been shown to be equivalent to the use of abdominal ultrasound in some patients; however, the technique is difficult to use in obese women, patients who cannot relax enough in order to be examined adequately, and elderly women with vaginal stenosis. Catheterization is the most commonly used method. The technique is inexpensive, but it does carry a small risk of infection (less than 2%). Routine catheterization for measurement of residual urine is best done using a short plastic self-catheterization catheter or the equivalent. Use of an elaborate Foley catheter is too expensive and may not empty the bladder completely.

Ultrasound has been advocated as a way of measuring elevated postvoid residuals. Because ultrasound is widely available and is not invasive, it has some attractiveness for this purpose; however, traditional ultrasound machines are expensive and may require the patient to be seen in another part of the clinic. A variety of complex equations must often be used in order to determine the final bladder volume measurement, and this can be cumbersome. Ultrasound is unreliable at small bladder volumes, but this is not much of a drawback since small residual urine volumes are generally not clinically significant. Recently, a number of small portable ultrasound units have been produced which are dedicated solely to the measurement of residual urine volumes. These units contain software which calculates bladder volume automatically using a predetermined equation and set ultrasound measurements which are made by the person using the machine. The results are displayed on a small screen or printed out automatically. The increasing availability of such units will make ultrasound a more popular technology for residual urine measurement, particularly in busy clinics that see large numbers of patients with urinary tract complaints.

It may be difficult for some patients to initiate voiding when the bladder volume is small; therefore, postvoid residuals obtained after voids of less than 150 ml may not be accurate. Likewise, in a busy clinic the patient may feel under pressure to "perform," and may have voiding difficulty as a result of an inability to relax. An *isolated* postvoid residual of greater than 100 ml is not necessarily diagnostic of a voiding disorder and should be confirmed before that diagnosis is given. In fact, a residual urine of 50 to 100 ml might be perfectly acceptable in some elderly patients. If the residual is greater than 100 ml in a younger woman, the test should be repeated at another time with the patient voiding in private with a comfortably full bladder.

Simple Uroflowmetry. Evaluation of a patient's voiding pattern can be extremely helpful and does not necessarily require the use of complex uroflow equipment. The sound of urination contributes greatly to an understanding of what is going on, particularly for clinicians who have extensive urodynamic experience. Total voiding time can be measured with a stopwatch and an audibly smooth voiding curve with no interruptions is a good screening test for voiding abnormalities. This pattern does not exclude the possibility of voiding with abdominal straining or voiding simply by pelvic relaxation. The clinician must also learn to listen discretely and without comment during micturition to avoid creating artificial interruptions during voiding. Patients who audibly grunt and strain, have a weak dribbling or tinkling flow, or take a prolonged amount of time to void, probably need further evaluation.

Documentation of Frequency, Incontinent Episodes, and Voided Volumes

Frequency/Volume Bladder Chart. The frequency/volume bladder chart is probably the single most useful simple urodynamic test. The importance of the bladder chart has already been emphasized in Chapter 3. This "urinary diary" is nothing more than a record of urinary output kept by the patient for several days, with the times of urination recorded along with each voided volume. A separate column can be used to record episodes of urine loss. Patients should be provided with detailed written instructions on how to keep a bladder chart, and an inexpensive plastic "hat" which fits over the toilet bowl rim is a convenient specimen collector which facilitates the recording of accurate information. The urinary diary should be kept for at least two days, preferably three to five days, in order to obtain an accurate baseline picture of the patient's bladder habits. The patient should not be instructed in "normal" and "abnormal" voiding patterns before this is done, since she may unconsciously change her habits and provide erroneous information.

Some clinicians ask the patient to record her intake as well as urinary output. Others feel that fluid intake may be accurately estimated by looking at urine production. It is not uncommon for the recorded voids to exceed the recorded fluid intake because patients omit the fluid intake which comes from eating solid food. If the time of fluid intake is not recorded, it is sometimes more difficult to judge its effects on voiding patterns, as in the case of the patient who drinks before bedtime or during the night. In our experience elderly patients are able to keep bladder diaries without difficulty, and even patients who are somewhat senile or have severe learning disabilities may be able to do this if they are assisted by their family or other caretakers.

A review of frequency/volume charts is extremely helpful in fluid management and bladder retraining. Such a chart is the only reliable method for determining the patient's functional bladder capacity (maximum voided volume), her average voided volume, and her daily fluid intake. This information is critical to the success of all bladder behavioral management schemes, particularly for the patient with a hypersensitive bladder or an overactive detrusor. The maximum voided volume also provides a reasonable goal for filling during cystometry, since there is no reason to think that a patient should hold more fluid in the laboratory than she does urine in normal daily life. Iatrogenic overdistension of the bladder is a common cause of "voiding difficulty" during urodynamic testing.

Exclusion of Other Diagnoses

The importance of examining the urine *itself,* as well as the patient, cannot be overemphasized. A urinalysis is important to exclude the presence of other disorders which might be overlooked. Urinary tract infection must always be ruled out as a potential etiologic factor in any patient with lower urinary tract complaints. Patients with recurrent or persistent urinary tract infections may be colonized by fastidious organisms which are not normally picked up by routine culture methods. A specific request to the microbiology laboratory to culture for fastidious organisms is appropriate in these cases. Similarly, the use of Kass's criterion of 10^5 colony-forming-units per ml of urine may not be an appropriate threshold for the diagnosis of infection in the *symptomatic* patient. These levels of colonization were originally developed to screen patients for *asymptomatic* bacteriuria using clean-catch urine specimens. Patients who have frequency, urgency, or dysuria in the presence of less than 10^5 colonies/ml may have a real infection which should be treated, especially if only one organism is present. Cystometric testing should not be performed in the presence of an acute urinary tract infection, since the presence of infection makes the bladder hypersensitive and may cause abnormal detrusor contractions which would not otherwise be present. Frequency/volume charts are also atypical and uninterpretable in the presence of an acute infection.

Hematuria must always be investigated further and is discussed elsewhere in this book. The acute onset of urinary tract symptoms in the elderly (particularly in association with hematuria) or the persistence of irritative symptoms at any age, should prompt the clinician to send a specimen for urinary cytology to screen for urinary tract malignancy.

In summary, simple urodynamic tests are widely available, require very little expertise to perform, and can add greatly to the information obtained from the history and physical examination. For many patients with urinary incontinence, these simple urodynamic tests are all that is needed to confirm a diagnosis. In the patient with pure stress incontinence of a mild nature who desires conservative management there is no need to proceed with a cystometrogram. Likewise, the patient with frequency, urgency, and possibly urge incontinence confirmed by frequency/volume charts, who has a minimal postvoid residual and a negative urinalysis, may be tried on simple bladder retraining and fluid management. Should these not be effective, simple or complex cystometry is indicated. Patients who have had previous surgery, patients in whom previous management techniques have not been useful, or patients in whom future surgery is contemplated, will benefit from further urodynamic testing as discussed below. Simple cystometry may be all that is required for the evaluation of some problems pertaining to incontinence or disordered sensation. Voiding difficulty generally requires further evaluation, often with complex urodynamics, pressure-flow voiding studies, EMG and fluoroscopy.

Cystometry and Voiding Studies

Cystometry means "to measure the bladder" and the paper tracing of pressures which is produced is a *cystometrogram* ("CMG"). Cystometry has been invaluable in enhancing our understanding of normal bladder mechanics and in defining abnormal function. During *simple cystometry*, bladder pressure *alone* is measured while the bladder is filled to capacity. In *complex cystometry*, multiple physiologic parameters are measured during the filling (and usually during the emptying) phases of the bladder cycle. These measurements usually include bladder pressure, "abdominal" pressure, "true" detrusor pressure, the rate of bladder filling, and the volume infused. "Abdominal" pressure is generally assessed by measuring either rectal or vaginal pressure. The "true" or "subtracted" detrusor pressure is obtained by measuring bladder and abdominal pressure simultaneously, and then subtracting abdominal pressure from bladder pressure by electronic technology. The pressure that is left is taken as the "true" detrusor pressure and is displayed as a separate line on the tracing. Electromyography may be performed simultaneously with filling, using either wire or surface electrodes placed in or on the urethral or anal sphincters to evaluate the response of the pelvic floor muscles to bladder filling and emptying. If radiographic contrast is used instead of sterile water or normal saline, a simultaneous fluoroscopic picture of bladder filling and emptying can be obtained. If voiding is studied, urine flow rate, volume voided, bladder pressure, abdominal pressure, and detrusor pressure are measured, either with or without fluoroscopy and EMG. All of these techniques have their place in helping us understand lower urinary tract complaints.

The Normal Bladder Cycle

As has been noted before, the bladder is a simple organ with a relatively simple function: to store the urine coming in from ureters without an appreciable rise in bladder pressure, and then to contract and expel that urine completely (but voluntarily) at a socially acceptable time and place. This is accomplished through a complex and as yet incompletely understood process which coordinates neuromuscular activity with bladder filling and emptying.

During the filling phase the bladder expands to accommodate the increasing volume without an appreciable rise in pressure. The bladder is normally a low-pressure system and that pressure must be lower than the pressure in the kidney and ureter in order for any urine to flow into the bladder. The normal first desire to void occurs when tension-stretch receptors in the bladder are activated, usually at a capacity of 150–250 ml. An early first desire to void may be produced either by abnormal detrusor activity or increased sensation. The bladder should fill to capacity without leaking. It should be able to retain its contents despite external physical stresses such as coughing, sneezing, or exercise, and the detrusor muscle should remain relaxed until a voluntary contraction is initiated. The normal bladder capacity for women will generally be between 450–650 ml. Although this can be evaluated during cystometry (''cystometric bladder capacity''), the most accurate way of measuring bladder capacity is through a frequency/volume bladder chart kept for several days. The largest voided volume recorded on this chart is the *functional bladder capacity,* and this volume should be known prior to urodynamic testing. There is no reason to expect a patient to hold more urine in the laboratory than she holds in daily life, although occasionally it is useful to press a patient with a suspected bladder sensory disorder to hold more than her functional capacity in order to demonstrate that there is no structural limitation which makes her bladder volume low.

During the emptying phase of the bladder cycle the pelvic floor and urethra should relax and the detrusor muscle should contract, causing effective bladder pressure to rise while outlet resistance decreases. This should result in smooth and complete bladder emptying. Urodynamic studies during the voiding phase can evaluate abnormal emptying mechanisms such as emptying without a detrusor contraction, outflow obstruction, or dyscoordination of detrusor contraction with sphincteric relaxation. Voiding studies may also identify patients at risk for postoperative voiding difficulty. While simple cystometry can provide much useful information regarding the filling phase of the bladder cycle, voiding dysfunction requires complex studies for proper evaluation. Patients with these symptoms need detailed investigation. Patients who have a large postvoid residual after simple bladder filling and subsequent voiding may also benefit from a more detailed evaluation.

7imple Cystometry

Simple cystometry is the technique of evaluating bladder function through simple measurement of bladder pressure alone. The setup for simple cystometry using a Y manometer is shown in Figure 4.1, and the technical procedure used is detailed in Table 4.3. This test is useful to confirm the diagnosis in patients with clear-cut symptoms of stress or urge incontinence, particularly those who are interested in conservative therapy and who have not yet had any form of management. Occasionally this technique is useful for the patient with mild mixed symptoms who is interested in conservative management, but simple cystometry should not be the first-line diagnostic test in patients with neurologic abnormalities, voiding disorders, previous bladder neck surgery, and complex problems—*especially* if they have already failed initial attempts at therapy. Patients with abnormal findings on simple cystometry may need complex urodynamic studies to delineate their disorders more fully.

Simple cystometry is useful for obtaining information on bladder sensation, bladder capacity, and in differentiating simple stress incontinence from urge incontinence due to detrusor overactivity. Abnormal findings on simple cystometry would include an early first desire to void at less than 100 ml, pain or incontinence during filling, or a bladder capacity of less than 400 ml or greater than 650 ml. Pressures during simple cystometry are measured by watching the level of fluid rise and fall in the manometer. These pressure changes must be

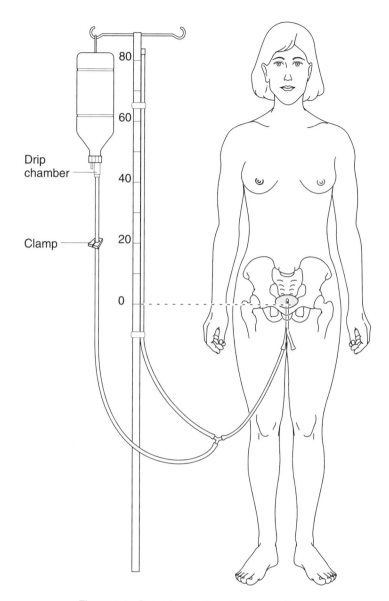

Figure 4.1 Setup for simple water manometry.

carefully observed and correlated with the patient's symptoms during the study. Examples of simple cystometrograms exhibiting a number of different findings are given in Figures 4.2 through 4.7. Although line drawings are used to demonstrate the changes which may be observed, it must be clearly understood that simple cystometry using a manometer does *not* generate any "hard copy" for later review. The clinician must evaluate all of these pressure changes as the study progresses and put them together at the end of the study. This means that the treating clinician should be present for the study and make these observations himself.

Pitfalls of Simple Cystometry

Care must be taken when diagnoses are based on simple cystometry. First of all, the technique can only be used for bladder filling. Voiding studies cannot be performed because of the large urethral catheter which is used for filling and for measurement of bladder pressure. Catheters of at least 12 Fr will be necessary

TABLE 4.3. Instructions For Performing Simple Cystometry

1. Place a three-way 16 or 18 Fr Foley catheter with a 10 ml balloon into the bladder after the patient voids.
2. Measure the residual urine.
3. Attach one port to the hanging bag of sterile water or saline which is to be used for bladder filling. Attach the second port to the manometer to record the intravesical pressure. The manometer should be zeroed at the pubic symphysis, with the patient in the position she will be in during filling (standing is best).
4. Fill the patient's bladder with fluid by gravity flow at a rate of 60–100 ml/min with the filling bag elevated approximately five feet in the air.
5. Record the volume infused at:
   First desire to void
   Strong desire to void
   Symptoms of urgency or pain
   Bladder capacity
6. Pressure elevations of more than 15 cm of water are suspicious for detrusor instability, particularly if they are associated with symptoms of urgency or urge incontinence.

Advantages: Inexpensive and readily available. Good screening technique for many patients.

Disadvantages: This technique only measures intravesical pressure. A "normal" study is useful in some cases, but this method may fail to provide enough provocation to elicit detrusor overactivity in many patients. The patient may be checked for stress incontinence during bladder filling, but coughing will produce enormous rises in the manometer. These should fall rapidly back to baseline. Fluctuations in bladder pressure during filling which are caused by straining or patient movement may confuse the diagnosis by simulating detrusor instability. Many manometers are calibrated in millimeters of mercury rather than centimeters of water, so conversions must be made. No permanent record of the bladder pressure tracing is made during simple cystometry.

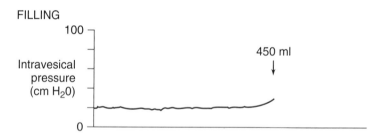

Figure 4.2 Normal simple cystometrogram. There are no fluctuations in bladder pressure and the capacity is 450 ml.

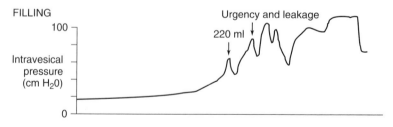

Figure 4.3 Simple cystometrogram showing phasic fluctuations in bladder pressure due to detrusor overactivity.

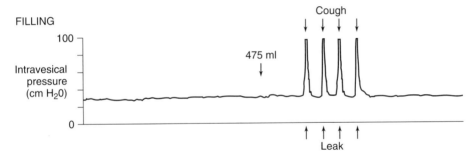

Figure 4.4 Simple standing cystometrogram in a patient with stress incontinence. Large pressure spikes are generated with each cough and each cough is accompanied by a spurt of urine leakage. The pressure spikes promptly return to baseline. Interpreting such phenomena by looking at a manometer can be tricky. The bladder capacity is normal.

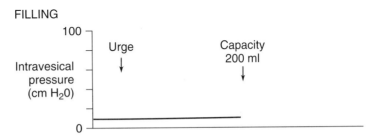

Figure 4.5 Simple cystometrogram showing a hypersensitive bladder with a reduced bladder capacity. In spite of the patient's complaints of urgency, there are no fluctuations in bladder pressure.

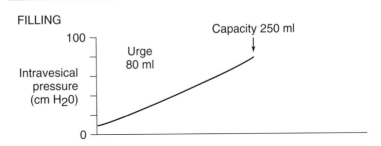

Figure 4.6 Simple cystometrogram showing a hypersensitive bladder with reduced compliance. Bladder pressure rises steadily but without phasic changes until capacity is reached. In this case, the capacity is also reduced (250 ml).

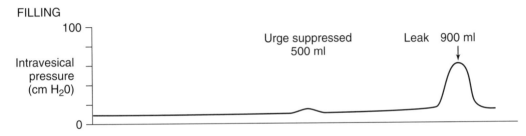

Figure 4.7 Simple cystometrogram showing a large capacity bladder. In this case the patient had transient urgency at a capacity of 500 ml, but lost control of her bladder at 900 ml as a result of overzealous bladder filling

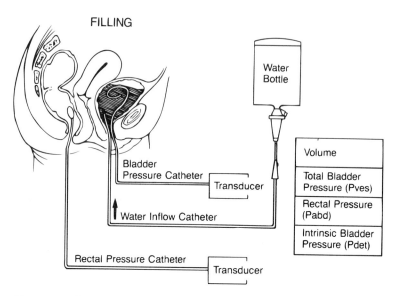

FILLING

Figure 4.8 Complex cystometry: Filling phase. Three catheters are generally used: A filling catheter through which sterile water will flow, a bladder pressure catheter, and a rectal pressure catheter. Intrinsic detrusor pressure (*Pdet*) is calculated electronically by subtracting rectal pressure (*Pabd*) from total bladder pressure (*Pves*). (From Wall and Addison, Postgrad Obstet Gynecol 1988; 8(26):1–7, with permission.)

for these studies, since filling is too slow with narrower catheters and may lead to a false impression of increased bladder pressure. A dual-lumen Foley catheter is ideal, but the balloon may cause irritability if it is pulled down into the bladder neck. A simple red rubber catheter can also be used, but must be taped carefully in position so that it does not become dislodged and fall out during the study. Increased abdominal pressure during simple cystometry may give the false impression that abnormal detrusor activity is occurring when in fact it is not, and could be a cause of false positive studies during simple cystometry. Increases in abdominal pressure which occur during the study may be missed unless the patient's abdomen is palpated during the examination. Simple filling cystometry may also not challenge bladder control very much. Provocation is often necessary to make the diagnosis of detrusor instability to be missed in some patients with unstable bladders. The use of simple cystometry to confirm a suspected diagnosis of detrusor instability is hampered by the fact that techniques such as change of position, heel-bouncing, and coughing which are normally used to provoke detrusor overactivity during complex cystometry will all produce changes in bladder pressure which may be mistaken for abnormal detrusor activity during simple filling studies. However, the use of stimuli such as the sound of running water or having the patient wash her hands under a tap are still practical. The patient who experiences urgency and empties her bladder during simple cystometry with no ability to control her urine flow may be presumed to have detrusor instability, even if the pressure changes are uninterpretable.

Probably the biggest drawback to the use of simple cystometry is that it requires significant expertise in the evaluation of abnormal bladder function in order to interpret it properly. Clinicians who are thoroughly comfortable with the performance and interpretation of complex urodynamic studies are usually quite good at making a diagnosis on the basis of simple cystometry alone. However, the physician who does not have this background and who evaluates only a few patients each year is at much higher risk of making a mistake until such expertise has been attained.

If simple cystometry confirms that the patient has abnormal sensation or if clear-cut urge incontinence has been demonstrated with an obvious sustained rise in bladder pressure at the time of leakage, therapy for the "urge syndrome" may be initiated using fluid management, bladder drill, and/or anticholinergic medication. If the test is normal in a patient with true symptoms of stress incontinence, and if that symptom is confirmed, then appropriate management may be initiated for this patient, including conservative therapy or, in some cases, primary bladder neck surgery, depending on her presentation and examination. If the results of simple cystometry are unclear, or if the study does not reproduce her symptoms, complex subtracted cystometry should be considered prior to proceeding with surgery.

Complex ("Subtracted") Cystometry

Whereas simple cystometry measures bladder volume and simple bladder pressure, complex cystometry measures multiple parameters simultaneously: bladder volume, filling rate, bladder pressure, abdominal pressure, and subtracted detrusor pressure (Fig. 4.8). Pressure-flow studies measure urine flow rate and the volume voided in addition to these pressures (Fig. 4.9). Additional parameters which may be measured in some tests include simultaneous urethral pressure, urethral closure pressure, and EMG activity, and all of these parameters may be measured under fluoroscopic control.

Because simple cystometry does not produce a hardcopy tracing which can be reviewed, the physician must be in the room when simple cystometry is performed if he is to understand what is going on. Complex cystometry, on the other hand, does produce hardcopy which can be stored, retrieved, and reviewed. It would be a mistake, however, to give the impression that interpreting complex urodynamic studies is like reading an electrocardiogram or a chest x-ray. Properly done urodynamic studies are the product of a continuous interaction between the patient and the urodynamicist. The patient's report of what is occurring during her study is absolutely critical for a proper interpretation of the results and the separation of relevant information from artifact. The tracing must be labeled with appropriate information on sensation of fullness, urgency, leakage, pain and any other relevant information if it is to have any meaning at all. The exact moment when these things occur must be clearly identified. As a result,

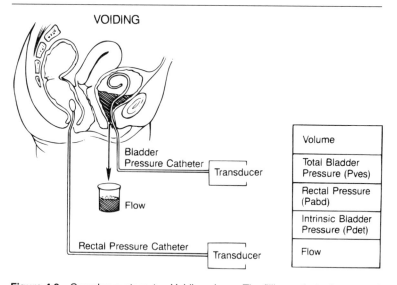

Figure 4.9 Complex cystometry: Voiding phase. The filling catheter is removed and the patient is placed over a urine flowmeter. Bladder and rectal pressure are measured during voiding, and the intrinsic detrusor pressure during voiding is calculated by subtracting rectal from bladder pressure. (From Wall and Addison, Postgrad Obstet Gynecol 1988; 8(26)1–7, with permission.)

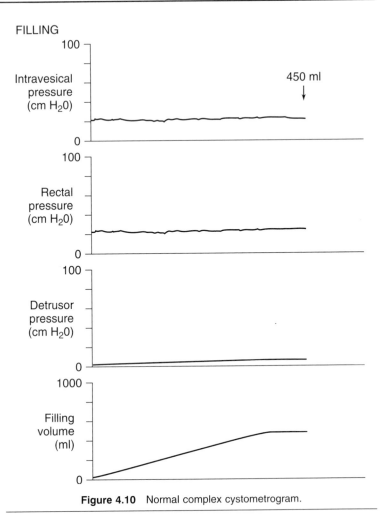

Figure 4.10   Normal complex cystometrogram.

studies are best performed by someone who has taken the patient's history and examined her. While it is admittedly easier to have a nurse perform urodynamic studies and let the doctor review them at a later date, this will work only if the doctor and the nurse have an excellent working relationship with clear communication and if both are fully familiar with the performance and interpretation of urodynamic tests. As Hulka has remarked, ''The magic is in the magician, not in the wand.'' It is next to useless to send a patient for urodynamic studies to someone who has an unclear understanding of the clinical problem. For this effort you will receive in return a computerized printout of meaningless physiologic information that has no relationship to the patient's symptomatology. If urodynamic referral results in test results which are no more helpful than this, the clinician should look for a new referral center.

Subtracted or complex cystometry is considered to be more reliable than simple cystometry because the technique avoids the problem of artifact produced by changes in intra-abdominal pressure. As a result, complex cystometry generally allows more provocative maneuvers to be carried out during the testing (such as change of position, heel-bouncing, bending over, etc.) and therefore is better for detecting unstable detrusor activity. Since special electronic equipment is necessary, subtracted cystometry is more expensive than simple cystometry and the complexities of recording multiple pressures require considerable expertise in both the performance and interpretation of these studies. Even with the best available equipment and an experienced clinician, however, subtracted cystometry is not infallible, since a patient's symptoms may vary from day to day and the urodynamics laboratory is far from being a "normal" setting. Urodynamic studies are not like indelible "fingerprints," unaltered by time or circumstance.

An outline of what is involved in performing complex subtracted filling cystometry is given in Table 4.4. It must be pointed out, however, that there are many different variations of cystometric technique and different authors mean different things when they refer to "urodynamic studies." The care with which the study is done is an integral part of its sensitivity and specificity. For example, a 2-minute fluoroscopic study of the bladder at cystometric capacity under conditions of coughing will have a high degree of accuracy in detecting genuine stress incontinence, but will not be nearly as precise in detecting detrusor instability as an hour-long study involving a supine fill followed by an erect fill with multiple provocative stimuli such as running water in the background, change of position, coughing, or even walking around the room. Long-term ambulatory urodynamic studies will provide even more sensitivity. This is not to say that any of these techniques are "wrong," but merely to point out that all tests do not necessarily provide the same information. A surgeon who reports a 100% success rate for his operation based upon objective postoperative "urodynamic studies," may not be including maneuvers which would be likely to produce stress incontinence reliably. The International Continence Society therefore suggests that the details of urodynamic technique should be reported in any publication utilizing urodynamic studies. The reader who needs to learn about urodynamic technique in detail should refer to any of the technical volumes listed at the end of this chapter.

The normal parameters for a complex subtracted cystometrogram are similar to those obtained during a simple cystometrogram as discussed previously, with the addition of more complex pressure measurements (Table 4.5). An example of a normal complex cystometrogram is given in Figure 4.10. Figure 4.11 shows the kind of tracing produced by a woman with incontinence due to detrusor overactivity (detrusor instability). Figure 4.12 gives an example of the cystometric findings in a woman who has genuine stress incontinence. The tracing clearly demonstrates that the pressure increases in the bladder seen with coughing are due to elevations of intra-abdominal pressure rather than detrusor instability.

Pressure Measurement
Bladder pressure is a summation of several factors, the most important of which are the pressure exerted by the activity of the bladder detrusor muscle and the pressure exerted on the bladder by surrounding intra-abdominal pressure. The amount of abdominal pressure will vary with position, coughing, straining and so forth. Simple cystometry only measures the total pressure in the bladder and cannot help us sort out these various components (Fig. 4.1). Complex cystometry, on the other hand, attempts to compensate for the contribution to bladder pressure made by surrounding intra-abdominal pressure by *subtraction*. In order to obtain the "true" detrusor pressure (that is, the component of total bladder pressure due to the activity of the bladder muscle itself), abdominal pressure is subtracted from the measured (total) bladder pressure. The pressure that remains is called the "subtracted detrusor pressure."

Bladder pressure is generally measured using a simple intravesical pressure catheter while abdominal pressure is approximated by measuring rectal or vaginal pressure with a catheter placed in one of these organs. The urodynamic equipment then electronically subtracts rectal/vaginal pressure from bladder pressure to generate a third pressure tracing on the cystometrogram (Fig. 4.8). Both rectal and vaginal catheters measure pressures in the same clinical range. Some women find the vaginal pressure catheter more comfortable, but these catheters tend to be held in position less reliably and will give erratic pressure readings in women with significant prolapse. Rectal pressures are subject to artifacts caused by compression or blockage of the pressure catheter tip by feces. A finger-cot or slitted balloon should be tied over the catheter tip to prevent

TABLE 4.4. Instructions For Performing Subtracted Filling Cystometry

1. The patient voids with a full bladder.
Record: voided volume, peak flow rate, voiding time, mean flow rate, and note the pattern (normal, interrupted, straining, etc.).
2. Place the patient in a modified lithotomy position, clean the urethral orifice, and catheterize her to measure the residual urine. This should be done using sterile technique. This may be done using either the filling catheter or a separate catheter. Microtip electronic transducer catheters are quite narrow and are poorly suited for this purpose.
Measure the residual urine and record it. Send a sterile urine specimen if one has not been obtained previously.
3. Insert the intravesical pressure catheter and tape it securely to the patient's thigh.
4. Insert the abdominal pressure catheter. This may be placed in the rectum or in the lateral fornix of the vagina. Secure this catheter with tape.
5. Connect the pressure lines to the pressure catheters and the filling line to the filling catheter. If fluid-filled pressure lines are used, they must be flushed with sterile water to eliminate any air bubbles and to establish a continuous column of water that will transmit pressure accurately.
6. Place the patient in the desired position for cystometry (supine, sitting, or standing). If fluid-filled lines are used for measuring pressure, adjust the transducers so that they are at the upper border of the pubic symphysis. Zero the detrusor pressure to baseline. Although the intravesical and intra-abdominal pressures may have an initial reading of 0–15 cm of water in the supine position, the machine should subtract the abdominal pressure from the bladder pressure to give the true detrusor pressure. Ask the patient to cough. The pen should deflect upwards equally in both the bladder and abdominal pressure tracings. The detrusor pressure tracing should move only slightly. If the detrusor pressure tracing moves significantly up or down with the cough, adjust the appropriate bladder or abdominal pressure catheter and flush the line again. The intravesical catheter may be against the bladder wall and filling the bladder with another 30 ml may help correct this. Abdominal pressure catheters placed in the vagina may become dislodged or kinked by a prolapse. Pressure catheters placed in the rectum may be trapped by stool or pushed up against the side of the rectum.
Note the initial pressures, especially intravesical pressure.
7. Once fine adjustments to the catheters have been made, begin filling at the desired rate (usually medium filling rates around 75 ml/min). The patient should be quiet and should concentrate on her symptoms during filling. Too much talking or joking or having a friend in the room may distract the patient and lead to an inadequate study.
Record the volume at which the patient notices her first desire to void (FDV).
The patient may notice the cool temperature of the filling liquid. This is different from the first desire to void, which can be described as the point in bladder filling when she would think about looking for a place to urinate at the next convenient opportunity, such as when the next commercial break comes on during her favorite television program.
Have the patient cough and listen to the sound of running water to see if detrusor instability can be provoked.
8. Continue filling. It is often useful to have the patient cough at intervals (such as every 100 ml of fluid infused) to attempt to provoke detrusor activity and to check for the presence of stress incontinence.
Note any symptoms of urgency or pain and record when they occur.
Record the volume at which the patient has a strong desire to void.
A strong desire to void can be defined for the patient as that point in bladder filling when she would stop what she was doing to urinate, such as getting up in the middle of her favorite television program to urinate without waiting for the commercial break.
Record the cystometric bladder capacity.
The cystometric capacity is reached when the patient tells you she cannot hold any more, either because of discomfort or because she feels that leakage is inevitable. Often a patient will complain of fullness but can hold considerably more fluid with encouragement. Knowing the patient's functional bladder capacity (largest voided volume on her bladder chart) is extremely helpful in performing cystometry. There is no reason to expect that a patient should be able to hold more fluid in the urodynamics laboratory than she does in daily life. Most patients will hold about the same, or slightly less, and there is nothing to be gained by overfilling a patient's bladder except iatrogenic voiding dysfunction. When filling has been completed, allow the pressures to equilibrate for one minute.
Record the detrusor pressure after equilibration to allow determination of bladder compliance.
9. Remove the filling catheter. The patient will be more comfortable and the catheter serves no function once filling has been completed.
10. Perform provocative maneuvers. During filling it is customary to ask the patient to cough or listen to running water at the first desire to void and again at capacity. If filling cystometry was performed in the sitting or supine positions, the patient should stand after cystometric capacity is reached and provocative maneuvers such as repetitive coughing, heel-bouncing, and washing her hands or listening to the sound of running water should be performed. Some patients may develop uninhibited detrusor contractions at capacity when they change position and empty their bladders completely. Unless stress incontinence has been tested for during filling by periodic coughing, the opportunity to demonstrate it may be lost if uncontrolled detrusor contractions occur with the change of position.
Record any response to provocation: urgency, incontinence, or any replication of symptoms.

TABLE 4.5.   Approximate Normal Parameters Of Female Bladder

- Residual urine less than 50 ml (ideally none)
- First desire to void occurs between 150 ml and 250 ml
- Strong desire to void does not occur until after 250 ml
- Cystometric capacity between 400 ml and 600 ml
- Bladder compliance between 20 ml/cm H_2O and 100 ml/cm H_2O measured 60 seconds after reaching cystometric capacity
- No uninhibited detrusor contractions during filling, despite provocation
- No stress or urge incontinence demonstrated, despite provocation
- Voiding occurs due to a voluntarily initiated and sustained detrusor contraction
- Flow rate during voiding is greater than 15 ml/sec with a detrusor pressure of less than 50 cm H_2O

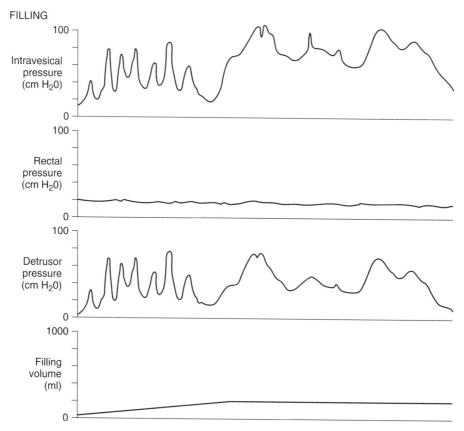

Figure 4.11   Cystometrogram demonstrating unstable detrusor contractions (detrusor instability) during bladder filling. Note that the bladder pressure and subtracted detrusor pressure rise together, whereas the abdominal pressure remains stable. If the rise in bladder pressure had been due to straining, the pressure elevations would have canceled each other out and the detrusor tracing would have remained stable while the other two tracings showed similar changes.

obstruction of the pressure channel, particularly if water-filled lines are used for rectal pressure measurement. Spontaneous rectal contractions may also cause pressure undulations which interfere with the subtracted pressure tracing. Subtraction artifacts caused by spontaneous rectal activity are often mistaken for unstable detrusor contractions by the inexperienced clinician.

Pressure measurements can be made with a simple fluid-filled pressure line linked to an external pressure transducer. This is essentially the same type of

FILLING

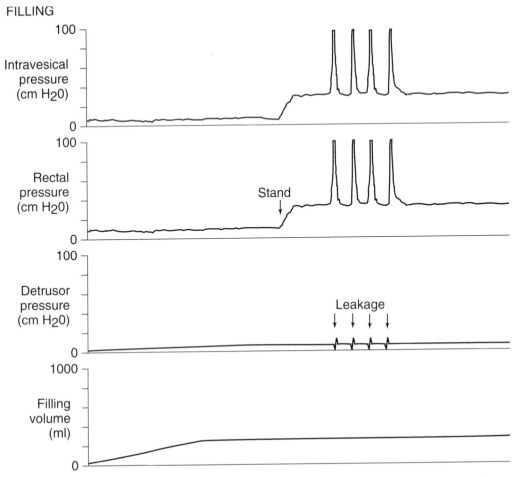

Figure 4.12 Cystometrogram demonstrating genuine stress incontinence. In this tracing the patient's bladder has been filled with her in the supine position. When she stands up, there is a rise in bladder and rectal pressure, but the subtracted detrusor pressure does not change. Coughing produces simultaneous increases in bladder and abdominal pressure which result in urine loss. Note that the detrusor pressure remains flat ("stable") during these episodes of coughing.

pressure measuring system which is used for monitoring internal uterine pressure during labor. If such systems are used in cystometry, the pressure transducers should be zeroed at the level of the pubic symphysis. If the patient changes position, the position of the external pressure transducer should also be changed to keep it at this level. If fluid-filled lines are used, care must be taken to flush all air bubbles out of the system because they may causing damping of the pressure tracing. Pediatric feeding tubes (5 Fr) make excellent sterile disposable pressure lines when connected to the longer piece of tubing that attaches to the external pressure transducer. Once the pressure lines have been inserted into the bladder and the rectum, they must be flushed with fluid to ensure patency and proper pressure transmission. When the lines are in place and have been flushed, care should be taken to make sure they transmit pressure properly by having the patient cough vigorously and checking the deflection on the bladder and abdominal pressure channels. The amount of the deflection should be the same in each channel. If they are not, the lines should be flushed and all connections checked before proceeding with the study. The pressure lines must be kept still during the study, as knocking or brushing the pressure lines will produce

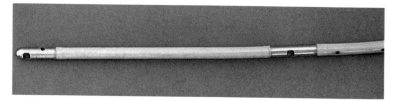

Figure 4.13 Electronic microtip transducer pressure catheter.

significant artifacts on the tracing which may render it unreadable. In spite of these drawbacks, urodynamic studies done using fluid-filled pressure lines are economical, practical, and serviceable for routine clinical use.

An alternative recording technique is to use electronic microtip transducer pressure catheters (Fig. 4.13). Originally developed for invasive cardiac pressure monitoring, this technology was introduced to urodynamic practice in 1975. The transducers involved in these catheters are very small and are placed at the end of the catheter itself where they generate an electronic signal which is transmitted down the catheter to an interface box linked to the urodynamic equipment. These catheters therefore measure absolute pressure from wherever they are located. This eliminates the need for frequent zeroing of the transducer to accommodate changes in patient position. Many of these electronic catheter systems include a separate 1 mm infusion port which allows both bladder filling and pressure measurement to be accomplished using a single catheter. Such systems generally require a special infusion pump to drive fluid through this small channel, and this increases the cost of the system. Electronic microtip catheters produce little artifact with movement and can record instantaneous pressure changes, which allows the patient to be even more active during studies performed with this equipment. The ambulatory urodynamic recording systems which are being developed for long-term monitoring all utilize some form of microtip transducer catheter system.

The drawback to this high technology approach is that these catheters are extremely expensive (costing as much as two thousand dollars per transducer) and are often very fragile. Hundreds of urodynamic studies must be done with an electronic catheter to amortize the cost down to a level comparable with that of disposable pressure tubing. Additionally, microtip transducer catheters must be calibrated and balanced at frequent intervals, and they must be handled with gentle, meticulous care. The transducer at the tip should NEVER be squeezed or tapped with a finger or any other object. Those who have good luck keeping these expensive catheters in working condition feel that their advantages outweigh their disadvantages. Those who have accidentally dropped or stepped on one may feel rather differently.

Filling Options
The bladder is usually filled with sterile water or saline during urodynamic studies. Radiocontrast dye or carbon dioxide may be used under special circumstances. Carbon dioxide gas is cleaner, neater, faster, and cheaper than water, but the reaction of this gas with urine produces carbonic acid which can be intensely irritating to the bladder. Measurement of cystometric capacity using carbon dioxide results in measurements which are only about 60% of the volume obtained by fluid instillation. Voiding studies are not possible if carbon dioxide is used, and because the gas is clear and odorless, leakage cannot be observed to occur. Gas cystometry is useful in picking up unstable detrusor contractions, but the irritation produced by the carbon dioxide and carbonic acid may produce false positive results in some patients.

Liquids, on the other hand, are more physiologic because the bladder normally holds urine, not gas. Voiding studies as well as filling studies can be done if a liquid filling medium is used, and leakage can be seen and therefore documented. If radiocontrast dye is used, the study can be done under fluoroscopy, which allows visualization of ureteral reflux, the outline of the bladder, and the configuration of the urethra and bladder neck. Liquids are generally used at room temperature (25° C) for provocative testing and at body temperature (37° C) for nonprovocative testing.

The bladder may be filled incrementally or continuously. Three rates of filling have been defined by the International Continence Society:

- *Slow filling.* This is filling which takes place at 10 ml/min or less. This is used almost exclusively for nonprovocative testing in neurologically impaired patients where detrusor hyperreflexia is probable or the risk of autonomic dysreflexia is present. Filling the bladder at a rate of 10 ml/minute is extremely time-consuming and is impractical for routine clinical use.
- *Medium filling* is used most commonly in routine urodynamic testing and encompasses filling rates of 11 ml/min to 100 ml/min. Most testing is done at around 75 ml/min. This can be achieved by a moderate flow of liquid under gravity from a suspended bag of fluid, and bladder capacity can be reached within a reasonable period of time. Medium fill cystometry using gravity flow can easily be done using a 12 Fr red rubber catheter connected to a filling line.
- *Fast filling* is filling at rates of greater than 100 ml/min. Depending on the characteristics of the system, a filling rate this fast may require an infusion pump to drive the liquid in at a constant pressure. This is a very provocative rate and may produce artifactual detrusor instability. In addition, the normal bladder may be overwhelmed by fluid entering it at this rate, and artificially high bladder pressures may result as the rate of bladder filling exceeds the ability of the bladder to relax and accommodate this load. Such pressure tracings generally demonstrate a progressive, steady rise in pressure as filling advances. If this is noticed, filling should be stopped and the bladder allowed to equilibrate. Many patients who are said to have "low compliance" bladders have merely had a technically flawed cystometrogram performed on them. If the pressure remains elevated after one minute of equilibration, there may be a genuine problem with bladder compliance.

Position

In real life patients rarely experience bladder symptoms while lying down, and performing cystometry on patients lying flat on an examination table is unlikely to be very sensitive in reproducing their symptoms. Urodynamic testing is therefore best done with the patient either sitting or standing. If cystometry is performed in the supine position, the patient should be tilted to the upright position on the examination table, or changed to a different position once bladder capacity has been reached. If fluid-filled pressure lines are used, the location of the transducer should be adjusted to the level of the pubic symphysis with each change of position. Use of a modified birthing chair is useful in performing urodynamic studies, since it allows easy access to the perineum for catheter insertion with the patient lying down and also allows the patient to be moved to the sitting position during the study. A flowmeter can also be placed under the chair for voiding studies; however, one should avoid the impression of conducting the test over a toilet, since it may be unreasonable to expect the patient to suppress detrusor contractions under these conditions when her bladder is extremely full.

Provocation

Under the close observation of strangers in the clinical laboratory setting, most patients will do their utmost to avoid the embarrassment of leakage, consciously altering their usual behavior by intense cortical suppression of bladder activity or by tightening the pelvic floor—both of which suppress detrusor activity. As a result, symptoms experienced outside of the laboratory will not always be demonstrated under study conditions. (As a rule, artifactual voiding difficulty is more common in this setting than is artifactual detrusor instability.) To help overcome these problems, a variety of "provocative" techniques are used to challenge the patient's ability to suppress detrusor activity. These techniques include rapid filling, filling with a cool liquid, changes of position, coughing, listening to running water, heel bouncing, and hand washing. These may be done during filling, at cystometric capacity, or under both circumstances. Idiosyncratic "triggers" for incontinence reported by the patient should also be explored if possible, such as singing, straining, bending over, or special positions. While some patients report uncontrolled micturition occurring during fits of giggling, the authors have been unable to induce uncontrollable laughter in patients during cystometry, in spite of their best efforts.

Recording and Record Keeping. The pressure tracings which comprise the actual cystometrogram are often the only record of a urodynamic study. These records have no meaning unless the events which take place during the study are carefully noted on the tracing *at the exact point at which they occur.* Typically the following events are marked: start of filling, the patient's first sensation of the bladder starting to fill, the patient's first desire to void (normal desire to void), a strong desire to void, the development of urgency (fear of leakage or pain), and cystometric capacity. The point at which any incontinence occurs should be carefully marked and the time at which any provocative maneuvers such as running water, change of position, coughing, etc., are carried out should also be noted. These may either be written by hand on a paper tracing, or marked and noted electronically on a computer-based system. This data can be entered into a computer database for report generation, or transferred onto a separate urodynamic record sheet along with the final diagnosis and any clinical comments (Fig. 4.14).

Social and Environmental Concerns

A good cystometric study depends on patient cooperation as well as technical proficiency. The urodynamicist as scientist can make technical improvements in procedures and measuring devices, but the urodynamicist as caregiver must still avoid the introduction of error from social and environmental factors by putting the patient at ease and being sensitive to her concerns. A supportive, private atmosphere is essential to obtaining good voiding studies. Insensitive observation by a crowd of clinicians can produce artificial straining or interrupted voiding patterns by inhibiting the patient. This can lead to erroneous conclusions based on a study which does not reflect the patient's normal voiding habits. Similarly, the patient must be alert and oriented enough to cooperate with the person performing the study. She must be able to indicate sensations of fullness, urgency, and pain, and she must understand the need to inhibit the micturition reflex and suppress detrusor contractions. Urodynamic studies will add little to the care of agitated, uncooperative, demented patients. Sensitivity to patient concerns and the need for patient cooperation in performing urodynamic studies crosses all technologic barriers—advances in urodynamic technique will never compensate for poor studies produced by an impatient, abrupt urodynamicist.

Interpreting Complex Cystometry

What makes a subtracted cystometrogram abnormal? The general parameters of a normal study are given in Table 4.5. A normal cystometrogram should demonstrate normal sensation, capacity, and compliance (change in volume with respect to change in pressure). Incontinence should not be demonstrated. The subtracted detrusor pressure tracing should remain flat, without phasic pressure changes. If incontinence is demonstrated during coughing with a flat detrusor tracing, the patient is said to have "genuine stress incontinence." If leakage is demonstrated due to abnormal detrusor contractions with an associated sense of urgency, the patient is said to have "motor urge incontinence due to detrusor instability/(hyperreflexia)." If a voiding study is done as well as a filling study, the patient should void by a sustained detrusor contraction with a pressure of less than 50 cm H_2O and a flow rate of more than 15 ml/sec. There should be little or no residual urine and the flow pattern should be normal.

Because cystometry is done under rather artificial conditions, it is important to emphasize that patients may be said to have a "normal" *cystometrogram* rather than a "normal" *bladder.* Since cystometry represents only a brief window on bladder function, there are patients whose symptoms are not reproduced within the confines of the urodynamics laboratory who nonetheless have significant problems. The patient who has many of the symptoms of detrusor instability (urgency, frequency, urge incontinence) but a normal, stable cystometrogram

URODYNAMICS DATA FORM

PATIENT_____   DATE_____

INDICATIONS FOR STUDY:_____

BLADDER CHART: Kept for _____ days   Min _____ ml   Max _____ ml   Av void _____ ml
Av. Frequency _____ /day   Av. Nocturia _____ / night   _____ Incontinent episodes in _____ days
Average daily urine output _____ ml

UROFLOWMETRY
Peak flow rate _____ ml/sec   _____ Nomogram percentile
Mean flow rate _____ ml/sec   _____ Nomogram percentile
Voided volume _____ ml   _____ ml Residual urine
Void typical for patient? Yes   No
Pattern: Normal   Straining   Intermittent   Poor flow   Other:_____

FILLING CYSTOMETRY
Filling medium: Sterile water   Normal saline   Contrast   Other: _____
Temperature: Room temperature   Body temperature   Chilled   Other_____
Filling position: Sitting   Standing   Supine
Filling rate: _____ ml/min   Slow   Medium   Fast
First desire to void _____ ml   Pdet _____ cm H20
Strong desire to void _____ ml   Pdet _____ cm H20
Cystometric capacity _____ ml   Pdet _____ cm H20   (End filling pressure after 60 seconds)
Bladder compliance (Vol ml/ P cm H20) _____   Low (<20)   Normal (21 - 100)   High (>100)

Detrusor Activity in the Filling Phase: Stable   Unstable   Symptomatic?   No   Yes   Urgency   Leakage
Detrusor instability provoked by: Filling   Coughing   Running Water   Standing   Other _____
Volume at first contraction _____ ml   Pdet _____ cm H20
Unstable leakage at _____ ml and Pdet of _____ cm H20
Height of maximum phasic detrusor contraction   Pdet_____ cm H20

Was Genuine Stress Incontinence Demonstrated?   No   Yes   Comments:_____
_____

PRESSURE/FLOW VOIDING STUDIES
Peak flow rate _____ ml/sec   Pdet at peak flow _____ cm H20   Max Pdet _____ cm H20
Stop test: Done   Not done   Unable to inhibit   Piso _____ cm H20
Voids by: Detrusor contraction   Straining   Combined   Relaxation
Volume voided _____   Residual urine _____   Not measured

CONCLUSIONS AND DISPOSITION: _____
_____
_____
_____
_____
_____
_____
_____
_____
_____, M.D.

Figure 4.14   Data sheet for recording the results of complex cystometric testing.

does *not* have a normal bladder in real life. What this means is that the test has failed to reproduce her symptoms. This in itself may have important therapeutic implications for patient management. Given two patients with identical symptoms of frequency, urgency, and urge incontinence, the one who cannot suppress detrusor contractions during cystometry may be managed best initially with anticholinergic medications, while the one who can suppress detrusor activity when forced to do so during testing may be more suited to bladder retraining and behavioral modification as an initial treatment strategy.

The correlation of symptoms with cystometric findings is especially important in making the diagnosis of detrusor instability. Although a detrusor pressure rise of 15 cm H_2O is generally considered the threshold at which detrusor activity becomes significant, this must always be judged within the context of the patient's symptoms. A detrusor contraction of 16 cm H_2O to which the patient remains oblivious and which produces no symptoms should not be considered abnormal. Small pressure rises of 10 cm H_2O accompanied by urgency or leakage *are* clinically significant in spite of their ''subthreshold'' nature. Technical details regarding the diagnosis of detrusor instability are dealt with in more detail in Chapter 8, ''Urge Incontinence and the Unstable Bladder.''

Voiding Studies

It is difficult to evaluate voiding function without the use of complex tests. Normal voiding should take place through a combination of pelvic floor and urethral relaxation accompanied by a sustained detrusor contraction. However, many women void primarily by abdominal straining or primarily by pelvic floor relaxation, without generating a sustained detrusor contraction. Although measurement of residual urine volumes after voiding is obviously of great importance, this by itself does not provide a complete evaluation of voiding since some patients with severe voiding problems may empty their bladders completely and leave no residual urine, even though they accomplish this only with great effort and perseverance. Simple uroflowmetry, which has already been discussed, can not provide more than a rough clinical screening for voiding dysfunction. More thorough evaluation requires either complex uroflowmetry using calibrated electronic instruments, or pressure-flow voiding studies, often performed with simultaneous EMG of the pelvic floor muscles and fluoroscopy of the urethra and bladder neck.

As has been emphasized previously, it is particularly important that patients be placed at ease during voiding studies. Psychologic inhibition is a major cause of voiding dysfunction in the urodynamics laboratory. Patients should be allowed to void with as much privacy as possible and should be questioned to make sure that the voiding pattern that they demonstrate is typical for them. It is also important to make sure that patients have adequate leg support during voiding, as this has been shown to be extremely important for pelvic floor relaxation and normal voiding. The patient who has to sit on an unfamiliar commode in a skimpy hospital gown with her feet swinging in the air and two doctors and a nurse watching her attempt to urinate, is very likely to put on a ''bad performance.'' For these reasons, one should be very careful about giving someone a diagnosis of voiding dysfunction based on an isolated study, particularly if they have no symptoms. While there are many women with occult voiding problems, there are also many women who have been studied hastily and with poor technique.

Complex Uroflowmetry

This is uroflowmetry performed by having the patient void while sitting on a special commode into a calibrated electronic flowmeter which generates a printed flow tracing (Fig. 4.15). Flowmeters are usually based on one of two types of technology: weight transducers, in which a special sensor detects the increasing weight of the urine flowing into the collecting container, and generates a printout on this basis; or a spinning disc, in which urine flows into the collecting container over the surface of a rotating disc which moves at constant speed. The inertia of the urine flowing over the disc increases the amount of power necessary to keep the disc spinning at a constant rate. This change in power is proportional to the urine flow and is then changed electronically into a flow rate tracing.

A third, and less common, form of flowmeter, called a capacitance flowmeter, has a metal strip suspended vertically in the collecting device. The solutes in the urine conduct electricity across the capacitor and as the urine volume rises the effective area of the capacitor decreases and the capacitance falls. The rate of change of volume in the collection device is then changed into a flow rate tracing. Rotating disc flowmeters are the most accurate and are not subject to kick artifact from the patient's foot striking the collection bucket during the flow study, which is a significant drawback of weight transducers.

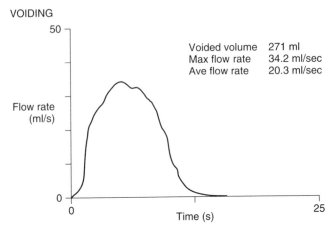

Figure 4.15 Normal complex urine flow study from an electronically calibrated urine flowmeter.

Depending upon the calibration of the equipment, complex urine flowmeters can measure peak flow rate, mean flow rate, voiding time, flow time, volume voided, and time to peak flow. It is customary to regard a ''normal'' urine flow rate as being a peak flow of at least 15–20 ml/sec with a voided volume of 150–200 ml. This is based on the idea that women unable to generate a peak flow of 15 ml/sec are likely to have some form of outlet obstruction, and this may serve as a useful ''rule of thumb'' for looking at flow rates. However, one of the most important facts which must be remembered about voiding is that urine flow is directly dependent upon voided volume. Therefore, flow rates cannot really be interpreted without reference to the voided volume.

A more meaningful way of looking at urine flow studies is to look at a nomogram where flow rate is compared to voided volume, and to figure out where the patient falls on the curve. Nomograms have been developed for both peak flow rate (Fig. 4.16) and mean flow rate (Fig. 4.17). It would seem logical to expect patients with lower nomogram centile rankings to have more significant problems and to be at more risk of developing voiding difficulty after surgery than patients with higher rankings. For this reason, use of nomogram centiles would seem to be a useful screening test for female voiding problems.

Of equal importance to the ''numbers'' provided by complex uroflowmetry is the voiding pattern produced on the uroflow tracing. Normal female voiding should be accomplished by pelvic floor relaxation accompanied by a sustained detrusor contraction. This will produce a bell-shaped curve on a urine flow study (Fig. 4.15). If the patient uses abdominal straining to assist a detrusor contraction, the flow study will show sharp ''spikes'' superimposed on the otherwise normal curve (Fig. 4.18). Patients with significant voiding difficulty often have an interrupted pattern punctuated by isolated sharp spikes (Fig. 4.19) These patients are voiding primarily by straining and their stream stops when they stop straining to catch their breath. Patients with low, flat, prolonged patterns are also particularly likely to have significant voiding dysfunction (Fig. 4.20). This pattern is often seen following bladder neck surgery and may represent the development of some degree of outflow obstruction.

It should be emphasized that complex uroflowmetry is mainly a screening test to pick up abnormal voiding patterns. They are often over-interpreted, but do provide useful information on voiding, particularly when analyzed in view of the volume voided and the residual urine.

Pressure-flow Voiding Studies

Pressure-flow voiding studies involve a combination of complex uroflowmetry with complex voiding cystometry. In these studies the uroflow trace is dis-

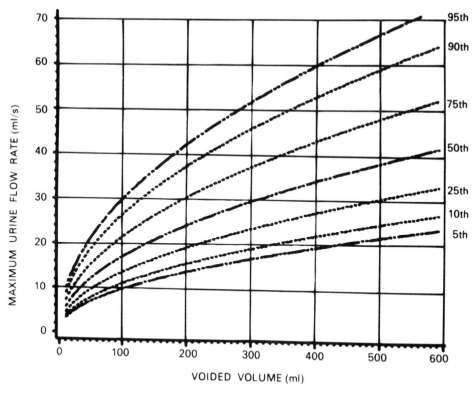

Figure 4.16 Liverpool nomogram for maximum (peak) flow rate. (From Haylen BT, et al., Br J Urol 1989; 64: 30–38, with permission.)

played on the multichannel tracing along with the bladder pressure, abdominal pressure and subtracted detrusor pressure tracings (Fig. 4.9). This allows simultaneous observation of all pressure activity in relationship to the urine flow pattern. Figure 4.21 shows a normal pressure-flow study in which the patient voids with a sustained detrusor contraction. An outline of a suggested technique for performing pressure-flow studies is given in Table 4.6.

Pressure-flow voiding studies provide an accurate means of differentiating detrusor contraction, straining, and pelvic relaxation as mechanisms of urination. They can also help separate poor flow or poor relaxation from true outflow obstruction. Outflow obstruction may be said to exist when a patient voids with a peak urine flow of 15 ml/sec or less with a voiding detrusor pressure of more than 50 cm H_2O. Outflow obstruction is very common in men due to the problem of benign prostatic hypertrophy, but is relatively rare in women unless they have undergone bladder neck surgery. Normal detrusor pressures during voiding in women are generally more than 20 cm H_2O. However, many women void primarily by relaxing the urethra and pelvic floor.

Patients who void by straining or by relaxation alone appear to be at substantially greater risk of postoperative voiding problems, especially if they have poor detrusor function. But if the bladder can be emptied completely by straining or urethral relaxation, how do you know if the detrusor is strong enough to overcome the changes in anatomy produced by an operation? If the patient is suddenly asked to stop her flow during a voiding study, there is often an immediate pressure rise noted on the subtracted detrusor tracing. This occurs because the detrusor is still contracting when the patient shuts off her urine flow by contracting the external urethral sphincter and closing the bladder neck. An isometric rise in detrusor pressure, called "Piso" or "Pdet(iso)" is thus pro-

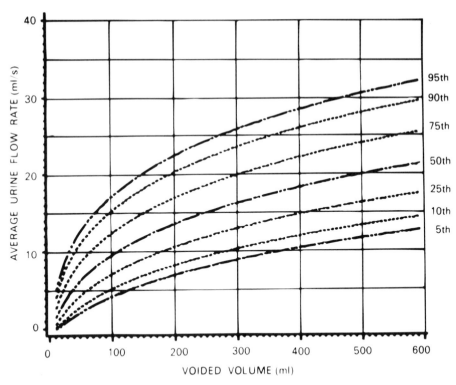

Figure 4.17   Liverpool nomogram for average flow rate. (From Haylen BT, et al., Br J Urol 1989; 64:30–38, with permission.)

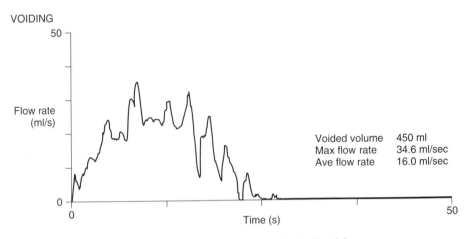

Figure 4.18   Voiding assisted by abdominal straining.

duced (Fig. 4.22). The isometric rise in detrusor pressure is regarded as a measure of reserve detrusor power or the maximum detrusor pressure that the muscle can generate. Patients who are unable to generate a Piso of more than 10 cm H_2O appear to be at greater risk of postoperative voiding trouble than patients who can generate a strong, healthy contraction.

When voiding has been completed there is often an "after-contraction," a detrusor contraction which continues to rise, sometimes higher than the maximum voiding pressure. The significance of an after-contraction is unknown, but

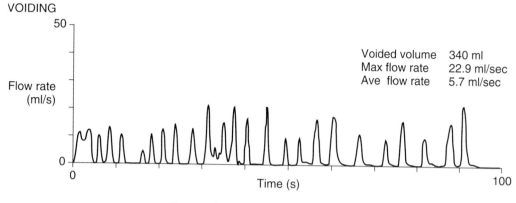

Figure 4.19   Voiding only by straining.

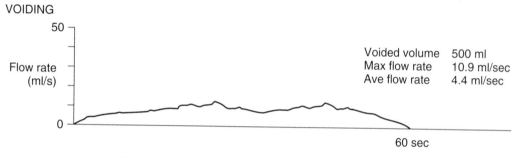

Figure 4.20   Poor flow after multiple bladder neck surgeries.

it is often seen in patients with detrusor hyperreflexia. It may represent the detrusor continuing to contract against a bladder neck which has now closed, or it may simply represent an artifact of catheter compression in an empty bladder in some patients. Examples of the findings that may be obtained during pressure-flow voiding studies are given in Figures 4.23–4.25.

Electromyography   A wide variety of electromyographic tests are used by neurophysiologists to assess the neuromuscular unit. These tests range from relatively nonspecific recording techniques using various types of surface electrodes, to invasive studies requiring special needles (concentric, single fiber) or electrical stimulators to obtain detailed, specific information about neuromuscular physiology and pathology. Urodynamic testing utilizes only crude surface electromyographic recording techniques which provide *kinesiologic* information about muscle contraction or relaxation during bladder filling or emptying. These studies can only determine whether or not a muscle group is contracting at a given moment in time. They cannot provide useful diagnostic information about the integrity of the neuromuscular unit or define precisely the location of a neurologic lesion which affects bladder function. To obtain information of this kind, special studies are required which need expensive electrophysiologic equipment and specialized technical skills for their proper performance and interpretation. These studies require referral to specialist centers and are beyond the scope of this book.

Electromyography is the technique of recording electrical potentials generated by the depolarization of muscle fibers. Although striated skeletal muscle can be relaxed to the point of complete electrical silence, the striated urethral sphincter must maintain a degree of continuous muscle activity to keep the urethra closed until voiding is initiated. Unlike the striated skeletal muscle in the rest of the body, which is composed of a mixture of Type I (slow-twitch) and Type II (fast-twitch) fibers, the striated urethral sphincter contains mainly

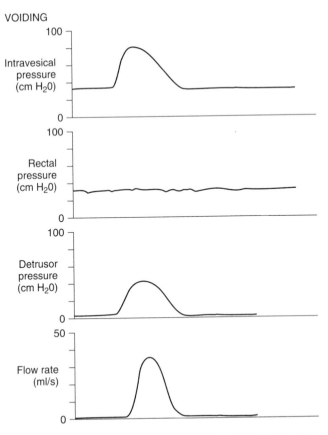

VOIDING

Figure 4.21   Normal pressure-flow voiding study. A normal flow rate is developed with a sustained detrusor contraction of appropriate pressure.

Type I fibers, which allows it to maintain this constant closure. EMG recordings made during urodynamic testing are an effort to evaluate the function of this muscle group. These recordings are made by applying surface patch electrodes to the perineum, usually on either side of the anal sphincter, or by inserting wire electrodes directly into the muscle of the external anal or urethral sphincter itself. These wires then run through the electromyography unit to a strip-chart recorder, where a visual signal is recorded, and through an amplifier to a speaker, where an auditory signal is produced which increases with increasing muscle activity and decreases with decreasing muscle activity. Experienced electromyographers rely more on listening to the signal than on watching it develop on a paper tracing or on an oscilloscope.

The rationale for obtaining electrical signals from the anal sphincter rather than the urethral sphincter is: (*a*) this muscle is far easier to find in women than the striated muscle around the urethra, and (*b*) the sphincters and the pelvic floor, for all practical purposes, act synchronously during bladder filling and emptying. Although this appears to be true for the vast majority of patients without overt neurologic disease, this may not be the case in patients with partial spinal cord lesions or multiple sclerosis. Care must therefore be taken in interpreting studies from such patients if this type of approach is used. Surface patch electrodes are convenient, but often stick to the perineum poorly, particularly in obese women. Wire electrodes are generally better, but must be inserted firmly and quickly because placing them can be painful. If electrodes are inserted around the urethra in women, this can cause a moderate amount of bleeding.

TABLE 4.6. Instructions For Performing Pressure-Flow Voiding Studies

1. The voiding cystometrogram (pressure-flow study) is performed at the end of the filling cystometrogram. After provocative measures have been completed, the patient is allowed to sit to void. If a separate filling catheter has been used, this should be removed prior to sitting and voiding. This leaves only the pressure catheter in place and facilitates voiding. The urine flowmeter should be positioned under the commode or birthing chair to record the urine flow. Some flowmeters must be zeroed prior to use.

2. The patient is asked to initiate voiding. If EMG is being performed, pelvic floor and urethral relaxation should be demonstrated by electrical silence during voiding. A detrusor contraction should occur, followed by the initiation of urine flow. It is not uncommon to see flow in the absence of a detrusor contraction in the female, since voiding may occur due to urethral relaxation or straining alone. Do not encourage straining.

Record the peak flow rate, average flow rate, and voiding time.
Record the maximum detrusor pressure during voiding.
Record the detrusor pressure at peak urinary flow.
Note any after-contraction.
Note the pattern of flow: Interrupted, straining, prolonged, and whether it was typical for the patient.

3. If the patient is unable to void, try running water, leaving the room with the machine on, and, if necessary, coughing or straining. Give the patient as much privacy as possible, particularly if she has a known voiding disorder.

4. An isometric detrusor test or "stop-flow" test, may be performed to help assess the risk of postoperative voiding difficulty, particularly for patients undergoing bladder neck surgery for stress incontinence. When approximately one-third of the bladder volume has been expelled by a detrusor contraction, the patient is asked to stop her urine flow abruptly. A transient rise in detrusor pressure should be seen after flow ceases, appearing as an additional "peak" or "cap" on the detrusor tracing. This additional rise in detrusor pressure is called the "Pstop" or "Pdet(iso)" and is regarded as a measurement of inherent detrusor power. Patients who void without an obvious detrusor contraction may be able to generate one under these circumstances. These patients seem less likely to have postoperative voiding problems than patients who are unable to generate an isometric detrusor contraction at all.

Record Pstop (change in detrusor pressure with sudden cessation of flow).
Record Pdet(iso) (the total detrusor pressure with sudden cessation of flow).

The stop test should be used selectively. It should not be performed as part of the initial urodynamic evaluation of patients who are being evaluated for voiding disorders. Although many of these patients will be able to stop their stream, many of them will not be able to start again afterwards, and the pressure-flow study will be far less useful than if they had been allowed to void to completion.

5. If the patient is unable to void after a reasonable attempt, remove the pressure catheters and perform a urine flow study only. If the patient still cannot void, have her urinate in private on a standard toilet and check the residual urine afterwards. In these cases it may be useful to place a plastic "hat" in the toilet to measure the volume voided.

Evaluation of muscle activity with these techniques has its greatest utility in the analysis of voiding disorders.

Electromyography during normal cystometry should demonstrate only slight muscle activity with the bladder empty and a slow, progressive increase in pelvic floor activity as the bladder fills (Fig. 4.26). This represents the normal recruitment of muscle fibers around the urethra which helps keep outlet resistance higher than the bladder pressure as filling takes place. If the patient coughs during bladder filling, this should be marked by a compensatory burst of increased EMG activity occurring simultaneously with the cough as the pelvic muscles contract (Fig. 4.26). During voiding, there should be a marked decrease in muscle activity as the pelvic floor relaxes, followed by the initiation of a detrusor contraction. Muscle relaxation should be maintained during voiding and should then increase when voiding has been completed (Fig. 4.27).

Dyscoordination of sphincteric relaxation with detrusor contraction is called

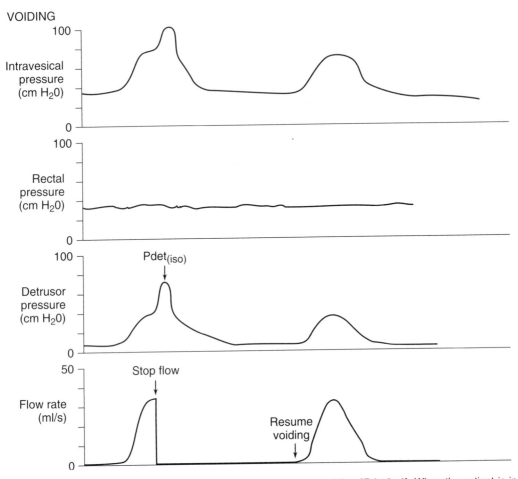

Figure 4.22 Generation of an isometric detrusor contraction during voiding [*Pdet(iso)*]. When the patient is instructed to stop her urine stream, she does so by contracting the striated muscles of the pelvic floor. This produces an immediate cessation of flow. But because the detrusor muscle is still contracting, an isometric rise in detrusor pressure should occur as the muscle contracts against the closed outlet. The resulting rise in pressure is regarded as a measurement of inherent detrusor power.

Fluoroscopic Monitoring During Complex Cystometry (Videocystourethrography, VCU)

"detrusor-sphincter-dyssynergia." This phenomenon is found most commonly in patients with multiple sclerosis, but it is usually overdiagnosed during urodynamic testing because poor relaxation of the urethra in nervous, inhibited patients produces tracings which look very similar to true neuromuscular dyssynergia. Practitioners who decide to utilize EMG for routine testing should beware of the pitfalls involved and should make sure that their equipment is electrically isolated and properly grounded. Interference from 60–cycle current is notorious for producing bizarre patterns on a strip-chart recorder and is often a cause for an incorrect diagnosis.

If the bladder is filled with radiocontrast dye as opposed to sterile water or saline during complex cystometry, the process of bladder filling and emptying can be observed radiographically through the use of fluoroscopy. This adds another dimension to the study and provides further information. If this is done, the study is typically recorded on videotape and displayed on a monitor that shows superimposed tracings of bladder, abdominal, and subtracted detrusor pressures, EMG activity, urine flow, and infused volumes. This type of study is therefore often called videocystourethrography or videocystometrography

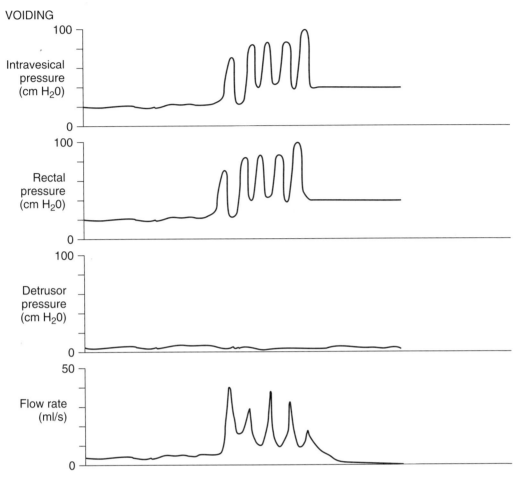

VOIDING

Figure 4.23 Voiding by abdominal straining. Note that bladder pressure rises during voiding but that this is accompanied by a rise in rectal pressure, rather than detrusor pressure. This shows that the patient is voiding by straining, not by detrusor contraction.

("VCU"), not to be confused with a "VCUG" or "voiding cystourethrogram" (see below).

Simultaneous fluoroscopic monitoring allows the clinician to look at the bladder outline during filling and emptying, detect vesico-ureteral reflux, and observe the position of the bladder neck in relationship to the surrounding bony structures (notably the pubic symphysis) during coughing. It allows detection of bladder and urethral diverticula, permits localization of urethral strictures during voiding studies, and provides a clear picture of bladder neck closure during resting and straining conditions. For these reasons, many specialists regard the VCU as the "gold standard" for urodynamic testing. On the other hand, fluoroscopic studies involve a quantum leap in expense, technical expertise, scheduling, and the number of variables that have to be juggled during the examination of a patient (Fig. 4.28). While these studies are indispensable for the evaluation of men with neuropathic bladder dysfunction, they are less useful in the examination of women with primary bladder complaints. These studies are most useful in evaluating complex problems at tertiary referral centers. Examples of such problems include severe voiding dysfunction, suspicion of vesicoureteral reflux, patients with complex neurourologic problems, patients with previous failed surgery, and patients with significant incontinence of unclear etiology.

VOIDING

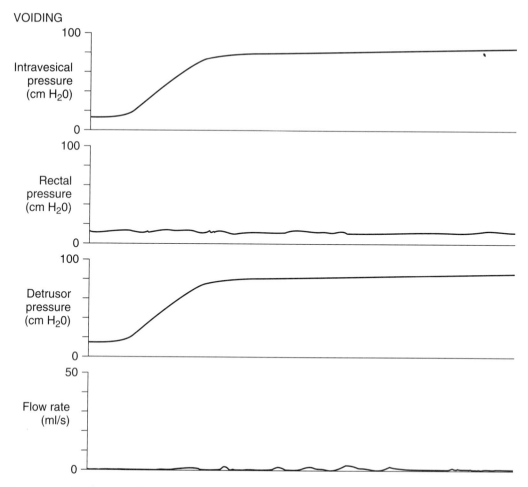

Figure 4.24 Obstructed voiding after bladder neck surgery. Note the extremely high intravesical and detrusor pressures need to generate minimal flow.

Other Urodynamic
Tests
Urethral Pressure Studies

Urethral function plays an important role in the maintenance of continence and the development of incontinence. Any technique that increases our understanding of urethral function should thereby improve our ability to help patients with urinary incontinence. This philosophy led to the belief that measurement of urethral pressure would lead to an enhanced understanding of urethral function and would allow easier diagnosis of many lower urinary tract complaints. A wide variety of techniques have now been developed to measure urethral pressure, under both static and dynamic conditions. Whether or not these techniques have led to an enhanced understanding of urethral function and have improved our diagnostic capabilities remains a matter of some controversy.

The static urethral pressure profile is obtained by pulling a pressure catheter through the urethra from the bladder to the external urethral meatus at a constant rate. It usually requires a special catheter-puller to do this and the patient cannot move during this part of the study. This may be done using a fluid-filled catheter which is perfused at a low but constant rate (Brown-Wickham technique) or by using a microtip transducer pressure catheter with two sensors spaced 6 cm apart. Figure 4.29 illustrates the parameters which are measured during urethral pressure profilometry.

The resting urethral pressure is the pressure measured in the urethra at rest, and this will vary with the position of the measuring catheter in the urethra as

VOIDING

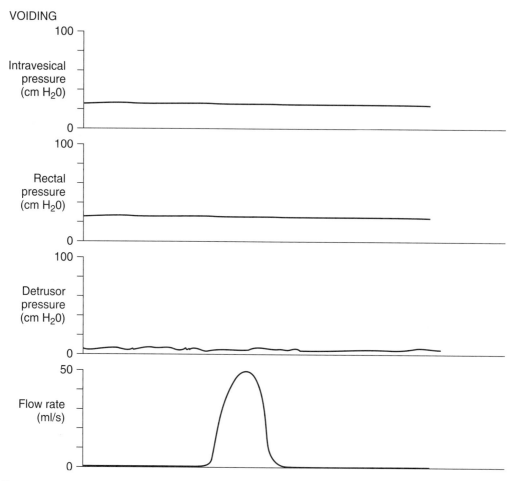

Figure 4.25 Voiding without significant detrusor contraction. This patient voids by relaxing the pelvic floor and letting the water drain out of the bladder. Note that there is almost no change in bladder, rectal, or detrusor pressures.

well as the position of the patient. The total profile length is the distance from where urethral pressure first exceeds bladder pressure to the point where the pressure falls to atmospheric pressure at catheter withdrawal. The total profile length is not clinically useful. The functional profile length represents the length of the urethra in which urethral pressure exceeds bladder pressure. This pressure difference is called the urethral closure pressure. Maximum urethral closure pressure is the largest pressure difference between the urethral pressure and the bladder pressure, whereas maximum urethral pressure is the largest pressure measured in the urethra with respect to atmospheric pressure. The differences between the two are important. Since continence is maintained by keeping urethral pressure higher than bladder pressure, the urethral closure pressure——that is, the pressure margin between the urethra and the bladder——is of more practical importance than the absolute pressure measured in the urethra.

The pressure measuring system should be zeroed to atmospheric pressure before the catheter is inserted for a urethral pressure study. The pressure catheter must be placed into the bladder before it is withdrawn, and the speed of the pulling mechanism and the speed of the paper in the strip-chart recorder should be synchronized before the study is begun. This is best done if both speeds are the same (e.g., 1 mm/sec).

A dynamic urethral pressure profile (or urethral closure pressure profile)

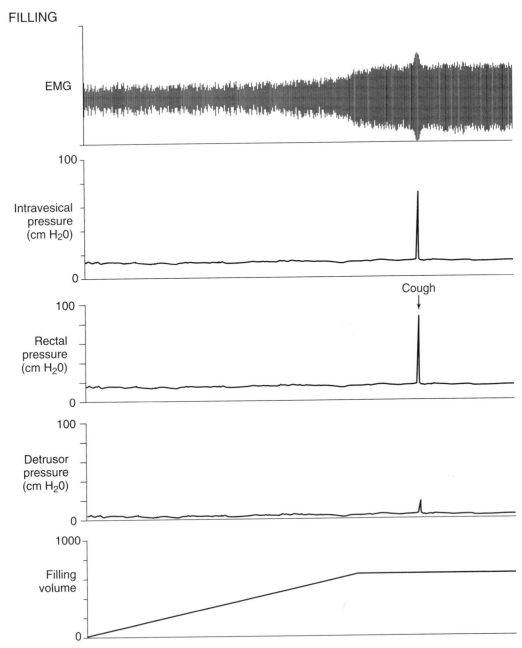

Figure 4.26 Normal EMG showing increasing recruitment of muscle fibers in the pelvic floor during bladder filling. Note the increased burst of EMG activity during coughing, as the pelvic floor muscles respond to the increased stress.

involves simultaneous measurement of urethral pressure and bladder pressure, and the calculation of urethral closure pressure. Urethral closure pressure is obtained by subtracting bladder pressure from urethral pressure throughout the test. During a dynamic urethral pressure profile the pressure catheter is pulled through the urethra while the patient coughs and a continuous recording of subtracted urethral closure pressure is made. At least one cough should be recorded in each quarter of the profile length. These coughs will appear as

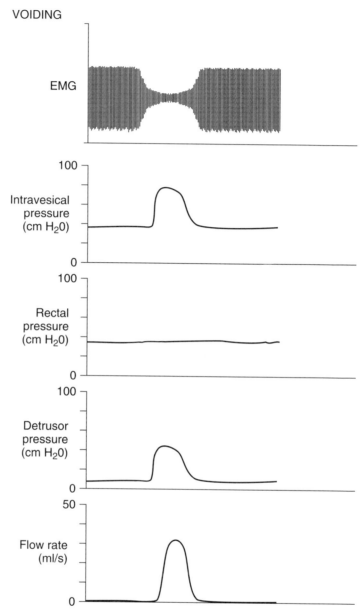

VOIDING

EMG

Intravesical
pressure
(cm H₂0)

Rectal
pressure
(cm H₂0)

Detrusor
pressure
(cm H₂0)

Flow rate
(ml/s)

Figure 4.27   Normal EMG showing appropriate relaxation of the pelvic floor during voiding.

pressure spikes on the tracing. If bladder pressure exceeds urethral pressure during a cough, the urethral closure pressure will demonstrate a negative deflection towards the baseline. Since urethral pressure must be higher than bladder pressure, some clinicians use this as a test for diagnosing stress incontinence. If *every* cough along the urethral closure pressure profile generates a negative spike *which reaches the baseline,* the study is said to be ''positive;'' that is, it ''demonstrates pressure equalization'' and therefore suggests a diagnosis of stress incontinence. Tracings in which only some of these negative deflections reach the baseline are said to be ''equivocal.'' Tracings in which no deflection reaches the baseline are ''negative,'' that is, pressure equalization has not been demonstrated.

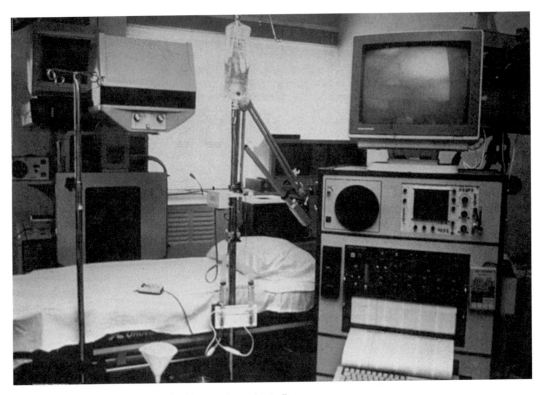

Figure 4.28 Setup for fluoroscopic video-urodynamic studies.

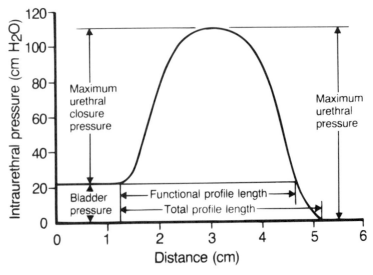

Figure 4.29 Parameters normally measured during urethral pressure profile studies.

The cough urethral pressure profile is highly susceptible to artifact. Positive tests depend entirely on the ability of the patient to cough forcefully, which not everyone can do under typical test conditions. The same patient may have positive, negative, and equivocal studies during the same testing session. In addition, the catheter tends to move with each cough, and many patients wiggle or change position each time they cough so that this test is plagued by movement artifact. Unless urine loss is seen to accompany a ''positive'' test, a diagnosis of stress incontinence has still not been made. Clinicians who make the diagnosis of stress incontinence on the basis of dynamic urethral pressure profiles alone—particularly without the benefit of directly observing urine loss—run a substantial risk of making a misdiagnosis due to artifact. The utility of this test seems marginal at best.

The ''pressure transmission ratio'' is defined as the increment in urethral pressure during coughing as a percentage of the simultaneously recorded increment in bladder pressure. The pressure transmission ratio was developed in an attempt to measure a common theoretical assumption about stress incontinence, namely that it develops because increases in intra-abdominal pressure are not properly ''transmitted'' to the urethra. While it is true that stress incontinence will not occur unless bladder pressure is higher than urethral pressure, it is a major assumption that passive transmission of the cough pressure is responsible for maintaining continence. It was hoped that surgical success in patients with stress incontinence would be confirmed by dramatic increases in the pressure transmission ratio. In fact, this has not occurred. There is little correlation between successful surgical outcome and pressure transmission ratios, and in some cases pressure transmission ratios of more than 100% have been recorded. This is clearly impossible if passive transmission of pressure is the key to continence.

Urethral pressure measurements have not fulfilled the hopes that early investigators placed in them. Although urethral pressures in stress incontinent women tend to be lower than the pressures in women who do not have this condition, there is no ''magic'' urethral pressure at which a diagnosis of ''genuine'' stress incontinence can be made simply on the basis of urethral pressure alone. There is a great deal of overlap between the urethral pressures of continent and incontinent women, and a great deal of overlap between the urethral pressures of stress incontinent women and women with detrusor instability. Furthermore, these ''pressures'' are not really pressures at all. They are obtained by dragging a stiff catheter through a compliant muscular tube (the urethra). If small balloon catheters which could accurately absorb force from all directions were used, a ''pressure'' measurement could be generated. Unfortunately, most of these measurements are made with microtip transducer pressure catheters which absorb and record only the force generated on the face of the transducer as it is dragged along the wall of the urethra. As a result, the orientation of the transducer within the urethral lumen is extremely important, and many investigators have shown consistent differences in readings made with anterior, posterior, or lateral orientations of the transducers. The problems are magnified further if the patient is moving, coughing, or contracting her pelvic muscles as the catheter is withdrawn.

Recently the concept of the ''low pressure urethra'' has received considerable attention. Some researchers have suggested that women with ''genuine'' stress incontinence and urethral closure pressures of less than 20 cm H_2O (measured with the patient in a sitting position and a full bladder) have a much higher rate of failure if they undergo ''standard'' bladder neck suspension operations, such as a Burch procedure, than patients with a higher urethral closure pressure who undergo the same operation. Some authors have suggested that sling operations should be done on such patients. Other researchers have not found the same failure rate and feel that urethral closure pressure is irrelevant if bladder neck hypermobility is present. It seems probable that urinary continence or incontinence is related not so much to passive urethral pressure per se as it is to how and where that pressure is exerted in relation to the other structures of the pelvic floor. At present, the significance of the "low pressure urethra" remains unclear. If urethral pressure studies are done on a patient with significant stress incontinence, and if these pressures are extremely low, the clinician should consider whether an alteration in the proposed surgery is merited based upon all the relevant factors in a given case.

Cystourethroscopy

Endoscopic examination of the bladder and urethra is most useful in the evaluation of patients with irritative bladder symptoms, especially those who have an acute onset of their symptoms, such as patients in whom these symptoms develop for the first time after surgery prompting a concern that a suture may have penetrated the bladder. Cystourethroscopy is primarily an anatomic examination of the bladder and urethra and its usefulness lies mainly in excluding tumors, stones, foreign bodies, and gross anatomic defects as causes of patient symptoms. Only a limited amount of useful physiologic information can be obtained by this technique, and cystourethroscopy does not have to be a routine test in the evaluation of patients with uncomplicated lower urinary tract symptoms. While some authors have emphasized the importance of "dynamic urethroscopy," that is, examining the closure of the bladder neck under conditions of stress, we have not found this especially helpful in most patients. If the bladder neck is observed to rotate downwards and outwards and to balloon open during coughing, this is useful information when added to a general clinical picture. However, movement of the patient and the urethroscope during these maneuvers can create an false impression. If the bladder neck is wide open and the urethra is heavily scarred, this may help make a diagnosis of intrinsic sphincteric dysfunction ("Type III" incontinence), but in general cystourethroscopy is only of limited value in diagnosing stress incontinence.

Cystourethroscopic examination of women can easily be accomplished in a clinic or office setting using topical 1% Lidocaine jelly injected into the urethra with a blunt syringe shortly before the procedure is performed. It is almost never necessary to perform this examination on women under general anesthesia unless biopsies are to be taken or other instrumentation done. The exception to this rule is the patient who must be examined under anesthesia to rule out interstitial cystitis and to obtain a measurement of the structural bladder capacity under conditions of deep muscular relaxation.

Our preferred medium for distending the bladder is water or normal saline, not gas. The reasons for this have been described earlier in the section on cystometry. Once the scope has been introduced, the obturator is removed and the residual urine is measured. A 30° or 70° lens is then introduced and the bladder inspected. This should be done in a systematic fashion which allows good visualization of all bladder surfaces. The ureteric orifices should be located on each side of the trigone. Careful observation will allow the endoscopist to note the opening and closing of the ureteric orifices with peristalsis and to see a stream of urine enter the bladder. The scope can be rotated easily once one ureter has been located, following the interureteric bar across the top of the trigone to find the other ureteric orifice. Because the trigone has a different embryologic origin than the rest of the bladder a whitish plaque is often seen covering this area, somewhat resembling early morning dew on a field of grass. While much has been made of "granular trigonitis" in women, these changes represent nothing more than squamous metaplasia of the urothelium and should cause neither undue alarm nor aggressive instrumentation. If a bladder diverticulum is encountered, its interior should be carefully inspected because it may contain a stone or a tumor.

Inspection of the urethra is best done with a 0° lens which allows a "straight ahead" view of the entire urethral lumen. It is important to examine the female urethra with a female urethroscope, *not* a male cystoscope (Fig. 4.30). The male instrument has a "gunsight" along its anterior surface which is neither necessary nor comfortable for examining the female urethra. In addition, the posterior surface of the male sheath is cut away to allow for the passage of instruments,

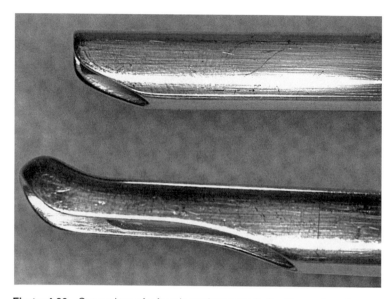

Figure 4.30   Comparison of a female urethroscope (top) with a male cystoscope (bottom). Note the elevated "gunsight" on the male instrument. If the male cystoscope is used to examine female patients, the large opening on the posterior aspect of the instrument will be outside the external urethral meatus long before the entire lumen has been examined. This prevents effective distension of the female urethra with fluid and results in an inadequate examination.

a design which prohibits adequate filling of the shorter female urethra. Use of a female urethroscope permits distension of the urethra with fluid during the examination and allows good visualization of the entire female urethra. Women should be examined with instruments designed for their anatomy, not made to adapt to male instruments which provide a second-rate view.

Skill in the use of a cystourethroscope should be part of the surgical armamentarium of all pelvic surgeons. Gynecologists will find this instrument most useful in assessing ureteral patency following pelvic surgery, particularly if intravenous indigo carmine dye is given 5 minutes prior to the examination. Cystoscopic examination of patients with hematuria or suspicious cytology in whom there is a concern about urologic malignancy, should have their examinations performed by the urologist who will continue to care for them. Bladder biopsies should be obtained by the urologic surgeon who will treat the patient, not the referring physician.

Radiographic Studies   An intravenous urogram (IVU, often called an IVP or intravenous pyelogram) is primarily an anatomic study of the urinary tract. Only limited information on function can be obtained by this technique. If information regarding renal function is needed, a wide variety of better tests are available, including renal perfusion studies and nuclear medicine scans. The intravenous urogram is most helpful in detecting structural anomalies of the urinary tract, which is important in the evaluation of continuous incontinence, recurrent urinary tract infections, hematuria (tumors), flank pain, and postoperative ureteral obstruction. The IVU is particularly helpful in the evaluation of a pelvic mass and in the workup of patients with congenital anomalies of the lower genital tract. Routine use of intravenous urography in the evaluation of patients with incontinence is not cost effective, and it appears to have little utility in the routine preoperative evaluation of patients undergoing most gynecologic surgery.

The voiding cystourethrogram (VCUG) is a fluoroscopic study of the bladder and urethra obtained during micturition. The bladder is filled with radiocontrast dye and pictures are taken both during filling and during voiding. The technique is especially useful for documenting vesico-ureteral reflux during voiding and for detecting urethral diverticula after voiding has been completed. Bladder stones, urethral stones, and bladder diverticula may also be seen with this technique. These studies are sometimes useful in detecting a vesico-vaginal or ure-thro-vaginal fistula which escaped detection by other means. The VCUG is a special study and is not used routinely in the evaluation of incontinent patients.

Bead-chain cystourethrography was popularized in the 1950's and 1960's as a way of looking at the bladder neck and the "posterior urethro-vesical angle." Green believed that stress incontinence could be divided into two subtypes based upon the results of a bead-chain study and that these studies would help determine whether a vaginal or abdominal surgical approach should be used in a particular patient. Subsequent research has led to the conclusion that there are no real differences between Green's two types of incontinence, both being manifestations of stress incontinence caused by anatomic hypermobility of the bladder neck which leads it to become displaced from its proper anatomic position during episodes of increased intra-abdominal pressure. Bead-chain cystourethrograms are no longer regarded as clinically useful studies and few clinicians utilize them for anything other than specialized research purposes any more.

Ultrasound is currently being investigated as a substitute for many radiologic techniques, generally to evaluate the position and mobility of the bladder neck. These studies are performed using either a perineal or transvaginal ultrasound probe. Some concern exists that use of a transvaginal probe which lies in direct contact with the bladder neck may alter lower urinary tract anatomy and give erroneous results. Ultrasound studies on the bladder neck usually require placement of a transurethral balloon catheter to help identify the anatomy, particularly if dynamic ultrasound studies are going to be performed. The role of ultrasound in the evaluation and management of lower urinary tract disorders remains investigational at the present time.

SUGGESTED READING

General

Abrams P, Blaivas JG, Stanton SL, Andersen JT. The standardisation of terminology of lower urinary tract function. Scand J Urol Nephrol Suppl 1988; 114:5–18.

Abrams P, Feneley R, Torrens M. Urodynamics. New York: Springer-Verlag, 1983.

Asmussen M, Miller A. Clinical Gynaecological Urology; Oxford: Blackwell Scientific, 1983.

Bock G, Whelan J (Eds). Neurobiology of Incontinence. New York: John Wiley, 1990. (Ciba Foundation Symposium, No. 151).

Drife JO, Hilton PA, Stanton SL (Eds). Micturition. New York: Springer-Verlag, 1990.

Hald T, Bradley WE. The Urinary Bladder: Neurology and Dynamics. Baltimore: Williams and Wilkins, 1982.

Krane RJ, Siorky MB (Eds). Clinical Neuro-Urology. Boston: Little Brown, 1991, 2nd ed.

McGuire EJ. Clinical Evaluation and Treatment of Neurogenic Vesical Dysfunction. Baltimore: Williams and Wilkins, 1984.

Mundy AR, Stephenson TP, Wein AJ (Eds). Urodynamics: Principles, Practice, and Application. New York: Churchill Livingstone, 1984.

Ostergard DR, Bent AE (Eds). Urogynecology and Urodynamics: Theory and Practice. Baltimore: Williams and Wilkins, 1991, 3rd ed.

Stanton SL (Ed). Clinical Gynecologic Urology. St. Louis: CV Mosby, 1984.

Thiede HA (Ed). "Urogynecology." Obstet Gynecol Clin NA 1990; 16:709–953.

Yalla SV, McGuire EJ, Elbadawi A, Blaivas JG (Eds). Neurourology and Urodynamics: Principles and Practice. New York: Macmillan, 1988.

General Cystometry

Aagaard J, Bruskewitz R. Are urodynamic studies useful in the evaluation of female incontinence? Prob Urol 1991; 5:11–22.

Arnold EP. Cystometry—postural effects in incontinent women. Urol Int 1974; 29:185–86.

Bhatia NN, Bergman A. Cystometry: Unstable bladder and urinary tract infection. Br J Urol 1986; 58:134–37.

Blaivas JG. Multichannel urodynamic studies. Urology 1984; 23:421–38.

Bump RC. The urodynamic laboratory. Obstet Gynecol Clin NA 1989; 16:795–16.

Enhorning G. Simultaneous recording of intravesical and intra-urethral pressure: A study on urethral closure in normal and stress incontinent women. Acta Chirurg Scand 1961; Suppl 276:1–68.

Haylen BT, Sutherst JR, Frazer MI. Is the investigation of most stress incontinence really necessary? Br J Urol 1989; 64:147–49.

Jorgensen L, Lose G, Andersen J. Cystometry: H_2O or CO_2

as filling medium? A literature survey of the influence of the filling medium on the qualitative and the quantitative cystometric parameters. Neurourol Urodyn 1988; 7: 343–50.

Massey A, Abrams P. Urodynamics of the female lower urinary tract. Urol Clin NA 1985; 12:231–41.

Millar H, Baker L. A stable ultraminiature catheter-tip pressure transducer. Med Biol Eng 1973; 11:86–89.

O'Donnell PD. Pitfalls of urodynamic testing. Urol Clin NA 1991; 18:257–68.

Perez LM, Webster GD. The history of urodynamics. Neurourol Urodynam 1992; 11:1–22.

Rowan D, James E, Kramer A, Sterling A, Suhel P. Urodynamic equipment: Technical aspects. J Med Eng Tech 1987; 11:57-64.

Sand P, Brubaker L, Novak T. Simple standing incremental cystometry as a screening method for detrusor instability. Obset Gynecol 1991; 7:453–57.

Stanton S, Cardozo L, Williams J, Ritchie D, Allan V. Clinical and urodynamic features of failed incontinence surgery in the female. Obstet Gynecol 1978; 51:515.

Stanton S, Krieger M, Ziv E. Videocystourethrography: Its role in the assessment of incontinence in the female. Neurourol Urodynam 1988; 7:172–73.

Sutherst J, Brown M. Comparison of single and multichannel cystometry in diagnosing bladder instability. Br Med J 1984; 288:1720–22.

Wall LL, Addison WA. Basic cystometry in gynecologic practice. Postgrad Obstet Gynecol 1988; 8(26):1–7.

Webster GD, Older RA. Value of subtracted bladder pressure measurement in routine urodynamics. Urology 1980; 16: 656–60.

Voiding Studies

Haylen BT, Ashby D, Sutherst JR, Frazer MI, West CR. Maximum and average urine flow rates in normal male and female populations—the Liverpool nomograms. Br J Urol 1989; 64:30–38.

Stanton SL, Ozsoy C, Hilton P. Voiding difficulties in the female: Prevalence, clinical and urodynamic review. Obstet Gynecol 1983; 61:144–47.

Massey JA, Abrams PH. Obstructed voiding in the female. Br J Urol 1988; 61:36–39.

Urethral Pressure Studies

Bump RC, Fantl JA, Hurt WG. Dynamic urethral pressure profilometry pressure transmission ratio determinations after continence surgery: Understanding the mechanism of success, failure, and complications. Obstet Gynecol 1988; 72:870–74.

Hilton P, Stanton SL. Urethral pressure measurement by microtransducer: The results in symptom-free women and in those with genuine stress incontinence. Br J Obstet Gynecol 1983; 90:919–33.

McGuire EJ. Active and passive factors in urethral continence function. Int Urogyn J 1992; 3:54–69.

Richardson DA. Value of the cough pressure profile in the evaluation of patients with stress incontinence. Am J Obstet Gynecol 1986; 155:808–11.

Versi E. Discriminant analysis of urethral pressure profilometry for the diagnosis of genuine stress incontinence. Br J Obstet Gynecol 1990; 97:251–59.

Sand PK, Bowen LD, Panganiban R, Ostergard DR. The low pressure urethra as a factor in failed retropubic urethropexy. Obstet Gynecol 1987; 69:399–402.

Ramon J, Mekras JA, Webster GD. The outcome of transvaginal cystourethropexy in patients with anatomical stress urinary incontinence and outlet weakness. J Urol 1990; 144:106–09.

Weil A, Reyes H, Bischoff P, Rottenberg RD, Krauer F. Modifications of the urethral rest and stress profiles after different types of surgery for urinary stress incontinence. Br J Obstet Gynecol 1984; 91:46–55.

Yalla S, Rossier A, Fam B, Gabilondo F. Dual pressure transducer catheter for evaluating vesicourethral function. Urology 1976; 8:160–63.

Electromyography and Electrophysiology

Blaivas JG. Sphincter electromyography. Neurourol Urodynam 1983; 2:269–88.

Barrett DM. Disposable (infant) surface electromyogram electrode in urodynamics: A simultaneous comparative study of electrodes. J Urol 1980; 124:663–65.

Chantraine A. EMG examination of the anal and urethral sphincters. In Desmedt JE (Ed). New Developments in Electromyography and Clinical Neurophysiology. Basel: S. Karger 1973: 421–32.

Fowler CJ, Fowler C. Clinical neurophysiology. In Torrens M, Morrison JFB (Eds). The Physiology of the Lower Urinary Tract. New York: Springer-Verlag, 1987, 309–32.

Nordling J, Meyhoff HH. Dissociation of urethral and anal sphincter activity in neurogenic bladder dysfunction. J Urol 1979; 122:352–55.

Vereecken RL, Verduyn H. The electrical activity of the paraurethral and perineal muscles in normal and pathological conditions. Br J Urol 1970; 42:457–63.

Perineal Pad Tests

Fantl JA, Harkins SW, Wyman JF, Choi SC, Taylor JR. Fluid loss quantitation test in women with urinary incontinence: A test-retest analysis. Obstet Gynecol 1987; 70: 739–43.

Frazer MI, Haylen BT, Sutherst JR. The severity of urinary incontinence in women: Comparison of subjective and objective tests. Br J Urol 1989; 63:14–15.

Jakobsen H, Vedel P, Andersen JT. Objective assessment of urinary incontinence: An evaluation of three different pad-weighing regimens. Neurourol Urodynam 1987; 6: 325–30.

Jorgensen L, Lose G, Andersen JT. One-hour pad-weighing test for objective assessment of female urinary incontinence. Obstet Gynecol 1987; 69:39–42.

Kromann-Andersen B, Jakobsen H, Andersen JT. Pad weighing tests: A literature survey on test accuracy and reproducibility. Neurourol Urodynam 1989; 8:237–42.

Richmond DH, Sutherst JR, Brown MC. Quantification of urine loss by weighing perineal pads: Observation on the exercise regimen. Br J Urol 1987; 59:224–27.

Sutherst J, Brown M, Shawer M. Assessing the severity of urinary incontinence in women by weighing perineal pads. Lancet 1981; 2:1128–30.

Versi E, Cardozo LD. Perineal pad weighing versus videographic analysis in genuine stress incontinence. Br J Obstet Gynaecol 1986; 93:364–66.

Victor A, Larsson G, Asbrink AS. A simple patient administered test for objective quantification of the symptom of urinary incontinence. Scand J Urol Nephrol 1987; 21: 277–79.

Walsh JB, Mills GL. Measurement of urinary loss in elderly incontinent patients. Lancet 1981; 2:1130–31.

Wilson PD, Mason MV, Herbison GP, Sutherst JR. Evaluation of the home pad test for quantifying incontinence. Br J Urol 1989; 64:155–57.

Other Studies

Bergman A, McKenzie C, Ballard C, Richmond J. Role of cystourethrography in the preoperative evaluation of stress urinary incontinence in women. J Repro Med 1988; 33(4):372–76.

Bhatia N, Bradley W, Haldemen S. Urodynamics: Continuous monitoring. J Urol 1982; 128:963–68.

Fantl J, Hurt G, Bump R, Dunn L, Choi S. Urethral axis and sphincteric function. Am J Obstet Gynecol 1986; 155: 554–58.

McInerney P, Vanner T, Harris S, Stephenson T. Ambulatory urodynamics. Br J Urol 1991; 67:272–74.

Richardson D, Bent A, Ostergard D. The effect of uterovaginal prolapse on urethrovesical pressure dynamics. Am J Obstet Gynecol 1983; 146:901–05.

Richardson D. Reduction of urethral pressure in response to stress: Relationship to urethral mobility. Am J Obstet Gynecol 1986; 155:20–25.

5 Understanding Stress Incontinence

Stress incontinence is urine loss that occurs when sudden increases in intra-abdominal pressure force urine past the urethral sphincter mechanism. This usually occurs during conditions of physical activity which stress the bladder outlet to such a degree that it can no longer remain closed. Urine loss then occurs because the abdominal pressure which is compressing the bladder exceeds the ability of the bladder outlet to withstand this extra pressure. Stress urinary incontinence is caused by factors which produce sudden increases in intra-abdominal pressure, such as coughing, sneezing, jumping, running, aerobic exercise, playing tennis, and so forth.

The term ''stress incontinence'' was coined by Sir Eardly Holland in 1928. At the present time the expression is used to refer to three separate, but related, entities. The differences between these three usages are important. ''Stress incontinence'' may refer to a patient complaint (a symptom), a physical finding (a sign), and a specific urodynamic diagnosis.

Symptom of Stress Incontinence

The patient's complaint of stress incontinence is her statement that she loses urine simultaneously with increases in intra-abdominal pressure. This problem may or may not be troubling to her and it may or may not be the type of incontinence which has led her to seek help. For example, a woman may present for evaluation because she has the sudden uncontrollable urge to urinate and loses large volumes of urine, but she may also have occasional small spurts of urine during severe coughing. Her major problem is probably unstable detrusor activity, but mild stress incontinence may also be present. Therefore the simple symptom—or even the simple demonstration—of stress incontinence does not mean that this is the patient's most significant problem. Symptoms, physical examination, and urodynamic investigation must all be used together to establish an accurate picture of the patient's problem. A symptom, per se, is only a starting point for further investigation.

Physical Sign of Stress Incontinence

Demonstration of urine loss occurring simultaneously with a cough during examination of the patient represents the *sign* of stress incontinence. As a sign, it represents a physical finding and is therefore different from the patient's complaint or symptom (though both of these may obviously coexist in the same patient). Although stress urinary incontinence may be suspected based on the patient's history, do not say the patient ''has stress incontinence'' unless you have seen it occur! As noted above, it is important to ask the patient during the examination if the urine loss which has just been demonstrated is troublesome to her and if it is the type of incontinence which has led her to seek medical help.

Patients who present with the complaint of stress incontinence must *always* be observed to leak before accepting that they have this problem. This is best accomplished if patients are examined with a comfortably full bladder. Patients coming for a urogynecologic examination should not be allowed to empty their bladders before being examined. This often requires breaking established habits with regard to pelvic examinations. If the patient's bladder is not full, it may be necessary for her to fill her bladder by having her drink several glasses of water before she is examined. If this is not feasible, an ordinary sterile red rubber catheter connected to a bag of sterile water or saline can be inserted into her bladder. This allows the bladder to be filled to a comfortable capacity easily and quickly so that her complaint can be verified.

Since most stress incontinence occurs during physical activity, it is useful to examine patients with this complaint in the standing position with their legs separated, watching for urinary leakage while they cough or strain. The patient's examining gown may be lifted to allow direct observation of the urethral meatus. It is useful to spread out an extra sheet or a large absorbent plastic-backed pad on the floor for her to stand on during this part of the examination, both for cleanliness as well as to see the urine loss more easily. The patient should be told that the purpose of this examination is to see her urinary leakage occur, and she should understand that no diagnosis can be made unless leakage can be demonstrated. This helps alleviate her embarrassment about being incontinent in front of others.

Remember, the first task of the examining physician in evaluating a patient complaining of the symptom of stress incontinence is to document that leakage does occur and to establish with her that this is her clinical problem.

Urodynamic Diagnosis of "Genuine Stress Incontinence"

The medical literature makes frequent reference to the term "genuine stress incontinence." This is a term defined specifically by the International Continence Society as "involuntary loss of urine occurring when, in the absence of a detrusor contraction, the intravesical pressure exceeds the maximum urethral pressure." As such "genuine stress incontinence" refers to a *specific urodynamic diagnosis*. Use of this term implies that the patient under consideration has undergone urodynamic testing and that these conditions have been met. Generally, this means that the patient has undergone subtracted cystometry with measurement of bladder and abdominal (usually rectal) pressure, and calculation of the subtracted detrusor pressure (Pdet = Pves − Pabd).

Since the diagnosis of "urinary incontinence" requires that urine loss be demonstrated objectively, use of the term "genuine stress incontinence" implies that urinary leakage has been seen during the test when bladder pressure was elevated due to an elevation of intra-abdominal pressure (e.g., coughing), and not because the bladder pressure was elevated by detrusor overactivity.

It is *not* necessary to measure urethral pressure or to perform complex subtracted urethral pressure measurements demonstrating "pressure equalization" in order to make this diagnosis. Since fluid can only flow from an area of higher pressure to one of lower pressure, if urine loss is demonstrated during a subtracted cystometrogram with stable detrusor activity at the moment of urine loss, the diagnosis of "genuine stress incontinence" has been established. Although some clinicians find these complicated urethral pressure measurements helpful, all current techniques for measuring urethral pressure are unphysiologic, are subject to significant artifact, and often result in marked differences of interpretation. The demonstration of urinary leakage is more important than "pressure equalization" on a strip chart recorder and it must be emphasized that *any* urodynamic test which does not reproduce the patient's symptoms should be considered a failed test. Beware of diagnoses made solely on the basis of a machine.

Some clinicians will give a patient the diagnosis of "genuine stress incontinence" if they have demonstrated urine loss clinically and the patient has a stable cystometrogram even though urinary leakage was not documented during cystometry. While this is technically incorrect, it is probably clinically accurate most of the time. Under these conditions, however, the diagnosis is by inference rather than by proof, and may be incorrect in some cases. Patients like this may still have incontinence due to cough-induced detrusor overactivity or some other factor. Since the object of cystometry is to reproduce the patient's complaint (i.e., incontinence) and correlate it with objective confirmatory data, failure to reproduce incontinence during cystometry is a technical failure of testing and therapeutic interventions which proceed on "assumptions" deduced from such testing may lead to problems later on, particularly if surgery is contemplated.

Use of the term "genuine stress incontinence" properly implies that urodynamic testing has been carried out, that urinary leakage under urodynamic test conditions has been observed, and that aberrant detrusor activity is not occurring during stress-induced leakage. This does not mean, however, that all stress incontinence is the same (in fact, it is not), nor does it give us any indication of what factors may be involved in producing this condition. Making the urodynamic diagnosis of "genuine stress incontinence" does not tell you how the condition should be treated.

Factors Contributing to Stress Incontinence

Why do women develop stress incontinence? The relatively short female urethra and the exposed and poorly supported female bladder neck make women particularly susceptible to this problem, at least compared with their male counterparts in whom stress incontinence is extremely rare unless the lower urinary tract has been damaged by surgery. Indeed, *occasional* stress incontinence in women is not abnormal. Several studies have shown that young, nulliparous women suffer from this complaint on a regular basis. This is not significant until it becomes socially or hygienically troublesome and crosses the line from occasional "subclinical" urine loss to "clinical" incontinence. Where this line is drawn in terms of lifestyle and discomfort varies for each woman.

What factors push some women across this clinical boundary? A list of risk factors is given in Table 5.1. The major culprits appear to be pregnancy, childbirth, and menopause. Although many people assume that childbirth is the major cause of stress incontinence, most studies which have looked at these risk factors have concluded that most stress incontinence begins before or during pregnancy, rather than in the puerperium. Francis, in classic studies published in 1960, found that 40% of primigravidae had occasional stress incontinence before pregnancy and that stress incontinence rarely presented for the first time following childbirth. In women who had postpartum stress incontinence, the condition was almost always present, if only in slight degree, either before the pregnancy began or it first appeared at some point during pregnancy. In women with stress incontinence prior to pregnancy, it nearly always worsened during pregnancy. Stress incontinence developing in pregnancy also tended to resolve during the puerperium, but to recur with subsequent pregnancies, ultimately remaining after delivery in some women to become a persistent, troublesome complaint. Studies by Iosif and Viktrup have confirmed these findings.

The risk factors listed in Table 5.1 all appear to be related to one or more of the three factors which, to the best of our current knowledge, interact to produce stress incontinence in women. The two major factors responsible for the two major types of stress incontinence are: (*a*) loss of support of the urethra and bladder neck which produces hypermobility of these structures and leads to stress incontinence due to bladder neck displacement during physically stressful conditions (Fig. 5.1), and (*b*) intrinsic sphincteric weakness, which may lead to stress incontinence due to sphincteric failure even though the outlet is well

---

TABLE 5.1.   Risk Factors For Stress Incontinence

1. Increasing parity, probably related to obstetrical trauma
2. Increased intra-abdominal pressure
   a. Medical factors [e.g., smoking, chronic bronchitis or other pulmonary problems, constipation with chronic straining at stool, obesity (?)]
   b. Environmental factors [e.g., jobs requiring heavy lifting or straining]
3. Pelvic floor trauma and denervation injury
   a. Obstetric trauma
   b. Nonobstetric trauma [e.g., pelvic fractures and radical surgery]
4. Hormonal status and estrogen deficiency
5. Connective tissue disorders

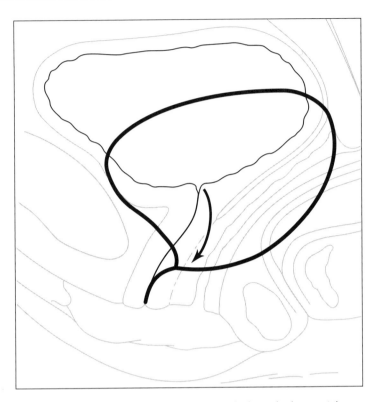

Figure 5.1 Stress incontinence due to failure of extrinsic urethral support. In normal continent women the urethra is supported by the endopelvic fascia and its attachments to the pelvic sidewalls and levator ani muscles. This provides support during periods of increased intra-abdominal pressure which allows urethral compression to occur, maintaining urinary continence. When support failure occurs, the bladder neck and urethra are displaced downwards (*heavy lines*), loss of compression occurs, and stress incontinence may result.

Failure of Extrinsic Support

supported (Fig. 5.2). These factors are not mutually exclusive and may coexist in the same patient. A third important factor in the development of stress incontinence appears to be neurologic damage to the pelvic floor, bladder neck, and urethra. Neurologic injury may be directly related to the other two factors and provides an attractive theoretical connecting link between them.

Normal support of the proximal urethra and bladder neck is maintained by the endopelvic fascia. This fascia lies underneath the urethra and is attached laterally to the arcus tendineus fascia pelvis (white line), the levator ani muscles, and the anterior vaginal wall (Fig. 5.3). The support that the pelvic floor provides for the bladder neck and urethra is dynamic, not static: The position of the vesical neck is under voluntary control. During radiographic studies such as voiding cystourethrography, it can be observed to elevate and descend. The same thing can be observed during a pelvic examination. The vesical neck is *not* normally fixed in a static position. In stress incontinent patients, the sudden burst of added pressure generated by coughing or sneezing overwhelms the resting urethral pressure and causes leakage. This usually occurs not because this pressure is distributed or "transmitted" unequally across the pelvic floor, but because loss of posterior support to the urethra and bladder neck prevents normal compression from occurring. In other words, the endopelvic fascial "platform" against which the bladder neck and urethra should be compressed closed by the force of abdominal pressure and the contraction of the levator ani muscles, has become unsteady and insecure (Fig. 5.4). The platform moves away from

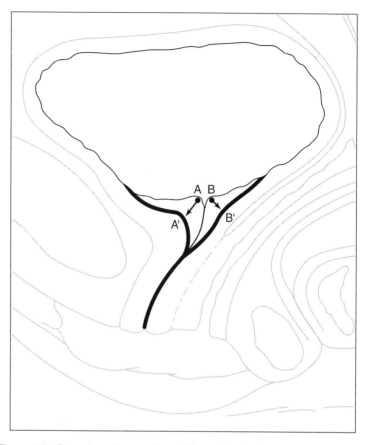

Figure 5.2   Stress incontinence due to failure of the intrinsic sphincteric mechanism. The bladder neck is normally closed at rest, providing the main barrier to urine leakage. If this intrinsic sphincteric unit is deficient for any reason, the bladder neck is open at rest (*heavy lines*) and stress incontinence may occur even if urethral support is good.

the force it is supposed to meet, rather than holding firmly against it. Compression (and hence continence) cannot occur when these two planes are moving away from each other, rather than moving against one another.

Clinically, patients with this type of stress incontinence are found to have increased mobility of the bladder neck and urethra. When such a patient is examined with a full bladder while coughing, the urethra and bladder neck are seen to rotate downward and outward—often dramatically—at the same time that urinary leakage occurs. Some investigators like to attempt to quantitate this mobility by inserting a lubricated sterile Q-tip into the urethra to the level of the bladder neck, watching it rotate upwards as the bladder neck descends. All this does is accentuate a physical finding which is observable with the naked eye. The necessity of performing a "Q-tip test" has been stressed too dogmatically by many authors. The important point is to document increased mobility of the urethra and bladder neck in this subset of stress incontinent patients.

An alternate way of evaluating bladder neck mobility is by erect fluoroscopic examination of the patient. Formerly this was done with lateral bead-chain cystourethrograms and formed the basis for Green's classification of patients into so-called "Type I" and "Type II" stress incontinence. "Type I" patients were those who had lost their "posterior urethro-vesical angle" but who maintained a normal "inclination to the vertical of the urethral axis," that is, they maintained

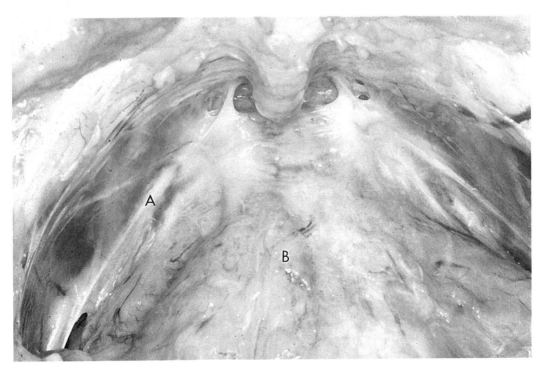

Figure 5.3 Normal relationships of the bladder (*B*) and endopelvic fascia, which is attached to the pelvic sidewall along the arcus tendineus fascia pelvis (*A*). When its normal attachments are maintained in this fashion, the endopelvic fascia provides resilient support for the urethra and bladder neck, allowing them to be compressed closed during increased intra-abdominal pressure.

some anterior bladder neck support. "Type II" patients had loss of the "posterior urethro-vesical angle" but also had "downward, backward, rotational descent of the urethra and bladder neck" with a "definitely abnormal angle of inclination to the vertical of the urethral axis," and had greater loss of support than "Type I" patients. However, numerous studies have shown that bead-chain cystourethrograms are not useful in diagnosing stress incontinence or categorizing patients into subtypes. Almost no one believes any longer that there is a significant difference between Green's Type I and Type II patients.

Since urethral hypermobility is often present in normal continent multiparous women, finding this is *not* the same thing as diagnosing stress incontinence. There are many women with severe stress incontinence who have no bladder neck mobility at all, and there are also many women with incontinence due to detrusor instability or other causes for whom the mobility of their bladder neck is irrelevant to their problem.

If a patient with genuine stress incontinence also has coexisting hypermobility of the bladder neck, correction of this problem will cure the stress incontinence in the overwhelming majority of cases. This does *not* mean, however, that all of these patients should have surgery or even that the best treatment for their condition is necessarily surgical in nature.

Many previous authors have felt that the contribution of anatomic hypermobility to the patient's incontinence could be evaluated by repositioning the urethra and bladder neck into a more normal position and seeing if the patient continued to leak under these circumstances. This is known as the "Marshall" or "Bonney" test. In this test the examiner demonstrates stress incontinence and then uses either two examining fingers or a rubber-shod clamp to push the bladder neck back into position and hold it there. The patient is then asked to

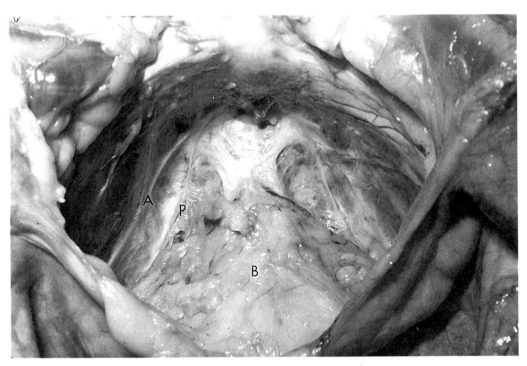

Figure 5.4   Development of a paravaginal defect in a stress incontinent patient. The pubocervical fascia (*P*) has been pulled away from its normal attachments to the pelvic sidewall along the arcus tendineus fascia pelvis (*A*), allowing the bladder (*B*) to sag below its normal position. Development of this paravaginal defect has disrupted the normal mechanisms of support and permits excessive bladder neck excursion during periods of increased intra-abdominal pressure, resulting in stress incontinence due to a failure of posterior support and urethral compression.

cough. If no leakage is demonstrated, the test is said to be "positive," and the assumption is that surgical repositioning of the bladder neck will cure the patient's stress incontinence. This test does give useful information, but it is absolutely critical that the urethra is not obstructed when it is performed! *Any* incontinence can be stopped if the urethra is forcefully occluded during the performance of such a test, and several authors have demonstrated this fact by making measurements of urethral pressure while this test is performed. If an *occlusive* test is performed it will be indiscriminately "positive" in most patients and will lose whatever diagnostic information it provides. The goal of the test should be to see if urine loss stops when the bladder neck is returned to a normal—not an occluded—position.

If this test is done at all, ring forceps or uterine dressing forceps should be used to support the vagina laterally, with one ring in each anterior lateral vaginal fornix. The anterior vagina should then be repositioned to its normal position along the level of the arcus tendineus fascia pelvis (Fig. 3.16*A-C*). If stress incontinence is no longer demonstrated when the bladder neck is supported laterally in its normal position during a careful exam, this is another piece of confirmatory evidence suggesting that the problem is loss of support. If stress incontinence is still demonstrable when this test is done correctly, this should be a clue that the vesical neck is not functioning normally and should mandate further investigation.

A related problem is stress incontinence in patients with a large prolapse. A large cystocele or vaginal vault prolapse can mask the presence of stress incontinence by swinging out below the urethra and kinking it closed during coughing or straining. This type of occlusion may result in "false negative" urodynamic tests unless some attempt is made to reduce the prolapse and check the patient for stress incontinence under these conditions. A pessary may be used to reduce the prolapse during urodynamic studies, if care is taken not to obstruct the urethra. The patient may also simply be examined with a full bladder and have her prolapse reduced by a Sims speculum or the posterior blade of an ordinary Graves speculum. A positive test of this type may alter the surgeon's choice of operative procedure in order to avoid the creation of "iatrogenic stress incontinence." If a large prolapse has been reduced by standard surgery, the patient with underlying weakness of the urethral closure mechanism may develop significant incontinence when the supporting prolapse is removed and the "latent" incontinence becomes overt. This new problem may be worse than the original complaint, unless the bladder neck is adequately supported, perhaps by a more extensive surgical operation than would otherwise have been envisioned. Examination of the patient with prolapse is covered in more detail in Chapter 14.

Intrinsic Sphincteric Weakness

The second important factor in maintaining urinary continence during conditions of physical stress is the strength and structural integrity of the urethral sphincteric mechanism itself, irrespective of its degree of support (Fig. 5.2). The tube of the urethra is normally held closed by several different structures, each contributing to keep the lumen shut. There are several components to this closure mechanism at the level of the bladder neck, as well as the more familiar striated external urethral sphincter. The proximal centimeter of the female urethra is normally held closed by a "loop" of detrusor smooth muscle under α-adrenergic control, and the trigonal ring. More distal to this, the striated external urethral sphincter acts as a "second line" of defense to prevent the escape of any urine which happens to enter the urethra. In addition to these smooth and striated muscular components, contributions to intrinsic urethral pressure are made by a number of other factors including the submucosal vascular plexus, the elastic properties of the urethral wall, mucosal coaptability, the amount of estrogenization present, and tonic input from the sympathetic nervous system, mediated by α-adrenergic receptors (Table 5.2). A genetic predisposition to developing stress incontinence may be hidden among these factors, influenced by such things as different types of connective tissue, the number of estrogen receptor present in the lower urinary tract, and so on. As yet we have little ability to evaluate these factors or to quantify their importance.

This intrinsic continence mechanism may fail either due to neuropathy—such as the open bladder neck seen in some patients with spinal cord injury—or trauma. This trauma may be the result of accident (such as automobile wrecks which produce direct physical trauma to the urethra or fracture the pelvic ring), difficult delivery, or surgery. In the latter case, the sphincteric unit may fail because part or all of it has been excised, as is sometimes the case in patients who have had a radical vulvectomy for vulvar carcinoma.

Patients who have undergone multiple surgical procedures for incontinence may eventually be left with a functionless, rigid tube in place of the supple, continent structure which existed before. A urethra of this kind may be in the

TABLE 5.2. Factors Contributing To Urethral Closure

A. Extrinsic Factors
  1. Endopelvic fascia and the integrity of its lateral attachments
  2. Levator ani muscles
    a. Strength of the levator muscle complex
    b. Connections of the levator complex to the endopelvic fascia
    c. Coordination of levator muscles contraction with coughing
B. Intrinsic Urethral Factors
  1. Autonomic (sympathetic) innervation and tone (α-adrenergic receptors)
  2. Striated muscle of the urethral wall
  3. Mucosal coaptation of the urothelium
  4. Vascular congestion of the submucosal venous plexus
  5. Smooth muscle of the urethral wall and blood vessels
  6. Elasticity of the urethral wall

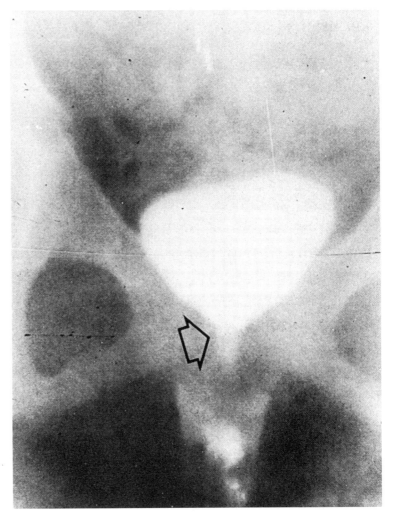

Figure 5.5   Fluoroscopic view of the bladder at rest in a patient with meningomye-locele. Note that the bladder neck is wide open (*arrow*). (From McGuire, Int Urogy-necol J 1992; 3:54–60.)

perfect anatomic location and yet remain useless. *Clearly, any operation de-signed to elevate or reposition the bladder neck in patients like this will be doomed to failure since it is intrinsic weakness—not location—that is responsible for their incontinence.* Fluoroscopic examination of the urinary tract in these patients will reveal a bladder neck which is wide open at rest, offering virtually no resistance to leakage when the pressure in the bladder is increased (Fig. 5.5). Many such patients will have "gravitational incontinence," with the fluid draining out of their bladders as the fluoroscopy table is raised from the horizon-tal to the vertical position. Urethroscopic examination will often reveal similar findings—a rigid, functionless tube which is nearly open from the bladder to the outside world. This condition is sometimes called the "drainpipe" or "lead pipe" urethra, or more commonly, "Type III" incontinence, to distinguish it from the "Type I" and "Type II" incontinence of Green's old classification. Recently, the term "intrinsic sphincter dysfunction" has been adopted for this problem.

Are urethral pressure studies helpful in making the diagnosis of Type III incontinence? A great deal of controversy exists in this area. If urethral pressure studies are done routinely in patients with lower urinary tract complaints, it is clear that women with stress incontinence tend to have lower urethral pressures as a group than women without genuine stress incontinence. It is also clear that urethral pressures tend to be lower in women with more severe incontinence and that urethral pressures tend to drop further in women who have had several previous unsuccessful operations. However, there is a great deal of overlap between these groups and this makes the interpretation of such results difficult in any individual case. For example, an older women who is continent may have a lower urethral pressure than a younger woman with severe stress incontinence. Furthermore, there clearly is no single urethral pressure measurement which can be used, by itself, to make the diagnosis of "genuine stress incontinence."

Some authors have suggested that patients with genuine stress incontinence who have urethral closure pressures of less than 20 cm H_2O are at higher risk of failure for "standard" retropubic incontinence operations than women who have higher urethral pressures. These authors have advocated treating such patients with a more radical operation, such as a sling procedure, irrespective of the presence or absence of urethral hypermobility. Other authors have had reasonable success in treating such patients with standard incontinence operations if bladder neck hypermobility was also present. It is likely that there are differences of surgical technique among some of these papers which may account for some of their differing results. It is therefore somewhat difficult at present to give clear guidelines about the usefulness of urethral pressure measurements in selecting patients for different types of operations. If a patient is found to have an extremely low urethral closure pressure, careful consideration should be given as to how this patient should best be treated, based upon the experience and clinical judgment of the physician involved.

Neurologic Damage to the Pelvic Floor

The third factor which appears to contribute to the development of stress incontinence is neurologic damage to the pelvic floor. In patients with severe central nervous system disease such as spinal cord injury or spina bifida who present with a wide open bladder neck and no history of previous localized trauma, the defect can be properly attributed to loss of autonomic adrenergic tone at the level of the bladder neck. These cases aside, increasing evidence suggests that denervation injury to the striated muscles of the pelvic floor is an important contributing factor in the genesis of stress incontinence. Studies using single-fiber electromyography, a sophisticated and sensitive technique for evaluating denervation injury and subsequent reinnervation, have consistently shown an increased fiber density in the pelvic floor musculature of women with genuine stress incontinence as compared to abnormal controls. The normal fiber density of a motor unit is low, but increases following denervation injury due to collateral sprouting of injured nerves as they attempt to reinnervate denervated muscle. The higher single fiber densities shown in stress incontinent women are direct evidence of associated neuromuscular injury.

Another piece of evidence suggesting a role for neuromuscular damage in the genesis of stress incontinence comes from studies of the motor terminal latency of the pudendal nerve which innervates both the external anal sphincter and the striated urethral sphincter. If a transrectal electrode is used to stimulate the pudendal nerve at the ischial spine and a second electrode is used to pick up the transmitted impulse at the anal sphincter, the latency time from stimulus to muscular response between these two points can be measured and compared from patient to patient. Several studies have now shown a prolonged latency time in stress incontinent women as compared to normal controls. One study has correlated prolonged latency time with decreased maximum urethral pressure in stress incontinent patients. Most of this injury appears to have been sustained during childbirth and probably is made worse in patients with chronic constipation who must habitually strain at stool. This type of denervation injury is also found in women with idiopathic anorectal incontinence.

What is the clinical significance of these findings? The most intriguing hypothesis is the one that links denervation injury both to outlet hypermobility and to sphincteric weakness. In the patient with an intact sphincteric unit, maintenance of continence during stress depends upon adequate support of the bladder neck and urethra, allowing compression of these structures during periods of increased intra-abdominal pressure. This allows a positive pressure gradient to be maintained so that outlet pressure remains higher than bladder pressure and urine is kept inside the bladder. If, as seems reasonable, the pelvic floor acts as a "trampoline" to provide constant resilient support and to "bounce" pressure across this area and thus to maintain the proper pressure gradient, then neuromuscular injury could contribute to failure of this mechanism by weakening muscular tone and decreasing the resiliency of the pelvic floor. If the injured muscles are unable to respond quickly enough, or are unable to maintain the constant tone necessary to provide a stable base for support, urinary incontinence could result. This could be likened to loosening the springs on a trampoline which attach it to the sides of its frame, making it "floppy" and creating "dead spots" which function poorly. Obstetrical injury which damages the connective tissue and fascial supports of the bladder neck and urethra could contribute to this process. Similarly, if stretch injury sustained during delivery or at other times damages the pudendal nerve, this damage could contribute to weakness of the intrinsic sphincteric unit itself, and further predispose a patient to developing urinary incontinence. The summation of these factors could ultimately diminish the patient's "margin for continence" and push her below the threshold for urinary leakage.

Stress Incontinence: A Philosophy of Management

What is our goal in treating stress incontinence or any other continence problem for that matter? Is it complete and total dryness at all times? If so, we are aiming for a condition that does not exist in the "normal" female population, since many studies have shown that nearly all women may develop isolated stress incontinence under the right conditions. Usually this is not clinically troubling to them, only an unusual and occasionally embarrassing accident. If this is not our goal, it must be something else. Because incontinence is a quality-of-life issue, our treatment programs should be aimed at helping the patient achieve as much control of her bladder as she wishes to obtain, to attain a level of dryness with which she is comfortable. Our goal should be to normalize lower urinary tract function as much as possible, consistent with the patient's own desires and willingness to put up with the costs—both financial and medical—of treatment.

Pelvic surgeons—both gynecologists and urologists—tend to think of stress incontinence and surgery almost as synonyms; however, surgery for genuine stress incontinence is always an elective procedure. It is a mistake to pressure a reluctant patient into having an operation about which she is uncertain. The complications of surgery can often be worse than the original condition, particularly for those patients who develop uncontrollable detrusor instability postoperatively or who are in chronic urinary retention and who must self-catheterize four to six times each day.

An operation should be carried out only: (*a*) when the patient thoroughly understands all of the treatment options open to her; (*b*) when she understands the possible complications of surgery; and (*c*) when she feels in her own mind that the problem is severe enough to warrant an operation. There is nothing wrong with several months of active conservative management for patients with stress incontinence. This will be sufficient either to control the problem to the patient's satisfaction or to convince her that surgery is her best hope of becoming dry.

Some women may not be bothered enough by the degree of their leakage to wish to undergo the expense and convalescence of surgery. Others may not have finished childbearing and, as a consequence, are reluctant to undergo an operation which might be damaged or undone by a subsequent pregnancy, labor, and delivery. Still other women may be in frail health and are fearful of the possible medical problems that surgery may exacerbate. All such women deserve consideration of a trial of conservative therapy and no patient should be persuaded to

TABLE 5.3. Common Myths About Stress Urinary Incontinence

Myth	Reality
Incontinent women have either stress incontinence or detrusor instability as the cause of their leakage	Urinary incontinence can be multifactorial and presents in many ways
A stable cystometrogram rules out detrusor instability as a cause for urinary incontinence	Cystometry represents only a limited look at bladder function and may not reproduce the conditions of daily life; unstable detrusor contractions may occur at other times, in other places, and in response to other provocations; stress incontinence and detrusor instability frequently coexist; the urodynamic findings must reproduce the patient's complaint in order to be helpful.
A stable cystometrogram establishes the diagnosis of genuine stress incontinence by exclusion, whether or not the patient leaks during the test	The diagnosis of incontinence is not confirmed until the patient is seen to leak under conditions that reproduce her complaint; a urodynamic test which does not do this is nondiagnostic
Since stress incontinence is always caused by loss of support, a positive "Q-tip" test establishes the diagnosis of stress incontinence	Patients may have stress incontinence without hypermobility of the bladder neck and urethra; conversely, there are many women with hypermobility of these structures who are perfectly dry
Visible demonstration of stress incontinence always means that the patient has this problem	Stress incontinence is not a problem until it bothers the patient or her caregivers; just because stress incontinence has been demonstrated does not mean that this is the origin of the patient's problem
Stress incontinence should always be treated with surgery.	Not only may stress incontinence not be the patient's problem, but there are many nonsurgical forms of treatment for this condition which are perfectly acceptable

have surgery simply because her operating surgeon is unfamiliar or uncomfortable with alternative management techniques. Physicians and surgeons who undertake the care of incontinent patients have a responsibility to become familiar with all available modalities of therapy and to refer patients appropriately if they are unable or unwilling to provide reasonable alternatives.

We do not, however, mean to imply that all patients with stress incontinence should be forced to undergo a prolonged period of conservative therapy prior to having surgery. A woman with severe stress incontinence who has been thoroughly evaluated and understands the risks and benefits of surgery should not be forced to put up with prolonged conservative therapy if she wishes to have the chance of cure that surgery provides. Therapy must be individualized and the appropriate plan of action developed for each patient.

In spite of all the papers which have been written about stress incontinence, many myths about this condition are still prevalent. Table 5.3 summarizes some of these misconceptions and points out why they are wrong. The development of good clinical judgment in the treatment of women with stress incontinence depends upon skill, practice, and a good fund of knowledge about this condition and its management. The next two chapters summarize the forms of treatment, both surgical and nonsurgical, which are currently available for stress incontinent women. Knowing when to operate and how to use nonsurgical management techniques are critical components of good clinical care for women with this problem.

SUGGESTED READING

General Considerations

Abrams P, Blaivas JG, Stanton SL, Andersen JT. The standardisation of terminology of lower urinary tract function. Scand J Urol Nephrol Suppl 1988; 114:5–18.

Beck RP, Hsu N. Pregnancy, childbirth, and the menopause related to the development of stress incontinence. Am J Obstet Gynecol 1965; 91:820–23.

Bent AE, Richardson DA, Ostergard DR. Diagnosis of lower urinary tract disorders in postmenopausal women. Am J Obstet Gynecol 1983; 145:218–22.

Crist T, Shingleton HM, Koch GG. Stress incontinence and the nulliparous patient. Obstet Gynecol 1972; 40:13–17

Dwyer PL, Lee ETC, Hay DM. Obesity and urinary incontinence in women. Br J Obstet Gynaecol 1988; 95:91–96.

Francis WJA. Disturbances of bladder function in relation to pregnancy. J Obstet Gynaecol Br Emp 1960; 67:353–66.

Feneley RCL, Shepherd AM, Powell PH, et al. Urinary incontinence: Prevalence and needs. Br J Urol 1979; 51: 493–96.

Francis WJA. The onset of stress incontinence. J Obstet Gynecol Br Emp 1960; 67:899–903.

Iosif S. Stress incontinence during pregnancy and in puerperium. Int J Gynaecol Obstet 1981; 19:13–20.

Iosif S, Ulmsten U. Comparative urodynamic studies of continent and stress incontinent women in pregnancy and in the puerperium. Am J Obstet Gynecol 1981; 140:645–50.

Nemir A, Middleton RP. Stress incontinence in young nulliparous women. Am J Obstet Gynecol 1954; 68:1166–68.

Nygaard I, DeLancey JOL, Arnsdorf L, et al. Exercise and incontinence. Obstet Gynecol 1990; 75:848–51.

Stanton SL, Kerr-Wilson R, Harris VG. The incidence of urological symptoms in normal pregnancy. Br J Obstet Gynaecol 1980; 87:897–900.

Thomas TM, Plymat KR, Blannin J, et al. Prevalence of urinary incontinence. Br Med J 1980; 281:1243–45.

Tapp A, Cardozo LD, Versi E, Montgomery J, Studd J. The effect of vaginal delivery on the urethral sphincter. Br J Obstet Gynaecol 1988; 95:142–46.

Van Geelen JM, Lemmesn WAJG, Eskes TKAB, Martine CB Jr. The urethral pressure profile in pregnancy and after delivery in healthy nulliparous women. Am J Obstet Gynecol 1982; 144:636–49.

Viktrup L, Lose G, Rolff M, Barfoed K. The symptom of stress incontinence caused by pregnancy or delivery in primiparas. Obstet Gynecol 1992; 79:945–49.

Wolin LH. Stress incontinence in young healthy nulliparous female subjects. J Urol 1969; 101:545–49.

Yarnell JWG, Voyle GJ, Richards CJ, et al. The prevalence and severity of urinary incontinence in women. J Epidemiol Comm Health 1981; 35:71–74.

The Urodynamics of Stress Incontinence

Aagaard J, Bruskewitz R. Are urodynamic studies useful in the evaluation of female incontinence? A critical review of the literature. Prob Urol 1991; 5:11–22.

Arnold EP, Webster JR, Loose H, et al. Urodynamics of female incontinence: Factors influencing the results of surgery. Am J Obstet Gynecol 1973; 117:805–13.

Byrne DJ, Hamilton SPA, Gray BK. The role of urodynamics in female urinary stress incontinence. Br J Urol 1987; 59: 228–29.

Cantor TJ, Bates CP. A comparative study of symptoms and objective urodynamic findings in 214 incontinent women. Br J Obstet Gynaecol 1980; 87:889–92.

Cardozo LD, Stanton SL. Genuine stress incontinence and detrusor instability: A review of 200 cases. Br J Obstet Gynaecol 1980; 87:184–90.

Castleden CM, Duffin HM, Asher MJ. Clinical and urodynamic studies in 100 elderly incontinent patients. Br Med J 1981; 282:1103–05.

Fall M, Erlandson BE, Pettersson S. Evaluation of history and simple supine cystometry as a preoperative test in stress urinary incontinence. Acta Obstet Gynecol Scand 1984; 63:241–44.

Farrar DJ, Whiteside CG, Osborne JL, et al. A urodynamic analysis of micturition symptoms in the female. Surg Gynecol Obstet 1975; 141:875–81.

Glezerman M, Glasner M, Rikover M, et al. Evaluation of reliability of history in women complaining of urinary stress incontinence. Eur J Obstet Gynecol Reprod Biol 1986; 21:159–64.

Hastie KJ, Moisey CU. Are urodynamics necessary in female patients presenting with stress incontinence? Br J Urol 1989; 63:155–56.

Haylen BT, Sutherst JR, Frazer MI. Is the investigation of most stress incontinence really necessary? Br J Urol 1989; 64:147–49.

Jarvis GJ, Hall S, Stamp S, et al. An assessment of urodynamic examination in incontinent women. Br J Obstet Gynaecol 1980; 87:893–96.

Korda A, Krieger M, Hunter P, et al. The value of clinical symptoms in the diagnosis of urinary incontinence in the female. Aust NZ J Obstet Gynaecol 1987; 27:149–51.

Lagro-Janssen ALM, Debruyne FMJ, Van Weel C. Value of the patient's case history in diagnosing urinary incontinence in general practice. Br J Urol 1991; 67:569–72.

McGuire EJ, Lytton B, Pepe V, et al. Stress urinary incontinence. Obstet Gynecol 1976; 47:255–64.

Maes D, Wyndaele JJ. Correlation between history and urodynamics in neurologically normal incontinent women. Eur Urol 1988; 14:377–80.

Moolgaoker AS, Ardran GM, Smith JC, et al. The diagnosis and management of urinary incontinence in the female. J Obstet Gynaecol Br Commw 1972; 79:481–97.

Ouslander J, Staskin D, Raz S, et al. Clinical versus urodynamic diagnosis in an incontinent geriatric female population. J Urol 1987; 137:68–71.

Susset JG, Dutaartre D, Leriche A, et al. Urodynamic assessment of stress incontinence and its therapeutic implications. Surg Gynecol Obstet 1976; 142:343–52.

Vereecken RL. Female incontinence: How much work-up is necessary? Eur J Obstet Gynecol Reprod Biol 1984; 18:351–60.

Walter S. Symptoms and signs in 300 consecutive female patients referred for urinary incontinence. Scan J Urol Nephrol Suppl 1981; 60:47–49.

Walter S, Olesen KP. Urinary incontinence and genital prolapse in the female: Clinical, urodynamic and radiological examinations. Br J Obstet Gynaecol 1982; 89:393–401.

Vereecken RL, Wouters M. Discrepancies between clinical

and urodynamical findings: Which are true? Urol Int 1988; 43:282–85.

Versi E, Cardozo L, Anand D, Cooper D. Symptoms analysis for the diagnosis of genuine stress incontinence. Br J Obstet Gynaecol 1991; 98:815–19.

Warrell DW. Investigation and treatment of incontinence of urine in women who have had a prolapse repair operation. Br J Urol 1965; 37:233–39.

Webster GD, Sihelnik SA, Stone AR. Female urinary incontinence: The incidence, identification, and characteristics of detrusor instability. Neurourol Urodynam 1984; 3: 235–42.

Bladder Neck Hypermobility

Bergman A. Koonings PP, Ballard CA. Negative Q-tip test as a risk factor for failed incontinence surgery in women. J Reprod Med 1989; 34:193–97.

Bergman A, MaCarthy TA, Ballard CA, et al. Role of the Q-tip test in evaluating stress urinary incontinence. J Reprod Med 1987; 32:273–75.

Bhatia NN, Bergman A. Urodynamic appraisal of the Bonney test in women with stress incontinence. Obstet Gynecol 1983; 62:696–99.

Bhatia NN, Bergman A. The pessary test in women with urinary incontinence. Obstet Gynecol 1985; 65:220-26.

Bump RC. The mechanism of urinary continence in women with severe uterovaginal prolapse: Results of barrier studies. Obstet Gynecol 1988; 72:291–95.

Crystle CD, Charme LS, Copeland WE. Q-tip test in stress urinary incontinence. Obstet Gynecol 1971; 39:313–15.

Drutz HP, Shapiro BJ, Mandel F. Do static cystourethrograms have a role in the investigation of female incontinence? Am J Obstet Gynecol 1978; 130:516–20.

Fantl JA, Beachley MC, Bosch HA, et al. Bead-chain cystourethrogram: An evaluation. Obstet Gynecol 1981; 58: 237–40.

Fantl JA, Hurt WG, Bump RC, et al. Urethral axis and sphincteric function. Am J Obstet Gynecol 1986; 155: 554–58.

Gardy M, Kozminski M, DeLancey J, et al. Stress incontinence and cystoceles. J Urol 1991; 145:1211–13.

Green TH, Jr. Development of a plan for the diagnosis and treatment of urinary stress incontinence. Am J Obstet Gynecol 1962; 83:632–48.

Greenwald SW, Thornbury JR, Dunn LJ. Cystourethrography as a diagnostic aid in stress incontinence. Obstet Gynecol 1967; 29:324–27.

Karram MM, Bhatia NN. The Q-tip test: Standardization of the technique and its interpretation in women with urinary incontinence. Obstet Gynecol 1988; 71:807–11.

Kitzmiller JL, Manser GA, Nebel WA, et al. Chain cystourethrogram and stress incontinence. Obstet Gynecol 1972; 39:333–40.

Migliorini GD, Glenning PP. Bonney's test—fact or fiction? Br J Obstet Gynaecol 1987; 94:157–59.

Montz FJ, Stanton SL. Q-tip test in female urinary incontinence. Obstet Gynecol 1986; 67:258–60.

Symmonds RE, Jordan LT. Iatrogenic stress incontinence of urine. Am J Obstet Gynecol 1961; 82:1231–37.

Steinhausen TB, Kariher DH, Sherwood CE, et al. Chain cystourethrogram before and after urethrovesical suspension for stress incontinence. Obstet Gynecol 1970; 35: 405–15.

Wall LL, Hewitt JK. Urodynamic characteristics of women with complete post-hysterectomy vaginal vault prolapse. Urology; In Press.

Walters MD, Diaz K. Q-tip test: A study of continent and incontinent women. Obstet Gynecol 1987; 70:208–11.

Walters MD, Shields LE. The diagnostic value of history, physical examination and the Q-tip cotton swab test in women with urinary incontinence. Am J Obstet Gynecol 1988; 159:145–49.

Intrinsic Urethral Sphincter Dysfunction

Allen TD. The surgical management of total urinary incontinence in the female patient. J Urol 1987; 138:521–24.

Blaivas JG. Treatment of female incontinence secondary to urethral damage or loss. Urol Clin NA 1991; 18:355–63.

Gierup HJW, Hakelius L. Free autogenous muscle transplantation in the treatment of urinary incontinence in children: Background, surgical technique and preliminary results. J Urol 1978; 120:223–26.

Henriksson L, Ulmsten U, Andersson KE. The effect of changes of posture on the urethral closure pressure in healthy women. Scand J Urol Nephrol 1977; 11:201–06.

Hilton P, Stanton SL. Urethral pressure measurement by microtransducer: The results in symptom-free women and in those with genuine stress incontinence. Br J Obstet Gynaecol 1983; 90:919–33.

Kadar N, Nelson JH Jr. Sling operation for total incontinence following radical vulvectomy. Obstet Gynecol 1984; 64: 85S–87S.

McGuire EJ, Lytton B, Pepe V, et al. Stress urinary incontinence. Obstet Gynecol 1976; 47:255–64.

McGuire EJ. Combined radiographic and manometric assessment of urethral sphincter function. J Urol 1977; 118: 632–35.

McGuire EJ. Urodynamic findings in patients after failure of stress incontinence operations. In Zinner NR, Sterling AM (Eds). Female Incontinence. New York: Alan R. Liss 1981:351–60 (Prog Clin Biol Res 78).

McGuire EJ. Mechanisms of urethral continence and their clinical application. World J Urol 1984; 2:272–79.

McGuire EJ. Active and passive factors in urethral continence function. Int Urogynecol J 1992; 3:54–60.

McGuire EJ, Wang CC, Usitalo H, et al. Modified pubovaginal sling in girls with myelodysplasia. J Urol 1986; 135: 94–96.

Morgan JE, Farrow GA, Sims RH. The sloughed urethra syndrome. Am J Obstet Gynecol 1978; 130:521–24.

Reid GC, DeLancey JOL, Hopkins MP, et al. Urinary incontinence following radical vulvectomy. Obstet Gynecol 1990; 75:852–58.

Rud T, Andersson KE, Asmussen M, et al. Factors maintaining the intraurethral pressure in women. Invest Urol 1980; 17:343–47.

Versi E, Cardozo L, Studd J, et al. Evaluation of urethral pressure profilometry for the diagnosis of genuine stress incontinence. World J Urol 1986; 4:6-9.

Versi E. Discriminant analysis of urethral pressure profilometry data for the diagnosis of genuine stress incontinence. Br J Obstet Gynaecol 1990; 97:251–59.

Woodside JR. Pubovaginal sling procedure for the management of urinary incontinence after urethral trauma in women. J Urol 1987; 138:527–28.

"The Low Pressure Urethra"

Bergman A, Koonings PP, Ballard CA. Proposed management of low urethral pressure type of genuine stress incontinence. Gynecol Obstet Invest 1989; 27:155–59.

Bowen LW, Sand PK, Ostergard DR, et al. Unsuccessful Burch retropubic urethropexy: A case-controlled urodynamic study. Am J Obstet Gynecol 1989; 160:452–58.

Koonings PP, Bergman A, Ballard CA. Low urethral pressure and stress urinary incontinence in women: Risk factor for failed retropubic surgical procedure. Urology 1990; 36:245–48.

Ramon J, Mekras JA, Webster GD. The outcome of transvaginal cystourethropexy in patients with anatomical stress urinary incontinence and outlet weakness. J Urol 1990; 144:106–09.

Ramon J, Mekras J, Webster GD. Transvaginal needle suspension procedures for recurrent stress incontinence. Urology 1991; 38:519–22.

Richardson DA, Ramahi A, Chalas E. Surgical management of stress incontinence in patients with low urethral pressure. Gynecol Obstet Invest 1991; 31:106–09.

Sand PK, Bowen LW, Panganiban R, Ostergard DR. The low pressure urethra as a factor in failed retropubic urethropexy. Obstet Gynecol 1987; 69:399–402.

Neuromuscular Damage in Genuine Stress Incontinence

Allen R, Hosker GL, Smith ARB, Warrell DW. Pelvic floor damage and childbirth: A neurophysiological study. Br J Obstet Gynaecol 1990; 97:770–79.

Anderson RS. A neurogenic element to urinary genuine stress incontinence. Br J Obstet Gynaecol 1984; 91: 412–15.

Gilpin SA, Gosling JA, Smith ARB, et al. The pathogenesis of genitourinary prolapse and stress incontinence of urine: A histological and histochemical study. Br J Obstet Gynaecol 1989; 96:15–23.

Smith ARB, Hosker GL, Warrell DW. The role of partial denervation of the pelvic floor in the aetiology of genitourinary prolapse and stress incontinence of urine: A neurophysiological study. Br J Obstet Gynaecol 1989; 96: 24–28.

Smith ARB, Hosker GL, Warrell DW. The role of pudendal nerve damage in the aetiology of genuine stress incontinence in women. Br J Obstet Gynaecol 1989; 96:29–32.

Snooks SJ, Swash M, Setchell M, et al. Injury to innervation of pelvic floor sphincter musculature in childbirth. Lancet 1984; 2:546–50.

Snooks SJ, Swash M. Abnormalities of the innervation of the urethral striated sphincter musculature in incontinence. Br J Urol 1984; 56:401–05.

Snooks SJ, Bedenoch DF, Tiptaft RC, et al. Perineal nerve damage in genuine stress urinary incontinence: An electrophysiological study. Br J Urol 1985; 57:422–26.

Snooks SJ, Swash M, Setchell M, et al. Injury to innervation of pelvic floor sphincter musculature in childbirth. Lancet 1984; 2:546–50.

Snooks SJ, Swash M. Abnormalities of the innervation of the urethral striated sphincter musculature in incontinence. Br J Urol 1984; 56:401–05.

Swash M, Snooks SJ, Henry MM. Unifying concept of pelvic floor disorders and incontinence. J Roy Soc Med 1985; 78:906–11.

Wall LL, DeLancey JOL. The politics of prolapse: A revisionist approach to disorders of the pelvic floor in women. Perspect Biol Med 1991; 34:486–96.

6 Conservative Management of Stress Incontinence

Both gynecologists and urologists are trained to think of stress incontinence as a surgical problem. This bias often leads practitioners to discourage nonsurgical management, either from a lack of familiarity with these techniques or because they lack the interest and motivation necessary to provide this type of patient care. Practitioners who reserve nonsurgical management only for patients who are poor candidates for surgery may unfairly reinforce their prejudice against conservative treatment methods and unfairly deny patients who are reluctant to have surgery the opportunity of successful nonsurgical treatment. For example, practitioners whose instruction to patients in pelvic floor muscle exercises consists only of a brief conversation should not be surprised when these women return after a few months requesting ''something more.''

Surgery for stress incontinence is *elective*. It is a ''quality of life'' decision, not an emergency, and this means that as in all treatment decisions regarding the incontinent patient, *the decision to operate is patient-driven*. It is a mistake to talk a patient into having an elective operation about which she is reluctant, and then to have a bad outcome either due to failure of the operation to correct the incontinence or the development of a complication such as voiding difficulty. The decision to operate should therefore be made when the diagnosis is clearly established, when there is a reasonable chance of success, when the patient understands the procedure and its potential complications, and when she has had the opportunity to consider other forms of therapy and either try them or reject them. Surgery should *not* be undertaken until the stress incontinence bothers the patient enough for her to wish to have it corrected. Many women with stress incontinence can be helped, often dramatically, by the effective application of conservative management principles. Surgeons who do not offer nonsurgical options to patients, either within their own practice or by referral to trained interested nurses or physical therapists, cannot really offer their patients an unbiased treatment plan for stress incontinence.

Review of the factors contributing to urethral closure listed in Table 5.2 suggests that both extrinsic and intrinsic factors contributing to continence can be improved by muscle re-education, exercise, hormone replacement, and drug therapy. In addition, the use of timed voiding regimens and fluid management techniques can reduce the urine load presented to the bladder, and improve the patient's clinical situation. Even if the patient's stress incontinence cannot be completely resolved using nonsurgical methods, these techniques still may have have a role to play in maximizing the benefit the patient achieves after an operation, particularly if the results are less than was hoped for.

Medical Management of Stress Incontinence

Most people would be happy if there were ''a pill'' they could take to make their stress incontinence go away. There are, in fact, a number of medications that can be used to minimize this problem, although they rarely will cure the condition completely. In many cases the degree of improvement that these medications can bring will be all that is necessary to control the patient's symptoms. Decreasing the frequency of stress leakage, so that it becomes an occasional annoyance rather than a major clinical problem, is a perfectly acceptable solution

TABLE 6.1. Drug Treatment of Genuine Stress Incontinence

Drug	Dose[a]
Pseudoephedrine	30–60 mg po TID/QID
Ephedrine	15–30 mg po BID/TID
Norephdrine	100 mg po BID
Norfenefrine	15–30 mg po BID/TID
Phenylpropanolamine	50–75 mg po BID
Imipramine	10–25 mg po BID/TID

[a] po = by mouth; BID = two times per day; TID = three times per day; QID = four times per day.

for many patients. The threshold at which this change occurs varies with each patient, so that an acceptable clinical response will occur with different amounts of urine loss in different women.

The tone of the urethra and bladder neck are controlled to a great degree by the sympathetic nervous system. This area around the bladder outlet contains large numbers of α-adrenergic receptors, and stimulation of these receptors by α-agonists will increase the tone, and hence the outlet resistance, of the bladder. Conversely, α-blockers can be used to lower outlet resistance and improve voiding dysfunction. In some cases use of these medications may even cause stress incontinence by dropping the resistance below the threshold for continence.

α-Stimulants

Table 6.1 lists the major medications with α-stimulating properties that have been used in the pharmacologic treatment of stress incontinence. These drugs appear to work by raising intraurethral pressure and improving closure of the bladder neck. They can be used in a number of ways. For example, women with exercise-induced incontinence may benefit by taking a dose of medication two hours before they exercise. If this is the only time that they experience stress incontinence, they do not need to take the medication on a continual basis. Similarly, most women will not require a dose before bedtime, since stress incontinence is seldom a problem during sleep.

Women with mild to moderate stress incontinence will probably obtain more relief from using these medications than women with severe stress incontinence, but the results are often surprising. Because these drugs are relatively quick-acting and have a relatively short half-life, the benefits that will be obtained from pharmacologic therapy alone will probably be manifest within a few days. However, since multiple factors are involved in urethral closure, most of these women will have concurrent problems which also need to be addressed. These include such things as urogenital atrophy from estrogen deprivation which can be improved by hormone replacement, and poor pelvic muscle tone which will respond to supervised pelvic muscle exercises. An improvement in estrogen status will take several weeks, and no significant improvement in pelvic muscle tone can be expected in less than two to three months, so attempts at conservative management should be given time to work before they are abandoned. As these factors impinging on urethral closure improve, the efficacy of drug therapy is also likely to improve. Therefore, it is usually best to adopt a multifaceted approach when treating stress incontinence conservatively, attempting to maximize the efficacy of each factor which contributes to urethral closure.

The predominant side effect of α-stimulant medications is hypertension, which may limit their usefulness in elderly patients. The vascular system is loaded with α-receptors and just as α-stimulating agents will increase urethral tone, so they will also increase vascular tone and hence may elevate blood pressure. If significant increases in blood pressure are going to occur they will usually do so within the first few days after starting the medication. Patients who are begun on these medications should have their blood pressure checked several times within the first week or so to make sure that they are not developing this problem. They should have their blood pressure rechecked periodically thereafter.

Pseudoephedrine is a common ingredient in many cold remedies and appetite-suppressant compounds, including such over-the-counter brands as Actifed, Sudafed, and Dexatrim. Phenylpropanolamine (Ornade spansules) and ephedrine are also commonly found in similar preparations.

Imipramine (Tofranil, Ciba-Geigy) has both α-stimulating effects on the urethra and bladder neck as well as relaxant effects on the detrusor. This drug is therefore useful in treating mixed incontinence, stress incontinence, or detrusor instability since its α-stimulating effects help the stress incontinence while its anticholinergic effects help the detrusor instability. It is usually given in doses of 10–25 mg TID. The lower starting dose is preferred for elderly patients. Once the patient has been started on the drug and had time to adjust to its effects, the dose may then be titrated to obtain optimal effects. Imipramine is more prone to cause orthostatic hypotension than hypertension, and may also cause cardiac arrhythmias in some patients. These side effects are not usually a problem at the lower doses used in treating urinary incontinence compared to the higher doses used in treating depression, but this should be kept in mind by the treating physician. It may be useful to obtain a baseline electrocardiogram in selected patients prior to starting long-term treatment. If the patient's incontinence worsens she may not be emptying adequately because of the anticholinergic effect. Measurement of the postvoid residual urine will confirm that this is happening, and the medication can be discontinued, or in selected cases, self-catheterization begun.

α-Blockers

Although understanding how α-stimulants can improve stress incontinence is important, it is equally important to understand how α-blockers can *cause* stress incontinence or make it worse. α-Blocking drugs are in widespread use as agents for treating hypertension because of their relaxant effects on vascular smooth muscle. The most common of these are prazosin (Minipress, Pfizer) and terazosin (Hytrin, Abbott). Phenoxybenzamine (Dibenzyline, Smith Kline and French) is less commonly used. These agents may relax the urethra and open the bladder neck enough to cause stress incontinence. Patients who are taking these drugs and present with a complaint of incontinence, particularly if the incontinence began after starting one of these medications, should be changed to another drug as part of their initial therapy. The incontinence may resolve spontaneously.

Estrogens

Estrogens in a variety of preparations have also been used as part of a therapeutic medical regimen for stress incontinence. Research in cell biology has clearly demonstrated that there are estrogen receptors in the lower urinary tract, particularly the urethra, and that the exfoliative cytology of the bladder in women changes in relation to their menstrual cycle. Postmenopausal women develop urogenital atrophy due to estrogen deprivation, and many of these women subsequently present with irritative lower urinary tract symptoms, urethral caruncles, and stress incontinence. All of these conditions can be improved, and sometimes cured, by appropriate hormone replacement therapy. Some evidence suggests that the number of α-receptors in the urethra increases in response to estrogenic stimulation and this should enhance the effects of concurrent medical therapy. Similarly, improvement in the integrity of the urethral mucosa by estrogen may enhance its coaptation and thus improve the continence mechanism by improving urethral closure. Local administration of estrogen through the use of vaginal estrogen cream provides the most rapid and profound changes. Although epithelial improvement can occur in a few weeks, it often takes two months or more for connective tissue changes to occur, so an assessment of the effectiveness of estrogen should not be made until after at least two months of treatment.

Muscular Rehabilitation by Physical Therapy

Since much of the support for the urethra and bladder neck comes from the pelvic musculature, particularly through the muscles of the levator ani complex and their connection to the endopelvic fascia, exercise of the pelvic musculature

Pelvic Muscle Exercises

could be expected to improve the continence mechanism in two ways. First, strengthening the striated urogenital sphincter might enhance its ability to constrict the urethral lumen. This could yield a higher resting urethral pressure or increase the amount of pressure generated in the urethra during a cough through active contraction of this muscle. Second, because the levator ani muscles are important for pelvic and urethral support, an exercise program might improve the support of the proximal urethra. Since these muscles might be activated during a cough, continence might be improved without a noticeable rise in resting urethral pressure measurements.

The periurethral levator ani muscles contain both Type I (slow twitch, 70%) and Type II (fast twitch, 30%) muscle fibers, making them capable of maintaining tone over a long period of time as well as increasing tone suddenly to compensate for the increased abdominal pressure which occurs with coughing, sneezing, straining and other activities. Loss of these two forms of muscular activity either due to nerve injury or stretching and tearing of the levator hiatus may weaken the continence mechanism enough to create urine loss. Programs of pelvic floor exercise are attempts to rehabilitate and strengthen the levator ani and striated urogenital sphincter muscles, increasing the tone and augmenting the contractile force which they can generate under conditions of stress, thereby improving the function of the continence mechanism.

The first person to investigate pelvic floor muscle strengthening exercises systematically was Arnold Kegel. Kegel clearly understood the role of the levator ani muscles in promoting and maintaining continence. He also understood that many women were unaware of these muscles and did not know how to exercise them. The most important point of Kegel's exercise regimen was his making patients aware of these muscles and teaching them how to exercise them properly. He did this by individual examination of each patient, carefully palpating the pubococcygeus muscle during a pelvic examination and teaching the patient to contract these muscles against his examining finger. Once he was satisfied that the patient knew where this muscle was and could contract it volitionally, she was instructed in the use of a simple pneumatic device called a "perineometer." The perineometer was a flexible rubber chamber connected by tubing to a manometer that was calibrated from 0–100 mm Hg. The rubber chamber was inserted into the vagina. When it was compressed by contraction of the levator sling it could measure the force of the contraction as well as demonstrate it to the patient simultaneously. The perineometer therefore functioned as a biofeedback device to reinforce patient compliance with the exercise program. The patient was instructed to exercise for 20 minutes three times a day and to record her progress on a chart. Kegel always stressed the importance of supervision and encouragement in the treatment of patients using this technique and recommended that they be seen every week. He eventually reported an overall "success" rate of 84% in the treatment of stress incontinence.

"Kegel exercises" have become very popular in childbirth education classes and are given widespread lip service as therapy by the medical profession. Unfortunately, they have degenerated into something very different from Kegel's original concept. When taught as part of childbirth education classes, these exercises are invariably taught in large groups without individual examination or instruction. When patient instruction in "Kegel exercises" is given in the office, it usually consists of a 30 second discussion in which the patient is instructed to "start and stop your stream a few times" each day while urinating. The patient is then told to come back in 6 months or a year for follow-up. Rehabilitation programs of this kind are worthless. This is like telling someone to "run around the block a few times each week" and come back for the Olympic track and field trials in the 1500 meters 6 months later. Bo has clearly shown that even with intensive individual instruction up to 30% of women still do these exercises incorrectly. Women who are instructed in these exercises during a brief office interview or in large groups during childbirth education classes are unlikely to perform them effectively.

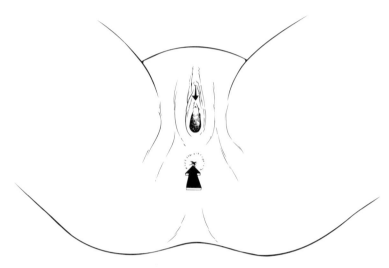

Figure 6.1 Proper contraction of the muscles of the pelvic floor causes descent of the clitoris (small arrow) and an upward and inward contraction of the anus (large arrow).

For any program of physical therapy or muscular rehabilitation to work, it must involve proper "hands on" instruction which clearly identifies the muscle groups that are to be exercised, supervision to make sure the exercises are being done properly, some form of monitoring to check on continuing compliance with the program, and some form of feedback by which the patient and therapist can gauge progress towards defined treatment goals. Kegel's original program included all of these elements.

The first task in teaching pelvic muscle exercises is to identify the muscles in question and make the patient aware of where these muscles are and what to do with them. This involves examining the patient and palpating the muscles while she is instructed in how to exercise them. Any program which does not do this is next to useless. Proper contraction of the muscles of the pelvic floor will cause the clitoris to descend and the anus to retract as the urogenital hiatus is closed (Fig. 6.1). The clinician should get into the habit of palpating the puborectalis and pubococcygeus muscles routinely during pelvic examination and asking the patient to contract them against the examining finger. These muscles can be located approximately 5 cm inside the vaginal introitus at the 5 o'clock and 7 o'clock locations. Palpation of these muscles is demonstrated in Figure 6.2. The strength of the muscular contraction can then be assessed subjectively on a scale of 0–5 (Table 6.2). If this is done routinely, clinicians will be surprised at the number of women who have no awareness of this muscle group and almost no ability to contract it voluntarily.

Because patients have so little awareness of these muscles, the absolute first priority in any regimen of muscular rehabilitation is careful education regarding what the patient is supposed to do and how she is supposed to do it. The patient must understand her tasks and goals clearly if any program of pelvic physical therapy is going to succeed. This is why verbal instruction alone in teaching these exercises gives such poor results: Patients do not clearly understand where the muscles are and how to contract them. These exercises *must* be taught in "hands on" fashion if patients are going to understand what is required of them. Bo's study showed that of the 30% of women who were performing Kegel exercises incorrectly, the most common mistake was contracting the gluteus muscles instead of the pelvic floor.

In addition to contracting these pelvic floor muscles against the examiner's finger, the use of a commercially available perineometer similar to the one designed by Arnold Kegel is often helpful in instructing patients in how to do

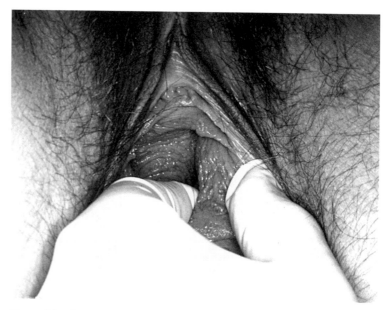

Figure 6.2   Correct palpation of the pelvic floor musculature.

TABLE 6.2.   Assessment of the Strength of Pelvic Muscle Contraction

0	No visible or palpable muscular contraction
1	A very weak contraction which is difficult to detect under the examining finger
2	A weak contraction that is nonetheless clearly perceived
3	A contraction that is well perceived but one which cannot be maintained against moderate opposition from the examiner's finger
4	A contraction with good force but one which cannot resist intense opposition from the examiner's finger
5	Maximum contraction; strong resistance to opposition

these exercises (Fig. 6.3). When the exercises are done correctly, squeezing on the inflatable vaginal probe will cause a pressure rise. Of course, abdominal straining can produce the same results if this type of device is used, so the instructor must ensure that the abdominal musculature is relaxed when these exercises are performed. The examiner's hand can also be used to palpate the patient's abdomen while the exercises are taught. Some biofeedback systems also include surface electrodes which can be applied to the anterior abdominal wall to help detect straining.

Several other types of vaginal perineometers are available commercially. Some of these contain a vaginal surface electromyography electrode which generates a reading of muscle contractility in microvolts on a screen or on a lighted scale. When displayed on a computer screen, EMG signals (or perineometer pressure measurements) can be used to set contractile goals for a patient and to chart her progress towards them. The patient then has a graphic depiction of her pelvic muscle contractility which can serve both as a marker of her current activity and a spur to greater heights of achievement. While surface EMG has some utility in measuring an *individual* patient's progress over time, the technique is unreliable for making comparisons from one patient to another. Surface EMG cannot be used reliably to quantitate muscle strength, nor can it be used as a reliable diagnostic tool for detecting denervation or pelvic myopathy.

Another extremely useful technique for patient education is electrical stimulation of the pelvic muscles. The levators can be made to contract by passing a

TABLE 6.3. Instructions for Patients: How to Do Pelvic Floor Muscle Exercises

Many women with urinary incontinence can decrease their urinary leakage during coughing, laughing, sneezing, or other activities by exercising the muscles of the pelvic floor. These exercises are often called "Kegel exercises," after the doctor who first described them.

To find the muscle you need to exercise, imagine that you have a tampon in your vagina that it is falling out and you must tighten your muscle in order to hold it in. The muscle you tighten is the muscle you should exercise. Another way to find the right muscle is to sit on the toilet, begin to urinate, and then stop your urine flow. The muscle you use to stop your stream of urine is the muscle you should exercise. Your doctor can help you determine which muscle to contract and make sure you are doing it properly by checking you during a pelvic examination.

Do not make a habit of doing these exercises by starting and stopping your urine flow while voiding! You can teach yourself bad bladder habits and develop voiding difficulty by doing this! Instead, you should practice your exercises at other times. Stopping your urine stream during voiding is only to help you find the correct muscle to contract.

Pelvic muscle exercises can be done in many different ways. We will give you instructions on how to do three types of exercises. We suggest that you do a mixture of all three exercises for the best results. Since continued vigorous exercise can lead to muscle soreness and fatigue, don't try to do your exercises all at one time. Spread them out over the course of the day: We suggest doing 100 muscle contractions divided into several sessions. If you do have muscle soreness, try doing the exercises vigorously every other day instead. This will allow your muscles to recover from the fatigue of exercise.

These exercises can be done anywhere and at any time. You may find it helpful to associate an activity with your muscles, such as doing them while stopped at a red light, during a TV commercial, talking on the phone, or doing various household chores such as ironing, washing dishes, cooking, etc. The important thing is to get in the habit of doing them!

TYPE A   Tighten the pelvic floor muscles for a count of 10 and relax. Repeat 25–50 times.

TYPE B   Tighten the pelvic floor muscles and relax in quick succession. Repeat 25–50 times.

TYPE C   Tighten the pelvic floor muscles as TIGHTLY as possible for 6–8 seconds, then contract the muscles quickly 3–4 more times. Relax, then repeat 5–10 times.

You may notice some soreness in the pelvic muscles and around the vaginal opening once you start exercising regularly. Do not worry about this: It is only soreness associated with increased muscle activity. ***The benefits of these exercises will continue ONLY as long as you do them!*** Use it, or lose it! You should expect to have to do these exercises regularly for three months before you notice an improvement in your urine loss.

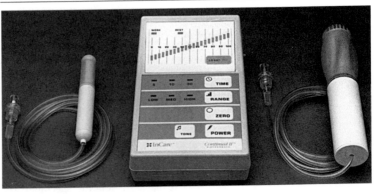

Figure 6.3 A contemporary perineometer which can be used with either a vaginal pressure probe or a rectal pressure probe (Hollister Corporation).

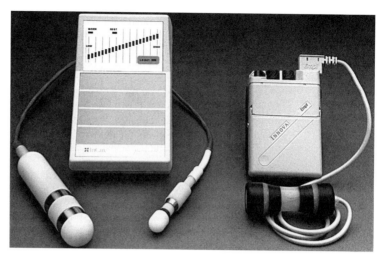

Figure 6.4 Two examples of commercially available electrical stimulators: the Microgyn II (Hollister), which can be used for vaginal or rectal electrical stimulation, and the Innova transvaginal electrical stimulator (Empi Corporation).

small electrical current through them. As the electrical stimulus causes these muscles to contract, the patient becomes more aware of where the muscles are located and how to contract them herself. A number of commercially available electrical stimulators are now available which can be used for therapy as well as patient education (Fig. 6.4).

Some awareness of the location and function of the levator muscles can be taught to women by having them stop their stream of urine during voiding. Stopping the flow of urine requires contraction of the levator muscles. If a woman can do this successfully, it helps reassure her that she is exercising the proper muscle groups, but successful exercise programs must be much more intensive than stopping the flow of urine a couple of times each day. In addition, teaching a patient to stop and start her urine stream time after time can create dysfunctional voiding in some patients and may create a new problem rather than solve an old one.

Once the patient and clinician have identified the muscle group under consideration, an exercise regimen must be developed (Table 6.3). The patient should be encouraged to develop both short-term "burst" contractions as well as longer tonic contractions. The goal here is to strengthen both the slow-twitch muscles which provide continuous support as well as the fast-twitch fibers which are recruited during periods of activity or exercise. She should be told to tighten these muscles maximally and to hold the contraction for 5 or 6 seconds, rest for 10–15 seconds, and repeat the process. She should aim to do around 100 of these exercises each day, divided into several separate sets. The exercises should be finished with several sets of sharp, hard, short contractions ("flicks") to develop the fast-twitch muscle fibers. Linking this exercise program to repetitive daily activities is useful: Have the patient do a set of exercises each time she stops at a traffic light while driving, or each time a commercial comes on while she is watching television. It is especially important for the patient to hold the contraction at maximal intensity for a full 5 or 6 seconds, as many patients will develop a good maximal contraction but will allow it to fade out fairly quickly.

As with any program of muscle exercise, it is possible to overexercise the muscles. Several good workouts spaced at regular intervals throughout the day are more likely to be beneficial than random occasional activity. Experience suggests that patients are unlikely to do exercises more than three or four times per day, in spite of their best intentions. Kegel suggested that patients should keep diaries documenting their compliance and their progress. Some form of monitoring is very important, and patients should be seen at regular intervals for encouragement and motivation, particularly in the early stages of therapy. As is true for any muscle group, the levators may become tender after a few days of exercise. This can cause mild dyspareunia in some patients. Women should be told that this will resolve and if it does occur it helps confirm that they are doing the exercises properly. Progress with these exercises can be judged in many ways. Patients will notice a subjective improvement in their ability to contract the pelvic muscles which will be accompanied by decreased frequency of urine loss and a gradual improvement in symptoms over time. Progress is slow, but with practice, steady.

One ingenious way of assisting women to exercise the pelvic muscles is by intravaginal weight training using specially designed ''cones.'' These vaginal cones consist of a set of five small (5 cm) tampon-like weights of equal volume but increasing weight (Fig. 6.5). Starting with the lightest weight, the patient places one cone into the vagina while she is standing. She then holds this in

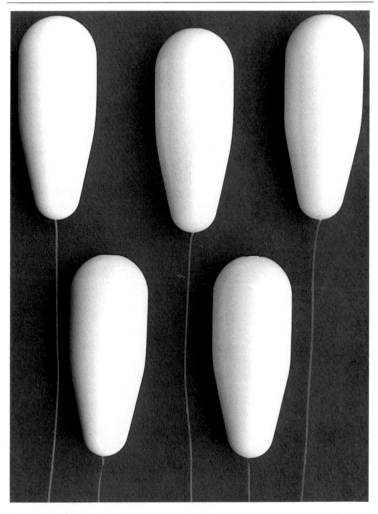

Figure 6.5 Vaginal cones for pelvic muscle weight training (Dacomed Corporation, 1701 East 79th Street, Minneapolis, MN 55425, toll-free telephone number 1–800–328–1103).

place by contracting her pelvic floor muscles for one minute while she walks around. When she is able to do this successfully, she moves on to the next highest weight in sequence until she finds one that cannot be retained for 60 seconds. A formal exercise program is then begun using this weight of cone. The patient places this weight in the vagina and attempts to retain it in place for 15 minutes, twice daily. When this goal has been achieved, she moves on to the next highest weight using the same exercise regimen.

The cones cannot be retained in place if the patient strains instead of contracting her pelvic muscles. Only proper contraction of the levator ani muscles will keep the cone in the correct position. The feeling that the cone is starting to slip out of the vagina provides a form of internal biofeedback and the patient must increase her muscular contraction to prevent this from happening. Her progress may be gauged not only by the improvement in her symptomatology, but also by the increasing weight of the cones which she is able to carry.

These weights are an excellent adjunct to a well-designed pelvic muscle rehabilitation program, but they are not a substitute for individual instruction in pelvic muscle exercises. Simply handing a patient a set of cones and telling her to "get to work" is not likely to be effective, particularly for patients who have poor pelvic muscle tone (Grades 0, 1, or 2). If given an initial task which they cannot handle, these patients may become discouraged unnecessarily. Patients with extremely poor muscle tone should be given careful individual instruction before moving on to more demanding tasks. This group in particular may benefit from electrical stimulation therapy as part of their initial rehabilitation program.

As with all muscle rehabilitation programs, continual exercise is needed to maintain muscular strength; you either "use it or lose it." Muscles maintain their tone and their strength only through regular periodic activity. Patients who obtain a clinical cure from their incontinence using this therapy must understand that they must continue to perform pelvic muscle exercises on a regular basis or they run the risk of relapsing. Since pelvic muscle exercise is virtually without side effects except some soreness and muscle fatigue, almost anyone with stress incontinence may benefit from this form of therapy—even those patients who have failed surgical intervention. Because pelvic floor disorders are so common among women, the authors believe that regular exercise of the muscles of the pelvic floor should be as much a part of the preventive health care routine for women as annual Pap smears and monthly breast self-examination. There is little chance of harm and much potential good to be gained from exercise of this kind.

Electrical Stimulation   Electrical stimulation therapy has already been mentioned briefly as a tool for helping patients identify the muscles of the pelvic floor that they need to exercise. In addition to making patients aware of these muscles, electrical stimulation can provide direct benefits to the muscles themselves, especially when used for extended periods of time. Electrical current causes striated muscles to contract, and in contracting over time they increase both their strength and tone by repetitive exercise. Electrical stimulation can be used to make the muscles contract involuntarily, thus providing a form of artificial muscle training. If an intermittent electrical current is passed through the musculature of the pelvic floor on a chronic basis, these muscles can be exercised until they are strong and resilient enough that incontinence is diminished or cured. In addition to providing a form of muscle exercise, electrical stimulation improves reinnervation of injured muscle and enhances axonal sprouting, as well as improves reflex activation of the muscles.

A number of studies have been undertaken to prove that chronic electrical stimulation of the pelvic floor is a viable treatment for incontinence. These studies have had with varying degrees of success. Some studies have used long-term chronic stimulation with a transvaginal or transrectal electrode (Fig. 6.3). Other studies have used intermittent electrical therapy, such as two 15 minute sessions each day. All of these studies have shown some success, but many of them have had problems with patient acceptance, device failure, or long-term compliance using electrical stimulation therapy.

Some commercially available electrical stimulation equipment combines the capability of performing electrical stimulation with the ability to monitor vaginal/rectal pressure or EMG activity. This allows a multifaceted approach to patient education and treatment and permits more individualization of care—an important consideration in any rehabilitation program. Electrical stimulation is quite effective in teaching patients which muscles they need to contract, since many women have almost no awareness of the musculature of the pelvic floor and how to manipulate it. Once they have been made aware of these muscles through electrical stimulation, they can be taught to contract them voluntarily and to exercise them on a routine basis. Once patients have reached this stage, they may benefit from a home perineometer or the use of vaginal cones. This may be a more logical and more promising way of utilizing electrical stimulation therapy than by passive electrical stimulation of muscles alone.

Mechanical Support Devices

Since stress incontinence so often stems from a defect in pelvic support, many people have hoped that some form of pessary or intravaginal support device could be developed that would solve the problem without resort to surgery or more exotic forms of therapy. Indeed, many younger women with mild, exercise-induced incontinence, find that they can alleviate their symptoms by putting an ordinary menstrual tampon in the vagina before exercising. This provides additional support for the urethra and is often remarkably effective in stopping stress incontinence. Many women will find that this is all the therapy they require for their problem; others, however, are not so fortunate. The continuous use of an absorbent menstrual tampon may cause significant vaginal dryness and irritation. Since a dry tampon can be quite difficult to remove, patients should be told to remove it while showering or bathing. Placing the tampon inside a condom which is then inserted into the vagina will also make it easier to remove.

Where stress incontinence is associated with varying degrees of uterine prolapse, particularly in elderly women, the use of a supportive pessary may cure their discomfort or render it tolerable. In some cases, however, continence is maintained by the prolapse: It kinks the urethra and bladder neck as it descends, preventing urine loss. Women with this type of problem may actually be made worse by the use of a pessary because it may elevate the prolapse and remove the last remaining barrier to urine loss. Other women, such as those with massive posthysterectomy vaginal vault prolapse and enterocele, may have such a large prolapse that no pessary can be retained successfully. If pessaries are used in an attempt to cure incontinence, care should be taken to make sure that they fit well, that the vagina is well estrogenized, and that these patients are seen periodically for examination, pessary removal, and cleaning. Curing incontinence by placing a pessary has not achieved much if it is neglected and erodes into the rectum or bladder, or becomes so entrapped that it must be removed surgically at a later date.

A variety of specialized devices have been developed to cure stress incontinence by simple mechanical support. None of these has been consistently successful. These include the Edwards spring, Bonnar's inflatable balloon, and the Biswas silastic vaginal pessary. All of these devices have the same drawbacks as standard pessaries: potential discomfort, potential erosion, potential urinary obstruction or the need to remove them before voiding, and the awkwardness of the device in elderly patients who may lack the dexterity to manipulate them.

Other Considerations

Finally, some common sense suggestions must be made about stress incontinence. For the most part women with stress incontinence have a good idea as to what activities are going to make them leak: coughing, lifting, straining, sneezing, and so on. Simple changes in body posture have been shown to be effective in decreasing urinary leakage under these circumstances. Have the patient squeeze her thighs together or cross her legs tightly if she is about to sneeze. Encourage women who do lots of lifting (such as nurses or factory workers) to tighten their pelvic floor muscles each time they lift something. This is often quite effective, but many patients have never been told to do this. If the patient knows she will have to do some lifting or if she is going to an aerobics class or out jogging, have her empty her bladder before engaging in these activities. Fluid management and proper voiding habits are very useful management techniques for nearly all types of incontinence, yet this basic advice is often overlooked.

SUGGESTED READING

Medical Management of Genuine Stress Incontinence

Beisland HO, Fossberg E, Moer A, et al. Urethral sphincteric insufficiency in postmenopausal females: Treatment with phenylpropanolamine and estriol separately and in combination: A urodynamic and clinical evaluation. Urol Int 1984; 39:211–16.

Diernas E, Rix P, Sorensen T, et al. Norfenefrine in the treatment of female urinary stress incontinence assessed by one-hour pad weighing test. Urol Int 1989; 44:28–31.

Dwyer PL, Teele JS. Prazosin: A neglected cause of genuine stress incontinence. Obstet Gynecol 1992; 79:117–21.

Ek A, Anderson KE, Gullberg B, et al. The effects of long-term treatment with norephedrine on stress incontinence and urethral closure pressure profile. Scand J Urol Nephrol 1978; 12:105–10.

Lose G, Rix P, Diernas E, et al. Norfenefrine in the treatment of female stress incontinence: A double-blind controlled trial. Urol Int 1988; 43:11–15.

Lose G, Diernas E, Rix P. Does medical therapy cure female stress incontinence? Urol Int 1989; 44:25–27.

Montague DK, Stewart BH. Urethral pressure profiles before and after Ornade administration in patients with stress urinary incontinence. J Urol 1979; 122:198–99.

Obrink A, Bunne G. The effect of alpha-adrenergic stimulation in stress incontinence. Scand J Urol Nephrol 1978; 12:205–08.

Wall LL, Addison WA. Prazosin-induced stress incontinence. Obstet Gynecol 1990; 75:558–60.

Wilson PD, Faragher B, Butler B, et al. Treatment with oral piperazine oestrone sulphate for genuine stress incontinence in postmenopausal women. Br J Obstet Gynaecol 1987; 94:568–74.

Estrogens and Urinary Incontinence

Batra S, Iosif CS. Female urethra: A target for estrogen action. J Urol 1983; 129:418–20.

Faber P, Heidenreich J. Treatment of stress incontinence with estrogen in postmenopausal women. Url Int 1977; 32:221–23.

Fantl JA, Wyman JF, Anderson RL, et al. Postmenopausal urinary incontinence: Comparison between non-estrogen supplemented and estrogen-supplemented women. Obstet Gynecol 1988; 71;823–28.

Hilton P, Stanton SL. The use of intravaginal oestrogen cream in genuine stress incontinence. Br J Obstet Gynaecol 1983; 90:940–44.

Iosif CS, Batra S, Ek A, et al. Estrogen receptors in the human female lower urinary tract. Am J Obstet Gynecol 1981; 141:817–20.

Schrieter F, Fuchs P, Stockamp K. Estrogenic sensitivity of alpha-receptors in the urethra musculature. Urol Int 1976; 31:13–19.

Smith P. Age changes in the female urethra. Br J Urol 1972; 44:657–76.

Tyler DE. Stratified squamous epithelium in the vesical trigone and urethra: Findings correlated with the menstrual cycle and age. Am J Anatomy 1962; 111:319–25.

Walter S, Wolf H, Barlebo H, et al. Urinary incontinence in postmenopausal women treated with estrogens: A double-blind clinical trial. Urol Int 1978; 33:135–43.

Wilson PD, Barker G, Barnard RJ, et al. Steroid hormone receptors in the female lower urinary tract. Urol Int 1984; 39:5-8.

Wilson PD, Faragher B, Butler B, et al. Treatment with oral piperazine oestrone sulphate for genuine stress incontinence in postmenopausal women. Br J Obstet Gynecol 1987; 94:568–74.

Pelvic Floor Muscle Exercises

Bemelmans BLH, Hankel M, Jackobs CHGM, Van Kerrebroeck PEV, Worm G, Debruyne FMJ. Pelvic floor reeducation and body posture correction for treatment of female urinary incontinence: Results of comprehensive pre- and post-treatment urodynamic testing. Neurourol Urodynam 1992; 11:209–18.

Benvenuti F, Caputo GM, Sandinelli S, et al. Reeducative treatment of female genuine stress incontinence. Am J Phys Med 1987; 66:155–68.

Bo K, Kvarstein B, Hagen R, et al. Pelvic floor muscle exercise for the treatment of female stress urinary incontinence: I. Reliability of vaginal pressure measurements of pelvic floor muscle strength. Neurourol Urodynam 1990; 9:471–77.

Bo K, Kvarstein B, Hagen R, et al. Pelvic floor muscle exercise for the treatment of female stress urinary incontinence: II. Validity of vaginal pressure measurements of pelvic floor muscle strength and the necessity of supplementary methods for control of correct contraction. Neurourol Urodynam 1990; 9:479–87.

Bo K, Hagen RR, Kvarstein B, et al. Pelvic floor muscle exercise for the treatment of female stress urinary incontinence: III. Effects of two different degrees of pelvic floor muscle exercises. Neurourol Urodynam 1990; 9:489–502.

Bo K, Larsen S. Pelvic floor muscle exercise for the treatment of stress urinary incontinence: Classification and characterization of responders. Neurourol Urodynam 1992; 11:497–508.

Burgio KL, Robinson JC, Engel BT. The role of biofeedback in Kegel exercise training for stress urinary incontinence. Am J Obset Gynecol 1986; 154:58–64.

Cammu H, Van Nylen M, Derde MP, et al. Pelvic physiotherapy in genuine stress incontinence. Urology 1991; 38: 332–37.

Ferguson KL, McKey PL, Bishop KR, Kloen P, Verheul JB, Dougherty MC. Stress urinary incontinence: Effect of pelvic muscle exercise. Obstet Gynecol 1990; 75:671–75.

Gosling JA, Dixon JS, Critchley HOD, et al. A comparative

study of the human external sphincter and periurethral levator ani muscles. Br J Urol 1981; 53:35–41.

Hahn I, Naucler J, Sommar S, et al. Urodynamic assessment of pelvic floor training. World J Urol 1991; 9:162–66.

Hahn I, Sommar S, Fall M. A comparative study of pelvic floor training and electrical stimulation for the treatment of genuine female stress urinary incontinence. Neurourol Urodynam 1991; 10:545–54.

Henalla SM, Kirwin P, Castleden CM, et al. The effect of pelvic floor exercises in the treatment of genuine urinary stress incontinence in women at two hospitals. Br J Obstet Gynaecol 1988; 95:602–06.

Jonasson A, Larsson B, Pschera H. Testing and training of the pelvic floor muscles after childbirth. Acta Obstet Gynecol Scand 1989; 68:301–04.

Kegel AH. Progressive resistance exercise in the functional restoration of the perineal muscles. Am J Obstet Gynecol 1948; 56:238–48.

Kegel AH. Physiologic therapy for urinary stress incontinence. J Am Med Assoc 1951; 146:915–17.

Klarskov P, Belving D, Bischoff N, et al. Pelvic floor exercise versus surgery for female urinary stress incontinence. Urol Int 1986; 41:129–32.

Moore K, Metcalfe JB. Effectiveness of vaginal cones in treatment of urinary incontinence. Urologic Nursing 1992; 12(2)69–72.

Mouritsen L, Frimodt-Moller C, Frimodt-Moller M. Long term effect of pelvic floor exercises on female urinary incontinence. Br J Urol 1991; 68:32–37.

Olah K, Bridges N, Denning J, et al. The conservative management of patients with symptoms of stress incontinence: A randomized, prospective study comparing weighted vaginal cones and interferential therapy. Am J Obstet Gynecol 1990; 162:87–92.

Peattie AB, Plevnik S, Stanton SL. Vaginal cones: A conservative method of treating genuine stress incontinence. Br J Obstet Gynaecol 1988; 95:1049–53.

Tchou DCH, Adams C, Varner RE, et al. Pelvic floor musculature exercises in treatment of anatomical urinary stress incontinence. Physical Therapy 1988; 68:652–55.

Wall LL, Davidson TG. The role of muscular re-education by physical therapy in the treatment of genuine stress incontinence. Obstet Gynecol Survey 1992; 47:322–31.

Wilson PD, Samarrai TA, Deakin M, et al. An objective assessment of physiotherapy for female genuine stress incontinence. Br J Obstet Gynaecol 1987; 94:575–82.

Electrical Stimulation Therapy

Eriksen BC, Eik-Nes SH. Long-term electrostimulation of the pelvic floor: Primary therapy in female stress incontinence? Urol Int 1989; 44:90–95.

Eriksen BC, Mjolnerold OK. Changes in urodynamic measurements after successful anal electrostimulation in female urinary incontinence. Br J Urol 1987; 59:45–49.

Erikson BC, Bergmann S, Mjolnerold OJ. Effect of anal electrostimulation with the Incontan device in women with urinary incontinence. Br J Obstet Gynaecol 1987; 94:147–56.

Fall M, Ahlstrom K, Carlsson CA, et al. Contelle: Pelvic floor stimulator for female stress-urge incontinence. Urology 1986; 27:282–87.

Fall M, Lindstrom S. Electrical stimulation: A physiologic approach to the treatment of urinary incontinence. Urol Clin NA 1991; 18:393–407.

Leach G, Bavendam T. Prospective evaluation of the Incontan transrectal stimulator in women with urinary incontinence. Neurourol Urodynam 1989; 8:231–36.

Laycock J, Green RJ. Interferential therapy in the treatment of incontinence. Physiotherapy 1988; 74:161–68.

Meyer S, Dhenin T, Schmidt N, De Grandi P. Subjective and objective effects of intravaginal electrical myostimulation and biofeedback in patients with genuine stress incontinence. Br J Urol 1992; 69:584–88.

Plevnik S, Janez J, Vrtacnik P, et al. Short-term electrical stimulation: Home treatment for urinary incontinence. World J Urol 1986; 4:24–26.

Mechanical Support Devices

Bhatia NN, Bergman A. Pessary test in women with urinary incontinence. Obstet Gynecol 1985; 65:220–26.

Biswas NC. A silastic vaginal device for the treatment of stress urinary incontinence. Neurourology Urodynamics 1988; 7:271–72.

Cardozo LD, Stanton SL. Evaluation of a female urinary incontinence device. Urology 1979; 13:398–401.

Edwards L, Malvern J. The control of incontinence of urine in women with a pubo-vaginal spring device: Objective and subjective results. Br J Urol 1971; 43:211–25.

Edwards L, Malvern J. Long-term follow-up results with the pubo-vaginal spring device in incontinence of urine in women: comparison with electronic methods of control. Br J Urol 1973; 45:103–08.

7

Surgical Management of Stress Incontinence

Philosophy of Surgical Management

The operative treatment of urinary incontinence has always held an important and venerable position in gynecologic surgery. Indeed, modern operative gynecology really began in the middle of the 19th Century when J. Marion Sims developed the first consistently successful approach for the cure of vesicovaginal fistulae resulting from obstructed childbirth. The amount of human suffering relieved as a result of his achievement over the last 150 years can scarcely be imagined. But many other gynecologic surgeons have also made substantial contributions to the surgical cure of female incontinence, particularly stress urinary incontinence.

Dr. Howard A. Kelly, of Johns Hopkins, developed the anterior vaginal repair with "Kelly plication" of the bladder neck at the beginning of this century and laid the basic foundations for all subsequent vaginal approaches to this problem. Shortly thereafter, in Germany, Goebel, Stoeckel, and Frangenheim—gynecologists all—developed the basic techniques for all subsequent suburethral sling procedures. The first attempts to cure incontinence by periurethral injection of chemical substances were made in Britain in the 1930's by Murless. The modern era of retropubic bladder neck surgery began in 1949 when urologists Marshall and Marchetti, working with Krantz, a gynecologist, published their paper on abdominal vesicourethral suspension. Further pioneering improvements in this operation were subsequently made in the 1960's by C. Paul Hodgkinson and John Burch. The needle suspension procedure was originally described by Armand Pereyra in 1957, and subsequently refined by him, working with Dr. Thomas Lebherz. Minor changes have since been made in this operation by countless surgeons who have attached their names to their own version of the original technique. The development of modern prosthetic materials and advanced reconstructive surgical techniques since the 1970's has opened a vast new array of sophisticated and highly technical operations for patients with complex incontinence, and this process is likely to continue into the 21st Century. Where does this leave the woman with relatively straightforward stress incontinence? What is the optimal surgical treatment for her condition?

The diagnosis of "genuine" stress incontinence and the principles of conservative, nonsurgical management have been discussed in the previous chapter. Before dealing with the technical details of various operative procedures and their complications, however, some basic questions must be considered: (*a*) Why should you operate for stress incontinence? (*b*) What are the objectives of surgical treatment? (*c*) How do you select the correct surgical procedure for a given patient?

Why Should You Operate for Stress Incontinence?

Surgery for stress incontinence is *elective*. It is a "quality of life" decision, not an emergency, and this means that, as in all treatment decisions regarding the incontinent patient, *the decision to operate is patient driven*. It is a mistake to talk a patient into having an elective operation about which she is reluctant, and then to have a bad outcome either due to failure of the operation to correct the incontinence or the development of a complication such as voiding difficulty. The decision to operate should be made when the diagnosis is clearly established, when there is a reasonable chance of success, when the patient understands the procedure and its potential complications, and when she has had the opportunity to consider other forms of therapy and either try them or reject them. Surgery should *not* be undertaken until the stress incontinence bothers the patient enough for her to wish to have it corrected. "Informed consent" is not a substitute for good judgment on the part of the surgeon.

What are the Objectives of Surgical Treatment?

Here again, these issues are patient driven. Making patients dry is *not* a problem. Almost every incontinent patient could be made dry by performing an obstructive sling procedure and an augmentation cystoplasty, having her empty her bladder thereafter by self-catheterization; however, the morbidity of such an approach would be extraordinarily high. There will be some patients desperate enough to pay the price—both financial and physical—to achieve dryness by this means; however, for most patients this is far more surgery than they wish (or need) to contemplate. What they are interested in is reducing their symptoms to a level that is tolerable for their lifestyle. For some, an active professional tennis player with stress incontinence, for example, complete dryness during exercise may be mandatory. For others, such as an elderly sedentary woman, reduction of continuous copious urine loss to the point where she must use only three pads per day may be life-transforming. Therapy must be individualized and patient directed.

There are three major objectives in surgery for stress incontinence: (*a*) patient objectives, (*b*) physiologic objectives, and (*c*) anatomical or structural objectives. In all three cases, the ideal is to restore normality: to alleviate symptoms, restore the normal physiology of bladder function (both storage and emptying), and to restore normal anatomical structure.

Assessing the outcome of operative procedures clearly must involve some form of evaluation of each of these three objective areas. Patient symptoms must be assessed subjectively, since symptoms are subjective complaints, and because there is no objective correlation between the amount of urine lost and the degree to which this bothers the patient. However, a good evaluation must at least include examination of the patient with a full bladder while she coughs or strains and a uniform method of recording responses, such as a standardized questionnaire or visual analog scale.

The outcome of surgery must be discussed objectively and candidly with the patient. The best person to obtain this information is usually not the operating surgeon, since patients will frequently not admit their dissatisfaction directly to their doctor. Surgeons have a vested personal interest in achieving successful outcome and are not always the best persons to evaluate "success." The medical literature on stress incontinence is full of individual series of "successful" operations reported by surgeons whose operations were successful because they said they were. The follow-up of patients in most of these papers is short, less than 2 years, sporadic, and superficial. In-depth analysis looking for complications, voiding difficulties, pain, prolapse, and so forth has generally been avoided, the operative philosophy here being "if the patient doesn't look bad, neither will I." Those patients "lost to follow-up" are not pursued with any vigor, often because these are the failed patients who were so unhappy that they either did not come back for return appointments or sought help from another doctor. "Subjective" cure rates in analyses of surgery for genuine stress incontinence are nearly always higher than "objective" cure rates.

Subjective cure of symptoms or patient "happiness" with the operation is always difficult to compare from one study to another, though some progress could be made by using a standardized methodology. Being completely dry after surgery is different from being happy with the surgical outcome. Pain, irritative voiding symptoms, the development of prolapse, or severe voiding difficulty can also be worse than the original problem for which the patient had her operation. How the bladder stores and empties urine before and after surgery is more easily evaluated through urodynamic studies. This represents the major rationale for preoperative urodynamic testing. Operations are carried out to correct abnormal physiology—urinary incontinence—which is causing significant symptoms in a patient, and which is usually linked to a structural defect of the continence mechanism. To do this properly a diagnosis must be established, the physiology evaluated, and a structural fault established which can either be restored to normal (a displaced bladder neck, for example) or corrected by creating a compensatory abnormality (such as partial obstruction by a sling procedure for a damaged urethra). It makes little sense to perform an operation for abnormal physiology (urinary incontinence) without evaluating that physiology either before or after surgery. Many patients will have abnormal structure (a hypermobile bladder neck), but will not suffer from significant incontinence.

Correction of abnormal anatomy that is not responsible for abnormal physiology is not particularly useful. In the best of all possible worlds, therefore, all patients would receive thorough preoperative urodynamic testing to evaluate their bladder physiology, and a thorough postoperative evaluation to see how that physiology had been altered by surgery. The best scientific papers do this, largely because the demonstration of incontinence before and after surgery, under controlled urodynamic conditions, provides us with about the only objective measurement of surgery which can be compared from series to series and operation to operation. Postoperative evaluation is particularly important in cases of surgical failure in order to identify the reason that the procedure was unsuccessful: misdiagnosis, failure of surgical technique, new pathophysiology, etc. Similarly, successful elimination of stress incontinence only to replace it with uncontrollable detrusor instability or disabling voiding difficulty is hardly a "success" in the eyes of the patient.

Do all patients need full urodynamic studies before undergoing surgery for stress incontinence? There is nothing wrong with this approach; however, it can reasonably be argued that a woman with no prior surgery and a complaint limited essentially to stress incontinence, who has a demonstrable anatomic defect (bladder neck displacement) *and stress incontinence which is objectively demonstrable on repetitive occasions*, may have an operation without full urodynamic studies. The surgeon who decides to operate in this way must be meticulous and systematic about performing a *complete* history and full physical examination (including simple retrograde bladder filling), and must not neglect any of the fundamental evaluations which we have described. Surgery represents a major life-event in terms of expense, morbidity, and recuperation. Urodynamic testing adds only slightly to the overall cost of surgery and may provide fundamental information about the patient that may modify the choice of surgical procedure, or reverse the decision to operate in the first place. The authors all agree that patients with prior failed surgery, unclear or complicated histories, and complex anatomic defects should have a thorough urodynamic investigation prior to an anti-incontinence operation.

Whether or not the anatomic or structural objectives of surgery have been achieved can be assessed by physical examination, perhaps in combination with imaging techniques such as fluoroscopy, ultrasound, magnetic resonance imaging, etc. Long-term follow-up is critical to look for new anatomical abnormalities—such as the development of an enterocele or vault prolapse after retropubic surgery—and to evaluate the long-term structural success of surgery. Determination of precisely which mechanical goals are to be achieved in a given patient—such as bladder neck elevation or urethral obstruction—will vary with the circumstances of each individual.

Which is the Best Operation for a Given Patient?

Approximately one paper per week is written in the world medical literature on the surgical treatment of stress incontinence. These papers describe nearly 200 operative approaches to managing this problem. Which operation is best? Which one should you choose for a given patient? Clearly some operations are idiosyncratic techniques of individual surgeons who report only their own subjective experiences. Others are well-established procedures which have been used and evaluated, to some degree at least, by many surgeons in many different countries. If we look at the operations which have been used successfully by many surgeons, and eliminate the "oddball" operations, we may classify surgi-

TABLE 7.1. Classification of Surgical Procedures for Genuine Stress Incontinence

I. Anterior colporrhaphy with Kelly plication
II. Abdominal bladder neck suspension operations designed to correct anatomic hypermobility
   A. Retropubic bladder neck suspension
      1. Marshall-Marchetti-Krantz operation
      2. Burch colposuspension
   B. Paravaginal bladder neck suspension
      1. Paravaginal repair
      2. Vagino-obturator shelf procedure
   C. Needle suspension procedures
      1. Pereyra procedure
      2. Subsequent minor modifications
III. Operations for intrinsic sphincteric weakness or dysfunction
   A. Sling operations
      1. Organic materials
         a. Autologous materials, e.g. rectus fascia, fascia lata
         b. Heterologous materials, e.g., procine dermis, ox dura
      2. Synthetic materials
   B. Periurethral injections
      1. Teflon past
      2. GAX collagen
IV. Salvage Operations
   A. Purposefully obstructive sling operations
   B. Periurethral injections
   C. Artificial urinary sphincter
   D. Urinary reconstruction and/or diversion

cal procedures into four broad categories: the traditional anterior colporrhaphy with ''Kelly plication,'' operations for bladder neck and urethral hypermobility, operations for intrinsic sphincteric dysfunction, and salvage operations (Table 7.1). The latter two categories are clearly different from the first two, and will be discussed separately.

As we mentioned in Chapter 5, there are two distinct types of stress incontinence: (*a*) that due to anatomic displacement of the bladder neck and urethra from their normal position during periods of increased abdominal stress (sometimes called ''hypermobility stress incontinence''); and (*b*) that due to intrinsic sphincteric dysfunction which leads to loss of effective urethral closure. The first task of the surgeon is to place the patient's problem into the appropriate category. If these points are not clear, the material in Chapter 5 should be reviewed before reading the rest of this chapter.

Let us begin by discussing management of the typical patient with stress incontinence who is presenting for the first time with urine loss caused by loss of normal urethral support. Which is the best operation for this patient? The best way to answer this question would be to take patients with comparable diagnoses, randomize them among a number of surgeons doing the same procedures with the same technique, and follow them over a prolonged period of time with objective measurements of outcome. Unfortunately, this has been very difficult to do. Only a handful of papers in the medical literature have done this (Table 7.2). In general, these comparative surgical studies have shown that retropubic bladder neck suspension operations, such as the Burch procedure, produce a better long-term objective cure of stress incontinence than do either needle suspension procedures or the anterior colporrhaphy. The reported success rates for anterior colporrhaphy are disturbingly low—so low that the choice of this operation for a patient with proven stress incontinence probably requires special justification. The reasons for this and their implications will be discussed later.

TABLE 7.2.   Comparative Surgical Studies of Operations for Genuine Stress Incontinence

Reference	Objective Cure Rates By Operations For Patients with Genuine Stress Incontinence				
	Number of Patients	Anterior Colporrhaphy	Needle Suspension	Burch Procedure	Length of Follow-up
Stanton and Cardozo	50	36%		84%	6 mos +
Mundy	51		40%	89%	12 mos
Weil et al.	86	57%	50%	91%	6 mos +
Van Geelan et al.	90	45%		85%	1–2 years
Bergman et al.[b]	289	69%	70%	87%	12 mos
Bergman et al.[c]	107	65%	72%	91%	12 mos

[a] From Wall LL. In: Thompson and Rock, TeLinde's Operative Gynecology, 7th ed. Philadelphia: Lippincott, 1991, with permission.
[b] Patients with concurrent prolapse.
[c] Patients without concurrent prolapse.

An Overview of Operations for Stress Incontinence

In this section we will survey the operations commonly employed for treating stress incontinence, discussing their fundamental characteristics, mechanisms of action, advantages, disadvantages, and the common errors made in their performance. The bibliography at the end of the chapter will provide the interested reader with access to technical discussions of specific operative procedures at a level beyond the scope of this book.

Anterior Colporrhaphy

The anterior vaginal repair operation for stress incontinence is the oldest surgical procedure for this condition, having been described by Howard Kelly in 1914. Kelly believed that stress incontinence was caused by an open vesical neck, not loss of urethral support, and described an operation to cure this condition by placing a lateral suture on each side of the bladder neck to pull it closed. He reported an initial subjective success rate of 90% with this operation, but subsequently found that this decreased to 60% over time. Because of its simplicity, this technique became popular all over the world. Kelly's operation represented a remarkable surgical achievement considering the general state of surgery at the turn of the century, with its high morbidity, lack of antibiotics, lack of blood transfusion, and crude suture materials. Kelly's patients undoubtedly had incredibly severe incontinence to undergo elective surgery under those conditions, but as a "patient driven" procedure, it was the best there was to offer at that time.

The fundamental problem with discussing the anterior colporrhaphy is that many substantially different operations have been lumped together under a single name. The major modifications of technique which have been described include: (*a*) plication of the bladder neck, where the bladder is simply imbricated under the urethra; (*b*) elevation of the urethra by plication of the endopelvic fascia under the vesical neck; and (*c*) fascial reattachment to bone, where a suture is placed lateral to the urethra and the needle is driven anteriorly into the posterior edge of the pubic symphysis to anchor the suture firmly (Fig. 7.1).

The mechanism of action of this operation is correction of bladder neck and urethral displacement under stress by stabilizing the fascial floor under the urethra to prevent downward motion. It is therefore an operation to correct stress incontinence due to hypermobility and lack of anatomic support. Its major advantages include its lower morbidity (particularly in older patients) because it avoids an abdominal incision, and the fact that it can easily be done in combination with other vaginal surgery, such as a vaginal hysterectomy and posterior colpoperineorrhaphy.

Although Kelly originally proposed his technique to narrow the vesical neck,

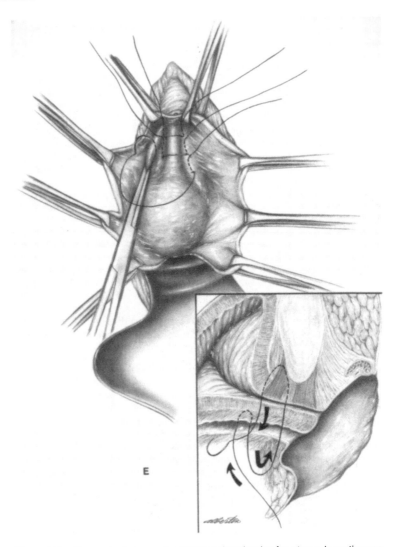

E

Figure 7.1 Proper technique of anterior colporrhaphy for stress incontinence. Beginning at the external meatus, successive vertical mattress stitches of No. 0 delayed-absorbable suture are placed in the mobilized paraurethral fascia. A Kelly clamp depresses the floor of the urethra as the sutures are tied to avoid necrosis of the wall of the urethra. The last suture at the bladder neck is anchored to the endopelvic fascia beside the urethra using No. 1 delayed-absorbable suture. This tissue is grasped with a straight Ochsner clamp. The suture passes deeply through the periurethral endopelvic fascia on the posterior aspect of the symphysis pubis (arrow). A second suture is placed on the opposite side of the urethra where it incorporates the same anatomical structures. Both sutures are tied, drawing the paraurethral fascia beneath the urethra and elevating the posterior urethra to a high retropubic position. (From Thompson JD, Rock JA (Eds). TeLinde's Operative Gynecology, 7th ed. Philadelphia: JB Lippincott, 1992, with permission.)

it must be remembered that the vesical neck is made of smooth muscle. Smooth muscle possesses a fundamental ability to undergo considerable elongation without a significant change in tension. This fact explains why Kelly's long-term results were so poor.

Several articles have been published reporting excellent success with specific technical modifications of the anterior colporrhaphy. These good results can only be achieved by using the specific techniques described in these papers.

Many of these modifications depend upon skillful dissection of the endopelvic fascia and bold placement of deep sutures into tissue directly on the pelvic sidewall or pubic bone (Fig. 7.1). If only simple plication of the endopelvic fascia under the bladder is performed, the immediate and long-term failure rates will be high.

Most surgeons who have sufficient experience with stress incontinence to know their failure rates choose not to use the anterior repair because its disadvantages outweigh its advantages when all factors are considered together. Subtleties of technique are of major importance in this operation. As a result, success with this operation is highly dependent on the skill of the operator and a hastily done repair is usually followed by the prompt return of stress incontinence. Furthermore, if the tissue is discovered to be inadequate during the dissection, there are few options available for turning this into a successful procedure except abandoning it altogether and starting an entirely different operation. If the endopelvic fascia is detached laterally, plicating it under the bladder neck will not achieve adequate support and elevation unless the dissection is carried out to include the pelvic sidewall. This is not particularly easy for most surgeons.

The major errors commonly made in performing the anterior colporrhaphy for stress incontinence are: inadequate assessment of the type of stress incontinence before surgery; commitment to a vaginal approach without careful consideration of possible alternatives which might serve the patient better in the long run; failure to perform an extensive anterior vaginal dissection; use of chromic catgut suture instead of delayed-absorbable suture; and failure to place anchoring sutures in strong supportive tissue either at the lateral pelvic sidewalls or underneath the pubic symphysis (Fig. 7.1). Mere plication of the bladder base upon itself under the urethra will not provide substantial long-term support.

The complications of anterior colporrhaphy include hemorrhage (particularly from the periurethral veins behind the pubic symphysis); laceration of the bladder and/or urethra; the development of periurethral fibrosis; and trimming excessive vaginal epithelium following the repair, with resultant vaginal narrowing, foreshortening, and the development of dyspareunia. Voiding difficulty following surgery is common, and many practitioners routinely place a suprapubic catheter to facilitate bladder drainage. If posterior colpoperineorrhaphy is combined with an anterior vaginal repair, voiding difficulty may be worse because plication of the levator ani muscles contributes to pain and spasm of the pelvic floor, with a subsequent inability to relax these muscles to initiate micturition. Osteitis pubis has been seen following anterior repair, and if the surgeon unwittingly unroofs a urethral diverticulum during the course of the dissection, a urethrovaginal fistula may occur.

It is clear that master surgeons can achieve good success with this technique. It is also clear, from looking at the literature, that the success rates for this operation vary greatly from one surgeon to the next. Because of the declining number of patients requiring vaginal surgery in any one surgeon's practice, few surgeons have the extensive experience that it takes to perfect these skill-intensive techniques. Fortunately, other surgical techniques are available that have proven to be reliable in the hands of many individuals. These provide the practitioner with alternatives which should prove to be more reliable for the average surgeon. Considering all factors together, we believe that the anterior vaginal repair is a poor choice of operation in the hands of most gynecologic surgeons, and that choosing this procedure for a patient with stress incontinence requires special justification based on individual circumstances.

Retropubic Operations
Marshall-Marchetti-Krantz Procedure

In 1949, Drs. Marshall, Marchetti, and Krantz, of Cornell University Medical Center, described a simple retropubic operation for the cure of stress incontinence by suturing the periurethral tissues to the back of the pubic symphysis. Interestingly, their first case was a 54-year old man who had severe incontinence following a radical abdominoperineal resection of the rectum and two subsequent transurethral resections of the prostate. Although initially an entirely empirical operation, this operation has since been well-studied and has become a standard part of both urologic and gynecologic surgery.

The operation works by stabilizing the suburethral fascia to prevent excessive displacement of the urethra during periods of increased physical stress. It also can induce an element of urethral obstruction by kinking the urethra.

In general, this operation is done with the patient in a modified lithotomy position (such as using Allen stirrups) to provide simultaneous access to the vagina and the abdomen. A low abdominal incision is made and the space of Retzius is entered and developed. Dissection of the space of Retzius must be carried out right up against the back of the pubic symphysis in order to avoid cystotomy. This is particularly important if the patient has had a previous retropubic operation, in which case scarring can be severe. The surgeon's hand is placed in the vagina to identify the bladder neck and urethra, aided by the placement of a Foley catheter. The periurethral fascia on each side of the urethra is exposed. Suture is passed through this region and then through the back of the pubic symphysis, elevating and kinking the urethra as the sutures are tied (Fig. 7.2).

The critical step of the procedure is placement of the sutures. The entire repair depends upon the strength with which the suture is anchored into the paraurethral fascia. It is very important to place the anchoring suture deeply, incorporating a large piece of tissue. This is easiest to achieve by elevating this tissue with a finger placed in the vagina, and driving the needle through the entire thickness of the fascia and vaginal wall. Placing the suture in a figure-of-eight fashion is helpful. The strength of this suture should be tested by pulling on it forcefully to make sure that it is anchored into the tissue before attaching it to the pubic bone. In reoperating on patients with recurrent stress incontinence after a previous MMK, the original suture is often found to have been placed only in the adipose tissue in the space of Retzius, and not anchored successfully into the periurethral fascia. The entire integrity of the repair depends upon anchoring this suture securely into the deep tissues around the vesical neck. This must not be neglected.

A number of modifications of this operation have been described over the years. These include variations in the point of attachment of the sutures, either directly to the pubic bone or to the symphyseal cartilage; additional plication of the vesical neck or the "crossover" technique in which sutures on one side are crossed over the urethra and sutured to the pubic symphysis on the contralateral side; the type of suture used (absorbable versus nonabsorbable); and the number of sutures placed (from one to three or more on each side). Some authors use a technique in which the dome of the bladder is opened and the level of the bladder neck is identified with a finger inside the bladder itself while the suspensory sutures are placed. This allows direct visualization of the bladder, ureters, and proximal urethra to make sure that sutures are not placed through any of these structures; however, it also increases the morbidity of the procedure.

The "MMK" operation has numerous advantages. It is straightforward, reliable, and relatively quick to perform. Its success depends upon direct attachment of the periurethral tissues to the back of the pubic symphysis rather than upon the integrity of intervening structures. Unlike the anterior colporrhaphy, there is relatively little variation in published success rates, and there has been widespread experience with the operation in many hands.

There are, however, difficulties with this operation. Urethral kinking or stricture can create severe postoperative voiding difficulties which may not resolve. Suture placement near or into the urethra can lead to chronic irritative voiding symptoms. Because the operation supports only the urethra, it cannot correct a significant coexisting cystocele and additional surgery may be necessary to correct this problem. Although the MMK operation does not provide enough elevation to correct a cystocele, it can still produce enough anterior elevation to change the axis of the vagina, pulling the cul-de-sac forward and open, and allowing a postoperative enterocele to develop. In patients who have had a hysterectomy, the MMK operation can predispose to the development of complete vaginal

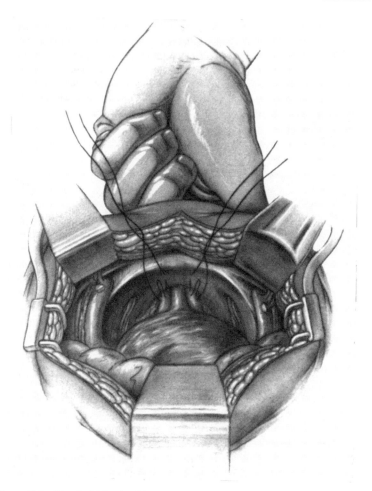

Figure 7.2 Marshall-Marchetti-Krantz procedure. The periurethral endopelvic fascia is elevated by the surgeon's finger and a "double-bite" stitch is placed through the full thickness of this tissue down to the vaginal mucosa. The initial suture is placed in the lateral margin of the periurethral fascia and an extra supporting bite is taken close to the urethra. The stitch is completed by an anchoring bite driven into the periosteum of the pubic symphysis. Two additional sutures may be placed proximally, on each side, up to the region of the urethrovesical junction. (From Mattingly RF, Thompson JD (Eds). TeLinde's Operative Gynecology, 6th ed. Philadelphia: JB Lippincott, 1985, with permission.)

vault prolapse. Obliteration of the cul-de-sac should therefore be considered at the time of surgery to prevent this from happening, if possible.

Among the most troublesome complications of the procedure is osteitis pubis, which may develop in up to 5% of patients undergoing this operation. This is a serious complication which can totally disable an otherwise healthy woman for months. These patients have severe pain in the region of the pubic symphysis which may radiate down the whole pelvic girdle. Characteristic x-ray findings have been described, but these are not present consistently and the diagnosis is usually made on clinical grounds alone. Some of these patients are merely uncomfortable; others may have to use a walker to move around; others may be bedridden. The condition usually remits spontaneously, but it can last for months, and may become chronic. Treatment consists primarily of reassurance, nonsteroidal anti-inflammatory drugs, and patience.

A number of errors are commonly made in the performance of this operation.

The most common of these is incorrect suture placement. Due to inadequate dissection or exposure, sutures are often placed into the bladder itself rather than in the periurethral fascia. This elevates the anterior bladder up against the pubic symphysis and does nothing to correct the underlying defect. The result is surgical failure. Similarly, sutures may be placed into or completely through the urethra, leading to the development of irritative, painful, postoperative symptoms. Inadequate anchoring of sutures is also a problem. Timidity on the part of the surgeon can lead to a failure to incorporate adequate tissue in the suture near the urethra or failure to fix the suture deeply enough into the pubic bone. Subsequent suture pullout can result in failure. Finally, use of absorbable suture, such as chromic catgut, rather than permanent or delayed-absorbable materials, can lead to failure if there is inadequate apposition of raw surfaces and subsequent formation of weak scar tissue. If permanent sutures are used, the surgeon must be sure that they have not penetrated the bladder or a stone will develop.

Burch Colposuspension
Operation

Faced with many of these problems in his own practice—particularly the problem of inadequate suture fixation and frequent suture pullout from the pubic periosteum—Dr. John Burch, of Nashville, Tennessee, set out to find an alternate location in which to anchor his periurethral sutures. After trying—and abandoning—suture placement into the fascia over the obturator internus muscle, he lit upon the ileopectineal ligament of Cooper as his preferred point of fixation. Since his original description of the procedure in 1961, the Burch operation (referred to as the "colposuspension operation" in British literature) has become one of the most commonly performed and best studied procedures for stress incontinence.

The operation works through two main mechanisms. Like the MMK operation, the Burch procedure stabilizes the suburethral fascia and urethra to prevent excess mobility under stress, thereby allowing the urethra to be compressed closed when abdominal pressure forces it against the underlying fascia. It also creates a different continence mechanism by repositioning the urethra and bladder neck so that the bladder base swings down below these newly elevated structures causing posterior compression. Depending on how high the bladder neck is elevated at the time of surgery, the operation can also introduce an element of obstruction.

Since the original description by Burch, a number of modifications of the operation have been introduced. These primarily involve the amount of bladder mobilization, the number and type of sutures placed, and the degree of suture bridging between the bladder neck and Cooper's ligament (Figs. 7.3–7.6). Some surgeons prefer merely to expose the perivesical fascia, pass sutures through it, and tie them under minimal tension. Other surgeons perform a thorough dissection of the lateral bladder neck, mobilizing the bladder and pushing it medially to expose the underlying fascia. While this increases the mobility of the bladder neck dramatically, allowing much greater elevation when the supporting sutures are tied down, it can also lead to significant hemorrhaging if the perivesical veins are lacerated. When it occurs, this bleeding can be difficult to control. Some surgeons place sutures along the urethra as well as at the lateral bladder neck; others avoid this, placing sutures only at the level of the bladder neck and then more proximally along the bladder edge to correct the cystocele, feeling that this reduces urethral kinking and diminishes postoperative voiding difficulty.

"Ideally," the Burch operation puts the edge of the vagina in direct apposition to Cooper's ligament; however, in some patients there is not enough vaginal mobility to permit this, and bridging or "bowstringing" of the sutures results. This may be especially marked in the postmenopausal woman with a stenotic vagina. There is no reliable marker for how tight to pull the sutures other than "feel" and experience. Bowstringing of the sutures by itself does not appear to matter very much if adequate elevation and stabilization of the bladder neck has been achieved, as long as permanent sutures have been used for the bladder neck suspension.

The Burch colposuspension has many advantages over the MMK. It can

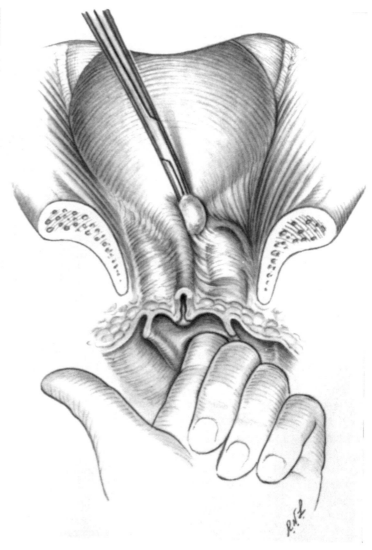

Figure 7.3   Burch colposuspension. The anterior vagina is elevated with the operator's finger as the bladder is mobilized medially to expose the underlying endopelvic fascia. (From Stanton SL, Tanagho EA (Eds). Surgery of Female Incontinence, 2nd ed. New York: Springer-Verlag, 1986, with permission.)

correct a coexistent cystocele, which the MMK procedure does not do adequately. The Burch procedure does not create osteitis pubis. Like the MMK operation it is direct, reliable, and straightforward and does not depend upon indirect attachments for success. There is widespread experience with this operation worldwide, and it has been subjected to more rigorous investigation than nearly any other operation for stress incontinence. The published success rates are consistently high, and in comparative surgical studies the colposuspension consistently has the highest objective cure rates at postoperative urodynamic testing of any "standard" operation for stress incontinence.

However, no operation is perfect, and neither is this one. Because the success of the operation depends upon elevating the vagina (hence, "colposuspension"), the operation is poorly suited to patients with reduced vaginal capacity and mobility, as is often the case in older women who may not be sexually active.

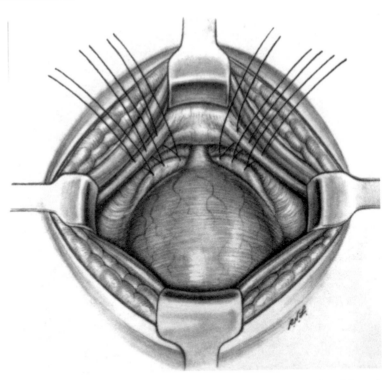

Figure 7.4 Burch colposuspension. Three permanent sutures are placed through the endopelvic fascia distal proximal to the bladder neck and passed through the ileopectineal ligament of Cooper. (From Stanton SL, Tanagho EA (Eds). Surgery of Female Incontinence, 2nd ed. New York: Springer-Verlag, 1986, with permission.)

On the other hand, successful surgery in women with normal vaginal capacity and mobility may lead to an altered vaginal axis. By placing the bladder neck in a high retropubic position the Burch colposuspension cures stress incontinence, but also pulls the anterior vagina forward (Fig. 7.6). Since the vagina is a muscular tube, pulling the anterior vagina forward also pulls the posterior vagina forward. Indeed, one can often feel a posterior vaginal "ridge" after surgery. Although this ridge usually relaxes over time, it may cause dyspareunia, particularly in the postoperative period. By altering the vaginal axis in this way, the cul de-sac is pulled open allowing potential enterocele formation and the worsening of previously asymptomatic rectoceles. Up to 28% of patients undergoing a Burch colposuspension may require an additional future operation for some type of prolapse.

The high success rate of the Burch procedure in curing stress incontinence also often comes at the expense of voiding function. The high success rate of this operation in curing stress incontinence is due, in part, to the fact that it is a partially obstructive procedure. Difficulty voiding, both short-term and long-term, can be a significant complication of this technique, particularly if the sutures are pulled tight to achieve maximal elevation of the bladder neck. Pre- and postoperative urodynamic studies of patients who have undergone this procedure clearly demonstrate altered voiding with lower mean and peak flow rates and higher voiding pressures. Some patients may have to use clean intermittent self-catheterization for an indefinite period of time following this type of surgery.

The common errors with this operation are similar to those encountered with the MMK. In particular, use of chromic catgut suture for bladder neck suspension of any type should be condemned as leading to an unacceptably high failure rate. In rare circumstances the elevating vaginal finger can be pushed through

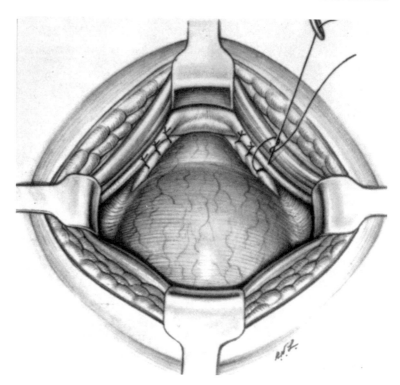

Figure 7.5   Burch colposuspension. The permanent sutures are tied down, elevating the perivesical endopelvic fascia and the bladder neck. If extensive mobilization is done, the anterior vagina can be brought into direct apposition to Cooper's ligament. If less extensive dissection is undertaken, the elevation achieved may not be as dramatic. "Bowstringing" of the sutures does not appear to affect surgical success rates very much, providing permanent sutures are used. (From Stanton SL, Tanagho EA (Eds). Surgery of Female Incontinence, 2nd ed. New York: Springer-Verlag, 1986, with permission.)

the vagina, creating an inadvertent colpotomy. This may simply be sutured over and the operation continued. There is no significant danger of infection from placing sutures through the entire thickness of the anterior vaginal wall. Without exception these sutures are re-epithelialized and do not cause problems, whereas fear of perforating the vagina with sutures (or fear of the surgeon suturing his own finger) may lead to inadequate anchoring of the supporting sutures with subsequent pullout and surgical failure. Although rare, it is possible to obstruct a ureter when lateral sutures are placed. Avoidance of this problem at the time of surgery is discussed in Chapter 16, "Urologic Injury in Gynecologic Surgery." It is advisable to establish ureteral patency and exclude suture perforation of the bladder by cystoscopy at the conclusion of this, or any other, anti-incontinence operation.

Paravaginal Repair (Vagino-Obturator Shelf)

Unlike the MMK and the Burch operations, which are empiric operations for stress incontinence, the paravaginal repair is based upon careful consideration of the anatomy of the continence mechanism in females. Support for the bladder neck is provided by the anterior vagina and endopelvic fascia, which attach on each side to the lateral pelvic sidewalls at the "white line" of the arcus tendineus fasciae pelvis and form a shelf of tissue underneath the bladder neck and urethra. This layer allows them to be compressed closed in an anterior-posterior fashion during periods of stress. When this supportive mechanism becomes loosened due to the trauma of childbirth, or for other reasons, the stability of this supportive layer of fascia diminishes and may ultimately fail, leading to increased bladder

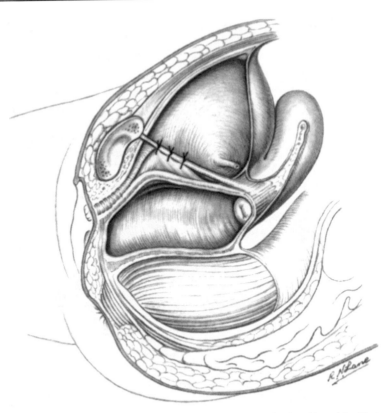

Figure 7.6 Burch colposuspension. Oblique view of the final position of the bladder neck following completion of the operation. Note the high tenting of the anterior vagina which can distort the vaginal architecture. (From Stanton SL, Tanagho EA (Eds). Surgery of Female Incontinence, 2nd ed. New York: Springer-Verlag, 1986, with permission.)

neck mobility and the development of stress incontinence (Fig. 7.7). The paravaginal repair operation reestablishes the lateral pelvic attachments of this layer of endopelvic fascia and restores the stability of this layer by correcting the fundamental anatomic defect which is present in most cases: lateral detachment of the vagina and endopelvic fascia from the arcus tendineus fasciae pelvis (Figs. 7.7–7.9).

In his 1961 article, where he described his search for a better point of suture attachment during retropubic cystourethropexy, John Burch states that he passed his sutures from the perivesical region to the fascia of the obturator internus muscle, but abandoned it as a technique because he felt that the attachment was not strong enough. He gave no follow-up on the patients so operated. Subsequently, Cullen Richardson described an operation in which defects where the endopelvic fascia had become separated from the arcus tendineus fascia pelvis could be identified on one or both sides in patients with stress incontinence. Repair of these defects could then be accomplished by reapproximating the endopelvic fascia and lateral vagina to the pelvic sidewall on each side, reinforcing and resuturing it. If necessary, this can be done along the entire length of the arcus from just below the pubic symphysis to the ischial spine. This operation, which is done through a low abdominal incision, restores continence by recreating the normal lateral suspensory mechanism of the anterior vagina and restoring the resiliency of the "trampoline" on which the bladder normally rests.

A similar operation was devised by the distinguished British urologist Richard Turner-Warwick. He called this operation the "vagino-obturator shelf" proce-

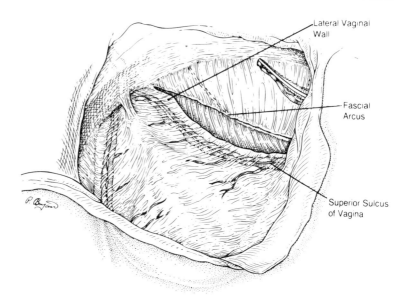

Figure 7.7   Paravaginal repair. Identification of a lateral paravaginal defect. The lateral vaginal wall and its accompanying endopelvic fascia have become separated from their normal attachments to the fascial arcus. (From Richardson AC. Contemporary Ob/Gyn 1990; 35(9):100–09, with permission.)

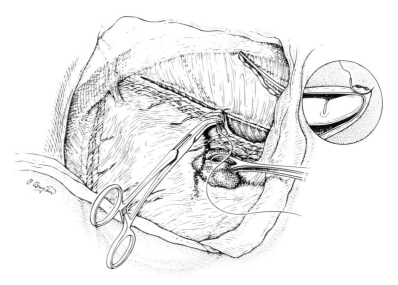

Figure 7.8   Paravaginal repair. Placement of the first medial bite or "key" stitch, which stretches the endopelvic fascia taut and anchors it back into place along the arcus tendineus fascia pelvis. (From Richardson AC. Contemporary Ob/Gyn 1990; 35(9):100–09, with permission.)

dure. This operation involves opening the space of Retzius, exposing and incising the lateral pelvic fascia at the level of the bladder neck, and then pulling the vagina through this incision and suturing it laterally to the fascia over the obturator internus muscle. Incising the endopelvic fascia to expose the underlying levator muscles and vagina allows the surgeon to take exceptionally firm bites of tissue without inadvertently incorporating the bladder into the suture. The

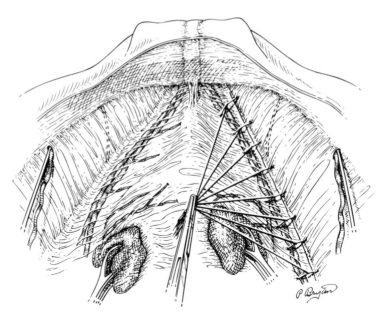

Figure 7.9 Paravaginal repair. Completed repair, showing re-attachment of the separated tissues to their normal supports along the fascial arcus. (From Richardson AC. Contemporary Ob/Gyn 1990; 35(9):100–09.)

fascial incision also creates raw surfaces which should form more scar tissue than would be the case if the fascia were simply pulled up, folded over, and reapproximated to the arcus tendineus fasciae pelvis. The functional results of this operation are almost identical to the paravaginal repair.

The main advantages of this type of procedure are that it restores normal or nearly normal anatomy, rather than creating some form of compensatory anatomic abnormality. The bladder neck is returned to its normal or near normal position without overelevation. As a result, postoperative voiding difficulty is greatly reduced. In fact, some surgeons have used this type of procedure with good results to correct obstructed voiding which has developed following a retropubic bladder neck suspension. Because high suspension of the bladder neck is avoided, the incidence of postoperative rectocele, enterocele, and vaginal vault prolapse seems to be much lower than with other operations. Since dissection of the bladder neck is largely avoided, the potential for significant hemorrhaging from the perivesical venous plexus is also diminished (but not eliminated).

The main disadvantage of this operation is that it does not yet have a proven track record. While certain individual surgeons have presented successful series, these results have not yet been duplicated by large numbers of other surgeons. There are, as yet, no good scientific evaluations of this operation, with pre- and postoperative urodynamic studies. The claims that stress incontinence is cured while maintaining normal postoperative voiding function have not yet been substantiated by objective urodynamic data, and neither has there been objective follow-up of patients who have undergone this operation to determine the long-term sustained cure rate.

Although the operation can be performed as a vaginal procedure, the paravaginal repair is currently almost always performed as an abdominal procedure. The operation involves extensive retroperitoneal dissection and surgery deep in the pelvis. Knowledge of the anatomy of this area is important to avoid damage to the ureters and the obturator neurovascular bundle. Chromic suture should not be used in the performance of this operation, as many of the tissue surfaces

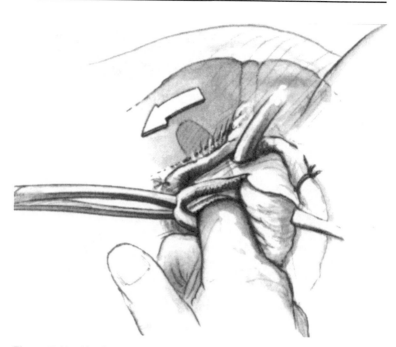

Figure 7.10 Needle suspension. The anterior vaginal wall is opened and the retropubic space is entered through blunt dissection. With the tip of the index finger flexed anteriorly against the posterior pubic symphysis, the paraurethral attachment to the pubic bone is perforated downward (in the direction of the *arrow*) toward the ischial spine, completely detaching the endopelvic fascia. (From Hurt WG (Ed). Urogynecologic Surgery. Gaithersburg, MD: Aspen Publications, 1992, with permission.)

**Needle Suspension
Procedures**

which are approximated along the arcus tendineus are not raw, and healing under these circumstances may not produce as firm a scar as would otherwise normally be expected. Permanent suture, such as Ethibond or Ticron, probably gives better, longer lasting results.

Needle suspension procedures for genuine stress incontinence attach long sutures from the periurethral tissues to the anterior abdominal wall by penetrating the space of Retzius with a long suture carrier (Figs. 7.10–7.13). These procedures require a combined abdominal and vaginal approach. These operations cure stress incontinence by stabilizing the suburethral fascia and urethra to prevent excess mobility.

The first needle suspension operation was developed by an American gynecologist, Armand J. Pereyra, in the 1950's, as a modification of the MMK operation which avoided the need to open the space of Retzius. The original procedure involved the use of a specially designed 10-inch suture carrier with two prongs—a needle cannula and a trocar—which allowed a double penetration of the anterior vaginal wall after the instrument had been inserted through an abdominal incision and advanced through the space of Retzius to a point just lateral to the bladder neck. After penetrating the anterior vaginal wall, the trocar and cannula tips were threaded with No. 30 stainless steel wire, which was pulled up through the carrier tract and tied over the suprapubic abdominal fascia, elevating the urethra and bladder neck. The technique has proved very popular and many surgeons have made minor modifications of this procedure and attached their names to them as ''unique'' operations; however, Dr. Pereyra devoted much of his surgical career to modifying and experimenting with this technique, and there are essentially no modifications in use today which were not first described by him.

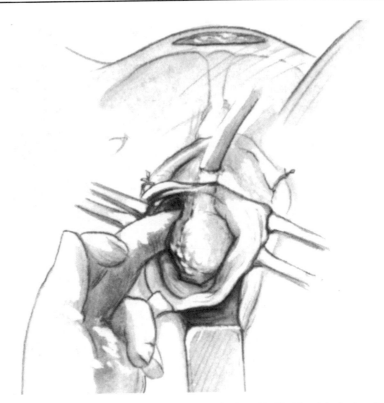

Figure 7.11 Needle suspension. One finger is placed behind the detached endo-pelvic fascia, mobilizing it into the vaginal operative field to facilitate placement of the helical anchoring sutures. (From Hurt WG (Ed), Urogynecologic Surgery. Gaithersburg, MD: Aspen Publications, 1992, with permission.)

The modifications which Dr. Pereyra and subsequent surgeons have made, can be grouped into five categories: the type of vaginal dissection, the method of suture anchoring, the way in which the space of Retzius is traversed, the method of abdominal fixation, and the use of endoscopy.

The operation is usually begun in a fashion similar to that of anterior colporrhaphy. An incision is made in the anterior vagina, which is thereafter dissected to expose the urethra and bladder neck. Needles are passed either transvaginally or transabdominally through the space of Retzius, and the suture fixed to the perivesical fascia at the bladder neck and to the abdominal fascia. Some authors prefer to use a midline vaginal incision, while others make an inverted "U" or inverted "T" incision in this area. Some authors carry the dissection out laterally through the endopelvic fascia and bluntly penetrate the space of Retzius from below; others do not, simply using the needle to "poke through." Many surgeons prefer to mobilize this area extensively prior to fixation, while others do not.

Because this operation depends almost entirely upon the integrity of the suture material and the permanence of tissue fixation for its success, the method of suture fixation to the perivesical fascia is of crucial importance. In patients with weak fascia or poor connective tissue, there is a tendency for many types of suture fixation to fail, either pulling out of the vaginal tissues or "cheese wiring" through them with the result that support is lost and incontinence recurs. This has proven to be a significant problem with the Dacron bolsters recommended by Stamey. In his technique the suture is passed through the tissues, a small bead or bolster of Dacron or silastic is threaded over the suture, which is then brought through the tissues again. This method of anchoring appears to be particularly susceptible to pull-through. A more secure way of fastening sutures

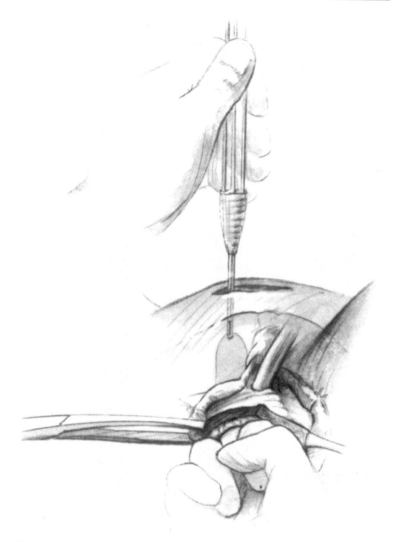

Figure 7.12   Needle suspension. With the vaginal dissection complete, a low suprapubic incision is made down to the level of the anterior rectus fascia. The long needle is passed under direct finger guidance. The vaginal finger is inserted to the posterior aspect of the rectus muscle (From Hurt WG (Ed). Urogynecologic Surgery. Gaithersburg, MD: Aspen Publications, 1992, with permission.)

to the tissues at the bladder neck is by incorporating wide helical bites of tissue which provide a more durable basis for secure support. Gittes recommends a ''no incision'' technique in which needles are passed through the abdomen and vagina without incision or dissection. The vaginal end is affixed with heavy through and through mattress sutures of nonabsorbable monofilament suture. The abdominal ends of the sutures are tied down into the abdominal fat. A success rate of 87% has been claimed with this technique, although no objective data have been presented to confirm this and the longevity of its results remains in doubt.

Techniques for traversing the space of Retzius include open or closed procedures and single- or double-pronged needle carriers. Closed procedures traverse the space of Retzius blindly by pushing the suture carrier from either the vaginal or abdominal end until it comes out on the other side. Great care must be taken not to penetrate the bladder or urethra if this is done. Most surgeons prefer an

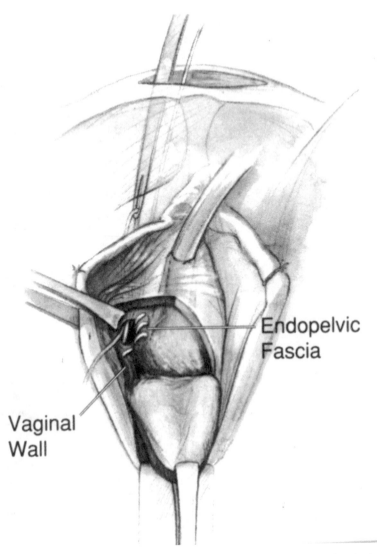

Figure 7.13   Needle suspension. A helical suture is placed through the detached endopelvic fascia and anchored in the full thickness of the vaginal wall, excluding the epithelium. (From Hurt WG (Ed). Urogynecologic Surgery. Gaithersburg, MD: Aspen Publications, 1992, with permission.)

open technique in which the endopelvic fascia is punctured and a finger is inserted into the space of Retzius and pushed up until it is just below the rectus fascia. The needle is then inserted through the abdominal fascia until it touches the surgeon's finger, which then guides it through the space of Retzius to the vaginal side. Several surgeons have modified Pereyras's double-pronged needle carriers to suit their own tastes. The double-pronged carriers are somewhat more cumbersome to use, but obviate the need for another puncture to bring the trailing end of the suture out so that the ends can be tied abdominally.

Abdominal fixation of the sutures can be attained by several techniques. They may be tied separately on each side of one long incision, or in separate stab incisions on each side of the abdomen, or tied together in the midline. They may be tied down over buttresses or not. Leach has developed a technique which exposes the periosteum behind the pubic symphysis and fixes the suture to the periosteum of the pubic tubercle.

Finally, the most important innovation in needle suspension procedures for stress incontinence was the addition of endoscopic control, advocated by Stamey. While this has not proved particularly useful in determining how much tension to use when tying down the sutures, it has proved invaluable in eliminating injury to the bladder and urethra. The suture carrier can either be passed under direct cystoscopic guidance to avoid bladder penetration, or cystoscopy can be carried out after the sutures are in place but before they are tied. It is essential to detect bladder injury by performing cystoscopy while the needles are in place, since the sutures may hide between folds in the bladder urothelium whereas the larger needle shaft is easily visible. Endoscopic evaluation of patients undergoing a needle suspension procedure is now the standard of care.

Needle suspension operations have many advantages. They are fast, often taking 30 minutes or less to accomplish. They are relatively easy to perform, even on obese patients, and they carry a low morbidity when properly done. They may be incorporated into many other kinds of vaginal operations as well.

However, there are also many distinct disadvantages to this kind of surgery. Success with this technique depends upon the integrity of a single suture—not tissue healing—and a single point of anchoring. If either of these two components fails, the chances of developing recurrent incontinence are high. There is no controlled endpoint for bladder neck elevation, so the tension on the sutures is variable. The results may range from failure to cure stress incontinence due to inadequate elevation to complete bladder neck obstruction. The operation is easily compromised by poor connective tissue, which allows suture pull-through. If buttresses are used on either side, there is potential for infection and erosion of foreign bodies, and this may occur years after the original operation. It is not uncommon for patients who have had needle suspension operations to develop postoperative pain or dyspareunia from the suture or buttresses. Many patients who have had these operations complain of pulling pain when they assume certain positions which cause twisting of the ''guy wires'' which support the bladder neck and urethra. There is a definite possibility of producing significant hemorrhage in the space of Retzius from lacerating the perivesical veins, and when this occurs it may be difficult to achieve hemostasis due to the poor surgical exposure. Similarly, in careless hands it is possible to do significant damage to the bladder and urethra from laceration and/or suture perforation which, if undetected, can lead to erosion, infection, and bladder stone formation. Overelevation of the bladder neck also predisposes the patient to enterocele formation by opening the posterior cul-de-sac of Douglas. In spite of the claims made by many surgeons, the long-term success of these operations has not been proven and objective urodynamic evaluation of outcome has generally not been carried out.

Several basic errors are commonly made in performing this operation. First among these is the use of absorbable suture material. Since there is no direct contact between raw tissues, scar tissue formation is minimal. If absorbable suture is used, when it dissolves nothing is left to support the repair and the incontinence will return. Inadequate anchoring of sutures has similar consequences. Many surgeons also omit to correct other pelvic relaxation such as a rectocele, enterocele, or uterine prolapse at the same operation, either from failure to understand the pathology involved or the inability to perform such operations. This leads to unnecessary postoperative complications and repeat surgery. Either over- or underelevation of the bladder neck can present with problems following surgery as noted above. Finally, inadequate cystoscopy and failure to detect suture perforation of the bladder and/or urethra remains a problem leading to the formation of stones.

We mention one final modification of the Pereyra needle suspension which has been found to create significant problems. A procedure called the ''four corner bladder suspension'' has been developed to correct large cystoceles using a needle suspension technique. This operation uses four sutures, two at the bladder neck and two placed proximally at the upper edges of the cystocele, all four sutures being brought out through the same abdominal incision and tied. This operation corrects the cystocele by standing the vagina upside down, pulling its axis forward and upward while elevating the vagina, uterus, and cul-de-sac up and away from the posterior supporting levator plate. This provides a wide open invitation for rapidly progressive genital prolapse and enterocele formation.

Sling Procedures

Sling procedures involve the placement of a strip of natural or synthetic material under the proximal urethra and bladder neck. This strap or ''sling'' is then attached to either the pelvis or the anterior abdominal wall. Sling operations can either be supportive or obstructive in nature. Supportive slings can cure stress incontinence by providing posterior urethral support which permits urethral compression during periods of increased intra-abdominal pressure. An obstructive sling creates intentional urethral obstruction to prevent urine loss and is used mainly as a ''salvage'' procedure. The main role of sling procedures is in the patient with adequate urethral support who has stress incontinence because of an open vesical neck or intrinsic sphincteric dysfunction.

Sling procedures are generally performed as combined abdominal and vaginal operations. Sometimes an additional procedure is also needed to harvest autologous tissue (such as fascia lata from the thigh) which is then used as the material for the sling. Adequate exposure of the proximal urethra and bladder neck must be obtained in order to perform a sling operation. Generally this is done by vaginal dissection, but it may also be accomplished abdominally by exposing the bladder neck and dissecting a tunnel beneath the proximal urethra. The space of Retzius is penetrated—either from above or from below—and the sling material is passed underneath the urethra, up through the incision on either side of the bladder neck, to the point of attachment where the strap is fixed into place. As with needle suspensions procedures, there have been many modifications of the sling procedure (Figs. 7.14–7.19). These involve choice of material used for the sling (Table 7.3), site of sling attachment, method of dissection, and the amount of sling tension.

Many natural and synthetic materials have been used for creating slings. The natural materials are either homologous materials—most often autologous tissues taken from other sites of the same patient's body—or heterologous tissues that have been taken from other animal species and processed to become suitable

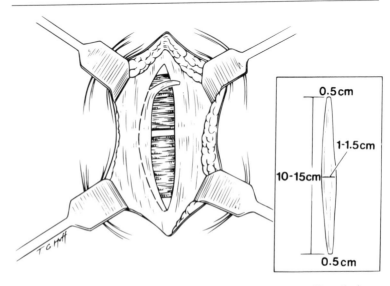

Figure 7.14   Pubovaginal sling. A strip of rectus fascia is harvested from the lower leaf of the fascial incision. The fascial incision runs to the lateral border of the rectus muscles. (From Hurt WG (Ed). Urogynecologic Surgery. Gaithersburg, MD: Aspen Publishers, 1992, with permission.)

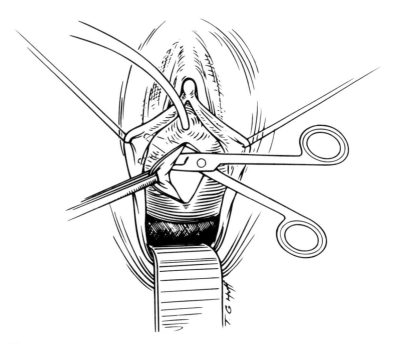

Figure 7.15 Pubovaginal sling. The anterior vagina has been opened at the level of the bladder neck, and the retropubic space is entered from below. The scissors are kept flat and parallel to the perineum. (From Hurt WG (Ed). Urogynecologic Surgery. Gaithersburg, MD: Aspen Publishers, 1992, with permission.)

for surgery. The most common heterologous tissues used in sling surgery are porcine dermis and ox dura mater. The most common autologous materials are fascia lata, which is harvested from the patient's lateral thigh, or abdominal fascia. If abdominal rectus fascia is used, the incision can be carried down to the pubic symphysis and the rest of the operation can be performed through the same incision. The development of synthetic fibers has led to the proliferation of many artificial materials of consistent strength and texture which have been used in sling procedures. The main drawbacks to the use of autologous materials are inconsistent strength, the necessity of performing an additional procedure to harvest them with its attendant risks, and the problem of scar tissue formation. The use of materials from other human donors runs the risk of tissue rejection in the recipient or transmission of serious viral infections. The use of animal tissues presents potential problems with supply, tissue rejection, and disease transmission. The main risks involved with synthetic materials are graft erosion and infection with a foreign body in situ. These have been particular problems when the material is inserted through a vaginal incision.

Variations also exist in the technique of dissection. It is possible to expose and dissect the bladder neck and create a suburethral tunnel solely through an abdominal incision. However, this procedure runs a greater risk of bladder or urethral perforation than when the dissection is done vaginally. The advantage of the abdominal technique is that the vagina is not opened into the space of Retzius, which diminishes the potential for contamination of the abdomen by vaginal flora. While this has not been a problem when natural materials have been used, it remains a serious drawback to the use of synthetic slings. Other sling procedures, such as the Aldridge rectus fascia sling, use a combined approach in which the abdomen and vagina are both opened, materials are passed from one side to the other, and then both are closed. Some surgeons perform a vaginal dissection to expose the urethra and bladder neck, but only open the abdomen down to the level of the rectus fascia. Sutures or sling materials are then passed

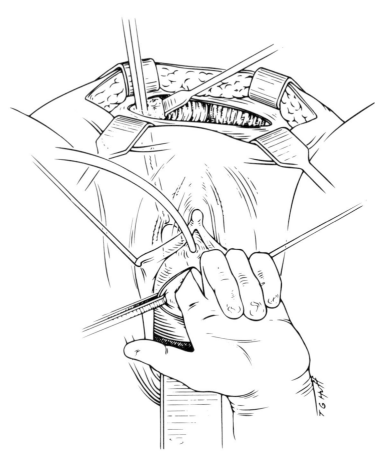

Figure 7.16   Pubovaginal sling. A long clamp is passed down through the abdominal incision under direct finger guidance. (From Hurt WG (Ed). Urogynecologic Surgery. Gaithersburg, MD: Aspen Publishers, 1992, with permission.)

from below upwards through small puncture incisions, much as in the fashion of a needle suspension procedure.

The anterior rectus fascia is the point of attachment most commonly used for a sling. The ends of the sling are commonly sewn to the rectus sheath on each side where they come up through the space of Retzius. Alternatively, there are ''patch'' techniques in which permanent sutures are placed on each side of the patch of sling material. These are then passed up to the rectus fascia and tied. Patch procedures are essentially sling modifications of needle suspension procedures. Less commonly, a sling may be attached to some other point of suspension, such as Stanton's silastic sling, which is placed below the urethra and bladder neck and then affixed to Cooper's ligament in much the same way as the sutures are placed for a Burch colposuspension procedure.

The most difficult part of a sling procedure is determining the amount of tension to place on the sling. Among the techniques which have been used to determine this are by evaluation of the axis of urethral inclination using a modified ''Q-tip test'' to obtain a Q-tip angle of 15° below the horizontal; by using a cystoscope to watch bladder neck closure and tying the sling at just the tension necessary to close the bladder neck; and by ''feel''—tying the sling so that it just ''feels right'' in the hands of an experienced surgeon. Measurement of the angle of urethral inclination will vary from patient to patient, technique to technique, and is cumbersome. It will also be different when the patient is awake

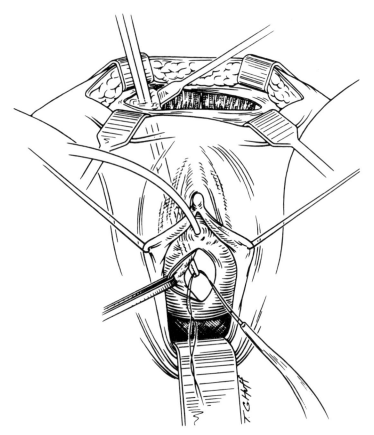

Figure 7.17 Pubovaginal sling. Permanent sutures have been placed on each end of the fascial strap. The ends of the sutures are grasped with the long clamp prior to pulling them up into the abdomen. (From Hurt WG (Ed). Urogynecologic Surgery. Gaithersburg, MD: Aspen Publishers, 1992, with permission.)

and ambulatory than when the patient is fully anesthetized. The point at which the bladder neck closes under tension is dependent upon cystoscopic technique and the point in the urethra at which the scope is placed during observation of the bladder neck. In the final analysis, it is the surgeon's skill and experience which determines how tight to make a sling.

Almost without exception the surgeon who is beginning to do sling procedures will make the sling too tight. The amount of tension necessary to provide support and compression for the urethra is far less than one would expect. As a general rule, one cannot make a sling too loose. Most experienced surgeons place a sling loosely enough to insert the index finger of the gloved hand between the sling and the bladder neck. If the sling is too tight, continence will be achieved at the expense of voiding function and the patient may have chronic urinary retention. In some cases, where slings are being used as salvage procedures, this is done intentionally; for the most part, however, the aim of the sling operation is to create support, not obstruction. The problem of postoperative bladder neck obstruction is compounded by the fact that some materials, such as Gore-Tex, appear to shrink significantly after insertion, increasing the amount of tension on the sling.

The main advantage of sling procedures is that they have a very high cure rate for genuine stress incontinence. They can cure stress incontinence due to intrinsic sphincteric dysfunction, whereas most other procedures can only cure

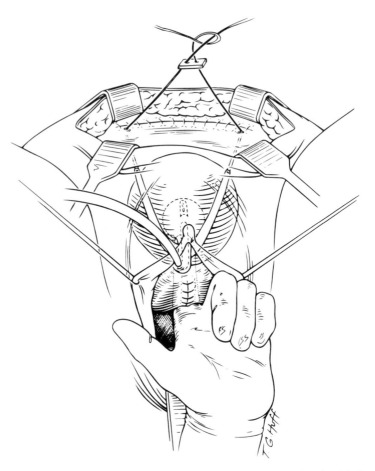

Figure 7.18 Pubovaginal sling. Once the sutures on both ends of the fascial sling have been pulled through into the abdomen, the tension on the sling must be checked. The sling sutures are passed through the lower fascial leaf and tied over a pledget. The fascial incision should be closed prior to tying the knot. (From Hurt WG (Ed). Urogynecologic Surgery. Gaithersburg, MD: Aspen Publisher, 1992, with permission.)

stress incontinence due to bladder neck displacement or hypermobility. Slings are generally independent of local tissue strength and have advantages where local tissues are weakened, scarred, or otherwise compromised by previous surgery or congenital anomalies.

The main disadvantage of the sling procedures is that there is *significant* potential for severe, long-term voiding dysfunction. This may require prolonged postoperative catheterization or clean intermittent self-catheterization, perhaps for life. If obstruction occurs, the chance of developing recurrent urinary incontinence due to detrusor instability is present and significant. This can make some patients wetter than they were before surgery and may be very difficult to control.

The most common errors that are made in performing sling procedures are (*a*) making the sling too tight, and (*b*) *making the sling too tight*. The end result is obstructed voiding and unstable bladder activity. In certain circumstances an obstructive sling with planned postoperative intermittent self-catheterization will be needed, but this should be the exception rather than the rule. Lower urinary tract damage may also occur either through direct penetration or injury at the time of surgery, or by subsequent sling erosion. Erosion and/or infection tends to be a much greater problem with artificial materials or heterologous tissue transplants than when the patient's own tissues are used.

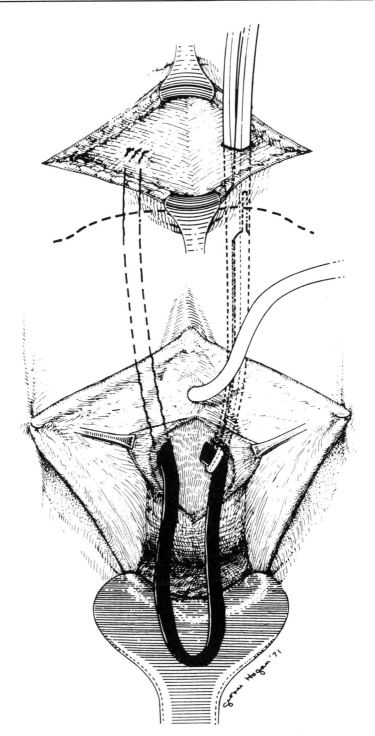

Figure 7.19   Fascia lata urethrovesical sling. In this type of sling a long strip of fascia lata, harvested from the lateral thigh, is passed up through the retropubic space with the aid of a long clamp. One end is sutured into position in the rectus fascia and the tension is adjusted before sewing the other end in place. (From Ridley JR (Ed). Gynecologic Surgery: Errors, Safeguards, Salvage, 2nd ed. Baltimore: Williams and Wilkins, 1981, with permission.)

TABLE 7.3. Materials Used for Sling Procedures

I. Organic Materials
  A. Autologous Tissues
    1. Fascia Lata
    2. Rectus Fascia
    3. Vaginal Patch
    4. Gracilis Muscle
    5. Round Ligaments
    6. Pyramidalis Muscle
  B. Heterologous Tissues
    1. Lyophilized Ox Dura Mater
    2. Porcine Dermis
	II. Synthetic Materials
	  A. Nylon
	  B. Marlex Mesh
	  C. Mersiline Mesh
	  D. Silastic
	  E. Gore-Tex

We cannot stress strongly enough the importance of proper patient selection before performing a sling procedure. A sling operation should not be performed on a patient without prior urodynamic investigation. Similarly, we feel that there are few indications for primary sling procedures. Patients who are candidates for sling operations are generally patients who have had multiple previous attempts at surgical cure of their stress incontinence, have significant congenital abnormalities of the urethra or bladder neck, or who have developed stress incontinence after radical surgery or pelvic trauma. Examples of patients in this latter category include women who have undergone radical vulvectomy with partial excision of the urethra, or women who have sustained fractures of the pelvic ring with avulsion of the urethra from its normal site of attachment.

Several authors have advocated using sling procedures for the treatment of stress incontinence based upon the finding of a "low pressure" urethra (maximum urethral closure pressure of less than 20 cm H_2O) during urethral pressure profilometry, irrespective of the degree of bladder neck descent or urethral mobility present. In several studies the failure rate for "standard" operations, such as the Burch colposuspension, has been reported to have been substantially higher than would have otherwise been expected where this urodynamic finding has been present. Other studies, however, have not found this to be the case. It seems likely that differences in surgical technique may account for some of these discrepancies. The authors of this book believe that a dogmatic approach to the use of sling procedures in patients with low urethral closure pressure cannot, at present, be justified. However, if urodynamic studies determine that a low urethral closure pressure is present, it seems prudent for the surgeon to consider carefully whether there may be other factors involved in an individual case that might alter the proposed choice of operation.

No patient should be subjected to a sling procedure unless she is prepared to accept the possibility of long-term voiding dysfunction and the need for clean intermittent self-catheterization. We recommend teaching patients this technique prior to embarking on sling surgery, and would suggest that patients practice catheterizing themselves for several weeks before any surgical intervention is undertaken. Doing this will allow them to see if they are physically able to carry out this technique and also to see if they can tolerate it psychologically. If they are unable to accomplish this, the surgeon should have second thoughts before performing a sling procedure.

Surgical Salvage Procedures

In addition to the procedures described above, there are several other options available for patients with complicated or refractory stress incontinence. Some of these are new and as yet unproven; others are effective, but more radical, operations. These options, which may be regarded as salvage operations, include obstructive sling procedures, periurethral injections of collagen or Teflon paste, the artificial urinary sphincter, and urinary diversion.

As noted in the previous section, the most common complication of sling operations for incontinence is voiding dysfunction due to outflow obstruction. This is usually inadvertent; however, in some cases obstruction may be planned deliberately and the sling pulled exceptionally tight in order to obtain dryness by sacrificing voiding function. Patients who are candidates for this type of surgery must be evaluated carefully (preferably with fluoroscopic video urodynamic studies), should have their upper urinary tracts evaluated to make sure there is no deterioration, and must be capable of performing self catheterization prior to undergoing surgery. These patients must have careful long-term follow-up. Surgeons who are unwilling to provide this should not perform this operation.

Since stress incontinence is due to dysfunction of the bladder neck and urethra—which are relatively accessible from the outside—clinicians have long sought for a substance that could be injected along these tubular structures to compress, support, rebuild, or narrow them so that urine loss would not occur. Early attempts in the 1930's to do this using sclerosing solutions were not very successful and often led to significant complications, such as sloughing of the urethra.

In the last 50 years improvements in the development of synthetic materials have led to renewed interest in this technology. Two major materials have been developed which seem to be useful in treating stress incontinence by periurethral injection: Polytef paste and GAX collagen. The mechanism by which injection of these materials improves continence in patients is uncertain. They may act to form a "washer-like" seal at the bladder neck. They might improve lateral urethral support, thereby restoring normal pressure vectors during periods of increased intra-abdominal pressure. They do not correct abnormal bladder neck displacement very well, and they probably do not work by increasing urethral closure pressure. Some element of urethral obstruction seems likely to play an important role in their success, since these injections appear to work better in patients who have good urethral support than in those with hypermobility of the urethra and bladder neck.

Both the Polytef and GAX collagen substances are injected submucosally at the vesical neck and along the proximal urethra. They can be injected transvaginally with a separate needle and syringe under cystoscopic guidance, or they can be injected transurethrally using a long needle passed through the operating port of a cystoscope. The main advantage of periurethral injection is that it is minimally invasive, and as a result has a low morbidity. Theoretically, this makes periurethral injections a useful adjunctive therapy for those disappointing patients whose stress incontinence persists after surgery which has stabilized the support of the bladder neck. Their problem might be solved by "topping up" the urethra with an injectable material to create a successful final watertight seal without the necessity of repeating a major operation. The major disadvantages of periurethral injections of these materials are their unproven long-term success and questions regarding their stability once they have been injected around the bladder neck and urethra. Overenthusiastic injection of these substances can lead to obstruction, while injection of inadequate amounts will lead to failure.

Polytef paste, a viscous liquid form of polytetrafluoroethylene (Teflon), achieved some notoriety as a treatment for stress incontinence in the late 1970's and early 1980's. Under anesthesia, this substance was injected into the periurethral tissues under cystoscopic guidance to narrow and resupport the urethra, particularly in patients with incontinence due to internal sphincter dysfunction or "Type III" incontinence. The paste is thick and difficult to inject without special instruments. Success with this technique has been modest, but substantial concern has arisen from the migration of the Teflon particles into the pelvic lymph nodes, lungs, kidneys, spleen, and brain of experimental animals.

More excitement has been generated by the recent development of GAX collagen, a glutaraldehyde cross-linked bovine collagen, which can be injected under local anesthesia with a small needle and syringe. The substance appears to be safe, nontoxic, does not produce an inflammatory response, and is replaced by natural host collagen over a period of several months. The material is easily

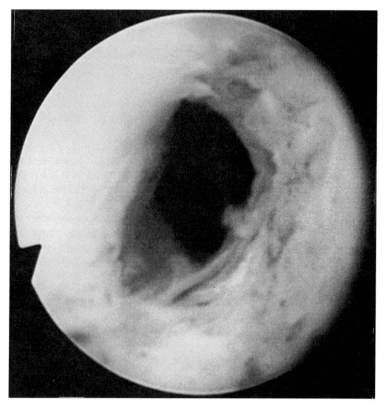

Figure 7.20 Cystoscopic view of an open bladder neck in a patient with "Type III" incontinence prior to injection of GAX collagen. Courtesy of Bard Urological, Inc.

injectable and the procedure can be performed in the office (Figs. 7.20–7.22). Approximately 17 ml of injected material is needed to attain continence, and patients may have to undergo repeated procedures, which are well tolerated. The procedure holds great promise of benefiting patients who are poor candidates for more extensive surgical operations, such as slings or implantation of an artificial urinary sphincter, but the results of the technique are preliminary and, as of this writing, the substance has not yet been released for general use by the Food and Drug Administration. The results are much better in patients with good urethral support but sphincteric weakness, than they are in patients whose main problem is excessive mobility of the bladder neck and urethra.

While their utility as primary procedures for stress incontinence remains doubtful for all but a handful of carefully selected patients, these procedures are likely to be useful adjuncts to other operations, particularly those cases where the bladder neck has been adequately resuspended but leakage persists due to a continuing problem with poor urethral function.

The American Medical Systems artificial urinary sphincter represents the "high technology" solution to bladder neck and urethral sphincter incompetence. After several prototypes, the Model 800 sphincter probably represents the final stage of development of the artificial sphincter. It is unlikely that these devices will become substantially better than they are now.

It must be stated emphatically at the outset, that these devices are not appropriate primary surgical treatment for stress incontinence. Appropriate candidates for this kind of surgery are women whose continence mechanisms have been destroyed by multiple surgical failures, trauma, congenital defects, or neuro-

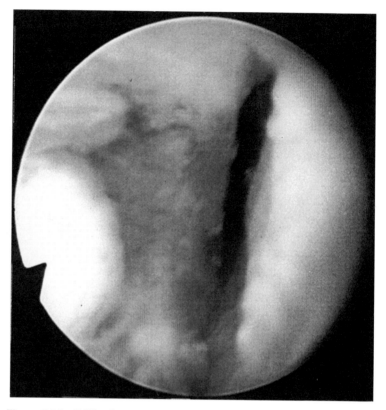

Figure 7.21   GAX collagen injection has been completed on the patient's right side. Note the bulging of the sidewall into the lumen. Courtesy of Bard Urological, Inc.

pathic disease processes. These patients represent only a tiny fraction of all women with stress incontinence. Artificial sphincters should only be implanted at tertiary care medical centers where an experienced surgical team can be assembled on a regular basis and patients may be given specialized follow-up care, for the rest of their lives if necessary.

The artificial sphincter itself consists of three components: a cuff, which is placed around the bladder neck and proximal urethra; a pump mechanism to deflate the cuff once it has been activated so that voiding may take place; and a reservoir for storing the medium which fills the device (Fig. 7.23). The cuff, which must be individually sized at the time of surgery, may be implanted through either an abdominal or vaginal incision. While the vaginal technique is easier, it has not gained widespread popularity due to the fear of infection around an artificial prosthesis. The pump mechanism is inserted into one of the labia majora, where it can be activated by the patient's hand. The reservoir is generally placed in the abdomen below the fascia.

The main problems with the artificial sphincter are cuff erosion at the bladder neck and technical failure of the device. In general, the artificial sphincter appears to function better in men than in women, due primarily to the longer male urethra and the presence of more tissue at the bladder neck. In women, the cuff must be inserted into the thin septum of tissue between the vagina and the bladder neck, which is prone to infection and erosion. Delayed activation of the cuff has been beneficial in preventing erosion. It should not be inflated with its filling mechanism until six weeks after it has been implanted. This decreases the risk of compromising the vascular supply around the healing bladder neck. Device

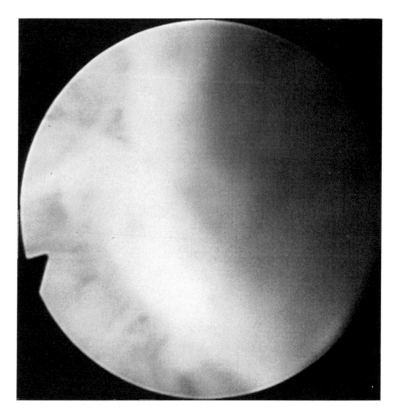

Figure 7.22   Completion of GAX collagen injection. The urethral lumen has been closed. Courtesy of Bard Urological, Inc.

failure can occur from multiple causes: incorrect sizing of the original cuff, failure to choose the proper pressure for the reservoir, failure to connect the parts properly, leakage of contrast material, air bubbles in the original pressure lines, etc. Many patients end up undergoing multiple surgical revisions of their sphincter before obtaining a successful result.

The bladder may be by-passed altogether by diverting the urinary stream into a segment of bowel which then empties into an external collection device attached to the skin surface. Better still, the urine stream may be diverted into a continent reservoir made of bowel which can then be emptied by the patient using intermittent external catheterization. Urinary diversion is rarely necessary for stress incontinence alone. Patients undergoing complicated bladder reconstruction with augmentation cystoplasty and various forms of continent urinary diversion, such as the Koch pouch or one of the increasing number of modifications of this technique, need comprehensive evaluation of both the upper and lower tracts prior to surgery, and treatment at a tertiary referral center. In general these will be patients who have suffered from malignancy, trauma, congenital defects, neurologic disorders, or combinations of the above. These cases require a high level of skill at a center which can provide excellent long-term follow-up.

Evaluation of Failed Surgery

Few things are as distressing to both patient and surgeon as an operation which has resulted in failure, with the patient remaining incontinent, sometimes worse off than before. The initial high hopes have been dashed and both parties may blame themselves, or attempt to fix blame upon the other, for what has

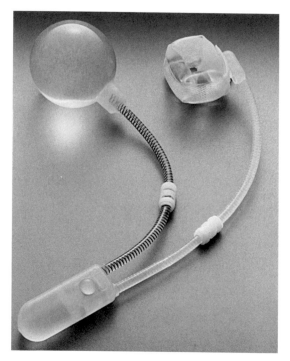

Figure 7.23   The AMS 800 artificial urinary sphincter. Courtesy of American Medical Systems, Inc. (Michael Schenk)

happened. Excellent doctor-patient communication and support is crucial under these circumstances, particularly in an increasingly hostile medico-legal climate. How should these cases be approached?

The most sensible way to evaluate failed surgery for stress incontinence is to begin afresh with a new, detailed history and physical examination. The urine should be analyzed and cultured at the outset and infection eliminated. The patient should be checked for persistent residual urine after voiding to rule out "overflow" problems. Symptoms should be correlated with objective findings, including urodynamic investigation. This is mandatory if further surgery is contemplated. Intravenous urography should be considered if the possibility of a fistula is present, particularly in patients who complain of "continuous" urinary leakage.

The most common reasons for surgical failure are: (*a*) misdiagnosis of the initial problem; (*b*) failure to achieve intended surgical goals; (*c*) development of a new problem; or (*d*) worsening of a previously minor problem.

Misdiagnosis of the initial problem can take many forms. Unfortunately, it is still all too common for physicians to assume that all female incontinence is "stress incontinence." An initial evaluation in which stress incontinence was never demonstrated, but was assumed to be present, still accounts for far too many cases of failed surgery. We know, from substantial experience, that a patient's history *by itself* is an unreliable guide to the final diagnosis. No patient should be subjected to surgery for stress incontinence on the basis of her history alone. Incontinence must be demonstrated. What is demonstrated must be confirmed by the patient as being representative of her problem. Some form of urodynamic testing is usually necessary to confirm the diagnosis. Unstable detrusor activity can be precipitated by physical activity—including exercise, coughing, sneezing, and change of position. This can mimic "stress incontinence" to a surprising degree, and an unwary practitioner can be fooled unless an objective patient evaluation is carried out. If detrusor instability is present postoperatively in a patient who has undergone surgery which fails on this basis, and no objective preoperative evaluation was obtained, it is hard to tell if this is a new complaint arising as a complication of surgery or an initial misdiagnosis.

Miscellaneous—and often unexpected—conditions, such as ectopic ureters, genitourinary fistulae, and urethral diverticula, may mimic stress incontinence. In the latter condition, the diverticulum fills with urine after the patient voids, and when she coughs urine loss occurs. Resuspension of the bladder neck will not cure any of these problems.

One of the major causes of failed stress incontinence surgery is still the assumption on the part of many practitioners that all stress incontinence is the same. It is clear that the major factor producing most stress incontinence is bladder neck displacement during periods of increased intra-abdominal pressure resulting in ineffective urethral closure. This is common, "garden variety," stress incontinence; however, it is also clear that some stress incontinence is due to intrinsic sphincteric weakness, often called "Type III" incontinence. These patients will demonstrate "genuine" stress incontinence during conventional cystometry, leak copiously during physical examination, and complain of stress incontinence. However, fluoroscopic examination will reveal a wide-open, patulous or tubular bladder neck, which is often frozen in position by multiple prior surgeries. Bladder neck incompetence of this type may also be hidden by a massive prolapse of the bladder or vagina. Patients with this type of problem will require a sling procedure or similar operation if they are to be cured. Failure from conventional surgery such as a needle suspension or a retropubic cystourethropexy is high in such cases.

Failure to achieve the desired surgical goals results in inadequate or insecure repositioning of the urethra and bladder neck, particularly when an anterior colporrhaphy has been performed. Long-term failures may occur in patients due to gradual loss of support over time, or, in some cases, due to an acute insult to the surgical site such as massive coughing with postoperative bronchitis. Many patients can report the exact instance of failure, when they felt something pop or rip and became wet again. Pull-out of sutures due to inadequate suture anchoring or the use of absorbable rather than permanent suture materials (especially chromic catgut) are very common reasons for surgical failure in patients whose initial problem was stress incontinence due to bladder neck displacement. All too often surgical failure results from sutures which are placed incorrectly at the time of surgery, particularly during retropubic operations. Since correct anatomic repositioning is of paramount importance in these operations, it cannot be stressed enough that the space of Retzius must be fully dissected and the bladder, vagina, and endopelvic fascia clearly identified, before sutures are placed. Failure to do this may result in inadequate elevation of the bladder neck or suturing of the bladder itself to the pubic symphysis. If you are in doubt about your location, do not hesitate to open the bladder dome when placing your sutures!

Aside from misdiagnosis and technical failures of surgery, the two most common causes for persistent incontinence are the development of a new problem or the worsening of an old one. These problems include major complications such as fistula formation, or less dramatic problems such as the development of a large postvoid residual or new onset detrusor instability which results in urge incontinence. The presence of voiding difficulty or mixed incontinence before the operation is undertaken should alert the surgeon that these patients may be at risk for persistence or worsening of these conditions following surgery, depending in part on the type of operation involved. Transient problems with large residual urine volumes are fairly common, and can be managed by a suprapubic catheter or a program of self-catheterization. Similarly, many patients report episodes of urge incontinence in the few days right after bladder neck surgery. Most of these symptoms resolve spontaneously given time. Persistent urge incontinence 6 weeks after surgery requires further evaluation and may require active intervention, particularly if it is severe.

In our opinion, successful correction of stress incontinence remains one of the most rewarding endeavors in pelvic surgery. However, the degree of success obtained is highly dependent upon careful preoperative evaluation of patients and attention to the details of each operation.

SUGGESTED READING

General

Hurt WG (Ed). Urogynecologic Surgery. Gaithersburg, MD: Aspen Publishers, 1992.

Stanton SL, Tanagho EA (Eds). Surgery of Female Incontinence, 2nd ed.; New York: Springer-Verlag, 1986.

Thompson JD, Wall LL, Growdon WA, Ridley JH. Urinary stress incontinence. In Thompson JD, Rock JA (Eds). TeLinde's Operative Gynecology, 7th ed. Philadelphia: JB Lippincott, 1992: 887–40.

Comparative Surgical Studies

Bergman A, Ballard CA, Koonings PP. Comparison of three different surgical procedures for genuine stress incontinence: Prospective randomized study. Am J Obstet Gynecol 1989; 160:1102–06.

Bergman A, Koonings PP, Ballard CA. Primary stress urinary incontinence and pelvic relaxation: Prospective randomized comparison of three different operations. Am J Obstet Gynecol 1989; 161:97–101.

Hilton P. A clinical and urodynamic study comparing the Stamey bladder neck suspension and suburethral sling procedures in the treatment of genuine stress incontinence. Br J Obstet Gynaecol 1989; 96:213–20.

Mundy AR. A trial comparing the Stamey bladder neck suspension procedure with colposuspension for the treatment of stress incontinence. Br J Urol 1983; 55:687–90.

Stanton SL, Cardozo LD. A comparison of vaginal and suprapubic surgery in the correction of incontinence due to urethral sphincter incompetence. Br J Urol 1979; 51: 497–99.

Van Geelen JM, Theeuwes AGM, Eskes TKAB, et al. The clinical and urodynamic effects of anterior vaginal repair and Burch culposuspension. Am J Obstet Gynecol 1988; 159:137–44.

Weil A, Reyes H, Bischoff, et al. Modifications of the urethral rest and stress profiles after different types of surgery for urinary stress incontinence. Br J Obstet Gynaecol 1984; 91:46–55.

Anterior Colporrhaphy

Bailey KV. A clinical investigation into uterine prolapse with stress incontinence: Treatment by modified Manchester colporrhaphy. J Obstet Gynaecol Br Emp 1954; 61:291–301.

Beck RP, McCormick S. Treatment of urinary stress incontinence with anterior colporrhaphy. Obstet Gynecol 1982; 59:269–74.

Beck RP, McCormick S, Nordstrom L. A 25–year experience with 519 anterior colporrhaphy procedures. Obstet Gynecol 1991; 78:1011–18.

Delaere KP, Moonen WA, Debruyne FM, et al. Anterior vaginal repair, cause of troublesome voiding disorders? Eur Urol 1979; 5:190–94.

Kelly HA, Dumm WM. Urinary incontinence in women

without manifest injury to the bladder. Surg Gynecol Obstet 1914; 18:444–50.

Low JA. Management of anatomic urinary incontinence by vaginal repair. Am J Obstet Gynecol 1967; 97:308–15.

Nichols DH, Milley PS. Identification of pubourethral ligaments and their role in transvaginal surgical correction of stress incontinence. Am J Obstet Gynecol 1973; 115: 123–28.

Richardson DA, Ostergard DR. Anterior vaginal repair versus retropubic urethropexy: A review of the literature. In Ostergard DR (Ed). Gynecologic Urology and Urodynamics: Theory and Practice, 2nd ed. Baltimore: Williams and Wilkins, 1985:469–77.

Stanton SL, Norton C, Cardozo L. Clinical and urodynamic effects of anterior colporrhaphy and vaginal hysterectomy for prolapse with and without incontinence. Br J Obstet Gynaecol 1982; 89:459–63.

Warrell DW. Anterior repair. In Stanton SL, Tanagho EA (Eds). Surgery of Female Incontinence, 2nd ed. New York: Springer-Verlag, 1986:77–85.

Marshall-Marchetti-Krantz Procedure

Lee RA, Symmonds RE. Repeat Marshall-Marchetti procedure for recurrent stress urinary incontinence. Am J Obstet Gynecol 1975; 122:219–29.

Lee RA, Symmonds RE, Goldstein RA. Surgical complications and results of modified Marshall-Marchetti-Krantz procedure for urinary incontinence. Obstet Gynecol 1979; 53:447–50.

McDuffie RW Jr., Litin RB, Blundon KE. Urethrovesical suspension (Marshall-Marchetti-Krantz): Experience with 204 cases. Am J Surg 1981; 141:297–98.

Mainprize TC, Drutz HP. The Marshall-Marchetti-Krantz procedure: A critical review. Obstet Gynecol Surv 1988; 43:724–29.

Marshall VF, Marchetti AA, Krantz KE. The correction of stress incontinence by simple vesicourethral suspension. Surg Gynecol Obstet 1949; 88:509–18.

Marshall VF, Segaul RM. Experience with suprapubic vesicourethral suspension after previous failures to correct stress incontinence in women. J Urol 1968; 100:647–48.

O'Leary JA. Osteitis pubis following vesicourethral suspension. Obstet Gynecol 1964; 24:73–77.

Parnell JP, Marshall VF, Vaughan ED Jr. Primary management of urinary stress incontinence by the Marshall-Marchetti-Krantz vesicourethropexy. J Urol 1982; 127: 679–82.

Parnell JP, Marshall VF, Vaughan ED Jr. Management of recurrent urinary stress incontinence by the Marshall-Marchetti-Krantz vesicourethropexy. J Urol 1984; 132: 912–14.

Persky L, Guerriere K. Complications of Marshall-Marchetti-Krantz urethropexy. Urology 1976; 8:469–71.

Raz S, Maggio AJ Jr, Kaufman JJ. Why Marshall-Marchetti operation works . . . or does not. Urology 1979; 14: 154–59.

Seski JC. Iatrogenic intravesical foreign body following Marshall-Marchetti procedure for stress urinary incontinence. Am J Obstet Gynecol 1976; 126:514–15.

Sjoberg B. Hydrodynamics of micturition following Marshall-Marchetti-Krantz procedure for stress urinary incontinence. Scand J Urol Nephrol 1982; 16:11–20.

Zimmern PE, Hadley HR, Leach GE, et al. Female urethral obstruction after Marshall-Marchetti-Krantz operation. J Urol 1987; 138:517–20.

Burch Colposuspension Operation

Burch JC. Urethrovaginal fixation to Cooper's ligament for correction of stress incontinence, cystocele and prolapse. Am J Obstet Gynecol 1961; 81:281–90.

Burch JC. Cooper's ligament urethrovesical suspension for stress incontinence: Nine year's experience—results, complications, technique. Am J Obstet Gynecol 1968; 100:764–74.

Cardozo LD, Stanton SL, Williams JE. Detrusor instability following surgery for genuine stress incontinence. Br J Urol 1979; 51:204–07.

Galloway NTM, Davies N, Stephenson TP. The complications of colposuspension. Br J Urol 1987; 60:122–24.

Hertogs K, Stanton SL. Lateral bead-chain urethrocystography after successful and unsuccessful colposuspension. Br J Obstet Gynaecol 1985; 92:1179–83.

Hertogs K, Stanton SL. Mechanism of urinary continence after colposuspension: Barrier studies. Br J Obstet Gynaecol 1985; 952:1184–88.

Hilton P, Stanton SL. A clinical and urodynamic assessment of the Burch colposuspension for genuine stress incontinence. Br J Obstet Gynaecol 1983; 90:934–39.

Langer R, Ron-El R, Neuman M, et al. The value of simultaneous hysterectomy during Burch colposuspension for urinary stress incontinence. Obstet Gynecol 1988; 72: 866–69.

Lose G, Jergensen L, Mortensen SO, et al. Voiding difficulties after colposuspension. Obset Gynecol 1987; 69: 33–38.

Stanton SL, Williams JE, Ritchie D. The colposuspension operation for urinary incontinence. Br J Obstet Gynaecol 1976; 83:890–95.

Stanton SL, Cardozo LD, Williams JE, et al. Clinical and urodynamic features of failed incontinence surgery in the female. Obstet Gynecol 1978; 51:515–20.

Stanton SL, Cardozo LD. Results of the colposuspension operation for incontinence and prolapse. Br J Obstet Gynaecol 1978; 86:693–97.

Stanton SL, Cardozo LD, Chaudhury N. Spontaneous voiding after surgery for urinary incontinence. Br J Obstet Gynaecol 1978; 85:149–52.

Wiskind AK, Creighton SM, Stanton SL. The incidence of prolapse after the Burch colposuspension. Am J Obstet Gynecol 1992; 167:399–405.

Paravaginal Repair (Vagino-Obturator Shelf)

Richardson AC, Lyon JB, Williams NL. A new look at pelvic relaxation. Am J Obstet Gynecol 1976; 126:568–73.

Richardson AC, Lyon JB, Williams NL. Treatment of stress urinary incontinence due to paravaginal fascial defect. Obstet Gynecol 1981; 57:357–62.

Richardson AC. How to correct prolapse paravaginally. Contemporary OB/GYN 1990; 35(8):100–14.

Shull BL, Baden WF. A six-year experience with paravaginal defect repair for stress urinary incontinence. Am J Obstet Gynecol 1989; 160:1432–40.

Turner-Warwick R. The female sphincter mechanisms and their relation to incontinence surgery. In Debruyne FMJ, Van Kerrebroeck PEVA (Eds). Practical Aspects of Urinary Incontinence. Boston: Martinus Nijhoff Publishers, 1986:66–75.

Turner-Warwick R. Turner-Warwick vagino-obturator shelf urethral repositioning procedure. In Gingell C, Abrams P (Eds). Controversies and Innovations in Urological Surgery. New York: Springer-Verlag, 1988:195–200.

Webster GD, Kreder KJ. Voiding dysfunction following cystourethropexy: Its evaluation and management. J Urol 1990; 144:670–73.

White GR. Cystocele: A radical cure by suturing lateral sulci of vagina to white line of pelvic fascia. J Am Med Assoc 1909; 53:1707–10.

White GR. An anatomic operation for the cure of cystocele. Am J Obstet Dis Wom Child 1912; 56:286–90.

Needle Suspension Procedures

Birhle W, Tarantino AF. Complications of retropubic bladder neck suspension. Urology 1990; 35:213–14.

Constantinou CE. Determinants of cure by endoscopic suspension of the bladder neck in the incontinent female patient. World J Urol 1986; 4:10–15.

Cornella JA, Pereyra AJ. Historical vignette of Armand J. Pereyra, MD, and the modified Pereyra procedure: The needle suspension for stress incontinence in the female. Int Urogynecol J 1990; 1:25–30.

Evans JWH, Chapple CR, Ralph J, EJG Milroy. Bladder calculus formation as a complication of the Stamey procedure. Br J Urol 1990; 65:580–82.

Gittes RF, Loughlin KR. No-incision pubovaginal suspension for stress incontinence. J Urol 1987; 138:568–70.

Handley-Ashken M, Abrams PH, Lawrence WT. Stamey endoscopic bladder neck suspension for stress incontinence. Br J Urol 1984; 56:629–34.

Karram MM, Bhatia NN. Transvaginal needle bladder neck suspension procedures for stress urinary incontinence: A comprehensive review. Obstet Gynecol 1989; 73:906–14.

Karram MM, Angel O, Koonings P, Tabor B, Bergman A, Bhatia N. The modified Pereyra procedure: A clinical and urodynamic review. Br J Obstet Gynaecol 1992; 99: 655–58.

Leach GE, Yip CM, Donovan BJ. Mechanism of continence after modified Pereyra bladder neck suspension. Urology 1987; 29:328–31.

Leach GE, Labasky RF. Bone fixation technique for transvaginal needle suspension. Urol Clin NA 1989; 16: 175–82.

Massey JA, Anderson RS, Abrams P. Mechanisms of continence during raised intra-abdominal pressure. Br J Urol 1987; 60:529–31.

Miyazaki F, Shook G. Ilioinguinal nerve entrapment during needle suspension for stress incontinence. Obstet Gynecol 1992; 80:246–48.

Peattie AB, Stanton SL. The Stamey operation for correction of genuine stress incontinence in the elderly woman. Br J Obstet Gynaecol 1989; 96:983–86.

Pereyra AJ. A simplified surgical procedure for the correction of stress incontinence in women. West J Surg 1959; 67:223–26.

Pereyra AJ, Lebherz TB. Combined urethral vesical suspension vaginal urethroplasty for correction of urinary stress incontinence. Obstet Gynecol 1967; 30:537–46.

Pereyra AJ, Lebherz TB. The revised Pereyra procedure. In Buchsbaum H, Schmidt JD (Eds). Gynecologic and Obstetric Urology. Philadelphia: WB Saunders, 1978: 208–22.

Pereyra AJ. Revise Pereyra procedure using colligated pubourethral supports. In Slate WG (Ed). Disorders of the Female Urethra and Urinary Incontinence. Baltimore: Williams and Wilkins, 1978:143–59.

Pereyra AJ, Lebherz TB, Growdon WA, Poers JA. Pubourethral supports in perspective: Modified Pereyra procedure for urinary incontinence. Obstet Gynecol 1981; 59: 643–48.

Ramon J, Mekras J, Webster GD. Transvaginal needle suspension procedures for recurrent stress incontinence. Urology 1991; 38:519–22.

Raz S, Klutke CG, Colomb J. Four-corner bladder and urethra suspension for moderate cystocele. J Urol 1989; 142: 712–15.

Stamey TA. Endoscopic suspension of vesical neck for urinary incontinence. Surg Gynecol Obstet 1973; 136: 547–54.

Stamey TA. Endoscopic suspension of the vesical neck for urinary incontinence in females. Ann Surg 1980; 192: 465–71.

Varner RE. Retropubic long-needle suspension procedures for stress urinary incontinence. Am J Obstet Gynecol 1990; 163:551–57.

Weiss RE, Cohen E. Erosion of buttress following bladder neck suspension. Br J Urol 1992; 69:656–57.

Zderic SA, Burros HM, Hanno PM, Dudas N, Whitmore KE. Bladder calculi in women after urethrovesical suspension. J Urol 1988; 139:1047–48.

Sling Procedures

Aldridge AH. Transplantation of fascia for relief of urinary stress incontinence. Am J Obstet Gynecol 1942; 44: 398–411.

Beck RP, Lai AR. Results in treating 88 cases of recurrent urinary stress incontinence with the Oxford fascia lata sling procedure. Am J Obstet Gynecol 1982; 142:649–51.

Beck RP, McCormick S, Nordstrom L. The fascia lata sling procedure for treating recurrent genuine stress incontinence. Obstet Gynecol 1988; 72:699–703.

Blaivas JG, Jacobs BZ. Pubovaginal fascial sling for the treatment of complicated stress urinary incontinence. J Urol 1991; 145:1214–18.

Gierup HJW, Hakelius L. Free autogenous muscle transplantation in the treatment of urinary incontinence in children: Background, surgical technique, and preliminary results. J Urol 1978; 120:223–26.

Horbach NS, Blanco JS, Ostergard DR, et al. A suburethral sling procedure with polytetrafluoroethylene for the treatment of genuine stress incontinence in patients with low urethral closure pressure. Obstet Gynecol 1988; 71: 648–57.

Jarvis GJ, Fowlie A. Clinical and urodynamic assessment of the porcine dermis bladder sling in the treatment of genuine stress incontinence. Br J Obstet Gynaecol 1985; 92:1189–91.

Karram MM, Bhatia NN. Patch procedure: Modified transvaginal fascia lata sling for recurrent or severe stress urinary incontinence. Obstet Gynecol 1990; 75:461–63.

Kersey J. The gauze hammock sling operation in the treatment of stress incontinence. Br J Obstet Gynaecol 1983; 90:945–49.

Kersey J, Martin MM, Mishra P. A further assessment of the gauze hammock sling operation in the treatment of stress incontinence. Br J Obstet Gynaecol 1988; 95: 382–85.

McGuire EJ, Lytton B. Pubovaginal sling procedure for stress incontinence. J Urol 1978; 119:82–84.

McGuire EJ. Urodynamic findings in patients after failure of stress incontinence operations. In Zinner NR, Sterling Am (Eds). Female Incontinence. New York: Alan R. Liss, 1981:351–60 (Prog Clin Biol Res 78).

McGuire EJ, Wang CC, Usitalo H, Savastano J. Modified pubovaginal sling in girls with myelodysplasia. J Urol 1986; 135:94–96.

McGuire EJ, Bennett CJ, Konnak JA, Sonda LP, Savastano JA. Experience with pubovaginal slings for urinary incontinence at the University of Michigan. J Urol 1987; 138: 525–26.

Morgan JE, Farrow GA, Stewart FE. The Marlex sling operation for the treatment of recurrent stress urinary incontinence: A 16 year review. Am J Obstet Gynecol 1985; 151:224–26.

Parker RT, Addison WA, Wilson CJ. Fascia lata urethrovesical suspension for recurrent stress urinary incontinence. Am J Obstet Gynecol 1979; 135:843–52.

Raz S, Siegel AL, Short JL, Snyder JA. Vaginal wall sling. J Urol 1989; 141:43–46.

Reid GC, DeLancey JOL, Hopkins MP, Roberts JS, Morely GW. Urinary incontinence following radical vulvectomy. Obstet Gynecol 1990; 75:852–58.

Rottenberg RD, Weil A, Brioschi PA, et al. Urodynamic and clinical assessment of the Lyodura sling operation for urinary stress incontinence. Br J Obstet Gynecol 1985; 92:829–34.

Stanton SL, Brindley GS, Holmes DM. Silastic sling for urethral sphincter incompetence in women. Br J Obstet Gynaecol 1985; 92:747–50.

Woodside JR. Pubovaginal sling procedure for the management of urinary incontinence after urethral trauma in women. J Urol 1987; 138:527–28.

Periurethral Injections

Appell RA. Injectables for urethral incompetence. World J Urol 1990; 8:208–11.

Appell RA. Periurethral collagen injection for female incontinence. Prob Urol 1991; 5:134–40.

Beckingham IJ, Wemyss-Holden G, Lawrence WT. Long-term follow-up of women treated with periurethral Teflon injections for stress incontinence. Br J Urol 1992; 69: 580–83.

Dewan PA. Is injected polytetrafluoroethylene (Polytef) carcinogenic? Br J Urol 1992; 69:29–33.

Kieswetter H, Fischer M, Wober L, Flamm J. Endoscopic implantation of collagen (GAX) for the treatment of urinary incontinence. Br J Urol 1992; 69:22–25.

Lewis RI, Lockhart JL, Politano VA. Periurethral polytetrafluoroethylene injections in incontinent female subjects with neurogenic bladder disease. J Urol 1984; 131: 459–62.

Lim KB, Ball AJ, Feneley RCL. Periurethral Teflon injection: A simple treatment for urinary incontinence. Br J Urol 1983; 55:208–10.

Lockhart JL, Sandord E. Periurethral Polytef and combined cystourethropexy for the management of difficult cases of urinary incontinence. Prob Urol 1990; 4:81–86.

Malizia AA, Reiman HM, Meyers RP, Sande JR, et al. Migration and granulomatous reaction after periurethral injection of Polytef (Teflon). J Am Med Assoc 1984; 251: 3277–81.

Mittleman RE, Marraccinni JV. Pulmonary Teflon granulomas following periurethral Teflon injection for urinary incontinence. Arch Pathol Lab Med 1983; 107:611–12.

Murless BC. The injection treatment of stress incontinence. J Obstet Gynaecol Br Emp 1938; 45:67–73.

Politano VA. Periurethral polytetrafluoroethylene injection for urinary incontinence. J Urol 1982; 127:439–42.

Schulman CC, Simon J, Wespes E, Germeau F. Endoscopic injections of Teflon to treat urinary incontinence in women. Br Med J 1984; 288:192.

Artificial Urinary Sphincter and Urinary Diversion

Diokno AC, Hollander JB, Alderson TP. Artificial urinary sphincter for recurrent female urinary incontinence: Indications and results. J Urol 1987; 138:778–80.

Donovan MG, Barrett DM, Furlow WL. Use of the artificial urinary sphincter in the management of severe incontinence in females. Surg Gynecol Obstet 1985; 161:17–20.

King LR, Stone AR, Webster GD (Eds). Bladder Reconstruction and Continent Urinary Diversion. Chicago: Yearbook Medical Publishers, 1987.

Kreder KJ, Webster GD. Evaluation and management of incontinence after implantation of the artificial urinary sphincter. Urol Clin NA 1991; 18:375–81.

Light JK, Scott FB. Management of urinary incontinent in women with the artificial urinary sphincter. J Urol 1985; 134:476–78.

Motley RC, Barrett DM. Artificial urinary sphincter cuff erosion: Experience with reimplantation in 38 patients. Urology 1990; 35:215–18.

Mundy AR, Stephenson TP. Selection of patients for implantation of the Brantley Scott artificial urinary sphincter. Br J Urol 1984; 56:717–20.

Nurse DE, Mundy AR. One hundred artificial sphincters. Br J Urol 1988; 61:318–25.

Rose SC, Hansen ME, Webster GD, Zakrzewski C, et al. Artificial urinary sphincters: Plain radiography of malfunction and complications. Radiology 1988; 168:403–08.

Scott FB. The artificial urinary sphincter: Review and progress. Med Instrument 1988; 22:174–81.

Stone AR. Neuropathic incontinence due to an incompetent outlet. Prob Urol 1989; 3:122–34.

Webster GD, Sihelnik SA. Troubleshooting the malfunctioning Scott artificial urinary sphincter. J Urol 1984; 131: 269–72.

Webster GD. Cystoplasty management of the intractable hostile neurogenic bladder. Prob Urol 1989; 3:102–21.

Webster GD, Perez LM, Khoury JM, Timmons SL. Management of type III stress urinary incontinence using artificial urinary sphincter. Urology 1992; 39:499–503.

8

Urge Incontinence and the Unstable Bladder

In simple terms the bladder is nothing more than a bag that holds urine. This bag is made up of interdigitated smooth muscle fibers, referred to collectively as the detrusor muscle. As the ureters slowly pump the bladder full of urine, the normal detrusor muscle gradually relaxes to accommodate this increasing urine volume without producing a significant rise in pressure. This process of *receptive relaxation* insures that the normal detrusor muscle remains compliant during bladder filling. As bladder volume increases, tension/stretch receptors in the bladder are stimulated and send afferent impulses to the cerebral cortex causing the first desire to void. In infancy and early childhood this first desire to void triggers a micturition reflex which leads to bladder emptying; however, with increasing physical and social maturity we learn to reset the threshold at which this micturition reflex occurs. Development of urinary continence requires learning how to suppress urination until we find a socially acceptable time and place for bladder emptying. Acquiring the ability to suppress the micturition reflex occurs during normal childhood toilet training. When the socially appropriate time for bladder emptying arrives, we are then able to relax the pelvic floor and generate a sustained contraction of the detrusor muscle until the bladder is completely empty.

In some individuals, however, the bladder does not behave this way. The detrusor muscle may contract inappropriately as the bladder fills, leading to urinary incontinence (Fig. 8.1). This can occur suddenly and without warning, or this event may be accompanied by a strong desire to void (urgency) followed by urine loss. In some instances the abnormal detrusor contraction may be caused by a change of position, sudden exposure to cold temperatures, the sound of water running in the sink, by activities such as coughing or laughing, or by hurriedly fumbling to get a key into the door lock upon returning home with a full bladder after shopping or running errands. The presence of a nearby bathroom may be all that is needed for some women to develop urgency which may result in incontinence. Women who have urinary incontinence as a result of abnormal detrusor contractions are often said to have "unstable" bladders; that is, their bladders do not respond to filling and normal activities by remaining quiescent, compliant, accommodating low-pressure systems. These bladders respond unpredictably to filling by developing high-pressure unstable contractions which produce incontinence, often with accompanying symptoms of frequency and urgency. Unstable bladder activity is a common cause of female urinary incontinence, often coexisting with stress incontinence, and it is the most common cause of urinary incontinence among the elderly.

A number of terms have been used in the past to describe this condition. Among them are "detrusor dyssynergia," "unstable bladder," "spastic bladder," "automatic bladder," "uninhibited bladder," etc. Because these terms have been used without precise definitions, they have led to more confusion than understanding in the literature. We will limit our terminology to the following words, which must be clearly defined before proceeding: urge incontinence, detrusor instability, detrusor hyperreflexia, unstable bladder, and hyperreflexic bladder.

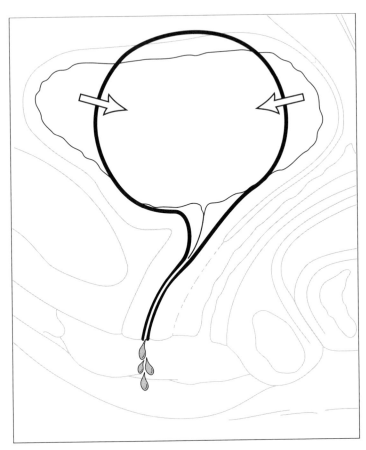

Figure 8.1 Urinary incontinence due to detrusor overactivity. Uninhibited contractions of the detrusor muscle cause urine loss, often in association with urgency.

The term *urge incontinence* refers to the *symptom* of urine loss that occurs in association with a strong desire to urinate (urgency). This is often—perhaps usually—associated with abnormal detrusor activity. A patient may have urinary urgency for two reasons: (*a*) the fear that urine loss is imminent so they must find a toilet immediately because they may not be able to control this urge; or (*b*) increasing pain or the fear that pain will develop as the bladder fills, causing them to rush to a toilet to get relief from these symptoms. Unstable detrusor contractions may cause the first type of urgency, but they rarely cause the second type, which is due to bladder hypersensitivity (see Chapter 12, ''Sensory Disorders of the Bladder and Urethra''). Unstable detrusor contractions may also cause sudden urine loss without the forewarning symptom of urgency. Since the only way to *prove* that the detrusor is contracting in any given patient is to measure detrusor activity, we cannot technically say for certain that an individual who complains of ''urge incontinence'' has these symptoms because of detrusor overactivity until this has been demonstrated during urodynamic studies, even though we may believe that this is what is happening. The term ''urge incontinence,'' therefore, refers to a specific patient symptom and does *not* represent a technical urodynamic diagnosis.

Detrusor activity can be measured by performing a subtracted cystometrogram in which bladder and abdominal (usually rectal) pressure are measured and the difference between the two is taken as the measure of detrusor activity [Pdet = Pves − Pabd]. Patients who demonstrate an abnormal pressure wave during the filling phase of a subtracted cystometrogram while they are attempting to inhibit micturition, are said to have urodynamically proven *detrusor instability*. This pressure change should be a "wave" that is, a rise in the subtracted detrusor pressure followed by some degree of relaxation (also called a phasic contraction or phasic pressure change). A slow, steady rise in detrusor pressure without these characteristics is a change in compliance, not a change in detrusor activity (see below). To be significant, detrusor contractions must produce symptoms. They do *not* have to be of any specific amplitude to be significant as long as they produce symptoms.

Patients with a diagnosed neurologic condition relevant to bladder dysfunction who develop detrusor contractions during cystometry are said to have *detrusor hyperreflexia*. The contractions which these patients develop are generally large in amplitude, reproducible, and predictable. They often occur at small bladder volumes. Common neurologic conditions associated with detrusor hyperreflexia include Parkinson's disease, multiple sclerosis, cerebrovascular accidents, spinal cord injuries, etc.

In the absence of neurologic disease, patients who produce unstable detrusor contractions during cystometry are said to have *idiopathic detrusor instability*. Idiopathic detrusor contractions are less predictable, of variable amplitude, and may be more difficult to elicit during cystometry. Because they refer to specific diagnoses based on the results of urodynamic testing, the terms "detrusor hyperreflexia" and "detrusor instability" are properly used only in patients who have had urodynamic studies which document symptomatic detrusor contractions. The use of these technical urodynamic terms implies that such tests have been carried out and these findings have been confirmed. The term "motor urge incontinence" is often used to describe the urodynamic finding of uninhibited detrusor contractions in a patient who develops urgency and leakage with these contractions during the urodynamic study.

The term "unstable bladder" will be used here loosely to refer to all bladders in which uncontrolled detrusor overactivity is suspected to be the cause of the patient's complaints. "Hyperreflexic bladder" will be used to refer to this condition when it results from a specific neurologic insult to bladder control. In using these terms we do not necessarily imply that the patients have had a "documented" urodynamic diagnosis.

Symptoms, Patient Evaluation, and Diagnosis

Patients with unstable or hyperreflexic bladders usually present with symptoms of urgency, frequency, and urge incontinence, often in association with nocturia and nocturnal enuresis. Typically they have complaints such as "When I need to go I can't hold my water and I wet all over myself," or "I'm always going to the bathroom—every 30 minutes—and sometimes I don't make it in time." Some patients do not have urgency, but merely state that "All of a sudden my water comes away and I can't control it." Patients with incontinence due to unstable detrusor activity are often among the most miserable of incontinent women. Unlike women with simple stress incontinence whose urine loss is associated with strenuous activities that they can avoid or prepare for, the woman with an overactive detrusor never knows when incontinence will strike. She is afraid to leave home unless she knows exactly where each toilet is along her route, and she plans her trips based upon this knowledge. She often goes out on errands padded and anxious, and frequently gives up previously pleasurable social activities such as shopping, going to church, attending musical events, etc. She may take up wearing only dark clothes to hide wet spots, and her worries about odor and embarrassment may eventually turn her into a housebound recluse. We have seen some women threaten to commit suicide if their bladder control could not be improved, and we have seen working women—particularly in factory assembly line jobs—whose continued employment was in jeopardy because of their constant need to rush to the company rest room. The social and emotional devastation caused by uncontrolled detrusor activity is very real.

How should these patients be evaluated? The first steps are simple. Since many of these symptoms can be related to urinary tract infection, a urinalysis and culture should be obtained initially. The physical examination should include a neurologic screening examination looking for previously unsuspected neuropathy which may require further evaluation. Most neurologic conditions resulting in a hyperreflexic bladder will be obvious; occasionally, however, an occult neurologic process will first manifest itself as urinary incontinence. The physician should always be aware of this fact. Atrophic urethritis/vaginitis should be treated with appropriate hormonal therapy, since estrogen deprivation can also produce many of the symptoms associated with detrusor overactivity. Finally, the patient should void and a residual urine should be checked. If this is elevated (over 100 ml), it must be investigated further. If the residual urine is persistent on several examinations, consideration should be given to instituting a program of self-catheterization. Patients with neuropathic conditions such as multiple sclerosis are prone to upper urinary tract deterioration as a late complication of their disease and should have sonography or intravenous urography every few years to rule this out. Patients with significant irritative bladder symptoms such as urgency, frequency, dysuria, pain, or hematuria should have urine sent for cytology and should undergo cystourethroscopy to rule out stones, tumors, or other local pathology as a cause for their symptoms.

Who should have sophisticated urodynamic studies prior to instituting treatment? If urodynamic testing is readily available, obtaining studies to confirm the initial clinical impression is quite reasonable, although this may not be absolutely necessary in all cases. The degree of diagnostic precision needed depends upon the consequences of treatment. Conservative treatment with behavioral modification or a trial of medication obviously requires less precision than the decision to perform radical surgery such as augmentation cystoplasty or urinary diversion. In a woman with urge incontinence who has a normal neurologic examination, a normal postvoid residual, a negative urinalysis, and no stress incontinence, it is perfectly reasonable to institute simple treatment prior to undertaking extensive urodynamic investigations. If the treatment fails, or it appears necessary to start using complex pharmacologic combinations to control her symptoms, or if the decision involves performing surgery for incontinence, then the patient should probably undergo formal urodynamic investigation.

Managing the Unstable Bladder

For practical purposes the treatment of the unstable bladder can be divided into simple and complex therapy. Simple therapy includes behavioral modification and drug therapy, while complex therapy encompasses electrical stimulation and radical surgery. These operations are performed either to denervate the bladder or augment its capacity. This discussion will deal principally with the more practical techniques of behavioral modification and drug therapy.

Behavioral Modification

Urinary continence is a learned behavior which develops in response to considerable social and cultural pressures brought to bear during childhood. The newborn infant has no control over the threshold at which a micturition reflex takes place, but empties more or less ''at will.'' By the time a child has reached the age of 2 or 3, daytime continence has been achieved and the child is able to suppress the micturition reflex until a socially acceptable time and place. Complete control of micturition during sleep usually follows somewhat later until full urinary continence has been established. The essence of this process is the establishment of cortical control over the rest of the neurourologic axis.

Behavioral modification techniques for treating detrusor instability are, in essence, based on the assumption that the underlying problem is the gradual ''subconscious'' escape of bladder function from previously established cortical control. As a means of teaching patients how to inhibit previously uninhibited detrusor contractions, bladder retraining programs are therefore nothing more than refresher courses in childhood toilet training for adults. The paramount role for bladder training is in treating idiopathic detrusor instability and the ''frequency-urgency syndrome.'' Timed voiding programs in which patients urinate at fixed time intervals are helpful in regulating bladder volume and in organizing bladder habits for patients with hyperreflexic bladder activity due to organic neurologic injury; however, these techniques will not abolish detrusor hyperreflexia in these patients. Timed voiding techniques in neurologically impaired patients will help regulate the circumstances under which hyperreflexic contractions occur and will minimize their consequences, but these patients usually need additional pharmacologic therapy as well. Bladder retraining is possible only if the neurologic pathways are intact and are subject to regulation by improving cortical suppression.

The most common form of bladder retraining is called "bladder drill." It is particularly effective in treating patients with urgency, frequency, and urge incontinence due to idiopathic detrusor instability. It is also very effective in treating the symptoms of urgency and frequency in patients with hypersensitive bladders who do not have detrusor instability, as well as in breaking bad toileting habits which may have developed in women with stress incontinence who strive to keep their bladders empty so that their leakage is less with activity or exertion. The success rate for this form of therapy approaches 85% and this can be maintained over time, although continuing patient reeducation may be necessary.

The goal of bladder drill is to break the cycle of frequency, urgency, and urge incontinence and to allow the patient to reestablish cortical control over her bladder function. The use of a frequency-volume bladder chart during the initial patient evaluation is very useful. The patient records all voided volumes and notes the time of each voiding or incontinent episode on this chart and brings it to her clinic appointment. This chart provides an objective record of bladder function and also helps make the patient aware of what her voiding pattern is really like. The guiding principle of bladder drill is to increase the time between voiding episodes gradually, so that the patient relearns to suppress the micturition reflex, raises the volume threshold at which that reflex occurs, and thereby increases her functional bladder capacity and prolongs the time interval between her voiding episodes.

The frequency/volume chart provides an objective record of how often the patient is going to the bathroom. Based on her record, she should start her bladder retraining program with a time interval that she can manage successfully, even if this means voiding as often as every 30 minutes. Patients can usually begin this process at hourly intervals. The patient is then instructed to empty her bladder every hour on the hour while she is awake; thus, she gets up and goes to the toilet at 6 AM, at 7 AM, at 8 AM, and so on throughout the day. It is important that she go at these times and *always* at these times, *whether she needs to go or not.* Thus, if it is 9 AM and she does not feel the urge to urinate, she should go to the toilet and urinate anyway, because the goal is to get her bladder to do what she tells it to do and not to have her bladder run her life. If it is 9:55 AM and she is desperate to urinate, she should try to wait 5 minutes and not go before 10 AM, even if this means considerable discomfort or even urinary leakage onto a protective pad. Distracting activities during this time may be helpful. Some adjustments in scheduling must obviously be made to conform to "real life" situations, particularly for working women. When the patient can manage a regimen like this for a week, she is instructed to increase the time interval by 15 minutes. She would then void at 6 AM, 7:15 AM, 8:30 AM, etc. The patient should *not* get up every hour during the night, but only void when she awakens from sleep and has to go. When she can maintain this schedule for a week, the time interval is again increased, and is increased on a weekly basis until the patient is voiding approximately seven times per day at intervals of approximately 3 hours.

This program works and works dramatically. The keys to success are patient motivation and *gradual* increases in the time interval between voids. Patients who try to progress too rapidly will exceed their capabilities and will fail, and this failure can be very demoralizing. Patients should be encouraged to keep a diary of voiding times which can be reviewed with them on a weekly basis, both to check compliance and to document progress. Frequent follow-up, either in person or by telephone, is extremely important to maintain motivation. Ready access to a sympathetic professional is important to incontinent patients and makes a big difference in the way they feel about themselves. This is should be a prime function for all doctors and nurses involved in taking care of incontinent patients.

Other forms of behavioral modification which have been tried with some success, include inpatient bladder drill (which requires a 2-week hospitalization and has the same success as outpatient therapy), hypnosis, and biofeedback. In the latter technique, the patient undergoes cystometry and receives feedback in the form of visual or auditory signals which are correlated with her rise in detrusor pressure. This is often done by having her watch the deflections of a pen on the strip-chart recorder of the urodynamic printout, or some other device. She then gradually learns to suppress the detrusor contractions which develop during cystometry and improve her bladder control. This method requires a vastly greater outlay of time and money than simple bladder drill, without significantly improved clinical outcome. In all cases, continuing patient motivation is a requirement for long-term success. Periodic office visits for these patients remain a useful way of instilling the confidence they need.

Drug Therapy

The use of drugs to treat detrusor instability represents a pharmacologic attempt to interfere with bladder smooth muscle contraction. Drugs may work at several different points in the physiologic pathway leading to detrusor contraction. Possible sites of action include modulating control mechanisms in the central nervous system, blocking the activity of acetycholine (which is the major neurotransmitter in the bladder), directly relaxing bladder smooth muscle, or regulating other substances believed to have a modulating effect on bladder contractile function. While the effects of a large number of drugs on detrusor contractility have been studied, the clinically useful, nonexperimental drugs may be broken down into six categories: anticholinergic drugs, antispasmodic or spasmolytic drugs, tricyclic antidepressants, calcium channel blockers, prostaglandin synthetase inhibitors, and estrogens (Table 8.1). It is important to realize that these drugs do not abolish detrusor contractile activity completely, but rather raise the threshold at which detrusor contractions take place. In some patients use of these drugs may precipitate urinary retention. This may actually worsen the incontinence if a large residual urine develops. Patients taking medications for the treatment of detrusor overactivity should be monitored to ensure this does not develop. Reducing the dose of the drug, or, in some cases, beginning intermittent self-catheterization, may be necessary to achieve optimum results.

Anticholinergic Agents

Since the main neurotransmitter involved in bladder contraction is acetylcholine, most drugs used in treating detrusor instability/hyperreflexia have significant anticholinergic properties, even if this is not their "main" mechanism of action when they are categorized pharmacologically. The prototypical anticholinergic drug is atropine, a powerful belladonna alkaloid, which exerts its effects through competitive antimuscarinic activity at parasympathetic neuroeffector

TABLE 8.1. Main Drugs Useful for Treating Detrusor Overactivity[a]

Drug	Dose
Anticholinergic agents	
Propantheline	15–30 mg po QID
Antispasmodic agents	
Oxybutynin	5–10 mg po TID/QID
Dicyclomine	20 mg po QID
Tricyclic antidepressants	
Imipramine	10–25 mg po TID
Calcium channel blockers	
Terodiline[b]	12.5–25 mg po BID

[a] BID = 2× per day; TID = 3× per day; QID = 4× per day.
[b] Not yet approved by the FDA for release in the United States

TABLE 8.2. Effects of Atropine in Relation to Dosage

Dose	Effects
0.5 mg	Slight cardiac slowing; some dryness of mouth; inhibition of sweating
1.0 mg	Definite dryness of mouth; thirst; acceleration of heart, sometimes preceded by slowing; mild dilatation of pupil
2.0 mg	Rapid heart rate; palpitations; marked dryness of mouth, dilated pupils; some blurring of near vision
5.0 mg	All the above symptoms marked; speech disturbed; difficulty in swallowing; restlessness and fatigue; headache; dry, hot skin; difficulty in micturition; reduced intestinal peristalsis
10.0 mg	Above symptoms more marked; pulse rapid and weak; iris practically obliterated; vision very blurred; skin flushed, hot, dry and scarlet; ataxia, restlessness, and excitement; hallucination and delirium; coma

[a] (From Weiner N. In: Goodman and Gilman's The Pharmacologic Basis of Therapeutics, 6th ed. New York: Macmillan, 1980, with permission.)

junctions in many organ systems, including the bladder. Because muscarinic cholinergic receptors are found in many parts of the body, the use of any anticholinergic drug will produce effects on many physiologic parameters, not just those related to bladder function. Different effects will become apparent at different dosage levels. The effects of atropine have been well-studied and the relationship of dose to physiologic response has been established (Table 8.2). Atropine is far more potent than any of the drugs used in the treatment of detrusor overactivity, but their side effect patterns will follow roughly the same dose-response pattern as atropine, since there has been little progress in developing anticholinergic drugs which act specifically on the bladder. The most common side effects which may be experienced include a dry mouth due to suppression of salivary and oropharyngeal secretions, occasional drowsiness, "constipation" due to decreased gastrointestinal motility, increased heart rate due to vagal blockade, and transient blurring of vision due to blockade of the sphincter of the iris and the ciliary muscle of the lens of the eye. Most of these side effects are mild at typical dosage levels. The most troublesome side effect is a dry mouth, which can usually be managed by instructing patients to suck on a piece of hard candy, chew gum, or eat a piece of moist fruit. Patients should be told specifically that this dry mouth is different from "thirst" and will not go away if they increase their fluid intake. If patients on anticholinergic drugs are not told this, they may increase their fluid intake dramatically. This will present an increased urine load to their bladders and may actually worsen their incontinence without eliminating their dry mouths!

These drugs are generally very safe. Even a massive dose of atropine is unlikely to cause death in an adult. The limiting factor in how large a dose the patient can be given usually depends on her tolerance of increasing side effects rather than toxic drug effects per se. Patients will eventually reach a point where the side effects of the medications trouble them more than their incontinence. All anticholinergic drugs should be used with caution in patients with pre-existing cardiac arrhythmias. Anticholinergic drugs are also contraindicated in patients suffering from narrow-angle glaucoma, who may experience a precipitous rise in intraocular pressure when given these drugs.

The major strictly anticholinergic drug in common use for treating detrusor instability is propantheline bromide (ProBanthine, Searle), usually given in a starting dose of 15 mg po QID. If patients' symptoms have not responded after 2 weeks on the drug, and they are not having intolerable side effects, the dose may be increased to 30 mg po QID. The dosage may be pushed higher than this, but most patients will find it difficult to tolerate side effects at a dose of 45 mg QID. Hyoscyamine sulfate (Levsin, Schwarz Pharma) is another anticholinergic agent, available as 0.125 mg tablets, which may be taken orally or sublingually up to 0.25 mg every 4 hours.

Many clinicians believe that patients are unlikely to be getting therapeutic benefit from these medications unless they are also getting some side effects, and the absence of any reported side effects when questioning the patient may be a clue that she is either not taking the medication or is taking an inadequate amount. Do not be fooled into thinking the drug ''doesn't work'' when in reality the patient is not taking it!

Antispasmodic Agents

Antispasmodic or spasmolytic drugs are so called because their direct relaxant effect on smooth muscle appears to be greater than their pure anticholinergic activity, at least when tested on bladder muscle strips in a pharmacology laboratory. There are three main drugs in this group: oxybutynin (Ditropan), dicyclomine (Bentyl), and flavoxate (Urispas).

Oxybutynin chloride (Ditropan, Marion Merrell Dow) is probably the most effective drug in this group. It is usually given in starting doses of 5 mg po TID. If the response is poor or incomplete, the dose may be increased to 5 mg po QID or even up to 10 mg po QID. Many patients have difficulty in tolerating the side effects of this drug, particularly the dry mouth and resultant dysphagia. Few patients will tolerate a dose of 10 mg po QID or higher. When beginning therapy in frail elderly women it is often wise to start with a much lower dose, such as 5 mg or even 2.5 mg po BID. The dose can gradually be increased if necessary. The short half-life of this drug means that it must be taken frequently, which many patients find annoying. However, its short half-life means that it can also be taken ''acutely,'' when patients feel they *must* have protection, such as before a special social event. Patients on oxybutynin should be encouraged to titrate the amount of the drug they take to their own levels of tolerance and comfort. Patients can be helped to do this by giving them an instruction sheet such as the one illustrated in Table 8.3. Ditropan is also available in a syrup form at a dose of 5 mg/5 ml.

Dicyclomine hydrochloride (Bentyl, Marion Merrell Dow) has probably been used more widely in the treatment of irritable bowel syndrome than in the treatment of detrusor instability. Since there seems to be a connection between these two disorders (both involve abnormal smooth muscle activity) this medication is especially useful in women with both problems. Dicyclomine hydrochloride in doses of 20 mg po QID appears to be useful in treating the unstable bladder, although there are few clinical trials in the medical literature.

Flavoxate hydrochloride (Urispas, Smith Kline & French) has been touted as an effective drug for treating detrusor instability, but the evidence from clinical trials does not support this contention. The usual dose of flavoxate is 200 mg QID. While it may occasionally be useful in patients with irritative bladder symptoms, it has little utility in treating the unstable bladder.

Tricyclic Antidepressants

Tricyclic antidepressants are so named because they all have a common three-ring molecular core and have similar therapeutic effects in the treatment of clinical depression. It has been known for some time that these drugs also have effects on the lower urinary tract. How these drugs affect the central nervous system to improve clinical depression is unknown. They have complex actions which potentiate the action of biogenic amines in the central nervous system by blocking their reuptake at nerve terminals. They also have variable antimuscarinic anticholinergic side effects which generate frequent complaints from psychiatric patients who take them for depression. These anticholingeric properties account for part, but not all, of the effects of these drugs on the urinary tract.

Imipramine (Tofranil, Ciba-Geigy) is the best known and best studied of these drugs. The psychiatric dose of imipramine used in treating depression is in the range of 150–300 mg per day, but urologic doses are much lower. The drug has anticholinergic properties which relax the detrusor muscle. It also increases the tone of the urethra and bladder neck by stimulating α-adrenergic

TABLE 8.3.   How to Take Ditropan (Oxybutynin) to Get the Best Results

During the first week take 1 table (5 mg) 3 times a day.

During the second week, take 2 tablets (10 mg) 3 times a day. (If your mouth is extremely dry on the first week's dosage and you are happy with the results the medicine is having on your bladder, there is no reason to increase the dosage to 2 tablets taken 3 times a day.)

At any time you are free to adjust your medication depending on your bladder symptoms. At times your incontinence may get better or may get worse. You can take up to 2 tablets 3 times a day or as little as 1/2 a tablet twice a day. Because the medicine does not stay in your system very long, if you take the medicine less than 3 times a day you may not get the results you want. You are free to adjust your dosage according to when your leakage is the worst or when you want to be sure you do not have a leakage episode.

This medicine will make your mouth dry. When you start taking the drug, we want to know that your mouth is dry so that we know you are taking enough medicine for it to work on your bladder. However, once you are happy with the effects of the medicine on your bladder, you may adjust the dose according to how dry your mouth is and what effect the drug is having on your bladder.

You will need to find the dosage that works best for you so that your mouth is not so dry that you cannot stand to take the drug. Each person is unique in the amount of medicine she may need.

Below is a list of things you can try to help with your dry mouth. If you find that something works well for you, please let us know so that we can share it with other patients. Remember, do not increase how much you drink to help with your dry mouth! The dryness that you have is not "thirst." Your mouth is dry because the drug makes the salivary ("spit") gland produce less fluid. If you drink more you will simply make more urine and will not make the dryness go away. This may actually make your leakage worse!

  1. Suck on hard candy (sour flavors may work best).
  2. Chew gum.
  3. Apply glycerin and lemon solution to the inside of your mouth.

Some possible dosage schedules may be:

Morning	Afternoon	Night	Possible Reasons for This Dose of Medicine
2 tablets	1 tablet	2 tablets	Mouth too dry on 2 tablets 3 times a day
1 tablet	2 tablets	2 tablets	Work in the evening
1 tablet	1 tablet	2 tablets	Have more leakage at night
2 tablets	1 tablet	1 tablet	Have leakage in the morning
2 tablets	2 tablets	1 tablet	Work during the day and must be dry
½ tablet	½ tablet	2 tablets	Dry mouth during the day but more leakage at night
½ tablet	½ tablet	½ tablet	Dry mouth less bothersome, still works on bladder

receptors at these sites. This makes imipramine a useful drug for treating patients with mixed incontinence (genuine stress incontinence and detrusor instability). The usual starting dose is 10 mg po TID and it may be increased up to 25 mg po TID or QID. Imipramine has long been used in the treatment of nocturnal enuresis. Patients with this complaint may benefit from doses of up to 75 mg at bedtime. Imipramine also has synergistic effects when used with other anticholinergic drugs, and can be added to pre-existing drug regimens with added patient benefit. Patients can learn to titrate their dose of imipramine to their own levels of tolerance and comfort, just as they can with other anticholinergic medications.

Limited experience in treating detrusor instability has also been reported using doxepin (Sinequan, Roerig), another tricyclic antidepressant, in doses of 50–75 mg at bedtime.

As noted above, tricyclic antidepressants produce typical anticholinergic side effects. In addition, however, they may produce orthostatic hypotension and cause cardiac arrhythmias, particularly in patients with pre-existing heart disease.

It may be useful to obtain a baseline electrocardiogram before initiating therapy if there is any question about the condition of the patient's heart, particularly if she is elderly. Because orthostatic hypotension can be a significant factor in precipitating hip fractures in elderly women, imipramine should be used with caution when treating geriatric patients. When treating these patients it is often helpful to start the drug at a dose of 10 mg twice a day for the first week, and increase it gradually thereafter, based on the clinical response which is obtained.

Calcium Channel Blockers

Calcium channel blockers have been used for a long time in the treatment of disorders of cardiovascular smooth muscle. Research has shown that these drugs also have effects on bladder smooth muscle. The cardiovascular potency of most calcium antagonists has limited their usefulness in treating detrusor instability. Terodiline hydrochloride, however, is a calcium channel blocker with selective action on bladder smooth muscle and limited cardiovascular side effects. From a pharmacologic viewpoint, this makes it an extremely interesting drug which has special potential for treating detrusor instability. At this writing, the drug is still pending approval from the Food and Drug Administration for release in the United States.

Terodiline has a long serum half-life (60 hours), which means that it can be taken as little as once or twice per day. The usual starting dose is 12.5–25 mg po BID. Some patients may have effective bladder control on as little as 25 mg once per day. The long serum half-life, however, means that it may take 10–14 days to produce clinical effects, so patients started on this drug should be warned that improvement in symptomatology will come slowly. Patients who are started on terodiline should, therefore, be given at least 1 month of therapy before deciding to change the dose or discontinue treatment due to lack of effectiveness.

The side effects of terodiline caused by its calcium channel blocking properties include ankle swelling due to dilation of veins in the legs, tremor or jitteriness, and headaches. Because the drug also has anticholinergic properties, patients may also experience dry mouth, blurred vision, and dizziness. In general, the side effects produced by terodiline appear to be better tolerated and of lower magnitude than those produced by other drugs. Some patients with pre-existing cardiac disease and prolonged Q-T intervals on their electrocardiograms have developed "torsades des pointes" ventricular tachycardia while on this drug, so it must be used with caution in patients who have cardiovascular risk factors.

Prostaglandin Synthetase Inhibitors

Prostaglandins cause smooth muscle to contract. Because of this action, some investigators have proposed using prostaglandin synthetase inhibitors to treat detrusor instability. In general, use of these drugs has not been very successful. They must be used in high doses to have any effect on the bladder and these high doses produce overpowering side effects. There are some women, however, who report increased urgency and frequency with exacerbations of urge incontinence around their menstrual periods. Anecdotal reports suggest that prostaglandin synthetase inhibitors are helpful in reducing symptoms in such patients, probably by decreasing the production and subsequent release of prostaglandins by the uterus. Since the bladder sits on top of the lower uterine segment, it is easy to see how increased uterine production of prostaglandins might affect bladder function in some women. Prostaglandin synthetase inhibitors are not first-line therapy for detrusor instability, but they may be useful adjuncts to treatment in some patients.

Estrogens

There is no clinical evidence that estrogens alone can return an unstable bladder to stability, but since genitourinary atrophy may produce substantial irritation in its own right, we recommend treating postmenopausal women with some form of hormone replacement therapy if they have symptoms of urgency, frequency, or urge incontinence, and have no contraindications to such therapy.

Other Forms of Therapy

The vast majority of patients with idiopathic detrusor instability can be treated successfully with a combination of bladder drill and drug therapy. Since few people wish to take medications frequently and for prolonged periods of time—particularly if those medications have unpleasant side effects—behavioral modification is usually the mainstay of long-term treatment for the unstable bladder. When drugs are used, they should be titrated to a patient's individual situation and tapered to low maintenance levels as soon as possible. Patients with detrusor hyperreflexia due to neurologic causes, however, will rarely (if ever) respond to behavioral modification alone and will probably need prolonged drug therapy. Refractory cases may benefit from electrical stimulation or radical bladder surgery.

Electrical stimulation has been used in the treatment of both genuine stress incontinence and detrusor instability for some years. Experimental evidence indicates that intravaginal or transrectal electrical stimulation activates inhibitory nerve fibers in the sympathetic hypogastric nerve while at the same time inhibiting parasympathetic excitatory neurons in the pelvic floor to produce a reflex inhibition of the detrusor. A variety of regimens, using either a vaginal or rectal plug electrode, have been used to deliver the electrical stimulus (Fig. 6.4). The results of such therapy have been mixed and some delivery systems have been plagued by device failure and poor patient acceptance. There is currently a renewed interest in this form of therapy, and new engineering approaches will probably eliminate many of the problems which plagued earlier devices. Unless they have a large number of incontinent patients and a special interest in this area, most clinicians in office practice will probably want to wait for new developments before employing this technology extensively.

Patients who have utterly intractable detrusor instability/hyperreflexia that has failed to respond to medical or behavioral therapy, will often benefit from surgical treatment. The operations available for treating this condition either denervate the bladder or augment its capacity. Surgical denervation can be created either centrally at the spinal cord or peripherally at the bladder. The capacity of the bladder can be increased by augmenting it with a patch of bowel or stomach. Because the interposed gastrointestinal segment does not contract when the rest of the bladder does, it acts to ''damp out'' unwanted vesical contractility, decreasing the force of the contraction produced so that continence can still be maintained. Augmentation cystoplasty currently appears to be the most effective operation for treating these difficult cases. It may be combined with reconstructive surgery on the bladder neck (such as a sling or artificial urinary sphincter), or it may be performed in conjunction with the creation of a continent catherizable urinary diversion. Surgery of this kind is never first-line treatment for patients and requires referral to a tertiary care urodynamics center where expert evaluation and follow-up can be provided.

It should be understood that everyone cannot always be rendered completely dry and totally continent. Detrusor instability is often a chronic disease process which waxes and wanes, with good periods and bad. The physician must bring sympathy, patience, and understanding to the care of these individuals, realizing all the while that although they may not all be cured, nonetheless they can nearly all be improved.

Which Therapy for Which Patient?

Given the array of drugs, behavioral techniques, electrical stimulators and complex surgical procedures which may be used in patients with incontinence caused by detrusor overactivity, how do you decide what to do? Which patients need which therapy? A few main patterns of urge incontinence can be described, based upon the clinical presentation of the patient. Each type of patient has her own needs, and therapy can be tailored to her specific situation.

"Frequent Flier"

Many women with urge incontinence present with a syndrome where they develop a sudden urge to urinate which sends them flying to the bathroom. They can suppress this urge briefly and sometimes they make it to the toilet in time, but sometimes they leak urine before they get there. Their lives are dominated by a pattern of frequency and urgency, intermixed with urge incontinence. These women are prime candidates for bladder retraining. Since they can suppress their urgency for a short period of time, therapy should be directed towards gradually lengthening the amount of time during which they can suppress detrusor contractions. It is sometimes useful to start a low-dose anticholinergic drug as well, and to taper this medication fairly quickly over a few weeks once their self-confidence begins to improve.

"Key-in-the-Lock"
Incontinence

One of the most common presentations of urge incontinence is urine loss that is triggered by specific social stimuli. Women with this problem often have trouble only under certain circumstances, such as in delaying urination once they get close to a bathroom when their bladders are full. The term was coined from the common situation described by many patients in which they arrive home from running errands with a full bladder and the need to urinate. As they fumble with their keys to get into the house, their urgency increases. As the door springs open, they make a mad dash for the bathroom but as they do so they start to leak urine. These patients have urine loss triggered by uncontrollable anticipation of bladder emptying. This may be the only situation in which urine loss occurs for them, but it may happen frequently. These patients need better bladder habits.

The first step in managing these patients is to explain that their problem is delaying urination once they have the urge to go. Often these women are chronic "holders," who urinate only three or four times per day. Once they do have to go, their bladders will not be denied. If they void regularly before the urge is present, however, this will often eliminate the incontinence. In women who have a reduced bladder capacity, anticholinergic medications may increase their capacity so that they do not have to void so frequently. Patients need to understand that medication will not alleviate their problem entirely and that they still need to urinate before they have an overwhelming urge to do so. Anticholinergic drugs can help make the time interval between voidings longer and therefore more convenient for them.

If these patients get into a situation where they develop symptoms of increasing urgency (such as getting into the house after being out for a while), they must not panic! The most important thing is to maintain control. They should slow down, stop, concentrate, cross their legs, or squeeze their thighs together (a very useful temporary continence mechanism), until the imminent urge to urinate subsides. Then they can proceed to the toilet *slowly and calmly.* Rushing will only make their symptoms worse! Women with situational urge incontinence under other circumstances, such as taking showers, swimming, washing dishes, and so forth, should be encouraged to find out what situations cause problems for them and to try to empty their bladders before engaging in such activities. If the urge to urinate hits them suddenly under these circumstances, they should likewise stop, concentrate, make the urge subside, and then proceed slowly and calmly to the bathroom. All behavioral therapy is simply an effort to get patients to control their bladder habits.

"Downpour Incontinence"

Downpour incontinence is a graphic description of the patient who has sudden, unexpected loss of large volumes of urine and gets soaked, just as the unexpected traveler out in the open can be drenched by an unexpected squall which blows up seemingly out of the blue. These patients experience urine loss without warning and once the leakage starts it cannot be controlled. They stand there helplessly while their bladder empties almost completely. Frequency and urgency may not be present. Their only symptoms are sudden, massive urine loss.

Patients with neuropathic bladders often present with this problem. These patients usually require anticholinergic medications, sometimes at high doses, to control their symptoms. Bladder retraining is not particularly useful for these patients, because prodromal urgency is often absent and the time from warning to leakage is so short. Cystometric studies often reveal a typical "trigger volume," a volume of urine which triggers a massive detrusor contraction. Rather than have patients with this problem attempt to prolong the intervals between voids, it is often useful for them to urinate on a rigorous schedule and to spread their fluid intake out throughout the day. This should help them keep their bladder volumes below the threshold which triggers a detrusor contraction.

DHIC

This refers to "Detrusor Hyperactivity with Impaired Contractility," a condition in which detrusor overactivity is combined with inefficient emptying. These patients develop motor urge incontinence along with a large residual urine. This condition is found most commonly in geriatric patients in whom the detrusor muscle has become both overactive and inefficient. These patients should be managed by removing the residual urine and treating any underlying urinary tract infection. Given the proper instruction and support, most elderly patients can manage to catheterize themselves. Removing the residual urine may be all that is required to restore continence in some patients. Others will require anticholinergic medications to stop the detrusor hyperactivity, after which they must catheterize to empty their bladders. Patients with this pattern can be extraordinarily difficult to treat, depending on their social circumstances and general medical condition. Many younger patients with neurologic conditions, such as multiple sclerosis, also present with detrusor hyperreflexia and elevated residual urines. These patients require time, skill, and multiple adjustments in their bladder management program as their condition often changes over time.

Urodynamics of Detrusor Instability: Technical Aspects

Clinically significant detrusor contractions cause changes in intravesical pressure which produce symptoms: urgency and/or incontinence. The urgency produced by these contractions may be associated with urinary frequency or incontinence. The incontinence produced by unstable detrusor contractions may occur when the patient is either awake or asleep, and it may or may not be associated with the forewarning symptom of urgency. The most accurate method we have at present for detecting changes in bladder pressure due to unstable detrusor contractions is subtracted cystometry. Although simple bladder pressure will rise when a detrusor contraction occurs, changes in bladder pressure may also be produced by coughing, straining, or changes of position. Measurement of simple bladder pressure alone is, therefore, not always very sensitive in detecting pressure increases due to detrusor activity, unless the patient is carefully observed by an experienced clinician.

The goal of urodynamic investigation is to reproduce the patient's symptoms. Simple filling of the bladder at a constant rate through a single catheter is all that is needed to evaluate sensation, first desire to void, and bladder capacity. Pressure measurements are not needed to do this. If the patient complains of urgency during bladder filling and leaks a large amount while lying quietly on the examination table without coughing or straining, this is sufficient to make the presumptive clinical diagnosis of "detrusor instability." If a simple manometer is attached to the system, a rapid rise in the column of water while leakage is occurring confirms that the bladder is contracting. The patient should again be observed to make sure she is not straining or moving when her leakage occurs.

Subtracted cystometry allows us to compensate for the extraneous rises which abdominal pressure produces on a simple tracing of bladder pressure. These extraneous pressure rises can sometimes mimic detrusor activity to a striking degree. The subtracted technique has some other advantages as well: it is more objective and requires less expertise than interpreting the rise and fall of a fluid column in a simple manometer. The subtracted cystometric technique utilizes simultaneous measurement of bladder pressure (Pves) and abdominal (usually rectal) pressure (Pabd) during cystometry. Pabd is then subtracted electronically from Pves to produce the "subtracted detrusor pressure" (Pdet). This may be expressed in the simple equation: Pdet = Pves−Pabd. The subtracted pressure technique thus "damps out" increases in intra-abdominal pressure to give us a clean "detrusor pressure" tracing. This "true" detrusor pressure is only the relative pressure difference between the rectum and the bladder and not an absolute measurement of a "real" physiologic pressure. It is, however, about as close as we can get to the true pressure exerted by the detrusor muscle under most clinical circumstances.

Detrusor contractions on a multichannel cystometrogram should manifest themselves as phasic contractions which produce a rise and fall in bladder pressure. This pressure change should be mirrored by a similar rise and fall in

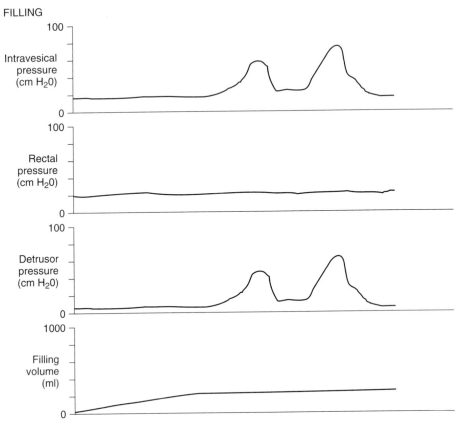

FILLING

Figure 8.2 Subtracted cystometrogram showing detrusor instability. Note that the bladder pressure rises along with the rise in detrusor pressure, while the abdominal pressure remains unchanged.

subtracted detrusor pressure. The abdominal (rectal) pressure tracing should remain stable while this occurs (Fig. 8.2). Almost any artifact on a cystometrogram can be resolved by comparing the three tracings carefully with one another and thinking about what is going on. All three pressure tracings should be consistent with each other. Straining, for example, will usually produce similar rises in bladder and abdominal pressure, but will be canceled out by the subtraction process to produce a relatively flat detrusor tracing (Fig. 8.3). Spontaneous rectal contractions, which are often stimulated by the initial insertion of a catheter into the rectum during cystometry, will produce phasic undulations on the abdominal pressure tracing. Because these rectal pressure changes are subtracted from the bladder pressure, their *mirror image* will appear on the detrusor tracing. Increases in rectal pressure will be subtracted to produce a downward deflection of the detrusor pressure tracing, and a sudden decrease in rectal pressure will produce an increase in the subtracted tracing which may mimic unstable detrusor activity (Fig. 8.4). Spontaneous contractions of this sort are present in about 50% of cystometrograms in which rectal pressure is used as the approximation of abdominal pressure; however, these contractions will fade away over the course of the study about 80% of the time. One cannot emphasize enough the importance of looking at all tracings simultaneously before rendering a diagnosis!

In urodynamic terms, the unstable detrusor can be defined as one that is shown objectively (i.e., by cystometry) to contract, either spontaneously or on provocation, during the filling phase of a cystometrogram while the patient is attempting to inhibit micturition. Without patient cooperation, it is impossible

FILLING

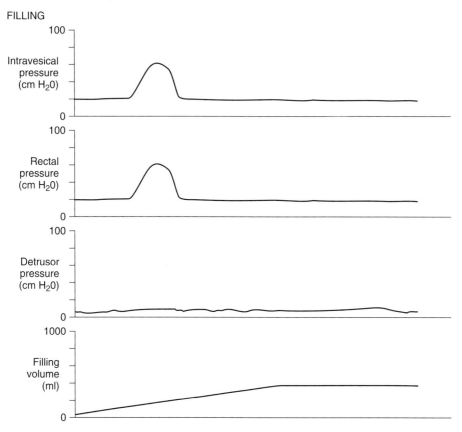

Figure 8.3   Artifactual rises in bladder pressure caused by abdominal straining. Note that bladder pressure and abdominal pressure increase together, while the subtracted detrusor pressure remains unchanged.

to differentiate involuntary detrusor contractility from voluntary micturition. This is one reason why it is difficult to perform urodynamic tests on uncooperative or mentally impaired patients.

A fundamental assumption of urodynamic testing is that the normal detrusor is stable and should remain stable even when provoked. When performing cystometry on patients suspected of having an unstable or hyperreflexic bladder, a major goal of the procedure is to provide enough provocative stimuli to cause the detrusor to contract. The normal individual should be able to suppress these contractions in spite of such stimuli, but the patient with detrusor instability will not be able to do so. We know that certain postural or environmental stimuli will trigger uncontrollable detrusor activity in some patients. Many patients will identify such stimuli if they are questioned carefully; hence, ''provocative cystometry'' refers to the technique of filling the bladder while using such stimuli in order to cause the hidden unstable detrusor to reveal itself. Numerous studies have shown that the more care that is taken to stimulate the bladder, the more detrusor instability will be uncovered. Thus, some detrusor instability will be uncovered by conventional supine filling cystometry, more by changing the patient's position after filling (e.g., from supine to upright), and still more by doing cystometry either in the erect position, or by doing two cystometrograms at the same session in rapid succession, such as filling first in the supine position and then in the erect position. The additional stimuli of heel-bouncing, coughing, listening to water running in the background, or even having the patient wash her hands while cystometry is being performed, will increase the diagnostic

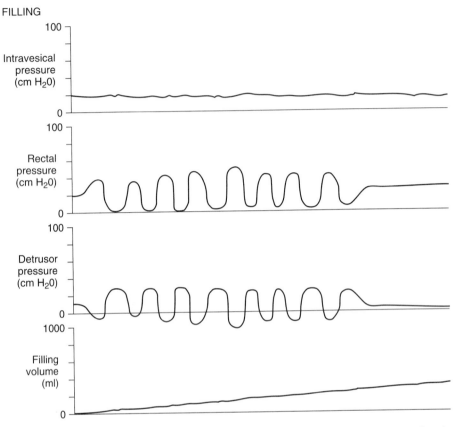

FILLING

Figure 8.4 Artifactual changes in detrusor pressure caused by subtraction of spontaneous rectal contractions. Note that bladder pressure remains unchanged. Artifact should be suspected when the detrusor pressure undulates below the baseline.

yield (Figs. 8.5 and 8.6). Care should always be taken to make sure that what is occurring during the study reproduces the problem the patient is complaining about. Artifacts and misinterpretations still occur.

The rate of filling is also important. Rapid filling uncovers more unstable bladders than does slow filling, and continuous infusion uncovers more instability than incremental filling. Filling is usually done at medium (10–100 ml/min) or fast (100 ml/min) rates, except in patients with profound neurologic impairment. Slow fill cystometry at rates of less than 10 ml/min are often used in these patients to gain a better appreciation of just how much their bladders can hold.

Slow filling in neuropathic patients is important for other reasons as well. Patients with spinal cord injuries, in particular, may develop autonomic dysreflexia if the bladder is filled too rapidly. This condition is characterized by profound systolic hypertension, sweating, piloerection, and paradoxical bradycardia. It usually occurs in patients who have cord lesions above T5/T6 with viable segments in the distal cord and an intact thorocolumbar outflow tract. These disturbances may be precipitated by bladder or rectal distension, or even skin lesions in some patients. The process may lead to convulsions, cerebrovascular accidents, and even death. Estimates suggest that up to 85% of paraplegics experience some degree of this syndrome from time to time. Should this occur during cystometry, the bladder must be decompressed immediately and pharmacologic agents given to lower the blood pressure. Clinicians who rarely treat patients with spinal cord injury are unlikely to see this complication, but must be aware of it.

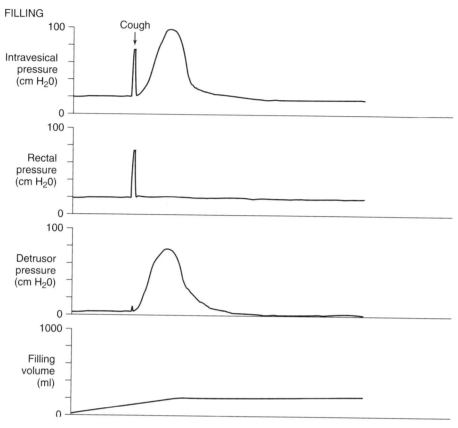

Figure 8.5 Unstable detrusor contraction provoked by coughing. The cough generates an immediate detrusor contraction. Leakage of this kind can be mistaken for simple stress incontinence unless a thorough evaluation of the patient is performed.

It should also be remembered that subtracted cystometry is only a *relative* approximation of true detrusor activity since cystometric data are obtained by measuring bladder pressure, assuming that bladder pressure represents the sum of the pressures produced by detrusor activity and the external forces acting on the bladder, then estimating intra-abdominal pressure indirectly by measuring rectal (or sometimes vaginal) pressure, and subtracting the latter from the measured bladder pressure. The detrusor pressure is the relative difference between these pressures. This is a calculation, an approximation, not a ''real'' pressure measurement. It will vary depending upon the cystometric technique used, the calibration of the equipment, patient position, whether vaginal or rectal pressure is used to approximate abdominal pressure, and whether electronic microtip transducer pressure catheters or fluid-filled pressure lines are used. In the latter case it is important that the transducers are positioned at the level of the upper border of the pubic symphysis at all times in order to avoid introducing artifactual changes into the study.

According to the early convention, adopted in 1976 by the International Continence Society in its first report on the standardization of terminology of lower urinary tract function, phasic detrusor contractions were considered significant if they were greater than an arbitrary threshold of 15 cm H_2O. However, it is clear that there are many patients with significant symptoms who have ''subthreshold'' detrusor contractions that do not reach this level of magnitude. The most recent terminology adopted by the International Continence Society (1988), recognizes this fact and has abandoned the 15 cm H_2O pressure threshold

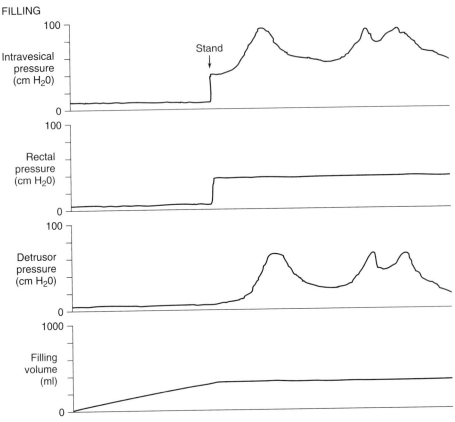

Figure 8.6 Detrusor instability provoked by change of position. The detrusor is stable during filling in the supine position, but assumption of an upright posture provokes an unstable contraction.

in the definition of unstable detrusor activity. The important point is always that cystometric findings *must* be interpreted within the context of the history and physical examination, because even low level contractions may be clinically significant if they produce symptoms. There is no magic number which must be obtained during cystometry to make the diagnosis of detrusor instability. The important thing is whether the patient says that what has happened during the change in pressure is what happens when she has symptoms. As a practical matter, contractions of less than 15 cm H_2O are much less likely to cause symptoms than high-pressure contractions; when they do cause symptoms, low-pressure contractions are generally easier to treat than high-pressure contractions.

Similar confusion exists regarding the relationship between bladder compliance and detrusor activity. Bladder compliance is a measurement of the volume/pressure relationship of the bladder. In most cases bladder compliance is a reflection of the viscoelastic properties of the bladder itself. Bladder compliance should be measured by filling the bladder to cystometric capacity and allowing the pressures to equilibrate for 60 seconds. The volume (in ml) is then divided by the end-filling detrusor pressure in cm H_2O obtained after equilibration. This produces a compliance index (Table 8.4). A normal bladder compliance index will be between 21 and 100 ml/cm H_2O. A low compliance bladder (that is, one which is poorly distensible and has a high end-filling pressure) will have a compliance index of less than 20 ml/cm H_2O. This is *not* the same thing as an unstable detrusor. If the compliance index is greater than 100 ml/cm H_2O, the bladder may be overly distensible. However, a patient cannot be given a diagno-

TABLE 8.4.   Bladder Compliance

$$\text{Bladder Compliance} = \frac{\text{Bladder Capacity (ml)}}{\text{Pdet at end of filling (cm } H_2O)}$$

Compliance Index	Significance
<21 ml/cm H_2O	Low bladder compliance
21–100 ml/cm H_2O	Normal bladder compliance
>100 ml/cm H_2O	High bladder compliance (Bladder capacity must be >650 ml)

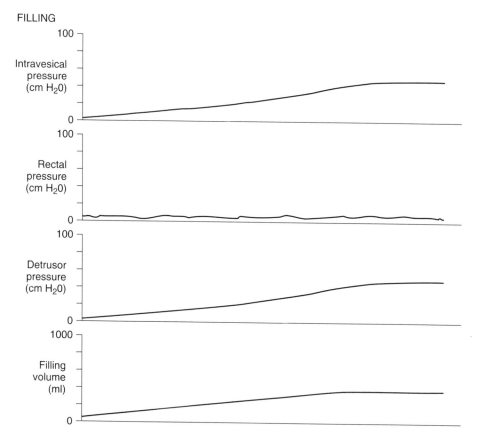

Figure 8.7   "Steep" cystometrogram showing low compliance and low bladder capacity. There is a slow steady rise in detrusor pressure without phasic activity.

sis of high bladder compliance unless the bladder capacity is greater than normal. Generally this means that a woman must have a high compliance index and a cystometric capacity of at least 650 ml to have this diagnosis.

Part of the confusion between "detrusor instability" and "low bladder compliance" originated in the arbitrary use of a 15 cm H_2O threshold for diagnosing detrusor instability. If the end-filling detrusor pressure was 15 cm H_2O, some clinicians labeled the patient as abnormal and gave her a diagnosis of "detrusor instability." In the absence of unstable contractions, the end-filling pressure must be interpreted in light of the bladder capacity. "Steep" cystometrograms with high end-filling pressures should be regarded as showing altered compliance rather than abnormal detrusor activity (Fig. 8.7). A steep or low compliance

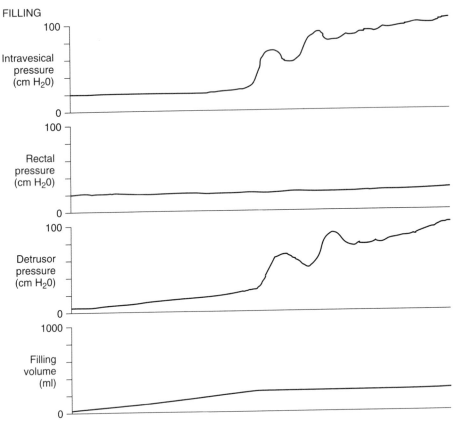

FILLING

Intravesical
pressure
(cm H₂0)

Rectal
pressure
(cm H₂0)

Detrusor
pressure
(cm H₂0)

Filling
volume
(ml)

Figure 8.8 Cystometrogram showing low compliance in association with detrusor overactivity (detrusor hyperreflexia).

cystometrogram can, of course, coexist with phasic detrusor instability (Fig. 8.8). This distinction is of critical importance, because low compliance may result from neurologic abnormalities or from changes in the viscoelastic properties of the bladder wall itself, such as fibrotic changes resulting from radiation therapy or vesical tuberculosis. Urodynamic studies of myelodysplastic children have shown that low compliance bladders with high resting intravesical pressures (over 45 cm H_2O) are associated with deterioration of the upper urinary tracts. Although the pediatric patient may be more vulnerable to high-pressure insults of this nature than an adult, prudent clinical practice would suggest screening women with these findings for the presence of ureteral reflux and upper tract damage.

"Low compliance" may also be an artifact, usually resulting from rapid bladder filling. If the bladder is filled at an unphysiologic rate, the bladder volume may increase more rapidly than the bladder muscle can relax to accommodate the increasing bladder volume. This generally produces a "steep" cystometrogram. Stopping the infusion and allowing the bladder to "catch up" with the fluid that is distending it will eliminate this artifactual "low compliance" (Fig. 8.9). This is another reason why the bladder should be allowed to equilibrate before compliance is calculated.

The object of cystometry is to reproduce the patient's symptoms and to correlate them with objective urodynamic data. Since cystometry represents only a twenty minute "window" on bladder activity that is observed under rather unphysiologic circumstances in a urodynamics laboratory, the patient's chief

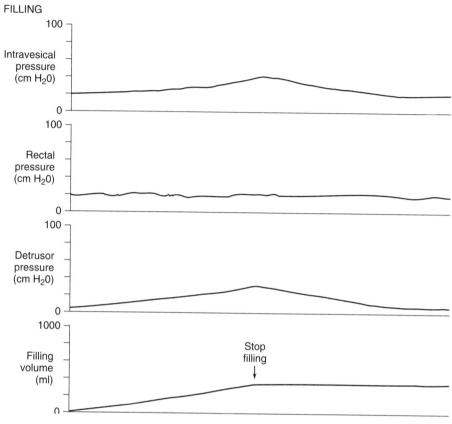

Figure 8.9   Artifactual low bladder compliance due to rapid infusion of fluid. Once bladder filling has been stopped, the bladder gradually accommodates to its fluid load and demonstrates normal compliance.

complaint may not always be reproduced by the study. There are some patients with an unstable bladder whose detrusor does not "misbehave" during a cystometric examination. Therefore, even if detrusor instability is *not* demonstrated one cannot speak of the patient having a "stable *bladder*," but only of having a "stable *cystometrogram*." The patient may still suffer from symptoms produced by unstable detrusor activity at other times and places! Similarly, bladder contractions which produce *no* symptoms at all have no significance. Urodynamic investigations should always take place within the context of patient's history and physical examination, and ideally should be performed by a physician who has taken the history and personally examined the patient.

To overcome the problems inherent in cystometry performed in an artificial laboratory environment, ambulatory urodynamic recording systems have been developed which can provide up to 24 hours of continuous monitoring of bladder, urethral, rectal, and detrusor pressures. These studies have advantages similar to those of a 24-hour Holter monitor over a 12-lead electrocardiogram in the diagnosis of cardiac arrhythmias. When analyzed by computer, these long-term urodynamic recordings allow a much more accurate assessment of detrusor activity. Systems such as these may ultimately replace conventional urodynamic studies in many situations. Ambulatory urodynamic monitoring of patients with symptoms suggestive of detrusor instability but "normal" conventional cystometrograms consistently shows a much higher rate of unstable detrusor activity when the bladder is monitored for a prolonged period of time.

SUGGESTED READING

Comprehensive Reviews

Freeman RM, Malvern J (Eds). The Unstable Bladder. London:Wright, 1989.

Wall LL. Diagnosis and management of urinary incontinence due to detrusor instability. Obstet Gynecol Surv 1990; 45:1S–47S.

General Considerations

Abrams P, Blaivas JG, Stanton SL, Andersen JT. The standardisation of terminology of lower urinary tract function. Scand J Urol Nephrol Suppl 1988; 114:5–18.

Arnold EP, Webster JR, Loose H, et al. Urodynamics of female incontinence: Factors influencing the result of surgery. Am J Obstet Gynecol 1973; 117:805–13.

Bates CP, Loose H, Stanton SL. The objective study of incontinence after repair operations. Surg Gynecol Obstet 1973; 136:17–22.

Booth CM, Whiteside CG, Turner-Warwick RT. A long-term study of the persistence of the urodynamic characteristics of the unstable bladder. Br J Urol 1981; 53:310–14.

Cantor TJ, Bates CP. A comparative study of symptoms and objective urodynamic findings in 214 incontinent women. Br J Obstet Gynaecol 1980; 87:889–92.

Cordozo LD, Stanton SL. Genuine stress incontinence and detrusor instability: A review of 200 cases. Br J Obstet Gynaecol 1980; 87:184–90.

Haylen BT, Sutherst JR, Frazer MI. Is the investigation of most stress incontinence really necessary? Br J Urol 1989; 64:147–49.

Rees DLP, Whitfield HN, Islam AKM, et al. Urodynamic findings in adult females with frequency and dysuria. Br J Urol 1975; 47:853–60.

Rees DLP, Whickham JEA, Whitfield HN. Bladder instability in women with recurrent cystitis. Br J Urol 1978; 50: 524–28.

Sand PK, Hill RC, Ostergard DO. Incontinence history as a predictor of detrusor instability. Obstet Gynecol 1988; 71:257–60.

Whiteside CG, Arnold EP. Persistent primary enuresis: A urodynamic assessment. Br Med J 1975; 1:364–67.

Whorwell PJ, McCallum M, Creed FH. et al. Non-colonic features of irritable bowel syndrome. Gut 1986; 27:37–40.

Whorwell PJ, Lupton EW, Erduran D, et al. Bladder smooth muscle dysfunction in patients with irritable bowel syndrome. Gut 1986; 27:1014–17.

Behavioral Therapy

Burgio KL, Whitehead WE, Engel BT. Urinary incontinence in the elderly: Bladder-sphincter biofeedback and toileting skills training. Ann Int Med 1985; 103:507–15.

Cardozo LD, Abrams PD, Stanton SL, et al. Idiopathic bladder instability treated by biofeedback. Br J Urol 1978; 50: 521–23.

Cardozo LD. Stanton SL. Biofeedback: A 5–year review. Br J Urol 1984; 56:220.

Fantl JA, Hurt WG, Dunn LJ. Detrusor instability syndrome: The use of bladder retraining drills with and without anticholinergics. Am J Obstet Gynecol 1981; 140:885–90.

Fantl JA, Wyman JF, McClish DK, et al. Efficacy of bladder training in older women with urinary incontinence. JAMA 1991; 265:609–13.

Freeman RM, Baxby K. Hypnotherapy for incontinence caused by the unstable bladder. Br Med J 1982; 284: 1831–34.

Frewen WK. Urge and stress incontinence: Fact and fiction. Br J Obstet Gynaecol 1970; 77:932–34.

Frewen WK. Urgency incontinence: Review of 100 cases. J Obstet Gynaecol Br Commonw 1972; 79:77–79.

Frewen WK. An objective assessment of the unstable bladder of psychosomatic origin. Br J Urol 1978; 50:246–49.

Frewen WK. Role of bladder retraining in the treatment of the unstable bladder in the female. Urol Clin NA 1979; 6:273–77.

Frewen WK. The significance of the psychosomatic factor in urge incontinence. Br J Urol 1984; 56:330.

Hafner RJ, Stanton SL, Guy J. A psychiatric study of women with urgency and urgency incontinence. Br J Urol 1977; 49:211–14.

Holmes DM, Stone AR, Bary PR. Bladder training—3 years on. Br J Urol 1983; 55:660–64.

Holmes DM, Plevnik S, Stanton SL. Bladder neck electrical conductivity in the treatment of detrusor instability with biofeedback. Br J Obstet Gynaecol 1989; 96:821–30.

Macaulay AJ, Stern RS, Holmes DM, et al. Micturition and the mind: Psychological factors in the aetiology and treatment of urinary symptoms in women. Br Med J 1987; 294:540–43.

Walters MD, Taylor S, Schoenfield LS. Psychosexual study of women with detrusor instability. Obstet Gynecol 1990; 75:22–26.

Drug Therapy

Awad SA, Bryniak S, Downie JW, et al. The treatment of the uninhibited bladder with dicyclomine. J Urol 1977; 117:161–63.

Baigre RJ, Kelleher JP, Fawcett DP, et al. Oxybutynin: Is it safe? Br J Urol 1988; 62:319–22.

Barker G, Glenning PP. Treatment of the unstable bladder with propantheline and imipramine. Aust NZ J Obstet Gynaecol 1987; 27:153–54.

Blaivas JG, Labib KB, Michalilk SJ, et al. Cystometric response to propantheline in detrusor hyperreflexia: Therapeutic implications. J Urol 1980; 124:259–62.

Bradley DV, Cozart RJ. Relief of bladder spasm by flavoxate: A comparative study. J Clin Pharmacol 1970; 10: 65–68.

Casteleden CM, Duffin CM, Gulati RS. Double-blind study of imipramine and placebo for incontinence due to bladder instability. Age Aging 1986; 15:299–303.

Finkbeiner AE, Bissada NK, Welch LT. Uropharmacology VI: Parasympathetic depressants. Urology 1977; 10: 503–10.

Fisher JP, Diokno A, Lapides J. The anticholinergic effects of dicyclomine hydrochloride in uninhibited neurogenic bladder dysfunction. J Urol 1978; 120:328–29.

Fisher-Rasmusen W, Korhonon M, Rossberg E, et al. Evaluation of long-term safety and clinical benefit of terodiline in women with urgency/urge incontinence: A multicentre study. Scan J Urol Nephrol 1984; Suppl 87:35–47.

Gajewski JB, Awad SA. Oxybutynin versus propantheline in patients with multiple sclerosis and detrusor hyperreflexia. J Urol 1986; 135:966–68.

Gerstenberg TC, Klarskov P, Ramierez D, et al. Terodiline in the treatment of women with urgency and motor urge incontinence. A clinical and urodynamic double-blind cross-over study. Br J Urol 1986; 58:129–33.

Glassman AH, Bigger JT, Jr. Cardiovascular effects of therapeutic doses of tricyclic antidepressants: A review. Arch Gen Psychiatr 1981; 38:815–20.

Holmes DM, Montz FJ, Stanton SL. Oxybutynin versus propantheline in the management of detrusor instability. A patient-regulated variable dose trial. Br J Obstet Gynaecol 1989; 96:607–12.

Kirkali Z, Whitaker RH. The use of oxybutynin in urologic practice. Int Urol Nephrol 1987; 19:385–91.

Lose G, Jorgensen L, Thunedborg P. Doxepin in the treatment of female detrusor overactivity: A randomized double-blind cross-over study. J Urol 1989; 142:1024–26.

Meyhoff HH, Gersternberg TC, Nordling J. Placebo—The drug of choice in female motor urge incontinence? Br J Urol 1983; 55:34–37.

Richelson E. Antimuscarinic and other receptor blocking properties of antidepressants. Mayo Clin Proc 1983; 58:40–46.

Tapp A, Fall M, Norgaard J, et al. Terodiline: A dose titrated, multicenter study of the treatment of idiopathic detrusor instability in women. J Urol 1989; 142:1027–31.

Thompson IM, Lauvetz R. Oxybutynin in bladder spasm, neurogenic bladder, and enuresis. Urology 1976; 8:452–54.

Thuroff JW, Bunke B, Ebner A, et al. Randomized, double-blind, multicenter trial on treatment of frequency, urgency, and incontinence related to detrusor hyperactivity: Oxybutynin versus propantheline versus placebo. J Urol 1991; 145:813–17.

Ulmsten U, Ekman G, Andersson KE. The effect of terodiline treatment in women with motor urge incontinence. Results from a double-blind study and long-term treatment. Am J Obstet Gynecol 1985; 153:619–22.

Wall LL, Warrell DW. Detrusor instability associated with menstruation—Case report. Br J Obstet Gynaecol 1989; 96:937–38.

Weiner N. Atropine, scopolamine, and related belladonna alkaloids. In Gilman AG, Goodman LS, Gilman A, Mayer SE, Melmon KL (Eds). Goodman and Gilman's The Pharmacological Basis of Therapeutics. 6th ed. New York: Macmillan, 1980:120–37.

Special Cases

Cardozo LD, Stanton SL, Williams JE. Detrusor instability following surgery for genuine stress incontinence. Br J Urol 1979; 51:204–07.

Jorgensen L, Lose G, Mortensen SO, et al. The Burch colposuspension for urinary incontinence in patients with stable and unstable detrusor function. Neurourol Urodynam 1988; 7:435–41.

Karram MM, Bhatia NN. Management of coexistent stress and urge urinary incontinence. Obstet Gynecol 1989; 73:4–7.

Koefoot RB, Webster GD. Urodynamic evaluation in women with frequency, urgency symptoms. Urology 1983; 6:648–51.

Langer R, Ron-El R, Newman M, et al. Detrusor instability following colposuspension for urinary stress incontinence. Br J Obstet Gynaecol 1988; 95:607–10.

McGuire EJ, Lytton B, Kohorn E, et al. The value of urodynamic testing in stress urinary incontinence. J Urol 1980; 124:256–58.

McGuire EJ, Savastano JA. Stress incontinence and detrusor instability/urge incontinence. Neurourol Urodynam 1985; 4:313–18.

McGuire EJ. Bladder instability and stress incontinence. Neurourol Urodynam 1988; 7:563–67.

Resnick NM, Yalla SV. Detrusor hyperactivity with impaired contractile function. An unrecognized common cause of incontinence in elderly patients. J Am Med Assoc 1987; 257:3076–81.

Steel SA, Cox C, Stanton SL. Long term follow-up of detrusor instability following colposuspension operation. Br J Urol 1986; 58:138–42.

Other Forms of Therapy

Fall M. Does electrostimulation cure urinary incontinence? J Urol 1984; 131:664–67.

Lindstrom S, Fall M, Carlsson CA, et al. The neurophysiological basis of bladder inhibition in response to intravaginal electrical stimulation. J Urol 1983; 129:405–10.

Mundy AR. The surgical treatment of urge incontinence of urine. J Urol 1982; 128:481–83.

Mundy AR. Long term results of bladder transection for urge incontinence. Br J Urol 1983; 55:642–44.

Mundy AR, Stephenson TP. ''Clam'' ileocystoplasty for the treatment of refractory urge incontinence. Br J Urol 1985; 57:641–46.

Torrens MJ. Bladder denervation procedures. Urol Clin NA 1979; 6:283–93.

Urodynamic Diagnosis of Detrusor Instability: Technical Aspects

Abrams PH, Blaivas JG, Stanton SL, et al. Standardisation of terminology of lower urinary tract function. Scand J Urol Nephrol Suppl 1988; 114:5–18.

Awad SA, McGinnis RH. Factors that influence the incidence of detrusor instability in women. J Urol 1983; 130:114–15.

Bates P, Bradley WE, Glen E, et al. First report on the standardisation of terminology of lower urinary tract function. Br J Urol 1976; 48:39–42.

Bhatia NN, Bradley WE, Haldeman S. Urodynamics: Continuous monitoring. J Urol 1982; 128:963–68.

Coolsaet BLRA, Blok C, van Venrouji GEFM, et al. Subthreshold detrusor instability. Neurourol Urodynam 1985; 4:309–11.

Coolsaet BLRA. Bladder compliance and detrusor activity during the collection phase. Neurourol Urodynam 1985; 4:263–73.

Griffiths CJ, Assi MS, Styles RA, et al. Ambulatory monitoring of bladder and detrusor pressure during natural filling. J Urol 1989; 142:780–84.

James D. Continuous monitoring. Urol Clin NA 1979; 6:125–35.

Kulseng-Hanssen S, Klevmark B. Ambulatory urethro cystorectometry: A new technique. Neurourol Urodynam 1988; 7:119–30.

McGuire EJ, Wagner FM, Weiss RM. Treatment of autonomic dysreflexia with phenoxybenzamine. J Urol 1976; 115:53–55.

McGuire EJ, Woodside JR, Borden TA, et al. Prognostic value of urodynamic testing in myelodysplastic patients. J Urol 1981; 126:205–09.

McGuire EJ, Woodside JR, Borden TA. Upper urinary tract deterioration in patients with myelodysplasia and detrusor hypertonia: A follow-up study. J Urol 1983; 129:823–26.

McGuire EJ, Rossier AB. Treatment of acute autonomic dysreflexia. J Urol 1983; 129:1185–86.

McInerney PD, Vanner TF, Harris SAB, et al. Ambulatory urodynamics. Br J Urol 1991; 67:272–74.

Macneil HF, Brading AF, Williams JH. Cause of low compliance in a guinea-pig model of instability and low compliance. Neurourol Urodynam 1992; 11:47–52.

Mayer R, Wells T, Brink C, Diokno A, Cockett A. Hand washing in the cystometric evaluation of detrusor instability. Neurourol Urodynam 1991; 10:563–70.

Nordling J, Steven K, Meyhoff HH, et al. Urinary incontinence in the female: the value of detrusor reflex activation procedures. Br J Urol 1979; 51:110–13.

Sizemore GW, Winternitz WW. Autonomic hyperreflexia—Suppression with α-adrenergic blocking agents. NEJM 1970; 282:795.

Trop CS, Bennett CJ. Autonomic dysreflexia and its urological implications: A review. J Urol 1991; 146:1461–69.

Van Waalwijk Van Doorn ESC, Remmers A, Janknegt RA. Conventional and extramural ambulatory urodynamic testing of the lower urinary tract in female volunteers. J Urol 1992; 147:1319–26.

Warrell DW, Watson BW, Shelley T. Intravesical pressure measurement in women during movement using a radio-pill and an air-probe. J Obstet Gynaecol Br Comm 1963; 70:959–67.

Webb RJ, Styles RA, Criffiths CJ, et al. Ambulatory monitoring of bladder pressures in patients with low compliance as a result of neurogenic bladder dysfunction. Br J Urol 1989; 64:150–54.

Webb RJ, Griffiths CJ, Ramsden PD, et al. Measurement of voiding pressures on ambulatory monitoring: Comparison with conventional cystometry. Br J Urol 1990; 65:152–54.

Webb RJ, Griffiths CJ, Zachariah KK, et al. Filling and voiding pressures measured by ambulatory monitoring and conventional studies during natural and artificial bladder filling. J Urol 1991; 146:815–18.

Webb RJ, Ramsden PD, Neal DE. Ambulatory monitoring and electronic measurement of urinary leakage in the diagnosis of detrusor instability and incontinence. Br J Urol 1991; 68:148–52.

Webster GD, Older RA. The value of subtracted bladder pressure measurements in routine urodynamic studies. Urology 1980; 16:656–60.

9   Mixed Incontinence

Many clinicians are under the mistaken impression that urinary incontinence is due *either* to detrusor instability *or* to stress incontinence, and that the only clinical problem lies in which pigeonhole to place the patient. **Mixed incontinence** occurs when a patient has *both conditions simultaneously.* Patients with mixed incontinence are often very difficult to manage, and the prevalence of a mixed etiology is more common than most practitioners realize.

Most patients actually present with mixed *symptoms.* Careful symptom studies have shown that if a detailed history is taken from all patients with urinary incontinence, most of them will be found to have mixed symptoms rather than pure complaints of either "stress" or "urge" incontinence. There are several reasons that this occurs. First of all, many women with stress incontinence void frequently in order to reduce the amount of urine that is in the bladder at any point in time, thus lessening the likelihood that they will leak if they cough or sneeze. This in turn often leads to poor bladder habits which result in increasing frequency and the development of urgency and occasional urge incontinence. Second, there are some women who have unstable detrusor activity precipitated by coughing, change of position, or physical activity. This condition can mimic stress incontinence to a remarkable degree and the patient may describe it as such. Third, there are some women who develop unstable detrusor contractions which cause urgency but which they can control unless they cough, sneeze, or provoke the bladder in some other way. The rise in intra-abdominal pressure which these activities creates is then more than the bladder can bear, and incontinence results.

Studies which correlate cystometric diagnoses with patients' symptom histories have shown that mixed *histories* are encountered far more often than mixed *urodynamic diagnoses.* That is, patients complain of mixed symptoms more often than both conditions can actually be demonstrated to coexist in an individual patient. For patients to be given a *urodynamic diagnosis* of mixed incontinence, the studies must demonstrate *both* stress incontinence and detrusor instability in the same patient. That is, the urodynamic testing must demonstrate urine loss occurring under conditions where intravesical pressure exceeds urethral outlet resistance in the absence of a detrusor contraction ("genuine" stress incontinence), and the studies must also demonstrate urine loss occurring during an unsuppressible detrusor contraction. The percentage of patients for whom this can be demonstrated in the urodynamic laboratory is considerably smaller than the number of patients who begin their evaluation with mixed symptomatology. As a result of this, most authors have concluded that the overlap in symptoms is so broad among patients with detrusor instability, "genuine" stress incontinence, and mixed incontinence, that the patient's history has little bearing on her final diagnosis. In all likelihood, however, detrusor activity and sphincteric function are probably linked closely with each other along a continuum of interrelationships, with "pure" stress incontinence at one end of the spectrum and "pure" detrusor overactivity at the other.

Continence is maintained by the sphincteric mechanism and the detrusor muscle working together: The bladder neck and urethra normally remain closed and the detrusor muscle remains relaxed during bladder filling. When this happens urinary leakage does not occur. Then, during normal voiding, the pelvic floor and urethra relax, the bladder neck opens, and a sustained detrusor contraction empties the bladder. When voiding has been completed, the detrusor relaxes, the pelvic floor regains its tone, and the urethra and bladder neck close again. Normal voiding, like normal bladder storage, is the result of the sphincteric mechanism and the detrusor working together.

It seems highly probable that many cases of incontinence are the result of defects in *both* of these components of the continence mechanism. Rather than being separate problems which occasionally occur together, it seems more likely that there is a broad continuum of interrelationships between detrusor behavior and normal sphincteric function. Conventional cystometry may not be the best way of sorting out these relationships and technically more sophisticated methods of looking at bladder neck function are probably needed to clarify this issue. For example, bladder neck electrical conductivity (BNEC) is a technique which evaluates bladder neck activity through a small ring electrode placed within the urethra right at the junction of bladder neck closure. If the bladder neck opens only slightly, the entrance of urine into the proximal urethra completes an electrical circuit which then causes a deflection on a monitor, indicating bladder neck opening. Holmes and colleagues found that abnormal bladder neck activity was closely associated with urinary urgency and that this technique was more sensitive in detecting detrusor instability than was conventional cystometry. This work suggests that subtle interrelationships between the detrusor and the urethra have more clinical significance that has usually been appreciated. Biofeedback training using BNEC to teach patients how to suppress bladder neck opening has been successful in treating urgency and urge incontinence.

Similarly, if intraurethral pressure is measured during urodynamic studies, as well as the more conventional parameters, a subset of patients will be found in whom a drop in intraurethral pressure occurs just before they develop an unstable detrusor contraction. Some studies have indicated that detrusor instability in such patients responds poorly to conventional anticholinergic therapy, but that much better results are obtained if α-adrenergic stimulants are used to increase urethral tone. This clinical observation also suggests that there is an integral relationship between urethral function and detrusor activity in some patients.

These findings confirm our belief that not all mixed incontinence is the same. There may be several subgroups of patients who present with similar findings, in spite of the fact that the underlying pathophysiology may be quite different. As yet, we are unable to separate these various subgroups clearly from one another. For the present it seems reasonable to view mixed incontinence as a spectrum of disorders ranging from almost pure stress incontinence with a small component of urgency/urge incontinence on the one end, to patients who have gross abnormalities of detrusor control and occasional sphincteric incompetence when the outlet is stressed on the other end. In between there are a large number of patients who have both problems equally, or one problem which is often made worse by a contribution from the other. The patient with an unstable bladder, for example, may find that detrusor overactivity raises intravesical pressure to such a level that the added pressure of a cough occurring during such an episode causes her to leak when she otherwise would not. These patients may report having stress incontinence "only if I cough when I really have the urge to go." The patient with a very weak bladder outlet may find that she cannot generate enough urethral resistance to counteract a relatively small detrusor contraction which she was able to suppress in the days when she had a normal sphincteric unit. Now, however, she wets herself with a very low "leak pressure." In cases such as these, which factor is most responsible for the patient's incontinence?

As has been mentioned, a fall in urethral pressure is sometimes seen just before the start of an unstable detrusor contraction in some patients. This, coupled with what we know of normal voiding, suggests that there may be a reflex arc involved in this process by which detrusor dysfunction is related to urethral dysfunction. It is well-known that some patients experience cough induced detrusor instability (Fig. 8.5), which may mimic stress incontinence to a considerable degree. In these patients, coughing or other physical activity serves as a trigger which causes a detrusor contraction. The forceful entry of urine into the bladder neck may, in some patients, cause both a stress leak as well as provoke a detrusor contraction which results in even worse incontinence. Although investigators have generally been unsuccessful in producing detrusor instability in patients by infusing fluid into the bladder neck, this experimental failure does not invalidate these clinical observations. Similarly, the sensation of urgency may develop in women with pure stress incontinence when urine enters an incompetent bladder neck. Mixed symptoms may therefore result from a single etiology.

How should patients with mixed incontinence be managed? Obviously, patients whose *sole* cause for incontinence is an unstable detrusor should not have bladder neck suspension surgery since repositioning the bladder neck does nothing to alter the pathophysiology which has led to their incontinence. A significant number of ''failed'' operations still occur because patients are improperly selected for surgery.

It is less clear whether surgery is contraindicated in patients who have both proven stress incontinence and detrusor instability. The surgical literature on stress incontinence as a whole strongly indicates that patients with *urodynamically proven* detrusor instability in addition to ''genuine'' stress incontinence, have a worse outcome after bladder neck surgery than patients who have ''genuine'' stress incontinence alone. However, in some patients pre-existing detrusor instability disappears following surgery. Detrusor instability may also appear de novo following surgery in up to 15% of patients in some series, depending upon the operation involved. If symptoms alone are investigated, however, patients who have the symptom of ''urge incontinence'' but do *not* have demonstrable detrusor instability at cystometry (i.e., they have ''sensory urgency'') seem to have a prognosis similar to patients with no symptoms of urge incontinence. This again suggests that unstable detrusor activity falls along a continuum of severity and that patients whose detrusor muscle is unstable enough to be provoked during cystometry may have a different prognosis after surgery than patients whose detrusor responds to filling cystometry by remaining stable, even though they may have symptoms of ''urge incontinence'' under other conditions (such as ambulatory urodynamic testing).

Because unstable detrusor contractions are preceded in many instances by relaxation of the urethra and pelvic floor, there may be a complex reflex pathway involving these two distinct sections of the lower urinary tract. Detrusor instability and stress incontinence are probably connected in many patients. It may be that, in some cases, an abnormal position of the urethra or bladder neck somehow establishes or facilitates detrusor overactivity. By repositioning these structures into a more normal anatomical relationship with each other, the trigger for abnormal detrusor contractions may be eliminated. Surgery for stress incontinence in these patients would, therefore, correct their unstable detrusor activity as well. Unfortunately, we have not yet been able to determine which patients fall into this category.

Finally, the amplitude of the detrusor contractions which are demonstrated during cystometry clearly has a bearing on both patient symptoms and prognosis. Coolsaet has shown that low-level detrusor contractions (under 15 cm H_2O) produce symptoms of urgency and frequency more often than they produce incontinence. Patients who demonstrate ''subthreshold'' contractions of this kind during cystometry but who have a relatively normal bladder capacity are quite different from patients with high amplitude detrusor contractions and a low bladder capacity.

In view of these considerations, we suggest that patients with mixed incontinence should be treated thoughtfully and their care individualized. Not only are the details of each case history different, but there appear to be several different etiologies for patient symptoms as well as several different etiologies for their bladder dysfunction. Mixed incontinence is a mixed bag in more ways than one.

A reasonable place to start is by attempting to make patients define their worst symptom. In some patients the urge incontinence resulting from detrusor instability is clearly the worst part of their problem. Other patients can clearly state that their stress incontinence is by far their major complaint. Other patients cannot begin to describe what is wrong with regard to either symptom. Patients with mixed and confusing symptoms will generally benefit from a full urodynamic investigation, particularly if surgery is contemplated. For those patients with demonstrated detrusor instability and proven stress incontinence, initial conservative therapy using bladder retraining, physical therapy, and pharmacologic agents should be started, particularly if urge incontinence is the predominant symptom. A conservative treatment plan should unquestionably be the rule if the patient has a small functional bladder capacity associated with high amplitude detrusor contractions during cystometry. Imipramine, possessing as it does α-adrenergic activity which increases the tone of the urethra and bladder neck while simultaneously relaxing the detrusor, is often very useful in patients with mixed incontinence, particularly if fluctuations in urethral pressure have been demonstrated during urodynamic investigation. Imipramine can also be added to a regimen which utilizes a major spasmolytic drug such as oxybutynin (Ditropan). α-Adrenergic drugs such as pseudoephedrine (Sudafed) or phenlypropanolamine (Ornade, Naldecon, Triaminic, Tavist-D) can also be used as part of a pharmacologic approach to this problem. Once a conservative management program has been initiated, the patient should be re-evaluated in a few weeks to see if her symptoms have improved. If her incontinence has been improved and she is happy with her new situation, nothing further needs to be done. If she still has significant incontinence and a relatively normal bladder capacity, consideration of surgery to correct proven stress incontinence may be appropriate.

Before surgery is carried out the patient must understand that although her stress incontinence is likely to be improved, not all of her leakage may go away. Many patients do quite well with surgery under these conditions; some, however, are worse off than they were before their operation. This is particularly likely to be true if patients undergo surgery which obstructs the bladder neck. Few women are more unhappy than those who have gambled on an operation to cure their problem and have ended up with worse leakage as well as voiding difficulty. Surgery is a reasonable option for women with severe stress incontinence and a small component of detrusor instability, and for women who have failed a trial of conservative management and who have significant persistent stress incontinence. These women should understand that while the chances of curing their stress incontinence are fairly good, the incontinence that is due to unstable detrusor activity may persist, and in some cases may worsen.

If the patient has severe stress incontinence which is clearly her major complaint, an obvious anatomic defect, and only suffers from occasional urge incontinence due to her detrusor instability, the options of medical and surgical therapy may be discussed with her. These patients generally have had incontinence for some time, and postponing surgery for a few weeks to determine the effects of pharmacologic treatment on their detrusor instability will certainly not make them worse. Nothing is lost by initiating such a plan even while the patient is awaiting admission for her operation, which could be canceled if her incontinence improved dramatically. On the other hand, some patients will prefer to have surgery as soon as possible, and to deal with any potential complications later. This is acceptable if these patients have a normal bladder capacity and relatively low-pressure detrusor contractions, provided they understand the risks and benefits of both options, and the somewhat unpredictable outcome of surgery. We merely wish to emphasize the point that the presence of stress incontinence is not a ''green light'' for surgery, particularly if other urinary tract prob-

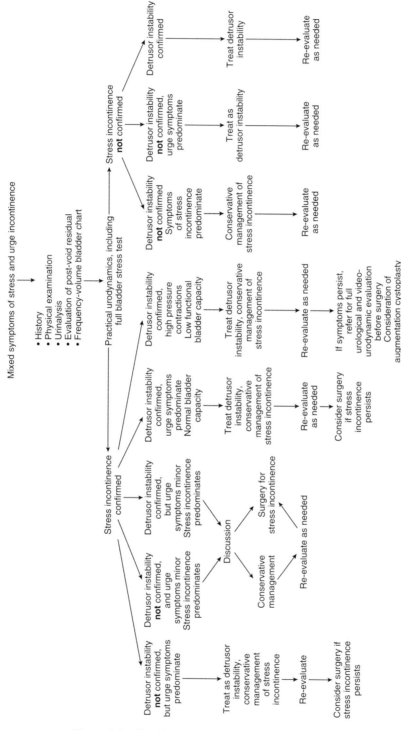

Figure 9.1   Algorithm for the management of mixed incontinence

lems are also present. "Informed consent" is not a substitute for good surgical judgment!

The patient who has a low functional bladder capacity and severe urge incontinence due to high-pressure detrusor contractions presents an especially difficult problem when significant stress incontinence is also present. The risk is that an obstructive bladder neck operation will worsen her detrusor instability, make bladder emptying more difficult, elevate intravesical pressure, and lead to recurrent urinary tract infections, upper tract dilation, and renal damage. These patients should always receive conservative treatment for detrusor instability before any consideration is given to surgery. The results are often surprising. A significant number of patients are completely cured once their detrusor overactivity has been regulated by pharmacologic therapy. For those patients with high amplitude detrusor instability in whom significant stress incontinence persists, particularly if the functional bladder capacity remains reduced, no surgery should be performed without a complete preoperative urologic and urodynamic evaluation. The work-up of such patients should include a full consultation with a competent urologist trained in reconstructive urology, as many of these patients will require augmentation cystoplasty combined with either an artificial urinary sphincter or an obstructive sling procedure.

A proposed algorithm for the evaluation and management of patients with mixed incontinence is given in Figure 9.1.

SUGGESTED READING

Arnold EP, Webster JR, Loose H, Brown ADG, Turner Warwick RT, Whiteside CG, Jequier AM. Urodynamics of female incontinence: Factors influencing the results of surgery. Am J Obstet Gynecol 1973; 117:805–13.

Bergman A, Koonings PP, Ballard CA. Detrusor instability: Is the bladder the cause or the effect? J Reprod Med 1989; 34:834–38.

Cardozo LD, Stanton SL, Williams JE. Detrusor instability following surgery for genuine stress incontinence. Br J Urol 1979; 51:204–07.

Clarke B. Urethral instability. Aust NZ J Obstet Gynaecol 1992; 32:270–75.

Fantl JA, Bump RC, McClish DK. Mixed urinary incontinence. Urology 1990; 36(Suppl):21S–24S.

Hindmarsh JR, Gosling PT, Dean AM. Bladder instability: Is the primary defect in the urethra? Br J Urol 1983; 55: 648–51.

Holmes DM, Plevnik S, Stanton SL. Bladder neck electrical conductivity in female urinary urgency and urge incontinence. Br J Obstet Gynaecol 1989; 96:816–20.

Holmes DM, Plevnik S, Stanton SL. Bladder neck electrical conductivity in the treatment of detrusor instability with biofeedback. Br J Obstet Gynaecol 1989; 96:821–26.

Jorgensen L, Lose G, Mortensen SO, et al. The Burch colposuspension for urinary incontinence in patients with stable and unstable detrusor function. Neurourol Urodynam 1988; 7:435–41.

Karram MM, Bhatia NN. Management of coexistent stress and urge urinary incontinence. Obstet Gynecol 1989; 73: 4–7.

Koefoot RB, Webster GD. Urodynamic evaluation in women with frequency, urgency symptoms. Urology 1983; 6: 648–51.

Koonings P, Bergman A, Ballard CA. Combined detrusor instability and stress urinary incontinence: Where is the primary pathology? Gynecol Obstet Invest 1988; 26: 250–56.

Langer R, Ron-El R, Bukovsky I, Caspi E. Colposuspension in patients with combined stress incontinence and detrusor instability. Eur Urol 1988; 14:437–39.

Langer R, Ron-El R, Newman M, Herman A, Caspi I. Detrusor instability following colposuspension for urinary stress incontinence. Br J Obstet Gynaecol 1988; 95: 607–10.

McGuire EJ, Lytton B, Kohorn E, et al. The value of urodynamic testing in stress urinary incontinence. J Urol 1980; 124:256–58.

McGuire EJ, Savastano JA. Stress incontinence and detrusor instability/urge incontinence. Neurourol Urodynam 1985; 4:313–18.

McGuire EJ. Bladder instability and stress incontinence. Neurourol Urodynam 1988;7:563–67.

Meyhoff HH, Walter S, Gerstenberg TC, Olesen KP, Nordling J, Pedersen PH, Hald T. Incontinence surgery in female motor urge incontinence. Acta Obstet Gynecol Scand 1983; 62:365–68.

Sand PK, Bowen LW, Ostergard DR, Brubaker L, Panganiban R. The effect of retropubic urethropexy on detrusor stability. Obstet Gynecol 1988; 71:818–22.

Stanton SL, Cardozo LD, Williams JE, Ritchie D, Allan V. Clinical and urodynamic features of failed incontinence surgery in the female. Obstet Gynecol 1978; 51:515–20.

Steel SA, Cox C, Stanton SL. Long term follow-up of detrusor instability following colposuspension operation. Br J Urol 1986; 58:138–42.

10

Atypical Causes of Incontinence

Most of the incontinence seen by gynecologists is stress or urge incontinence, or combinations of the two. However, there are other, less common, forms of incontinence which must be considered when evaluating the incontinent female patient. In general, these forms of incontinence consist of urine loss under special circumstances, or represent unusual conditions which mimic common forms of urine loss. Unless these special situations are recognized, the clinician may miss the diagnosis, or worse, proceed with an incorrect and potentially harmful therapy, such as surgically suspending the bladder neck of a patient with a urethral diverticulum or a fistula.

Many of the disorders discussed in this chapter are atypical forms of stress or urge incontinence which merit special attention because of their unique characteristics. For example, it is important to understand the difference between stress incontinence that occurs while laughing and so-called ''giggle incontinence.'' The former type of urine loss is merely simple stress incontinence which happens to be provoked by the increased intra-abdominal pressure of a good hearty laugh. ''Giggle incontinence,'' on the other hand, is a form of uncontrolled detrusor behavior in which complete bladder emptying is provoked by fits of laughter. The conditions can be confused with one another if a clear history is not taken from the patient.

Similarly, the first thought that leaps to the clinician's mind when seeing a patient who complains of ''continuous incontinence'' after childbirth or pelvic surgery is that she may have a genitourinary fistula. While this is sometimes true, it is far more common for the patient to describe stress or urge incontinence as ''continuous'' in order to emphasize the severity of her problem. With a little probing it is soon obvious that the patient has frequent—but intermittent—episodes of incontinence, rather than the constant debilitating leakage produced by a vesicovaginal fistula. When the presence of a fistula seems to be a likely possibility, special diagnostic tests may be needed to clarify the situation and locate the fistula.

The major goal of this chapter is to familiarize clinicians with some of the less common diagnostic entities that may confound and confuse them. Understanding that these conditions exist and how they may present will let the gynecologist give them thoughtful consideration during patient evaluation. Unless these less common causes of incontinence are considered in the differential diagnosis of the patient's problem, the correct diagnosis may be missed. These conditions include unusual anatomic causes of urinary incontinence (diverticula, fistulae, and congenital anomalies), special disorders of storage and emptying (overflow incontinence, detrusor hyperactivity with impaired contractility, nocturnal enuresis, and functional incontinence), and activity-related incontinence (giggle, coital, and exercise incontinence.)

Special Anatomic Causes of Incontinence

The most common ''anatomic'' cause of female urinary incontinence is inadequate support of the urethra leading to hypermobility of this structure and stress incontinence. This has been treated at length elsewhere in this book. However, there are some less common anatomic causes of incontinence which are often unrecognized because the symptoms they produce mimic other kinds of incontinence. Cursory physical examination may not suggest the diagnosis immediately. Most anatomic causes of incontinence are correctable with surgery if the proper diagnosis has been made.

Urinary Tract Diverticula   Urethral diverticula may produce urinary incontinence which typically presents as stress incontinence occurring immediately after voiding, or as postmicturition dribbling. Typically the patient reports that she has no trouble until after she urinates. Then, when she stands up, a small amount of urine runs into her underwear. Sometimes this occurs only if she coughs as she is pulling up her clothing. The urine loss is generally small but noticeable, and rarely ever enough to soak the patient's clothing. If the patient's *only* complaint is stress incontinence occurring under these conditions, a diverticulum should be suspected. These symptoms must clearly be distinguished from the patient who voids, stands up, and then has the sudden urge to go again and voids only a few drops. Patients with this complaint are more likely to have a sensory bladder disorder or unstable detrusor activity as the cause of these symptoms. It should also be remembered that while many patients with urethral diverticula complain of postmicturition dribbling, most postmicturition dribbling is *not* due to the presence of a urethral diverticulum. Many women have these symptoms as a variant of normal micturition.

The pathophysiology of ''stress incontinence'' after voiding or postmicturition dribbling in women with urethral diverticula is as follows. During voiding the urethral diverticulum fills with urine, but this urine is retained in the diverticulum sac due to the patient's position. When she stands up after micturition, the change of position empties the diverticulum, causing the release of a small amount of urine. This kind of incontinence is most likely to be produced by diverticula in the distal portion of the urethra, distal to the point of maximum urethral pressure. Fortunately, diverticula in this location are the easiest to detect clinically. They generally appear as a mass in the anterior vaginal wall which fills with a small amount of urine. Massage of this structure will often result in the expression of urine or pus from the urethral orifice. Urethral diverticula may produce symptomatic incontinence, but more commonly they are associated with a vaginal or urethral mass, pain, urethral discharge, dyspareunia, dysuria, or recurrent urinary tract infections. They may also be completely asymptomatic. A bladder diverticulum is unlikely to produce incontinence, but sometimes shows up as a fluid-filled mass in the anterior portion of the vaginal vault. Bladder diverticula which do not empty completely form reservoirs of stagnant urine that are often associated with recurrent urinary tract infections. They may also harbor bladder stones or tumors. Unless bladder diverticula present in an unusual manner, they are unlikely to be detected on physical examination and must be picked up by cystoscopy or cystography.

Urethral diverticula develop primarily in the posterior wall of the distal urethra in region of the periurethral glands. There are many theories regarding their etiology. Most clinicians believe they result from trauma, infection, or blockage of the periurethral glands. Others believe that these small sacs are congenital in origin. It has been suggested that up to 5% of women have a urethral diverticulum, most of which are asymptomatic. The most attractive theory is that repeated infection and obstruction of the periurethral glands results in the formation of cystic structures. When these become filled with urine or inflammatory exudates, they may become still more obstructed and enlarged until they are symptomatic. Because so many symptomatic diverticula are inflamed, it is usually wise to culture such patients for sexually transmitted diseases such as gonorrhea and chlamydia.

Urethral diverticula are often missed during physical examination because the anterior blade of the vaginal speculum obscures the anterior vaginal wall. Use of a half-speculum (such as a Sims' speculum) or the posterior blade of a Grave's speculum to examine the anterior and posterior vagina separately, will overcome this difficulty. The urethra should be palpated routinely for tenderness

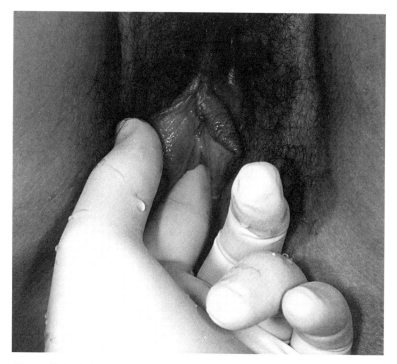

Figure 10.1 Palpating the urethra to detect the presence of a urethral diverticulum.

or the presence of a mass during examination of all incontinent patients (Fig. 10.1). Even under these circumstances, however, the diverticulum sac may be missed. Gentle massage of the urethra may empty the diverticulum, resulting in a discharge of urine or pus. Office urethroscopy will sometimes detect a diverticulum if it is large and has an open neck, but many diverticula have such a narrow orifice opening into the urethra that they cannot be distended without the use of positive pressure. Radiographic screening for diverticula can be accomplished by a voiding cystourethrogram or positive-pressure double-balloon urethrography (Fig. 10.2). If a voiding cystourethrogram is ordered, the radiologist must clearly understand that the clinician is looking for a urethral diverticulum, otherwise the study may focus only on the bladder and the films will be shot too high, leaving the pubic arch and the urethra uninvestigated. The postvoid films are the most important.

Double-balloon urethrography is also highly effective in demonstrating a urethral diverticulum. A Trattner or Davis-Telinde catheter is used for this study. The balloon at the bladder neck is inflated first, followed by the balloon at the urethral meatus, using 30 ml of saline. This assures a tight seal at both ends of the urethra to prevent leakage of the contrast material. Several milliliters of radiopaque dye are then instilled into the urethral lumen during fluoroscopy while films are taken. A voiding cystourethrogram is usually performed at the end of the study.

Many diverticula are asymptomatic. These should be left alone. Minor incontinence may not require surgical treatment if it is the patient's only complaint. These patients can be taught to "strip" the urethra with a finger after voiding to empty the diverticulum and this may well be the only therapy they need. If the diverticulum presents as a painful mass, or if the patient has recurrent urinary tract infections, surgical management may be required. Surgical procedures on a urethral diverticulum should not be undertaken lightly, because some diverticula are extremely complex, corkscrewing around the urethra or connecting with

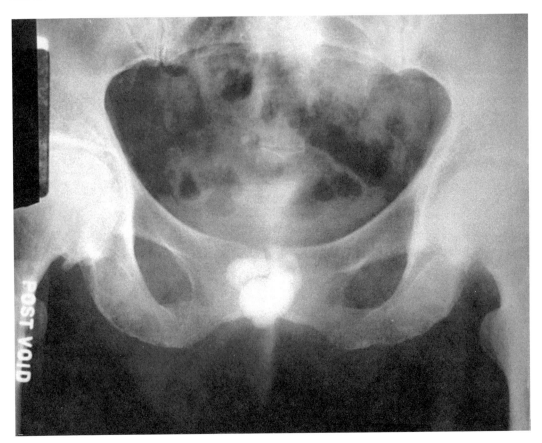

Figure 10.2 Urethrogram demonstrating multiple urethral diverticula in a 76-year old woman. Her only complaint was a slight amount of urinary leakage after voiding, and this was solved by having her "strip" her urethra with a finger after urinating but before she stood up. (Courtesy Dr. Leonard A. Wall.)

a series of other unsuspected diverticula in other locations. Such cases can turn into surgical nightmares and result in substantial damage to the urethra. The most common cause of urethrovaginal fistulae is attempted repair of a urethral diverticulum. Such a fistula occurs in between 5%–25% of attempted repairs.

If surgical repair is required, the patient should have a urethrogram to delimit the diverticulum completely and to rule out complex pathology. Marsupialization should be the primary procedure for symptomatic distal urethral diverticula. This assures complete emptying of the sac without compromising the innervation or muscular layers of the urethra. The technique has been described in detail by Spence and others. Complete excision of a urethral diverticulum requires surgical skill. Several techniques have been described. The entire diverticulum including the neck of the mass should be removed, generally through a vaginal approach. If the orifice of the diverticulum can be seen urethroscopically, it may be possible to insert a small Fogarty embolectomy catheter into the sac, inflate the balloon, and use this to aid in the dissection. Some clinicians will also inject methylene blue dye through such a catheter, to help identify the sac during the dissection. If rupture of the diverticulum occurs during excision, a small pediatric Foley catheter may be inserted into it, inflated, and used to help identify the sac during the procedure. The defect should be closed with fine suture in layers, avoiding superimposition of suture lines whenever possible. Failure to remove the entire sac including its neck and its opening into the urethra may result in recurrence of the diverticulum.

Genitourinary Fistulae

The most miserable forms of incontinence are due to fistulae. The patient

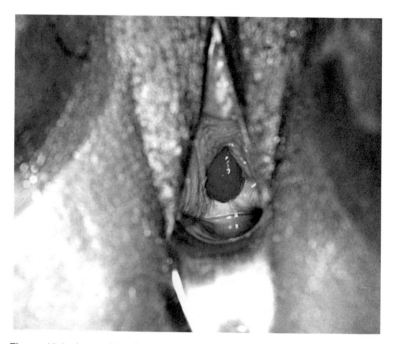

Figure 10.3   Large (5 cm) vesicovaginal fistula in a 20-year old, primiparous, woman from Ghana. She delivered a stillborn child following a prolonged obstructed labor, after which the base of her bladder sloughed off to create a massive fistula. The large mass seen protruding in this photograph is the anterior wall of the bladder which has prolapsed through the fistula into the vagina. (Courtesy Dr. Tom Margolis.)

presents with a history of constant urinary leakage from which she can never escape. Leakage occurs in all positions but is often worse when she is moving or ambulating, and is improved when she is lying down. Other symptoms depend on the size and location of the fistula. Patients with a large vesicovaginal fistula may never void at all because the urine runs out into the vagina as soon as it flows into the bladder, which never fills. Patients with a fistula do not usually experience urgency, and often have low voided volumes when they urinate. An occasional patient will have a small fistula tract which is closed until the bladder reaches a certain volume. When the bladder becomes distended to a certain size, the fistula tract opens and the patient develops a leak. This can be mistaken for ''urge incontinence'' if the patient says she doesn't leak ''until she has to go.''

Worldwide, the most common cause of vesicovaginal fistula formation is obstetric trauma. Over 80% of the urogenital fistula in developing countries are due to obstetric causes, primarily unattended prolonged obstructed labor. This should not be surprising in parts of the world where, due to poor childhood nutrition, infections, and early childbearing, a quarter of the childbearing population is at risk for cephalopelvic disproportion. Because access to modern operative obstetrics is so poor, particularly in rural areas, it is not unusual for women to labor for 2, 3, or 4 days in outlying areas with no medical intervention. These women usually deliver a stillborn child, after which the base of the bladder sloughs due to tissue necrosis induced by the constant pressure of the fetal head. Constant urinary incontinence then develops and the woman's life is destroyed, as she is no longer fit to live with her family and has become unattractive to her husband. Since in many parts of the world girls are married and become pregnant by the age of 13 or 14, the development of a fistula destroys their lives (Fig. 10.3). This is a major unaddressed healthcare problem for women around the globe and needs more publicity. In some parts of northern Nigeria, for example, gynecology clinics see upwards of 300 vesicovaginal fistulae each *month.* In more industrialized countries, such as the United States, most urinary fistulae occur after surgery, after pelvic irradiation, or due to pelvic malignancy.

It should be repeated that most women who complain of "constant leakage" *do not* have urinary fistulae but severe stress and/or urge incontinence; nevertheless, the diagnosis of fistula should be considered in such patients. A history of the onset of symptoms after pelvic surgery, especially after extensive procedures or operations complicated by hemorrhage, malignancy, or infection, is particularly suspicious for a fistula. Genitorurinary fistulae may be classified as follows: bladder to vagina (vesicovaginal, 35%), ureter to vagina (ureterovaginal, 25%), urethra to vagina (urethrovaginal, 20%), and fistulae involving other pelvic organs (vesicocervical, 5%; vesicouterine, 5%).

Evaluation of the patient in whom a urinary fistula is suspected should begin with the physical examination. After voiding, the patient should be catheterized to check the postvoid residual urine volume. This should be negligble. The same catheter may then be used to instill either sterile milk (easily obtained as sterile infant formula) or indigo carmine dye. A 60 ml syringe with the plunger removed, attached to the end of the catheter, forms a suitable receptacle for pouring in the dye. A vesicovaginal fistula may be diagnosed by seeing milk or dye pooling in the vagina. Careful inspection of all parts of the vagina should be undertaken and the position of the speculum should be changed several times to avoid the possibility that the instrument is obstructing the fistula tract; however, the opening of the fistula is sometimes so small that it cannot be located, even though dye is definitely escaping into the vagina.

When the position of a fistula is uncertain, a triple swab test may help locate it, and will also help determine if the leakage is from a ureterovaginal, vesicovaginal, or urethrovaginal fistula. The patient is given 200 mg of oral phenazopyridine hydrochloride (Pyridium) several hours prior to the test so that the urine entering the bladder is orange. The patient should void prior to the test to make sure that her urine has been colored by the drug. Next, the vagina and external urethral meatus are carefully cleaned and dried, and the vagina filled with several folded 4″ x 4″ gauze sponges or cotton balls. Care should be taken to cover the apex, middle, and lower portions of the vagina. The patient's bladder is then filled with 250–300 ml of sterile water or saline in which 2 ml of indigo carmine dye has been mixed. She should then undergo a pad test for an hour or so to allow the sponges to become stained with dye. When enough time has elapsed, the sponges are removed in the opposite order from which they were inserted. Each sponge should be carefully observed as it is removed. If the swab at the top of the vagina is stained orange, this is highly suggestive of a ureterovaginal fistula, since pure orange urine should be found only in the ureter. Orange urine entering the bladder will be obscured by the indigo carmine dye present there. If the top or middle sponge is stained blue, this suggests a vesicovaginal fistula. If the lowest sponge alone is stained, this may suggest a urethrovaginal fistula; however, staining on this sponge may occur due to leakage of urine through the urethra.

Cystourethroscopy should be part of the preoperative evaluation of patients with a fistula to help determine the location of the fistula in relation to the ureters, urethra, and trigone. Small fistulae may be as difficult to see during cystourethroscopy as they are during vaginal examination. A lacrimal duct probe may be useful in locating the fistula, and this may be passed gently through the fistula tract to see its openings in both the bladder and the vagina. Remember, just because one fistula has been found does not mean that others are not present!

Intravenous urography is commonly used to evaluate the urinary tract in patients with a fistula. This may help locate an otherwise undiscoverable fistula, and also helps assure the surgeon that the rest of the urinary tract is normal. When an intravenous urogram is performed on a patient with a fistula, she should be turned 45° from the anteroposterior position to avoid confusing urethral with vaginal passage of radiopaque dye. A ureterovaginal fistula detected by intravenous urography usually requires confirmation by retrograde pyelography.

How a fistula is treated depends upon when it is detected. If the fistula is small and is discovered immediately after surgery or parturition, continuous bladder drainage with a catheter for 6–8 weeks may result in spontaneous closure in some cases. Most fistulae will require surgical repair. Obvious urinary tract injuries should be discovered and repaired at the time of their occurrence. Most fistula develop in the first 10 days following a hysterectomy. Some authors recommend immediate repair, while others are adamant that repair of a vesicovaginal fistula which occurs a week or two after hysterectomy should be deferred for up to 6 months to allow scar tissue formation, a decrease in inflammation, and to obtain maximal postoperative healing. Waiting is not easy for either the patient or the physician. Patients with postoperative vesicovaginal fistulae should be seen regularly and provided with encouragement and emotional support. Management of their incontinence may be facilitated by inserting a Foley catheter through a hole made in the center of a contraceptive diaphragm and gluing it in place to create an intravaginal urinary collection device. Other external collection devices may be helpful during this period, but none are entirely acceptable.

Operative technique for fistula repair is covered in several reviews listed at the end of this chapter. The basic principles of fistula repair have not changed since the days of J. Marion Sims: excision of the fistula tract and surrounding scar tissue, close approximation of tissue planes without tension, avoidance of overlapping suture lines, and prolonged catheter drainage to prevent overdistension of the bladder while it heals. A transvaginal or transabdominal surgical approach may be used, depending on the location of the fistula and the skill of the surgeon. Vaginal excision of the fistula tract is aided by inserting a small Foley catheter through the fistula, inflating the balloon, and excising the scarred fistula while gentle traction is placed on the catheter. The incision should then be closed in multiple layers. At the conclusion of the repair, it is good practice to irrigate the bladder copiously to remove all clots and debris so that the catheter will not become blocked. The bladder should be drained continuously for at least 10 days after surgery to encourage healing. Meticulous attention to catheter care and bladder drainage is imperative! Otherwise excellent surgical repairs have failed because of postoperative mismanagement. Patients should not be sent home to manage their catheters after repair of a fistula in an ambulatory surgical unit! Because of the emotionally devastating nature of a urinary fistula in an otherwise healthy woman, surgical repair of these problems is best performed by an experienced surgeon. Referral of these cases is often necessary.

Congenital Anomalies

Two main congenital anomalies produce incontinence in women: bladder exstrophy and ectopic ureter. Bladder exstrophy occurs due to incomplete fusion of the mesonephric tubules. Mild forms of this condition are seen as epispadias in women. Epispadial defects include incomplete fusion of the genital tubercles and labia minor, and development of a bifid clitoris from incomplete midline fusion of that structure. Complete exstrophy of the bladder is immediately recognized at birth, and requires complex reconstructive surgery by a pediatric urologist. Occasionally a patient with epispadias will reach adulthood before her history of lifelong urinary incontinence is recognized (Fig. 10.4). Along with incomplete midline fusion of genitalia, absent pubic hair in the center of the mons pubis is almost pathognomonic of epispadias.

The diagnosis of ectopic ureter is made easily with intravenous urography, but requires an astute clinician because the findings on physical examination are subtle (Fig. 10.5). Since the hallmark of an ectopic ureter is continuous incontinence since birth, the condition is almost always detected in childhood. Adults who present with a history of *continuous* incontinence since childhood should be suspected of having an ectopic ureter until proven otherwise. The ureter may empty into the uterus, vagina, labia, or urethra.

Patients with bladder exstrophy, epispadias, or an ectopic ureter should be referred to a urologist skilled in the appropriate reconstructive surgery. However,

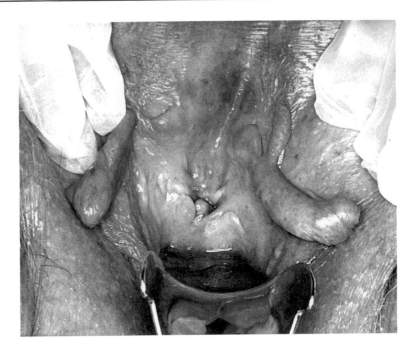

Figure 10.4 Bifid clitoris in an elderly woman with epispadias. This patient had a lifelong history of urinary incontinence and had had an unsuccessful anterior repair as a young woman. She subsequently had two additional Marshall-Marchetti-Krantz procedures, both of which failed, before the significance of her bifid clitoris and its relationship to epispadias was recognized. She was cured of her incontinence by a pubovaginal sling procedure.

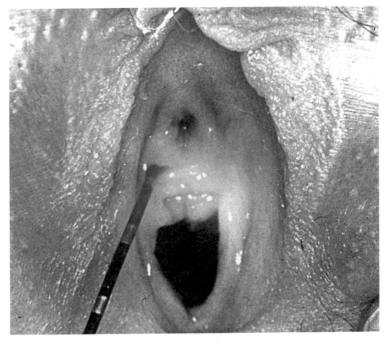

Figure 10.5 Ectopic ureter. A ureteral catheter has been placed through the ectopic orifice which opens into the vestibule.

many of these patients will also have coexistent Müllerian anomalies that may require reconstructive gynecologic surgery at the time of their urologic operation.

Disorders of Storage and Emptying

Aside from the anatomic causes of incontinence mentioned above, a number of special forms of incontinence exist which are due to incomplete emptying or detrusor overactivity under special circumstances. All of these conditions can be overlooked or misdiagnosed, with resultant mismanagement. For example, the patient who has giggle incontinence should not be taken to the operating room for bladder neck surgery because her problem is detrusor dysfunction, not stress incontinence. Similarly, treatment for urge incontinence may *produce* overflow incontinence, and upper tract damage may result if the problem is not recognized and treated.

Overflow Incontinence

The International Continence Society defines overflow incontinence as any involuntary loss of urine associated with overdistension of the bladder. The source of the overdistension may be bladder outlet obstruction or detrusor under-activity in association with neurologic disorders or medications. In patients with overflow incontinence, intravesical pressure gradually rises as the bladder fills, and incontinence occurs when bladder pressure finally exceeds urethral pressure (Fig. 10.6). This may occur for several reasons: An increase in intra-abdominal pressure from a cough or sneeze may raise intravesical pressure higher than outlet resistance and result in stress incontinence. The bladder may be filled to such an extent that the detrusor contracts involuntarily, causing incontinence but not resulting in efficient or complete bladder emptying (see below). Other patients may simply distend the bladder to such an extent that its limits of compliance have been reached and the urine leaks out continuously, much like rainwater running out the bunghole of a rain barrel which has been filled to capacity and has no more room.

Overflow incontinence is always cited as one of the three etiologies of urinary incontinence, along with stress and urge incontinence. In practice, overflow incontinence is relatively uncommon unless one is dealing with a special patient population, such as elderly patients or those with neurologic problems. Patients with lower motor neuron disorders are usually managed by specialists in rehabilitation medicine or urology. Occasionally some of these patients present to gynecologists for care. Measurement of postvoid residual urine will pick up those patients who are at risk of overflow incontinence. This should be done routinely in the evaluation of patients with lower urinary tract symptoms. The absolute volume of residual urine is less important than its relationship to the volume voided. In some cases, residuals of 50 ml are pathologic in neurologically compromised patients who void volumes of 25 ml or less. In neurologically intact patients, the diagnosis of overflow incontinence is usually not considered until the residual volume is over 150 ml on several occasions *and incontinence occurs.*

Patients with overflow incontinence in gynecologic practice will usually have the condition as a result of medical therapy, primarily the use of anticholinergic drugs. Patients with a suspicious neurologic history (i.e., poorly documented past transient ischemic attacks) and the elderly should have a postvoid residual checked within a week or so of initiating anticholinergic therapy. The clinician should be careful to look for symptoms of neuropathy or outflow obstruction in these patients prior to starting anticholinergic drugs, since it is important to treat underlying problems.

Treatment of overflow incontinence should be directed towards facilitation of bladder emptying. If a precipitating pharmacologic agent can be identified, it should be stopped and the patient should be re-evaluated. If this was the sole cause for the overflow incontinence, bladder emptying may return to normal and the problem may be solved. Further treatment depends upon the type of incontinence that has developed in association with bladder overdistension. If stress incontinence or distension-overflow incontinence was the problem, regular bladder emptying by intermittent catheterization may suffice to cure the problem. If the patient has detrusor overactivity with impaired emptying, two courses of

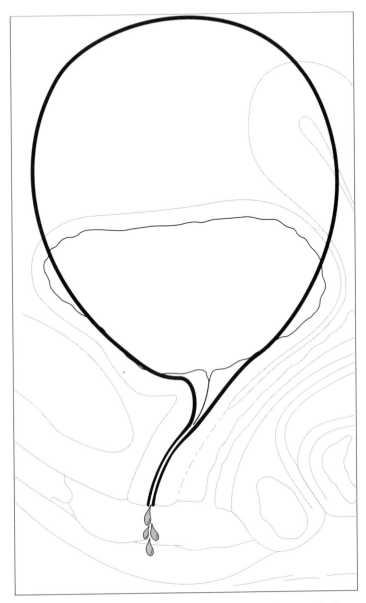

Figure 10.6   Overflow incontinence. The heavy black lines show a markedly over-distended bladder leading to urinary leakage. Incontinence may result from stress incontinence, detrusor contractions provoked by overdistension, or by gradually rising intravesical pressure as the bladder wall reaches its limits of compliance and will not stretch any farther.

therapy may be indicated. Regular intermittent catheterization may keep the bladder volume below the threshold at which uncontrolled detrusor contractions occur and this may be all that is necessary.

Alternatively, the problem can be controlled by vigorous use of anticholinergic medications which paralyze bladder contractility, after which the flaccid bladder can be emptied by a regimen of intermittent catheterization. Medications such as bethanechol chloride (Urecholine) and prostaglandins have been used in attempts to increase detrusor activity and promote bladder emptying, but the clinical results have been very disappointing. Urethral relaxants such as valium or prazosin have been shown to be effective in some cases, but may cause side effects. Occasionally a patient will be able to improve her bladder emptying with the voiding techniques outlined in Chapter 13. For most patients, clean intermittent self-catheterization is the best solution, either as the initial therapy or in combination with anticholinergic medications.

Detrusor Hyperactivity with Impaired Contractility (DHIC)

Detrusor hyperactivity with impaired contractility ("DHIC") is a special diagnosis described recently in elderly patients. Because the International Continence Society defines overflow incontinence as *any* incontinence associated with overdistension of the bladder, DHIC will be considered here as a separate entity. The authors, however, regard DHIC as a subset of overflow incontinence where increased residual urine is found in association with detrusor overactivity.

In 1986, Resnick and Yalla pointed out that many elderly patients with detrusor hyperreflexia have a concomitant impairment of detrusor contractility, resulting in both incontinence and incomplete emptying. It had generally been thought prior to this observation that abnormal detrusor contractions would result in total evacuation of the bladder contents. In their group of elderly men and women, these investigators found that age-related detrusor hyperreflexia (i.e., an age-related neuropathology leading to detrusor overactivity) produced incontinence but often left residual volumes of 200–500 ml. These patients suffered from a reduced functional bladder capacity since their threshold for triggering an uncontrolled detrusor contraction was only 50–100 ml above their residual urine volume. Standard medical therapy for detrusor hyperreflexia with anticholinergic or antispasmodic agents in these patients would only compromise their emptying powers further. Management of patients like these, therefore, is difficult and requires close follow-up. Initial therapy should make use of non-pharmacologic techniques such as biofeedback, fluid management, bladder retraining, and maneuvers to improve bladder emptying. Anticholinergic or antispasmodic drugs used in combination with clean intermittent self-catheterization will often result in a reduction of urinary frequency and urge incontinence. These patients need not catheterize themselves after each void. Often they can manage well by catheterizing after their first morning void and before going to bed at night, with one to two additional catheterizations during the day if needed.

The possibility of DHIC requires that a careful neurologic and voiding history be taken in all elderly patients presenting with incontinence, as well as measurement of postvoid residual urine volumes on several occasions. Many clinicians advocate formal urodynamic testing in women over 60-years of age because of the possibility of DHIC. Urodynamic studies are appropriate when simple treatment methods fail and should include both filling and voiding studies.

The abnormality in patients with DHIC may be failure of the pontine micturition center to augment and sustain the detrusor contraction initiated by the sacral reflex. When elderly patients are started on anticholinergic medications, they should be seen again within a week to check their postvoid residual urine volume. A history of initial improvement in incontinence on anticholinergic drugs followed by a worsening of their condition is suspicious for drug-induced retention. This is one reason why anticholinergic medications should be started at reduced doses in elderly patients, and increased under close supervision. Some clinicians feel that anticholinergic drugs should be a secondary treatment for detrusor overactivity in the elderly, since bladder retraining and fluid management are unlikely to compromise emptying.

Giggle Incontinence

Although incontinence associated with laughing is usually considered to be a common form of stress incontinence, laughter may sometimes induce reflex bladder emptying. In "giggle incontinence," or "giggle micturition" as it is sometimes called, laughter provokes a sudden uncontrollable emptying of the bladder, usually in young women who do not otherwise experience stress incontinence. The laughter which precipitates incontinence in these cases is not just a few chuckles, but rather is sustained—almost uncontrollable—hysterical laughter. This is the type of laughter which gives rise to the expression "I laughed so hard I almost wet my pants."

Giggle incontinence is most common in teenagers and young women. Urodynamic investigation of these patients is usually unrewarding, for three reasons. First, it is almost impossible to get patients to laugh uproariously enough to reproduce their symptoms during a urodynamic study. Second, because the incontinence occurs only under very special circumstances it appears that it involves some form of central nervous reflex activity which precipitates a normal micturition event, rather than an isolated aberration of detrusor behavior. Urodynamic studies on these patients are usually normal, unless they have other urologic symptoms such as giggle incontinence in association with frequency, urgency, urge incontinence and nocturnal enuresis. Finally, it appears that giggle micturition is a time-limited phenomenon. The vast majority of these patients outgrow their problem as they get older, implying that some form of delayed maturation of detrusor control is involved—or perhaps we simply lose our sense of humor as we age.

Coital Incontinence

Coital incontinence refers to incontinence which occurs during sexual intercourse. An attempt should be made to ascertain if leakage occurs with orgasm or with penetration. Incontinence related to orgasm is generally a form of provoked detrusor instability due to rhythmic parasympathetic discharge, while incontinence with penetration is more likely to be stress incontinence related to pressure from the penis on the bladder base. Some women also report that they leak urine during sexual relations if they strain or perform Valsalva maneuver.

One of our colleagues has seen a patient with explosive stress incontinence occurring during sexual intercourse. She complained of "jet-like" urinary leakage, even though she emptied her bladder before coitus. Further investigation revealed that she had a chronic residual urine of nearly 300 ml and always had sex lying supine under her partner. The combination of the large residual urine and the weight of her partner on her bladder caused massive spurting of urine during sexual activity (Dr. Inder Perkash, personal communication).

Coital incontinence is more prevalent than most physicians suspect, because most patients find it intensely embarrassing and are reluctant to discuss it with anyone. The problem is intensely personal and affects one of the most intimate aspects of patients' lives. For example, one of the authors has seen a woman who developed coital urge incontinence following a ureteral reimplantation after a surgical injury. She had no other urinary symptoms or leakage at other times. She developed urgency during intercourse even though she always emptied her bladder beforehand, and this urgency was often enough to make her interrupt coitus and run to the toilet. Her worst problem, however, was enuresis with orgasm, which caused her to lose enough urine to soak the sheets of her bed. One of her greatest sexual pleasures had been having her partner stimulate her to orgasm through cunnilingus, and since her leakage had begun he refused to continue to participate. Few women will volunteer information of this kind to a physician they do not know well.

Specific enquiries about coital incontinence should always be made when the history is taken from an incontinent patient. The devastating emotional consequences of coital incontinence may be the real reason that she has finally decided to seek help. It is often useful to "give permission" to the patient to discuss coital incontinence by initiating the discussion with a statement such as "Many of my patients say that they often lose urine during intercourse. Does this ever happen to you?" Although difficult to accomplish, orgasm-induced detrusor instability has been reproduced by masturbation during urodynamic testing. For practical reasons, the diagnosis is generally made on the basis of the history alone.

Treatment of orgasm-related detrusor instability is difficult. The most practical method utilizes an anticholinergic drug such as 5 mg of oxybutynin (Ditropan) or 50 mg of imipramine (Tofranil) several hours prior to intercourse. This assumes, of course, that sexual intercourse is planned in advance, which it usually is not. The patient with coital incontinence should also be instructed to empty her bladder prior to having intercourse.

Patients occasionally present with orgasm-induced incontinence alone. These patients appear to have detrusor overactivity associated only with the powerful autonomic stimulus of sexual release. On the other hand, patients rarely present with stress incontinence during sexual intercourse alone. Invariably, these patients also have stress incontinence with other activities, such as coughing, sneezing, walking, or exercising. Surgical repair of stress incontinence usually alleviates the sexual component of the problem. Nonsurgical management of stress incontinence occurring with penetration is more difficult, but vigorous pelvic muscle exercises may control this problem over time and may even enhance the patient's sexual enjoyment. The use of a tight fitting diaphragm may also be helpful.

Coital incontinence seems to bother the sexual partner far less often than it bothers the patient. Reassurance alone may be sufficient for some women, and many patients seem relieved to know that the condition occurs in other couples, but it is inappropriate to advise the patient just to "lie back and enjoy it." Surgery for coitally-related stress incontinence is unwise unless the stress incontinence occurs under other circumstances and is otherwise troublesome for the patient.

Incontinence with Exercise

Approximately one-third of all women who engage in vigorous exercise will experience some degree of incontinence associated with these activities. The incontinence produced by exercise is usually, but not exclusively, stress incontinence, and it is unusual for the incontinence to occur only with exercise. Confirming the diagnosis of stress incontinence, and assessing the degree to which it interferes with her quality of life, should be the main priorities in patient evaluation. Nygaard and colleagues have shown that repetitive bouncing activities such as high impact aerobics or jogging are more likely to produce incontinence than other forms of exercise. Women who experience stress incontinence during exercise will often benefit from switching to activities less likely to produce large increases in intra-abdominal pressure, such as swimming, walking, and cycling. Changing exercise patterns should always be discussed as part of the initial treatment. Incontinence which occurs only during trampoline jumping can be managed by simply avoiding this activity, but an aerobics instructor who leaks urine while leading her class may not be able to quit aerobics.

All patients who complain of exercise-induced incontinence should be given initial conservative management. Placing a tampon in the vagina prior to exercise is often very helpful. The tampon appears to reduce bladder neck hypermobility during exercise and probably helps compress the urethra during periods of increased intra-abdominal pressure. Since a dry tampon can be difficult or even painful to remove from the vagina, the patient should wait to remove it until she has bathed or showered after exercising. Placing the tampon inside a condom or finger cot prior to insertion will also make it easier to remove. Many women will find that emptying their bladders or wearing a simple perineal pad will be all that they require, although many women have already tried these measures before seeking medical advice. Phenylpropanolamine (as Ornade spansules) or ephedrine (as Dexatrim or Sudafed) taken 1 hour prior to exercise may also be helpful, since these drugs increase urethral closure pressure by stimulating α-receptors at the bladder neck. Finally, regular performance of pelvic muscle exercises are to be commended as an effective adjunct to physical fitness programs for women. These may even be performed during group exercises as substitutes for certain activities which tend to produce incontinence, such as sit ups and "jumping jacks." Individually tailored exercise programs with weighted vaginal cones would also appear to be useful in improving pelvic muscle tone in women with exercise-induced incontinence. Surgery for stress incontinence which occurs *only* during exercise should be approached cautiously.

Nocturnal Enuresis

Nocturnal enuresis refers to urine loss during sleep. The patient is usually awakened by the sensation of urine passing into the bed or wakes up to discover that the bed is wet. A patient who awakens with a sense of urinary urgency and leaks while trying to get to the bathroom has *not* just had an episode of nocturnal enuresis; she has suffered urge incontinence which occurred during the night. Nocturnal enuresis may be primary or secondary. *Primary nocturnal enuresis* refers to bedwetting which began in childhood and has persisted into the adult years. This is a very different condition from *secondary nocturnal enuresis,* which is bedwetting which developed for the first time in adulthood or has returned after a prolonged period of nighttime dryness.

The presence of other urinary tract symptoms is also extremely important. The adult with persistent primary enuresis and no other urinary tract symptoms is likely to have either a congenital defect in antidiuretic hormone secretion or a defect in the neuroregulation of the micturition reflex; that is, these patients have incomplete inhibition of normal micturition reflex activity during sleep. Studies in children with primary nocturnal enuresis have shown that what occurs in most cases is the development of a normal micturition reflex event which produces a sustained detrusor contraction leading to complete bladder emptying while they are asleep, rather than isolated small leaks due to phasic unstable rises and falls in detrusor pressure (detrusor instability). Adults who have daytime symptoms of frequency, urgency, and urge incontinence in addition to nocturnal enuresis are very likely to have detrusor instability. The presence of nocturnal enuresis in association with these conditions has a high positive predictive value for the urodynamic finding of detrusor instability. Central nervous control of bladder reflex activity develops in stages, with daytime bladder control being achieved much earlier than nighttime control. For this reason, evaluation of children with nocturnal enuresis can be deferred until the age of 10 or 12, unless other urinary tract symptoms are present.

Adult patients complaining of nocturnal enuresis should be evaluated for the presence of detrusor instability and overflow incontinence. Special attention should be given to the times that diuretic medications are taken, fluid intake in the evening hours or at night, and whether or not the patient uses alcohol or hypnotic drugs at bedtime. A frequency/volume chart is an important part of the investigation. One of our patients was cured of nightly enuresis occurring at 2 AM when she stopped drinking her double bourbon nightcap at 11 PM.

The initial treatment of nocturnal enuresis should include fluid management with avoidance of fluids several hours before bedtime, mobilization of dependent edema earlier in the day, and changes of medications which may be contributing to the problem. The patient with a chronically elevated residual urine may benefit from a single catheterization prior to going to bed. If the timing of the incontinence episode is predictable, some patients set an alarm approximately 1/2 hour before the incontinence is expected to occur. This allows them to wake up and void before they are wet. Regular toileting including one or two night trips may resolve the problem in certain elderly patients.

Childhood nocturnal enuresis often responds to the use of an enuresis alarm. Many varieties of these devices have been developed and some are sold through regular mail-order houses. Enuresis alarms usually consist of a pad which is placed under the sheets. The pad is attached to a buzzer or bell. When urine hits the pad, it completes an electrical circuit causing the alarm to sound, waking the patient. The idea is that this will train the patient to awaken when the bladder is being distended so that micturition can take place in the toilet, not in the bed. These devices are often useful in bringing about the final maturity of the developing neuroregulatory mechanisms of bladder control in children. Little data exists on their use in adults with secondary enuresis. Imipramine 50 mg at bedtime has been shown to reduce episodes of enuresis in many patients. Patients with overt detrusor instability will benefit from this drug, perhaps used in combination with oxybutynin (Ditropan) 5 mg three or four times per day. Many patients with nocturnal enuresis, and particularly patients with persistent primary enuresis or patients in whom nocturia and nocturnal enuresis are the only complaints, get dramatic relief with desmopressin. Desmopressin (DDAVP) is a synthetic analog of antidiuretic hormone (ADH) which increases renal tubular fluid resorption and thus decreases nighttime urine production. It is usually given as a nasal spray at bedtime, 10 μcg in each nostril, for a total nightly dose of 20 μcg. The drug has been shown to be safe and effective, but patients must be cautioned not to use it during the daytime as well.

Urethral Instability

"Urethral instability" has not been defined in generally accepted technical terms, but it can be thought of as urine loss due to uninhibited urethral relaxation which lowers urethral resistance below the prevailing bladder pressure. Since effective urine storage requires that outlet resistance remain higher than the pressure in the bladder if continence is to be preserved, involuntary urine loss can occur due to two factors. Either bladder pressure may rise higher than urethral resistance, as in the case of genuine stress incontinence or detrusor instability, or urethral resistance can fall lower than bladder pressure. In normal micturition both of these processes occur together: The pelvic floor and urethra relax while a sustained detrusor contraction develops to empty the bladder contents.

The term "urethral instability" has not been formally defined by the International Continence Society, and there is some controversy as to whether such a phenomenon actually exists as a discrete entity. The urodynamic definition of urethral instability usually requires pressure fluctuations of more than 15 cm H_2O in urethral pressure during the filling phase of a cystometrogram. Urinary incontinence due to urethral instability would be expected to occur in patients in whom the urethral pressure suddenly fell below bladder pressure, generating a leak. The data on this phenomenon are limited and contradictory. In most studies, a fall in urethral pressure is followed by a detrusor contraction, indicating a reflex link between the two processes. Occasional studies simply show a fall in urethral pressure which produces incontinence. There are probably some women with incompetent bladder necks who maintain urinary continence mainly by contraction of the external striated urethral sphincter. Since striated muscles are poorly suited to sustaining constant loads over time, these patients will ultimately develop episodes of "sphincter fatigue," and may leak urine when this occurs. Since the interplay between bladder pressure and outlet resistance is in constant flux throughout the day as patients undertake various activities from exercising to sleeping, it makes sense to assume that urethral pressure will be higher at some times and during some activities than others. The variations sometimes seen in urethral pressure during a multichannel cystometrogram may be nothing more than a reflection of normal variations in physiology. The clinician should be aware that some patients may have incontinence due to an "unstable" urethra, but these will be encountered rarely and will probably have associated stress or urge incontinence. Further research may clarify the role that urethral instability plays, if any, in the development of urinary incontinence.

Functional and Transient Incontinence
General Considerations

Continence depends upon the patient's ability to understand that control over bladder function is socially necessary. Incontinence may arise in patients who lose the perception that bladder control is important, either because of transient medical conditions or the development of a chronic problem such as dementia. Transient medical causes of incontinence are covered in Chapter 15, "Special Considerations in the Elderly," since these problems are more prevalent in the elderly. Functional or transient incontinence can also occur, however, in younger patients, particularly those with mental illness or emotional disturbances. One reason that incontinence is more prevalent in mentally disturbed women is the use of antipsychotic drugs. Although many patients clearly need this type of therapy, if incontinence develops it may be amenable to improvement through a change of medications. Drugs such as haloperidol have less effect on the bladder than other antipsychotics. Patients who do not perceive the benefits of bladder control may still be able to maintain continence through the use of timed voiding regimens. Prompted voiding schedules, which require these patients to empty their bladders at regular intervals, may be all that is necessary to prevent frequent incontinent episodes. Use of a wristwatch with a programmed beeper or alarm may be all that is necessary to motivate these patients to void regularly. Use of chronic indwelling catheters should be avoided whenever possible.

Incontinence in Pregnancy

It is a common belief that incontinence first presents following childbirth. In fact, the available data suggest otherwise. In pioneering studies which have not been repeated, Winifred Francis found that stress incontinence rarely, if ever, appeared for the first time during pregnancy. Approximately 40% of primigravidae reported that they had occasional stress incontinence before pregnancy; and in women who had developed stress incontinence before becoming pregnant, their incontinence invariably worsened during pregnancy. Stress incontinence which appeared during pregnancy tended to disappear in the puerperium, only to recur during subsequent pregnancies until, in some women, it remained after delivery to become a persistent and often progressive complaint. Francis concluded that women who develop stress incontinence in middle life are ''destined to do so from an early age,'' but that pregnancy itself, rather than parturition, revealed the underlying defect and made it worse. These findings were confirmed by Iosif, who interviewed 1411 newly-delivered women in Sweden and found that 22% of them had complaints of stress incontinence. Of the women with stress incontinence, 8.5% had the onset of their problem during puberty prior to pregnancy; 23% developed permanent stress incontinence which had its onset during pregnancy; 50% developed temporary, mild ''physiologic'' stress incontinence during the second half of pregnancy which disappeared on its own within 3 months of delivery; but only 19% of stress incontinent patients developed their problem in conjunction with or following parturition. Alterations in hormone levels and mechanical pressure from the enlarging uterus probably play a significant role in the development of incontinence during pregnancy, but the exact etiology is unclear. Van Geelen found that the urethral pressure profile was not altered by increasing uterine size, engagement of the fetal head, or serum levels of estrogen and progesterone, but these findings may simply reflect the inadequacy of urethral pressure measurements as tools for clinical investigation. Urge incontinence appears to be less prevalent during pregnancy than stress incontinence, but this has not been well studied.

The relationship between pregnancy and stress incontinence appears to be something like this. The anatomy of the female urethra and bladder neck makes women more susceptible than men to stress incontinence. The greater vulnerability of these structures in women means that some women will have intrinsically weaker sphincteric mechanisms than others. These women will develop some degree of stress incontinence even before they become pregnant. High levels of progesterone, a potent smooth muscle relaxant, develop during pregnancy and cause muscular support of the urethra and bladder neck to become ''softer,'' further predisposing some women to the development of stress incontinence. The additional pressure from the enlarging uterus further contributes to this problem. At delivery, additional stretching of muscles, fascia, and pelvic ligaments takes place. This may cause transient stress incontinence until the acute trauma is healed, but an element of neuromuscular damage may remain. In some women this is enough to lead to progressive stress incontinence. In others, however, the margin to continence is preserved until the additive effects of subsequent pregnancies finally tip the balance over and a clinical problem with incontinence develops.

There is scientific evidence to support this picture. Snooks and colleagues found that pelvic floor denervation was greater in patients who had undergone vaginal, as compared to cesarean, delivery. Primigravidae who had been delivered vaginally had evidence of immediate postpartum neurologic damage to the pelvic floor, but there was little evidence of residual damage 2 months after delivery, whereas multiparae showed persistent evidence of denervation 8 weeks after parturition. This probably represents the cumulative effects of delivery-induced damage to the pelvic floor musculature. Norton used weighted vaginal cones and Kegel exercises to rehabilitate the pelvic floor muscles in primiparous women who had had a normal vaginal delivery, and found that, although these techniques improved vaginal tone more rapidly than a group of matched controls, all women had improved to approximately the same level of pelvic floor strength

6 months after delivery. The evidence therefore suggests that postpartum stress incontinence should not be treated surgically for the first 9–12 months, since many of these patients will improve on their own.

Although "Kegel exercises" are widely taught in childbirth education classes, they are almost never monitored for correct performance or taught individually. Exercises taught in this manner, and performed without supervision, have not been shown clearly to improve either vaginal squeeze pressure or to prevent postpartum stress incontinence. The best studies on muscular rehabilitation for stress incontinence, by Bo and others (Chapter 6), suggest that vigorous individual instruction and close supervision are necessary in order to obtain maximum benefit with muscular rehabilitation therapy.

Vaginal Discharge

A small group of patients present with a complaint of stress incontinence that the clinician cannot verify. Typically these women complain of perineal dampness rather than copious leakage of urine. Often this dampness is noted later in the day and gets progressively worse the longer the patient is on her feet. Sometimes the incontinence is described only as discoloration or staining of her underwear or panty-liner. At cystometry, these patients invariably have a stable cystometrogram with no incontinence demonstrated. Physical examination, however, often reveals a copious vaginal discharge, either in the form of significant cervical mucus, a large amount of desquamated epithelial cells, or an otherwise asymptomatic vaginal infection. These are patients who have self-diagnosed their problem as urinary incontinence when in fact they have a vaginal discharge. Because they describe their symptoms as related to leakage of urine, the uncritical physician can be swept up in this line of thinking and make a major mistake by accepting the patient's story without independent confirmation. Mistakes of this kind are a powerful example of why the clinician must demonstrate urinary leakage and confirm with the patient that it reproduces her symptoms before accepting a clinical diagnosis of urinary incontinence. Reassurance and appropriate treatment for the underlying condition are all these patients need, not surgical suspension of the bladder neck.

Patients who remain unconvinced by the statement that they do not have urinary incontinence should undergo a Pyridium pad test. The patient is given 200 mg of phenazopyridine hydrochloride (Pyridium) about 2 hours before the test. Her perineum and urethra should be carefully cleaned prior to applying the perineal pad. At the end of the test period, a negative pad test in which no orange discoloration is present should convince her of the correctness of the diagnosis.

SUGGESTED READING

Congenital Abnormalities

Allen FJ, de Kock MLS. Asymmetric bilateral genital ureteric ectopy. Br J Urol 1990; 65:300–01.

Blakeley CR, Mills WG. The obstetric and gynaecological complications of bladder exstrophy and epispadias. Br J Obstet Gynaecol 1981; 88:167–73.

Huffman JW, Dewhurst CJ, Capraro VJ. Congenital anomalies of the female genitalia. In The Gynecology of Childhood and Adolescence. 2nd ed. Philadelphia: WB Saunders, 1981:141–74.

Lew B, Brant H. Obstetric and gynecologic complications associated with muellerian duct abnormalities. Obstet Gynecol 1966; 28:315–22.

Mitchell RJ. An ectopic vaginal ureter. J Obstet Gynaecol Br Commw 1961; 68:299–302.

Ritchey ML, Kramer SA, Benson RC Jr, Kelalis PP. Bilateral single ureteral ectopia. Eur Urol 1988; 14:41–45.

Stanton SL. Gynecologic complications of epispadias and bladder exstrophy. Am J Obstet Gynecol 1974; 119:749–54.

Wallingford AJ, Gabriels AG Jr. Ectopic ureter: A cause of female urinary incontinence Reports of four cases. Obstet Gynecol 1957; 10:95–100.

Weed JC, McKee DM. Vulvoplasty in cases of exstrophy of the bladder. Obstet Gynecol 1974; 43:512–16.

Urethral Diverticula

Appell RA, Suarez BC. Experience with a laterally based vaginal flap approach for urethral diverticulum. J Urol 1982; 127:677–78.

Coddington CC, Knab DR. Urethral diverticulum: A review. Obstet Gynecol Surv 1983; 38:357–64.

Davis B, Robinson DG. Diverticula of the female urethra: Assay of 120 cases. J Urol 1970; 104:850–53.

Ginsburg D, Gendary R. Suburethral diverticulum: Classification and therapeutic considerations. Obstet Gynecol 1983; 61:685–88.

Greenburg M, Stone D, Cochran S, Bruskewitz R, Pagan J, Raz S, et al. Female urethral diverticula: Double-balloon catheter study. Am J Radiol 1981; 136:259–65.

Houser LM, Von Eschenbach AC. Diverticula of female urethra: Diagnostic importance of postvoiding film. Urology 1974; 3:453–55.

Lee RA. Diverticulum of the female urethra: Postoperative

complications and results. Obstet Gynecol 1983; 61: 52–58.

Peters WA III, Vaughan ED Jr. Urethral diverticulum in the female: Etiologic factors and postoperative results. Obstet Gynecol 1976; 47:549–52.

Spence H, Duckett J. Diverticulum of the female urethra: Clinical aspects and presentation of a simple operative technique for cure. J Urol 1970; 104:432–37.

Stewart M, Brietland PM, Stidolph NE. Urethral diverticula in the adult female. Br J Urol 1981; 53:353–59.

Willis AJ, Gross PL. Utilization of Fogarty arterial embolectomy catheter in urethral diverticulectomy. Urology 1980; 16:205–06.

Woodhouse CRJ, Flynn JT, Molland EA, Blandy JP. Urethral diverticulum in females. Br J Urol 1980; 52:305–10.

Genitourinary Fistulae

Ampofo EK, Omotara BA, Otu T, Uchebo G. Risk factors of vesicovaginal fistulae in Maiduguri, Nigeria: A case-control study. Tropical Doctor 1990; 20:138–39.

Azia SA. Urinary fistula from obstetrical trauma. J Obstet Gynaecol Brit Commw 1965; 72:765–68.

Bird GC. Obstetric vesicovaginal and allied fistulae. J Obstet Gynaecol Brit Commw 1967; 74:749–52.

Coetzee T, Lithgow DM. Obstetric fistulae of the urinary tract. J Obstet Gynaecol Brit Commw 1966; 73:837–44.

Davits RJAM, Miranda SI. Conservative treatment of vesicovaginal fistulas by bladder drainage alone. Br J Urol 1991; 68:155–56.

Drutz HP, Mainprize TC. Unrecognized small vesicovaginal fistula as a cause of persistent urinary incontinence. Am J Obstet Gynecol 1988; 158:237–40.

Elkins TE, Drescher C, Martey JO. Vesicovaginal fistula revisited. Obstet Gynecol 1988; 72:307–12.

Kursh ED, Morse RM, Resnick MI, Perskey L. Prevention of the development of a vesicovaginal fistula. Surg Gynecol Obstet 1988; 106:409–12.

Landes R. Simple transvesical repair of vesicovaginal fistula. J Urol 1979; 122:604–13.

Lawson J. Vesicovaginal fistula—A tropical disease. Trans Roy Soc Trop Med Hygiene 1989; 83:454–56.

Lee RA, Symmonds RE, Williams TJ. Current status of genitourinary fistula. Obstet Gynecol 1988; 72:313–19.

Mustafa AZ, Rushwan HM. Acquired genitourinary fistulae in the Sudan. J Obstet Gynaecol Brit Commw 1971; 78: 1039–43.

Naidu PM. Vesicovaginal fistulae: An experience with 208 cases. J Obstet Gynaecol Brit Commw 1962; 69:311–16.

Patil U, Waterhouse K, Laungani G. Management of eighteen difficult vesicovaginal and urethrovaginal fistulas with modified Ingelman-Sundberg and Martius operations. J Urol 1980; 123:653–56.

Sims JM. On the treatment of vesicovaginal fistula. Medical Classics 1938; 2:677–712.

Symmonds R. Ureteral injuries associated with gynecologic surgery: Prevention and management. Clin Obstet Gynecol 1976; 19:623–35.

Tahzib F. Epidemiological determinants of vesicovaginal fistulas. Br J Obstet Gynaecol 1983; 90:387–91.

Tahzib F. An initiative on vesicovaginal fistula. Lancet 1989; 1:1316–17.

Tancer L. The post-total hysterectomy (vault) vesicovaginal fistula. J Urol 1980; 123:839–45.

Tancer ML. Vesicouterine fistula—A review. Obstet Gynecol Surv 1986; 41:743–53.

Thompson JD. Vesicovaginal fistulas. In Thompson JD, Rock JA (Eds). TeLinde's Operative Gynecology. 7th ed. Philadelphia: Lippincott, 1992:785-817.

Yenen E, Babuna C. Genital fistula: A study based on 197 consecutive cases. Obstet Gynecol 1965; 26:219–24.

Zacharin RF. Obstetric Fistula. New York: Springer-Verlag, 1988.

Overflow Incontinence and DHIC

Resnick N, Yalla S. Detrusor hyperactivity with impaired contractile function. An unrecognized but common cause of incontinence in elderly patients. JAMA 1987; 257(22): 3076-81.

Richardson D. Overflow incontinence and urinary retention. Clin Obstet Gynecol 1990; 33:378–81.

Giggle Incontinence

Arena MG, Leggiadro N, Arcudi L, Ruello C, D'Amico D, Deodato M, Meduri M. "Enuresis risoria:" Evaluation and management. Functional Neurology 1987; 2:579–82.

Cooper CE. Giggle Micturition. In Kolvin I, MacKeith RC, Meadow SR (Eds). Bladder Control and Enuresis. Clinics in Developmental Medicine; 48/49:61–65. Philadelphia: JB Lippincott, 1973.

Glahn BE. Giggle incontinence (enuresis risoria): A study and an aetiological hypothesis. Br J Urol 1979; 51: 363–66.

MacKeith RC. Micturition induced by giggling. Guys Hosp Reports 1964; 113:259–60.

Rogers M, Gittes R, Dawson D. Giggle incontinence. JAMA 1982; 247:1446–48.

Coital Incontinence

Hilton P. Urinary incontinence during sexual intercourse: A common, but rarely volunteered symptom. Br J Obstet Gynaecol 1988; 95:377–80.

Khan Z, Bhola A, Starer P. Urinary incontinence during orgasm. Urology 1988; 31:279–82.

Sutherst JR. Sexual dysfunction and urinary incontinence. Br J Obstet Gynaecol 1979; 86:387–88.

Nocturnal Enuresis

Cantor TJ, Bates CP. A comparative study of symptoms and objective urodynamic findings in 214 incontinent women. Br J Obstet Gynaecol 1980; 87:889–92.

Forsythe WI, Butler RJ. Fifty years of enuretic alarms. Arch Dis Child 1989; 64:879–85.

Hindmarsh JR, Pyrne PO. Adult enuresis—A symptomatic and urodynamic assessment. Br J Urol 1980; 52:88–91.

Norgaard J. Urodynamics in enuretics I: Reservoir function. Neurourol Urodynam 1989; 8:199–212.

Norgaard J. Urodynamics in enuretics II: A pressure/flow study. Neurourol Urodynam 1989; 8:213–18.

Rew DA, Rundle JSH. Assessment of the safety of regular DDAVP therapy in primary nocturnal enuresis. Br J Urol 1989; 63:352–53.

Poussaint A, Ditman K. A controlled study of imipramine (Tofranil) in the treatment of childhood enuresis. J Pediatr 1965; 67:283–87.

Torrens MJ, Collins CD. The urodynamic assessment of adult enuresis. Br J Urol 1975; 47:433–40.

Whiteside CG, Arnold EP. Persistent primary enuresis: A urodynamic assessment. Br Med J 1975; 1:364–67.

Urethal Instability

Constantinou CE. Urethrometry: Considerations of static, dynamic, and stability characteristics of the female urethra. Neurourol Urodynam 1988; 7:521–39.

Low JA, Armstrong JB, Mauger GM. The unstable urethra in the female. Onstet Gynecol 1989; 74:69–74.

Sand PK, Bowen LW, Ostergard DR. Uninhibited urethral relaxation: An unusual cause of incontinence. Obstet Gynecol 1986; 68:645–48.

Sorensen S, Norgaard JP, Knudsen LM, Rittig S, Djurhuus JC. Urethral pressure variations in healthy females during rest and sleep. J Urol 1987; 137:1287–90.

Ulmsten U, Hernirksson L, Iosif S. The unstable female urethra. Am J Obstet Gynecol 1982; 144:93–97.

Vereecken RL, Das J. Urethral instability: Related to stress and/or urge incontinence? J Urol 1985; 134:698–701.

Incontinence in Pregnancy

Francis W. The onset of stress incontinence. J Obstet Gynecol Br Commw 1960; 67:899–903.

Iosif S, Ulmsten U. Comparative urodynamic studies of continent and stress incontinent women in pregnancy and in the puerperium. Am J Obstet Gynecol 1981; 140:645–50.

Iosif S. Stress incontinence during pregnancy and in puerperium. Int J Gynaecol Obstet 1981; 19:13–20.

Norton P, Baker J. Randomized controlled trial of vaginal cones versus Kegel exercises in postpartum primiparous women. Neurourol Urodynam 1991; 9:434–35.

Stanton S, Kerr-Wilson R, Harris G. The incidence of urological symptoms in normal pregnancy. Br J Obstet Gynaecol 1980; 87:897–900.

Van Geelen J, Lemmens W, Eskes T, Martin C. The urethral pressure profile in pregnancy and after delivery in healthy nulliparous women. Am J Obstet Gynecol 1982; 144:636–49.

Viktup L, Lose G, Rolff M, Barfoed K. The symptom of stress incontinence caused by pregnancy or delivery in primiparas. Obstet Gynecol 1992; 79:945–49.

Other

Nygaard I, DeLancey J, Arnsdorf L, Murphy E. Exercise and incontinence. Obstet Gynecol 1990; 75:848–51.

Wall LL, Couchman GM, McCoy MC. Vaginal discharge as a confounding factor in the diagnosis of urinary incontinence by perineal pad testing. Int Urogynecol J 1991; 2:219–21.

11   Urinary Tract Infection

Acute cystitis is one of the most common diagnoses made in general clinical practice and accounts for some 5 million office visits each year. The diagnosis is often made by the patient herself, or by listening to her symptoms over the telephone. Commonly, no diagnostic testing is performed and empiric treatment is begun immediately based on the presumptive clinical diagnosis of urinary tract infection. If this condition is so common and so easily diagnosed, why devote an entire chapter to it? The reason is simple: Common things are sometimes mismanaged and sometimes common symptoms turn out to represent an uncommon—and sometimes serious—underlying problem. While many patients can indeed be treated empirically, some patients do require a more extensive evaluation, such as women with recurrent infections or atypical symptoms. Sometimes inappropriate testing is ordered or appropriate tests are misinterpreted. Finally, some patients' symptoms mimic urinary tract infection but are actually due to other syndromes which will not respond to antibiotic therapy. To continue treating these women by phoning in prescriptions for different antibiotics may miss an important underlying problem.

Physician training in the management of urinary tract infections is often inadequate. During residency training, gynecologists may treat urinary tract infections based on a urine culture and antimicrobial sensitivity testing, without understanding what these tests actually mean. For example, use of a colony count of "greater than 10^5 colony forming units per ml" as a diagnostic criterion for clinical infection is not always reliable. This clinical threshold was developed in studies designed to detect bacteriuria in clean-catch urine samples from asymptomatic women. This is a completely different situation from the patient with acute onset dysuria, urgency, and frequency. This chapter will examine the conditions which contribute to the development of urinary tract infections in women and will outline a logical approach to the clinical evaluation of acute cystitis, recurrent urinary tract infection, and related diagnoses, and their treatment.

Etiology and Evaluation of Urinary Tract Infection
Physiology of Bladder Resistance to Infection

The urine delivered to the bladder through the ureters is almost always sterile. Urine contains important elements which help it to resist infection: an acidic pH, a high concentration of urea, and immunoglobulins. Although pathogens are able to make their way from the urethra to the bladder, regular bladder emptying washes these organisms away and prevents the development of an infection. In one study, 10^5 bacteria were introduced into the bladders of male volunteers, but infection did not occur as long as the bladder was emptied, refilled with urine, and emptied again. Although bacteria may also be spread by hematogenous or lymphatic pathways, these factors are not usually as important in the development of lower urinary tract infections as they are for the development of pyelonephritis. The bladder epithelium itself is also highly resistant to bacterial invasion. A protective layer of mucus-like protein called glycosaminoglycan acts as a barrier to prevent invasion by bacterial species. Tamm-Horsfall protein, a glycoprotein commonly found in urinary casts, is secreted by the kidneys, and also appears to inhibit bacterial adherence to the bladder

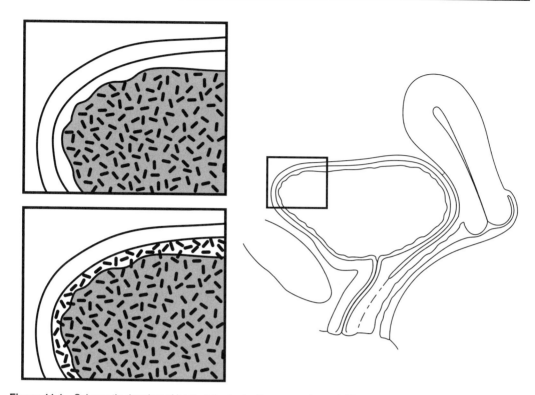

Figure 11.1   Schematic drawing of bacterial colonization versus bacterial invasion. The bladder is colonized with bacteria *(top)*, but symptoms are not produced until the bladder wall is invaded by these organisms *(bottom)*.

Pathogenesis of Urinary Tract Infection

wall, lessening the chance of infection. Unless bacteria attach themselves to the urothelium, the ability of the bladder to flush itself clean during emptying is remarkably efficient.

Why do women get urinary tract infections? There may be as many reasons as there are women, but several factors are clearly associated with the disruption of bladder defense mechanisms and the development of urinary tract infections. Women are eight times more likely to develop urinary tract infections than are men, perhaps in part because of the shorter length of the female urethra and the close proximity of large numbers of potentially pathogenic bacteria in the vagina and the bowel. The incidence of urinary tract infection increases with age, and certain anatomic conditions may predispose women to infection. The mere introduction of organisms into the bladder from the urethra will not lead to infection by itself. *Colonization* is the term used for the presence of organisms in the normally sterile urine. *Invasion* of organisms into the bladder epithelium constitutes acute cystitis (Fig. 11.1). Recurrent symptoms may be due to recurrence of a previously acquired infection, or, more commonly, from reinfection. These concepts have important implications for evaluation and treatment. Each of these conditions will be examined separately in this chapter.

Bacterial Invasion

Twenty-five percent of all women of reproductive age develop a urinary tract infection at some time in their lives, and of these half will develop recurrent problems with infection. This suggests that once the host defense mechanisms have been disrupted, urinary tract infection is more likely.

Organisms gain entry into the urothelium by several mechanisms. The glycosaminoglycan layer of the bladder may be disrupted. This may occur from instrumentation, toxins, bladder stones or other foreign bodies, or invasion by a tumor. There are several reports of prevention of bacterial adherence in vitro as well as the prevention of experimentally induced urinary tract infections by supplementing endogenous glycosaminoglycan with sodium pentosanpolysulfate (Elmiron). Invasion is made more likely by bacteria which have adapted to increase their adherence to bladder epithelial cells. The more adherent the bacteria, the more likely they are to cause infection. The ability of bacteria to adhere to epithelial cells is made more likely by special adhesive structures called *pili*. Pili have been grouped into two types. Bacteria with Type I pili have been isolated from patients with acute cystitis. These pili attach to mannose receptors on the urothelium. Type II pili are mannose-negative and appear to be found on more virulent bacteria. Pili are common in coliform bacteria; other kinds of bacteria may have developed different mechanisms for promoting adherence.

Once bacterial invasion has occurred, the bladder epithelium reacts to the infection by releasing kinins and cytokines, which produce local pain and inflammation. The bladder becomes more sensitive to bladder wall distension and symptoms of urgency, frequency, and suprapubic pain develop as the bladder fills. The organisms most commonly associated with urinary tract infection include *Eschericia coli* (80%, usually from the gastrointestinal tract); *Staphylococcus saprophyticus* (10%); *Klebsiella pneumoniae* (5%); *Enterobacter sp.* (2%); and *Proteus sp.* (2%). Certain bacteria—such as *Serratia marcessans* and *Pseudomonas aerugenosa*—are usually hospital acquired. *Staphlyococcus epidermidis* is most often seen in catheterized patients. More fastidious organisms may also be seen as bladder pathogens, including *Ureaplasma urealyticum* and other types of mycoplasma, and *Chlamydia trachomatis*. Anaerobic bacteria rarely cause urinary tract infection due to the high oxygen tension which normally exists in urine.

Reproductive Tract Factors   Approximately 1% of girls develop urinary tract infections in the first year of life. This suggests that there is an intrinsic protective immune resistance to infection, and possibly a minor benefit from estrogen. The incidence of infection declines every year thereafter until sexual intercourse begins. With the onset of sexual activity there is a sudden increase in the incidence of urinary tract infections, most likely due to the introduction of pathogenic bacteria into the urethra during coitus. The relative risk of developing a urinary tract infection is increased sixty-fold in women who have had intercourse within the previous 48 hours, compared to those who have not. The infecting organisms in such patients are those which have colonized the vagina, e.g., women with coliform bladder infections have coliforms in the vagina. The use of a contraceptive diaphragm has also been shown to be associated with an increased incidence of urinary tract infection, probably because voiding may be relatively obstructed during the 8 hours in which the diaphragm must be kept in place after coitus. There may also be a genetic component present in women who develop urinary tract infections. Women with ABO blood groups A and AB, and HLA type A_3 seem to have an increased risk of recurrent urinary tract infections compared to other groups. Nonsecretors of immunoglobulins also have an increased risk of infection. The prevalence of bacteriuria increases to as high as 20% in women aged 65-years or older. This may be due in part to loss of estrogen effects on the epithelium, decreased urethral vascularity, or impaired bladder emptying. In addition, there is an increased prevalence of other medical conditions in this age group which predispose patients to urinary infection, such as diabetes mellitus and renal disease. Because of the risk of developing urosepsis, the consequences of bacteriuria are also higher in this age group.

Anatomical Considerations   Any anatomical defect which promotes urinary stasis predisposes the patient to urinary tract infection. Examples of such defects include ureteral duplication in which one ureter empties incompletely, an ectopic ureter which empties into the vagina or urethra, and bladder or urethral diverticula which allow bacterial colonization of retained urine. Indwelling catheters and bladder instrumentation predispose patients to cystitis, both by introducing organisms into the bladder and by aiding bacterial adherence to the urothelium. Other foreign bodies, such as stones, or tumors, or sutures which penetrate the bladder wall, provide a ready nidus for infection.

Many women with voiding dysfunction develop recurrent urinary tract infections because they develop turbulent flow at the level of the bladder neck which washes urine from the midurethra back into the bladder, interfering with effective bladder washout. Fluoroscopically, these patients present with a so-called "spinning top" deformity of the bladder neck during voiding, with an open bladder neck but a constricted distal urethra. Some women with detrusor instability also develop recurrent infections because of the constant opening and closing of the bladder neck associated with ineffective emptying. High intravesical pressures due to detrusor hyperreflexia or low bladder compliance promote vesicoureteral reflux and are often associated with upper tract deterioration and recurrent pyelonephritis from ascending bacterial infection. The association of abnormal anatomy with urinary tract infection is the main reason that cystoscopy and intravenous urography have been used so frequently in the evaluation of recurrent urinary tract infections. These tests are particularly important in patients at high risk of an anatomic abnormality.

Bladder Habits.

Bladder habits also predispose some women to urinary tract infection. Infrequent voiders—the so-called "nurse's bladder," "teacher's bladder," or "professional bladder"—who have developed the habit of holding their urine for prolonged periods of time and void only a few times each day, are predisposed to stasis, voiding dysfunction, and infection. Organisms from the vagina come into close contact with the urethra during sexual intercourse, and women should be encouraged to void after coitus to wash bacteria out of the lower urinary tract and thereby help diminish the risk of infection.

Perineal hygiene is also important. Infection is often increased in elderly women with arthritis or other conditions that limit their manual dexterity and prevent them from cleaning their perineums. Women with frequent fecal soilage or staining are more likely to have urinary tract infections than others, and women who wipe their perineums from the rectum towards the urethra may be at higher risk of introducing colonic bacteria into the urethra than those who wipe themselves in the other direction after voiding.

Clinical Evaluation of Urinary Tract Infection
General Considerations

In many cases the diagnosis of acute cystitis can be made on symptoms alone and therapy initiated without an examination or clinical testing. The most common complaint is the acute onset of dysuria or pain with urination. It is unclear why micturition produces the acute pain associated with acute cystitis. Pain becomes pronounced when urine passes through the urethra and is often worse during the final moments of bladder emptying, especially if gross hematuria is present. Other frequent complaints in patients with acute cystitis include frequency, urgency, nocturia, and suprapubic pain or cramping.

Occasionally patients will experience urge incontinence in association with urinary tract infection. If related to the infectious process, such incontinence invariably resolves with antibiotic therapy. Gross hematuria is relatively uncommon in a simple urinary tract infection. Many of the symptoms of acute cystitis are nonspecific and may be produced by other pathophysiologic processes. Chronic frequency, urgency, or dysuria should make the clinician consider other possibilities, particularly in patients with persistently negative urine cultures or those who fail to respond to adequate antibiotic therapy. One study by Rees and colleagues, for example, found that 28% of women attending a clinic for chronic urinary tract infections actually had detrusor instability as the cause of their symptoms. Chemical irritants, such as soaps, douches, perfumes, and bubble baths may all cause chronic irritation which may be mistaken for recurrent urinary tract infection.

In patients with acute cystitis, the relationship of their symptoms to sexual intercourse, diaphragm use, menstrual cycles, and the menopause should be explored. Any history of recent or remote infections should be elicited, along with any recent urinary tract instrumentation or catheterization. Because vulvovaginitis may produce acute onset dysuria when urine comes into contact with

TABLE 11.1.   Patient Instructions for Obtaining a Clean-Catch Urine Specimen

1. Wash your hands with soap and water before starting.
2. Sit backwards on the toilet: This gives you more room to work. If you are wearing trousers, you may need to remove them completely.
3. Open the cleansing towelette and specimen jar provided for you and place them on the back of the toilet.
4. Use your left hand to separate the labia (the "lips" around the opening to the urethra) which need to be cleaned before obtaining the specimen. Use your right hand to cleanse this area with the towelette. Your left hand should continue to separate the labia until the urine has been obtained.
5. Now use your right hand to pick up the specimen jar. Do not touch the inside of the jar! Begin to urinate. When a good stream has developed, briefly place the specimen jar in the stream to obtain a urine sample. The jar does not need to be filled more than one-third full.
6. Place the lid on the jar, again without touching the inside of the container, and bring the specimen out of the toilet with you.

an inflamed or irritated vulva, symptoms of vaginal discharge should be investigated.

The physical examination in patients with acute cystitis is usually normal, except where vulvovaginal conditions or urethral abnormalities are responsible for their symptoms.

Pyelonephritis represents an acute inflammation of the upper urinary tract and typically presents with fever, flank pain, and malaise. It is often, but not necessarily, preceded by symptoms of acute cystitis. In acute pyelonephritis costovertebral angle tenderness (CVAT) can often be elicited by placing the palm of one hand over the kidneys and striking firmly but gently with the other hand. The underlying inflammation will often produce sharp pain as this is done. It is often useful to begin this part of the physical examination near the scapula and move caudally to determine the patient's baseline response to such pressure. There are many other causes of flank pain (Table 3.6), which should not be forgotten in the differential diagnosis.

Diagnostic Tests

Analysis of a clean-catch urine specimen is the basic test used in the clinical diagnosis of acute cystitis. Although clean-catch specimens are more difficult to collect in women than in men, careful instruction of the patient in proper technique should result in an adequate specimen (Table 11.1). The patient should carefully clean her external urethral meatus and begin voiding. A small specimen should be caught in a sterile cup during the most forceful part of urination. The British call this a "midstream urine" (MSU) to emphasize the optimal technique for specimen collection. Urine which is not collected meticulously in such a manner may flow over the labia or perineum and become contaminated by exogenous bacteria and epithelial cells. Clean-catch urine specimens can be collected in menstruating women if they carefully clean the perineum and use a vaginal tampon to halt the flow of blood. In the experience of the authors, simply sending the patient into the toilet to read the instructions for specimen collection without verbal reinforcement by the nursing staff usually results in poorly collected urine samples. Some patients may find it easier to collect a sterile specimen if they sit backwards on the toilet because this increases their access to the vulva. Urine specimens should be refrigerated immediately to prevent bacterial proliferation.

Immediate examination of the urine may be performed in the office on a split portion of the specimen. The urine sample should be examined for color. Cloudiness may indicate crystal formation in urine which has been in the bladder for some time, but also may indicate the presence of pyuria. Gross hematuria may be present, although this is rare in acute cystitis. Urine color alone is not reliable in diagnosing infection, as many patients increase their fluid intake prior to coming for an examination in an effort to dilute the urine and reduce their symptoms. Clear urine produced on this basis may still be infected and result

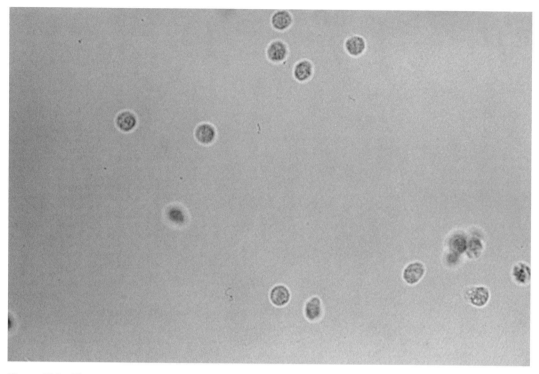

Figure 11.2   Photomicrograph of an unspun urine specimen from a patient with acute cystitis. Note the bacteria and multiple white blood cells.

in a false sense of security. The smell of urine may also be important and sweet or foul smelling urine may be encountered.

Microscopic examination of the urine specimen should be performed on an *unspun* sample, looking for bacteria, white blood cells, and red blood cells (Fig. 11.2) The presence of one or more bacteria per high-power field has a good correlation with significant urinary tract infection. Gram staining will improve the diagnostic accuracy, with an overall sensitive of 80% and a specificity of 90%. Counting red or white blood cells is facilitated by the use of a hemocytometer, a glass slide marked off into squares which is examined under high power magnification. The number of white or red cells can be determined by counting the number of cells in each of nine squares, dividing the number obtained by nine to find the average, and multiplying by 10 to calculate the number of cells per ml. The presence of white blood cells is less predictive of infection than is the presence of bacteria. A large number of squamous epithelial cells is indicative of vulvar or vaginal contamination of the specimen and renders it nearly worthless for diagnosis. Alternatively, the urinalysis and microscopic examination can be performed by clinical laboratory personnel, but it is to the clinician's advantage to become experienced in the examination of unspun urine. Just as gynecologists look at vaginal discharge microscopically, clinicians interested in the lower urinary tract should get used to looking at unspun urine specimens. A *spun* urine sample, on the other hand, collects the urinary sediment and is usefully examined for antibody coated bacteria (indicative of renal involvement), and various casts such as granular casts, broad casts, and casts of red or white cells. In patients with nephropathy, examination of the urinary sediment is the next best diagnostic test to a renal biopsy.

Bacterial culture of urine specimens can be reserved for patients in whom the diagnosis is obscure or who have recurrent symptoms. Antimicrobial sensitivities are useful mainly in instances where there is a high suspicion of antibiotic resistance. Examples of such situations include patients in whom relapse or inadequate treatment is suspected, patients who have persistent symptoms despite antibiotic therapy, infections acquired through catheterization or instrumentation in a clinic or hospital where resistant organisms may be prevalent, and in patients on antibiotic therapy for the treatment of other infections elsewhere in the body.

Determination of microbial sensitivity to antibiotics is expensive, currently costing approximately $20 per antibiotic tested. Laboratories often use a set combination of antibiotics for testing, depending upon whether the organism in question is gram-negative or gram-positive, and it may save money to request sensitivities only for certain antibiotics. For example, it is probably not useful to test sensitivities to sulfa drugs or penicillin in patients with allergies to these drugs. Patients who are on prophylactic antibiotics should generally be given another drug for treatment of cystitis as the likelihood of having an infection with an organism resistant to their usual drug is high. A culture which grows mixed flora has probably been contaminated, particularly if it was a "clean-catch" specimen. Culture for fastidious organisms such as *Mycoplasma* or *Chlamydia,* requires special arrangements. Cultures which grow organisms such as *Candida* or *Gardnerella* should not necessarily be dismissed out of hand, since these organisms can cause lower urinary tract complaints. This is especially true if the culture was obtained with good technique and is relatively pure.

Kass has published extensively regarding the microbiology of urinary tract infection. His work established the diagnostic threshold of 10^5 colony forming units per ml of urine (cfu/ml) as indicative of infection. However, these studies were performed to evaluate "significant" bacterial growth in the urine of women who had *asymptomatic* bacteriuria using clean-catch urine specimens in an attempt to find those women who were at risk for developing pyelonephritis. This criterion cannot, therefore, be applied unthinkingly to *symptomatic* women with frequency, urgency, or dysuria, nor should it be applied to cultures of urine obtained by sterile catheterization. Colony counts of 10^2 cfu/ml may be highly significant in patients with symptoms suggestive of urinary tract infection. This must always be kept in mind in dealing with any given clinical situation. Some microbiology laboratories will, in fact, report any culture of less than 10^5 cfu/ml as "negative" unless the specimen is specially labeled as a sterile catheter specimen or from a symptomatic patient. If the local laboratory is known to use this practice, it should be notified that the clinician wants to be informed of lower colony counts.

Office kits have recently become available which allow for the rapid diagnosis of urinary tract infection. These kits utilize specially treated dipsticks which change color if certain substances are present in the urine specimen. Urinary nitrates are converted to nitrites by certain bacteria, and these are then detected by the chemical reaction in the dipstick, indicating potential infection. *Enterococcus* infections will not be detected by this test, since these bacteria do not produce nitrites as metabolic by-products. A large number of white blood cells in the urine (pyuria) can be detected by a dipstick which detects the presence of the enzyme leukocyte esterase. The sensitivities of both of these tests are greatest when large bacterial concentrations are present. As a result, the tests may be negative if infection is present but the urine is dilute. Analysis of a specimen brought in promptly by the patient from her first morning void will therefore probably be the most accurate. Dipstick tests will not detect the presence of squamous cells and will overdiagnose infections in patients who are unable to collect an adequately clean specimen. Azo dyes such as Pyridium (phenazopyridine) will interfere with the interpretation of these tests, which complicates the diagnosis in patients who may have begun taking medications before being seen in the clinic. Although dipstick screening tests provide rapid chemical information which may help in the diagnosis of infection, microscopic examination of the unspun urine still appears to be the best rapid screening test for infection. Commercially available chemical urine test strips include Chemstrip (Boehringer Mannheim), N-Multistix (Ames Division, Miles Laboratories),

Bact-T-Screen (Marion), and Kyotest (Kyoto Diagnostics). The sensitivities of these assays in detecting significant bacteriuria range from 50%–91%; unfortunately, no one test has both a high sensitivity and specificity.

Other Diagnoses to Consider

Several other conditions may mimic symptomatic urinary tract infection closely and are discussed elsewhere in this book (see Chapter 12, "Sensory Disorders"). These diagnoses should be considered if a patient is suspected of having cystitis but the history or laboratory findings are not consistent with this diagnosis. The diagnosis of urethral syndrome, for example, depends upon the exclusion of urinary tract infection. In this case, dysuria is the prominent symptom, accompanied by frequency and urgency. Patients with urethral syndrome differ from those with acute cystitis in that they often complain of urethral pain at times other than during urination, while patients with acute cystitis usually only have pain with voiding. Cystitis often produces more pain at the end of voiding than does the urethral syndrome, and patients with the latter condition do not usually have hematuria. Many patients with urethral syndrome often improve for a time with antibiotic therapy, further confusing their diagnosis. Urethral infection with fastidious organisms such as *Ureaplasma urealyticum* or *Chlamydia* has been suspected as being the etiology of many cases of urethral syndrome.

Interstitial cystitis is a syndrome characterized by chronic bladder pain which is worsened by bladder filling and relieved by voiding. The suprapubic pain experienced by these patients is often mistaken for a urinary tract infection, but invariably they have a negative urinalysis and culture and generally they do not have dysuria. Many patients who are finally given a diagnosis of interstitial cystitis report that their initial symptoms began with a documented acute urinary tract infection, further clouding the picture.

Vulvar conditions may mimic acute urinary tract infections. Vulvovaginitis, especially that due to fungal organisms, can produce dysuria due to the irritative effect of urine on an inflamed vulva. Estrogen deprivation in postmenopausal women leads to atrophic changes in the urethra, vulva, and vagina which can result in dysuria, as can urethral caruncles, urethral prolapse, or urethral polyps. Some of the worst dysuria a patient can ever experience is due to herpetic infection of the vulva. This will not be detected unless the vulva is inspected in patients with this symptom.

Urethral infections are generally due to sexually transmitted diseases, most commonly *Neisseria gonorrheae* and *Chlamydia trachomatis.* Urethral cultures for these organisms should be taken in patients with refractory, persistent, or unexplained dysuria.

Toxic substances can also produce dysuria and/or vulvitis, including irritating bubble baths, deodorant soaps, and feminine "hygiene" deodorant sprays. These should be discontinued in patients with dysuria.

The passage of a urinary stone may produce many symptoms in both the upper and lower urinary tracts. These include acute infection associated with urinary stasis or chronic infection in the stone, dysuria, hematuria (85% of cases), and flank pain. The pain in such circumstances may be severe, far in excess to that experienced with cystitis or pyelonephritis.

Treatment of Urinary Tract Infection
General Considerations

Antibiotic therapy is the mainstay of treatment in urinary tract infections. The choice of antibiotics should aim at complete eradication of the organism without promoting new infections or the development of antibiotic resistance. The most common antimicrobial drugs used in the treatment of urinary tract infections, their indications and common side effects, are given in Table 11.2 The use of antibiotics such as nitrofurantoin, which is excreted almost exclusively in the urine and does not affect bowel or vaginal flora, should therefore to be encouraged. The drug is commonly given in doses of 50 mg or 100 mg four times per day (QID) for 5–10 days. The macrocrystalline form of nitrofurantoin (Macrodantin) appears to create less gastrointestinal upset than generic forms. This drug has become available in a twice-daily dose form (Macrobid), equiva-

TABLE 11.2. Commonly Prescribed Antimicrobial Agents for Urinary Tract Infection

Drug	Dosage: Prophylaxis/Treatment[a]	Toxicity/Side Effects
I. Uncomplicated urinary tract infection in adult women (Note: Quinolones are *not* indicated for the treatment of uncomplicated UTI)		
Nitrofurantoin	50 mg QD; 50–100 mg 3d QID ×	GI upset, peripheral neuropathy; long-term use associated with pneumonitis
Trimethoprim-sulfamethoxazole	½ tablet QD; DS BID × 3d	Allergic rash, peripheral neuropathy
Sulfisoxazole	500 g QID × 3d	Allergic rash, peripheral neuropathy
Ampicillin	500 mg QID × 3d	Fungal vaginitis, GI upset, allergic reaction
Cephalexin	500 mg QID × 3d	Same as ampicillin; hepatic dysfunction
II. Single dose therapy in adult women		
Trimethoprim-sulfamethoxazole	2 DS tablets	
Ampicillin	3 g	
Nitrofurantoin	200 mg	
Sulfisoxazole	2 g	
III. Treatment of complicated urinary tract infection (Upper Tract Involvement or Recurrence) (Check culture and sensitivity, treat accordingly.) Severe pyelonephritis may require hospitalization and intravenous administration of a third-generation cephalosporin, an aminoglycoside, or a combination of penicillin and an aminoglycoside.		
Trimethoprim-sulfamethoxazole	DS BID × 10–14d	
Cephalexin	500 mg QID × 10–14d	
Norfloxacin	400 mg BID × 10–14d	
Ciprofloxacin	250 mg BID × 10–14d	
Ofloxacin	200 mg BID × 10–14d	
IV. Treatment of uncomplicated urinary tract infection in pregnancy		
Nitrofurantoin	50–100 mg QID × 7d	
Ampicillin	500 mg QID × 7d	
Contraindicated: Sulfa-containing drugs, tetracyclines		

[a] QD = 1× per day; BID = 2× per day; QID = 4× per day; DS = double strength tablet.

lent to 50 mg QID, which makes it even more attractive as a drug. Other popular antibiotic regimens include single dose therapy with trimethoprim-sulfa, which is reported to have an 80% clinical efficacy in the treatment of uncomplicated cystitis. Single dose therapy with amoxicillin (3 g) appears to have comparable efficacy, but may result in irritating fungal vaginitis. Single dose therapy is attractive because many patients fail to complete a 7- or 10-day course of antibiotics once their symptoms begin to resolve. Recurrent infections should be treated for 7–10 days, as should cases of pyelonephritis. A culture and sensitivity profile is most useful in cases of recurrent infection, poor response of symptoms to therapy, or cases which are acquired in hospital or in patients who have been on antibiotics for other infections. In these cases the presence of a resistant organism should be suspected.

Recently, synthetic quinolone derivatives have been introduced and marketed aggressively by pharmaceutical companies. These medications are extremely effective in the treatment of urinary tract infections, particular against bacteria which have classically developed resistance to other agents. These drugs include norfloxacin, ciprofloxacin, and ofloxacin. These drugs are also extremely expensive, costing up to $2 per tablet. There is some evidence that quinolone resistance is already starting to emerge. These drugs should not be used in the treatment of uncomplicated cystitis, but should be reserved for refractory cases or infections with unusual organisms.

In addition to antibiotic therapy, several other therapeutic measures will make the patient more comfortable and will hasten resolution of her infection. Patients should be encouraged to drink large amounts of fluids to dilute their urine and help flush bacteria out of the bladder. Some patients are reluctant to do this if they have severe dysuria, since each micturition is so painful. These patients can be helped by the addition of phenazopyridine hydrochloride (Pyridium) to their treatment, given in doses of 100 mg or 200 mg three times per day for 2 days. This drug has a local anesthetic effect which provides a great deal of pain relief. As an azo dye, it also turns the urine bright orange, and patients should be warned that this will occur. Patients must understand that this drug is an anesthetic agent, not an antibiotic, and use of Pyridium alone will not cure their infection! Some patients who are short of funds have been known to purchase Pyridium only, since it is the "orange stuff" that clearly relieves their pain. The dye can also stain clothing, so special care must be taken during urination. The drug is contraindicated in patients with renal insufficiency, and the lower dose (100 mg TID) should be used in elderly patients. Patients with G–6–PD deficiency may develop hemolytic anemia while taking Pyridium. Massive acute overdosage may produce methemoglobinemia. A formulation which includes hyoscyamine and butabarbital (Pyridum Plus) is especially useful for patients with severe pain or cramping associated with infection. Like Pyridium, it should not be used for more than 2 days. Because of the butabarbital, chronic use of this medication can lead to dependence.

Urised is a combination of antiseptics (methenamine, methylene blue, phenyl salicylate, and benzoic acid) and anticholingeric parasympatholytic drugs (atropine sulfate, hyoscyamine) which is often used to relieve lower urinary tract discomfort and inflammation. Methenamine hydrolyzes in acid urine (less than pH 6) to produce formaldehyde, which has bacteriostatic activity. This drug should not be used with sulfonamides because they may react with the formaldehyde which is produced and form insoluble precipitates. Patients should be aware that the drug turns the urine a light blue or light green. The drug is probably less effective than Pyridium for the discomfort produced by acute cystitis, but is a better choice for treating chronic irritative symptoms as in the urethral syndrome. Acidification of the urine with cranberry juice or ascorbic acid (four or five 500 mg tablets taken throughout the day) is a common home remedy for acute cystitis and will enhance the efficacy of Urised by keeping the pH of urine low. Drinking cranberry or orange juice or taking large amounts of ascorbic acid is probably most effective in patients with chronic or recurrent urinary tract infections and as a prophylactic measure very early in the course of symptoms. The increased fluid intake such regimens promote may be as important as the substances themselves.

Treatment of Specific Conditions

Asymptomatic Bacteriuria

This condition is diagnosed in patients without any irritative symptoms of the lower urinary tract but who have two consecutive clean-catch urine cultures which grow at least 10^5 cfu/ml. Many of these patients will clear their bacteriuria without any intervention at all. Asymptomatic bacteriuria should be treated in pregnant women. In elderly patients bacteriuria may produce unusual symptoms which are atypical in other age groups, such as respiratory or gastrointestinal distress (see below). Asymptomatic bacteriuria should *not* be treated in women with chronic indwelling catheters or in women on clean, intermittent self-catheterization. These patients will always be colonized and repetitive treatment of *asymptomatic* bacteriuria or the use of "suppressive" or "prophylactic" antibiotics will not eradicate bacterial colonization and will only produce resistant strains of organisms. Patients being evaluated for urinary incontinence or irritative voiding symptoms are not included in the category of asymptomatic bacteriuria. Except as noted above, patients with asymptomatic bacteriuria have not clearly been shown to benefit from antibiotic treatment.

Acute Cystitis

If a woman has never had acute cystitis, or if she has had only occasional episodes of cystitis, treatment is straightforward. In the reliable patient, a simple history of symptoms consistent with acute urinary tract infection is sufficient. If any element of the history is unusual, or if the patient is unknown, she should probably be seen in the clinic. Examination of a fresh unspun urine specimen, along with a directed physical examination, is sufficient to begin treatment. The main decision then becomes whether to treat her with single dose therapy or a longer course of antibiotics. Patients often discontinue antibiotics as soon as their symptoms improve and single dose therapy with two double-strength trimethoprim-sulfamethoxazole tablets is relatively inexpensive, well tolerated, and treats approximately 80% of acute uncomplicated cases of cystitis effectively. Comparisons of this method with routine 7-day treatment initially showed a higher relapse rate 2 weeks after therapy, but the relapse rates after 6 weeks were virtually identical. Single dose therapy is less successful if penicillin derivatives are used. Another well tolerated and inexpensive form of treatment is nitrofurantoin 50 mg QID for 3–7 days, preferably in its macrocrystalline form. Single dose trimethoprim-sulfamethoxazole or 3–7 days of Macrodantin should be the first-line treatment of most cases of acute cystitis. Patients with debilitating diseases such as diabetes, the elderly, and patients with a history of pyelonephritis or recurrent infections should be treated for 7–10 days.

What follow-up should there be for acute cystitis? Many clinicians have advocated obtaining a urine culture several weeks after therapy has been completed. This is expensive and is probably unnecessary in the uncomplicated patient. However, patients should be warned that approximately 20% of cases will relapse within several weeks of treatment. This does not necessarily mean that the antibiotic therapy was unsuccessful. Most ''recurrent'' infections are reinfections rather than relapses, with the offending organism being reintroduced from a persistent colony in the vagina, in the bowel, or on the perineum. If symptoms recur, a 7–10 day course of antibiotics should be initiated after obtaining a urine culture with antibiotic sensitivities to make sure the pathogen is being treated appropriately. Patients who have persistent symptoms during treatment should be evaluated to determine if a resistant organism is present, or to see if another diagnosis is causing their symptoms.

Recurrent Cystitis

One-quarter of all women who develop acute cystitis will develop a recurrence. Women who develop recurrent cystitis average three urinary tract infections per year—a source of considerable discomfort and personal morbidity. A relapse of a previously treated infection is rare, occurring in less than 1% of patients. The vast majority of recurrent infections are reinfections originating with vaginal or colonic bacteria. Patients with recurrent cystitis need a more complex evaluation than do women with occasional acute cystitis, with an emphasis on measures to prevent further infections. Such patients may benefit from urine culture and antibiotic sensitivity determinations, to determine whether or not resistant organisms are present. Intravenous urography and cystoscopy have frequently been performed as part of the evaluation of such patients, looking for abnormalities which will explain their problem. Review of the literature shows controversy in this area, although the best studies show that these procedures are not cost effective for the majority of patients. One large study found that 97.5% of women with recurrent urinary tract infections had a normal intravenous urogram. It would seem, therefore, that radiographic studies should be reserved for patients at high risk of having anatomic abnormalities, such as those with a history of urinary infections in childhood, evidence of Müllerian anomalies, patients colonized or infected with unusual organisms, patients with a history of urinary stones, and patients with hematuria (Table 11.3).

TABLE 11.3.   Indications for Cystoscopy and Intravenous Urography in the Evaluation of Recurrent Urinary Tract Infection in Women

I. Situations in which duplicated or abnormal anatomy is suspected
   - Recurrent infections in childhood which were never evaluated fully
   - Concurrent Müllerian anomalies in the genital tract, i.e., septate uterus
   - History of pyelonephritis, especially in pregnancy
II. Situations in which other associated conditions may be detected by these tests
   - Painless hematuria
   - History of urinary tract stones
   - History of continuous incontinence, suggestive of fistulae
   - Inflammatory bowel disease, or Crohn's disease, because of possible enterovesical fistulae
   - Presence of pneumaturia, unless this is only associated with coitus

Patients with two to four documented infections in a single year are often treated with prophylactic antibiotics. The cost of such therapy is quite reasonable. Wu and colleagues have shown that the expenses incurred over the course of a year may be comparable to the cost of treating a single case of acute cystitis when physical examination, urinalysis, culture, and a week's worth of antibiotics are considered. Prophlyaxis usually consists of a single trimethoprim-sulfamethoxasole tablet or 50 mg of nitrofurantoin macrocrystals at bedtime. In cases involving resistant organisms, ciprofloxacin or other synthetic quinolone derivatives may be indicated, but these drugs should be used only for very vulnerable patients with a history of urosepsis. Prophylactic antibiotics are not useful for patients on long-term self-catheterization or patients in whom chronic indwelling catheters are used. The use of prophylactic antibiotics in these patients does nothing except promote the development of resistant organisms.

Urinary Tract Infections in Pregnancy

Pregnancy itself produces physiologic changes in the urinary tract which predispose patients to urinary stasis and the development of infection. Asymptomatic bacteriuria in pregnancy has been associated with preterm labor and birth in several studies. Both the morbidity and costs associated with these conditions mean that asymptomatic bacteriuria in pregnancy should be treated. Pregnant patients with a positive, well collected clean-catch urinalysis should be treated for asymptomatic bacteriuria. Because urinary tract infections may occur without urgency or dysuria, and because frequency is so common in pregnancy, obstetricians should have a low threshold for examining the urine of their patients. The antibiotic treatment of choice for the pregnant patient is nitrofurantoin. Sulfa drugs should be avoided if possible, particularly in the third trimester, when they may displace protein-bound bilirubin and increase the risk of neonatal jaundice. Acute cystitis in pregnancy should be managed aggressively with 7–10 days of antibiotics and close follow-up for the remainder of pregnancy. All pregnant patients who develop pyelonephritis should be hospitalized, treated with intravenous antibiotics, and observed for the development of preterm labor. After the acute episode has been resolved, they should be placed on prophylactic antibiotics (nitrofurantoin 50 mg daily) for the duration of their pregnancies and followed with regular urine cultures to check for the presence of asymptomatic bacteriuria. Postpartum intravenous urography should be considered in these patients to look for anatomic abnormalities which may have contributed to their problem, but radiographic studies should be deferred for at least 12 weeks after delivery to allow resolution of the physiologic changes in the urinary tract which have been produced by pregnancy.

Urinary Tract Infections in the Elderly

Asymptomatic bacteriuria is present in 20% of women aged 65–70 years, and in 25%–50% of women over the age of 80. Bacteriuria in the absence of symptoms does not require treatment; however, symptoms in this age group may be very subtle. Elderly women may not complain of dysuria, or may dismiss symptoms of frequency and urgency as part of the aging process. Urinary tract infection in the elderly may present instead as lack of well-being, altered sensorium or cognition, and respiratory or gastrointestinal distress. Elderly people with bacteriuria are more likely to die than those without bacteriuria, but this appears to be due to concomitant debilitating or fatal diseases and is not in itself a reason to treat otherwise asymptomatic bacteriuria.

Symptomatic bacteriuria should always be treated in elderly patients. Many of the host defense mechanisms such as complete bladder emptying, acidity of the urine, and the secretion of Tamm-Horsfall protein, are altered or lost in elderly people. Although *E. coli* is the most common cause of urinary tract infection in the elderly population, these women are more likely to have infections with gram-negative bacteria such as *Proteus, Klebsiella,* and *Pseudomonas* species. Elderly patients as a group often require hospitalization with these infections because of the likelihood of urosepsis and upper tract involvement. A 3–day course of therapy is probably adequate for treating most of this age group. Elderly women who develop reinfections should be evaluated for the presence of voiding dysfunction and the presence of residual urine, which is often due to the effects of medications. Decreased manual dexterity from arthritis is often a problem for older women, and this may lead to poor perineal hygiene which can contribute to the development of recurrent infections. Since coliform bacteria are often resistant to sulfonamides and penicillins, recurrent infections should be treated with trimethoprim or a quinolone derivative (norfloxacin, ciprofloxacin).

Sexual Intercourse and Urinary Tract Infections

The association between sexual activity and urinary tract infections has been immortalized in the expression "honeymoon cystitis." The link between the two is clear and convincing. One study showed that up to three-quarters of urinary tract infections in women occur within 24 hours of coitus. Voiding after intercourse will help wash out bacteria that may have entered the urethra and is a useful prophylactic measure. Coitus with a full bladder is uncomfortable for most women and emptying the bladder before sexual relations may mean that some women are unable to void afterwards. If this is a problem it can be avoided by urinating some time prior to having intercourse so that the bladder is relatively empty, but drinking enough fluid to ensure that some urine accumulates in the bladder and can be expelled after coitus. Having sexual relations in the morning may help some women with these problems because they can then get up for the day and will not be asleep all night with bacteria in their bladders.

Women with recurrent infections that are clearly related to intercourse should be especially careful about emptying their bladders after coitus and should avoid diaphragms as contraceptive devices, since the risk of infection is increased in women who use this method of birth control. Some patients will benefit from taking prophylactic antibiotics after intercourse, usually given as one trimethoprim-sulfamethoxazole tablet or 50 mg of nitrofurantoin. This approach seems be as effective as the daily use of prophylactic antibiotics, and much cheaper.

Catheterization and Urinary Tract Infections

Half of all patients performing clean, intermittent self-catheterization will have urine colonized by bacteria by the end of 1 year. These patients are generally asymptomatic. Unless the patient has been instrumented in a hospital setting, most acute infections developed by these patients will be due to urothelial invasion by their normal colonized bacteria. Diagnosis of acute cystitis should be based on the development of symptoms such as frequency, urgency, and dysuria, since examination of the urine in these patients will always reveal bacteria and white blood cells. It is important that patients performing self-catheterization understand this, since they may be seen by other physicians who will treat them unnecessarily. Frequent use of unnecessary antibiotics in this patient population will lead to the development of resistant organisms in the urinary tract of these patients and may replace a relatively innocuous bacteria with a more virulent strain. Treatment of recurrent symptomatic infections should begin with a review of the patient's catheterization technique and any deficiencies should be corrected. It is often useful for patients to have a supply of antibiotics at home which they can take for no more than 3 days when they feel like symptoms of an acute infection are developing. This is often enough to eliminate the problem.

Short courses of prophylactic antibiotics may be used in some patients and are particularly useful in patients who are just beginning to learn self-catheterization.

The use of chronic indwelling catheters should be avoided if at all possible. Whenever a catheterized patient is seen, the first question the clinician should ask is "Why does this patient have an indwelling catheter?" Development of strategies that will allow catheter removal should always be encouraged, particularly in nursing homes. Although condom catheters have been relatively successful in avoiding indwelling catheterization in men, none of the external devices for urine collection in women are as effective. This means that most women requiring long-term catheterization receive a transurethral balloon catheter. Infections developing in these patients are usually due to invasion of colonic bacteria which migrate up the catheter tubing. The infecting organisms generally can be cultured from the urethra several days before bacteriuria begins, but there appears to be no benefit derived from the application of topical antibiotic ointment to this area. Bladder irrigation with antimicrobial or antiseptic solutions likewise appears to have little usefulness in preventing infection.

The most important part of preventing urinary tract infection in patients with long-term indwelling catheters is meticulous aseptic technique and good catheter care at all points of catheter connection. The urine collecting bag should be kept in a dependent position to prevent retrograde flow of urine back into the bladder, and the bag should not be allowed to rest on the floor. If possible, the patient should be switched to intermittent self-catheterization by a nurse or family member. If self-catheterization is not a feasible option, the patient may benefit by placement of a chronic indwelling suprapubic catheter because it is easier to keep the catheter site clean. A 16 Fr Foley catheter can be placed into a distended bladder under local anesthesia. After 6 weeks the catheter tract will be epithelialized and the catheter can be deflated, removed, and replaced by a fresh catheter through the same site. Silicone or silicone coated catheters will last longer than ordinary catheters, although they are more expensive. Chronic catheterization generally leads to catheter encrustation and mucus production which eventually will block the catheter lumen. This blockage can be resolved temporarily by forceful flushing of the catheter, but generally the catheter will need to be replaced. Prophylactic ingestion of large doses of ascorbic acid (3 g TID) may decrease mucus production, reduce encrustation, and prolong catheter life.

Sterile Pyuria Sterile pyuria is defined as persistent white blood cells in urine that does not grow organisms on culture. Usually this represents infection with a fastidious organism or an organism that is not usually grown in the culture medium which has been used. Tuberculosis can produce this picture; more commonly, however, a chlamydial infection is responsible.

SUGGESTED READING

General Review

Johnson J, Stamm W. Diagnosis and treatment of acute urinary tract infections. Infect Dis Clin NA 1987; 1:773–96.

Kunin CM. Detection, Prevention and Management of Urinary Tract Infections. 4th ed. Philadelphia: Lea and Febiger, 1987.

Parsons L. Urinary tract infections in the female patient. Urol Clin NA 1985; 12:355–67.

Etiology

Cox C, Hinman F. Experiments with induced bacteriuria, vesical emptying, and bacterial growth on the mechanism of bladder defense to infection. J Urol 1961; 86:739–43.

Fihn S, Latham R, Roberts P, Running K, Stamm W. Association between diaphragm use and urinary tract infection. JAMA 1985; 254:240–45.

Kraft S, Stamey T. The natural history of symptomatic recurrent bacteriuria in women. Medicine 1977; 56:55–59.

Lindsay N, Harding G, Preiksaitis J, Ronald A. The association of urinary tract infection with sexual intercourse. J Infect Dis 1982; 146:579–83.

Reid G, Sobol J. Bacterial adherence in the pathogenesis of urinary tract infection: A review. Rev Infect Dis 1987; 9: 470–79.

Patient Evaluation

DeLange E, Jones B. Unnecessary intravenous urography in young women with recurrent urinary tract infection. Clin Rad 1983; 34:551–53.

Engle G, Schaeffer A, Grayhack J, Wendel E. The role of excretory urography and cystoscopy in the evaluation and management of women with recurrent urinary tract infection. J Urol 1980; 123:190–91.

Kass E. Bacteriuria and the diagnosis of infections of the urinary tract. Arch Int Med 1957; 100:709–14.

Rees DLP, Whitfield HN, Islam AKM, et al. Urodynamic findings in adult females with frequency and dysuria. Br J Urol 1975; 47:853–60.

Rees DLP, Whickham JEA, Whitfield HN. Bladder instability in women with recurrent cystitis. Br J Urol 1978; 50: 524–28.

Schaeffer A. The office microbiology laboratory. Urol Clin NA 1986; 7:463–81.

Wu T, Williams E, Koo S, MacLowry J. Evaluation of three bacteriuria screening methods in a clinical research hospital. J Clin Micro 1985; 21:796–99.

Management

Fihn S, Johnson C, Roberts P, Running K, Stamm W. Trimethoprim-sulfamethoxazole for acute dysuria in women: A single-dose or ten-day course. Ann Int Med 1988; 108: 350–57.

Greenberg R, Reilly P, Luppen K, Weinandt W, Ellington L, Bollinger M. Randomized study of single-dose, three-day, and seven-day treatment of cystitis in women. J Infect Dis 1986; 153:277–82.

Hanno P. Cystitis: A management guide to recurrent cases. Female Patient 1987; 12:55–67.

Stamm W, McKevitt M, Counts G, Wagner K, Turck M, Holmes K. Is antimicrobial prophylaxis of urinary tract infections cost effective? Ann Int Med 1981; 94:251–55.

Vosti K. Recurrent urinary tract infection: Prevention by prophylactic antibiotics after sexual intercourse. JAMA 1975; 231:934–37.

Urinary Tract Infections in the Elderly

Baldassarre J, Kaye D. Special problems of urinary tract infection in the elderly. Med Clin NA 1991; 75:375–90.

Brocklehurst J, Dillane J, Griffiths L. The prevalence and symptomatology of urinary infection in an aged population. Gerontol Clin 19; 10:242–45.

Nordenstam G, Brandberg A, Oden A, Eden C, Svanborg A. Bacteriuria and mortality in an elderly population. New Eng J Med 1986; 314:1152–56.

12

Sensory Disorders of the Bladder and Urethra: Frequency/Urgency/Dysuria/Bladder Pain

Sensory disorders are among the most distressing conditions affecting the lower urinary tract. Patients with these problems live within a cycle of pain or urgency that may repeat itself every 20 or 30 minutes. As a result, these patients' lives often revolve around voiding and the brief intervals between voiding episodes. While urinary incontinence is often embarrassing and inconvenient, it is not usually painful. Sensory disorders, on the other hand, may be very painful and may command the patient's full-time attention so that embarrassment and inconvenience become minor issues. There are many specific conditions which may produce these symptoms, and these are addressed in the second section of this chapter, "Specific Conditions and Their Treatment." Many of these symptoms have nonspecific causes, but may nonetheless respond to general management suggestions, which are discussed in the third section of this chapter, "Management of Nonspecific Conditions." The purpose of the first section of this chapter, "Triage of Patient Symptoms," is to discuss the major symptoms related to disorders of lower urinary tract sensation and to guide the clinician in searching for their etiology so that treatment may be initiated.

Triage of Patient Symptoms

The same sensory symptom may have many different causes, and many patients who are lumped together as having one clinical syndrome probably suffer from several distinctly different disorders which we are unable to separate from one another at the present time. How is the clinician to differentiate "interstitial cystitis," which presents with pain, frequency, and urgency, from "urethral syndrome," which also presents with pain, frequency, and urgency? A careful history must be taken from any patient with a sensory disorder of the lower urinary tract in order to characterize the nature and severity of the abnormal sensation. Patients with "classic" interstitial cystitis will complain of constant suprapubic or bladder pain which is transiently relieved by voiding, while patients with urethral syndrome will have variable pain symptoms which are usually exacerbated by voiding. Patients must be pinned down and made to describe *precisely* what they mean by "discomfort" in the bladder. Careful questioning often reveals that some patients mean that they are experiencing urgency, while others mean they are experiencing actual pain in the bladder. Always try to make the patient identify her worst symptom: Patients with painful bladder syndrome and patients with sensory urgency both complain of frequency, urgency, and suprapubic discomfort. In painful bladder syndromes, pain is a far more compelling symptom than frequency or urgency. Associated signs and symptoms are also important: A patient who presents with frequency and urgency may also have hematuria, a finding that is suspicious for malignancy or infection. Finally, remember that "common disorders are common." Urinary tract infection must be excluded in any patient presenting with these symptoms before another diagnosis can be considered.

Dysuria

Dysuria is defined as pain with micturition. Usually this pain is experienced as a burning sensation in the urethra, which may radiate into the suprapubic area. This should be distinguished from suprapubic pain which originates in the pelvis and is not primarily associated with voiding. The pain may occur with the initiation of voiding, or may peak as voiding is completed. Pain which is external and not urethral is likely to be due to vulvitis. Pain with micturition which radiates into the flanks is not dysuria, but may rather indicate ureteral reflux, which may be demonstrated on a filling and voiding cystogram. Dysuria may cause hesitancy and interrupted voiding patterns due to pain; this should be distinguished from patients who have abnormal voiding patterns due to urethral obstruction or other causes.

The most common source of dysuria is urinary tract infection. Often clean-catch urine samples are split into the initial voided specimen (presumed to reflect urethral organisms) and the midstream specimen (presumed to reflect intravesical organisms). Infections may be caused by fastidious organisms which are difficult to culture using standard techniques, and these patients often end up with an inappropriate diagnosis of ''urethral syndrome.'' Patients with urge syndromes experience relief with voiding, while patients with painful bladder syndromes usually experience extreme pain with filling, dysuria while voiding, and subsequent relief when micturition is complete.

Because it is both common and treatable, vulvitis must be excluded in patients with dysuria. Vulvar pain during voiding is not dysuria and the location of the pain should be carefully elicited. Acute onset of dysuria is usually associated with: (a) inflammation from soaps, perfumed or colored toilet paper, vaginal deodorant sprays, fabric softeners, or other chemical products used in the perineal area; (b) sexually transmitted diseases such as herpes or chlamydia; or (c) urinary tract infection.

Any patient with dysuria should be carefully examined for the presence of a urethral diverticulum, urethral or bladder stones, urethral discharge, urogenital atrophy, urethral caruncle, vulvitis, and hematuria. Urethroscopy may be useful, but other urodynamic tests are of lesser value.

Frequency and Urgency   Frequency is defined as voiding more than seven times per day, assuming a normal fluid intake of 1500–2000 ml per day. For patients who are awake 16 hours per day, this works out to voiding approximately once every 2 hours or so. Urgency is the sudden need to micturate. Patients may relate this as ''I have to rush to the bathroom,'' ''I cannot wait after I first feel I need to go,'' or even ''When I gotta go, I gotta go *now*.'' Patients will void frequently to avoid the sensation of urgency or to try to keep the bladder empty to avoid being incontinent. Frequency may occur without urgency, as with patients who carry a large residual urine and therefore have a small functional bladder capacity. Occasionally urgency will present without frequency, usually in association with urge incontinence.

Although increased detrusor activity is often the cause of frequency and urgency, they may also occur due to bladder hypersensitivity caused by inflammation, infection, or other factors. The sudden onset of irritable bladder symptoms raises the possibility of malignancy, particularly in patients over 50-years of age. Frequency and urgency may reflect a urinary tract infection in any patient. Chronic symptoms of frequency and urgency may be seen with sensory urgency, detrusor instability, low bladder compliance (usually secondary to radiation changes or chronic inflammation), estrogen deficiency, pregnancy, and medical conditions which involve excessive diuresis, such as diabetes mellitus, diabetes insipidus, hypercalcemia, or in patients with dependent edema who mobilize excessive amounts of fluid at night. Patients with painful bladder syndromes usually have frequency and urgency, but the dominant symptom is suprapubic pain with bladder filling.

Because voiding intervals are dependent in part upon fluid intake and individual whim, frequency and urgency should be evaluated with a frequency/volume bladder chart (see Chapter 3, ''Evaluating Symptoms''). Most people will have frequency and urgency if they are drinking 6 liters of fluid per day! It is surprising how many patients with lower urinary tract symptoms of all types—even incontinence—drink large quantities of fluid every day, thinking that this will improve their symptoms. This behavior probably stems from the common practice of telling patients with acute urinary tract infections to increase their fluid intake in order to dilute their urine. Excessive fluid intake is easy to diagnose with a bladder chart, and simple to treat. Patients must reduce their fluids to a reasonable level and understand the relationship between what they drink and what happens to the urinary tract; but they should not be chastised for failing to realize the source of their symptoms. In addition to keeping a frequency/volume chart and checking for an elevated postvoid residual, cystometry is valuable in diagnosing detrusor instability.

Nocturia

Nocturia is defined as being awakened by the need to micturate more than once per night. This increases with age, and two trips to the toilet per night is not abnormal in an 80-year old woman. Patients who have trouble sleeping and consequently get up to void because they are awake anyway do *not* have nocturia. Nocturia is also not the same as nocturnal enuresis (urine loss during sleep). Although nocturia may result from the same conditions that lead to daytime frequency and urgency, there are a few special considerations associated with nocturia. Because the patient is awakened from sleep, nocturia often represents true pathophysiology rather than patient whim or poor bladder habits. Diabetes should always be excluded in these patients. Elderly patients with dependent edema often experience a nighttime diuresis which leads to nocturia. Nighttime diuresis should be suspected particularly in the patient who does not experience daytime frequency, and this may be documented easily with a bladder chart. If associated with frequency, urgency, and urge incontinence, the symptom of nocturia is often a manifestation of detrusor overactivity, particularly if nocturnal enuresis is also present.

Bladder Pain

Pain originating in the bladder is usually experienced as suprapubic pain. Painful bladder syndromes are usually characterized by pain with bladder filling, although this is sometimes also associated with malignancy or infection. Urinary tract infection usually produces pain *with* voiding. *Constant* pain unaffected by the voiding cycle is uncommon if the bladder is the source. The quality of pain may be sharp or dull. Cramping pain is more likely to be related to the bowel or a gynecologic problem than to the bladder; however, cramping and urgency may both be caused by unstable or hyperreflexic detrusor contractions. Patients with irritable bowel syndrome also have a high incidence of detrusor instability. Patients with painful bladder symptoms should be screened for urinary tract malignancy with urinary cytology and should undergo cystoscopy to exclude the presence of foreign bodies or malignancy. This may require general anesthesia in order to obtain adequate filling, proper visualization, and the procurement of bladder biopsies. Cystometry is helpful in differentiating the hypersensitive bladder from the unstable bladder caused by detrusor overactivity. In general, however, urgency is more commonly associated with detrusor instability than is bladder pain.

Urethral Pain

Patients can usually distinguish urethral pain from bladder or vulvar pain. Pain during voiding (dysuria) should be distinguished from urethral pain that is present even when the patient is not voiding. Patients with urethral pain should be examined for the presence of abnormalities such as a diverticulum, discharge, urethral caruncle (Fig. 12.1) or a thrombosed urethral prolapse (Fig. 12.2). Urethral carcinoma is uncommon but may be misdiagnosed as a caruncle, urethral prolapse, or diverticulum. Urethral cultures for sexually transmitted diseases such as gonorrhea and chlamydia should be taken. Occasionally, urethral pain will be due to the presence of a foreign body. Careful examination of the urethra should be undertaken, including ''milking'' the urethra for discharge from the periurethral glands. Imaging studies such as voiding cystourethrography, or urethrography using a double-balloon catheter to occlude the urethral lumen while it is filled, will help determine the presence of a urethral diverticulum.

Associated Signs and Symptoms: Hematuria, Infection, Discharge, Vulvar Pain, and Urethral Mass

Gross hematuria may represent a malignancy or urinary tract stone, even in the presence of an infection, and requires radiologic and cystoscopic evaluation. Since most conditions which cause blood in urine will ultimately be treated by a urologist, hematuria should be evaluated by this specialty. However, it is completely appropriate for other physicians to initiate the work-up by obtaining

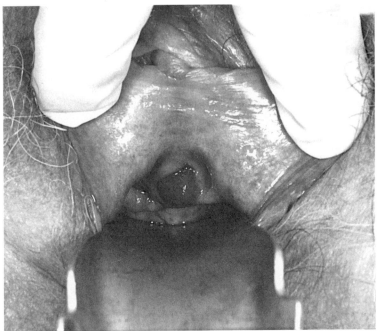

Figure 12.1   Urethral caruncle in an elderly, postmenopausal patient who is not taking estrogen supplementation.

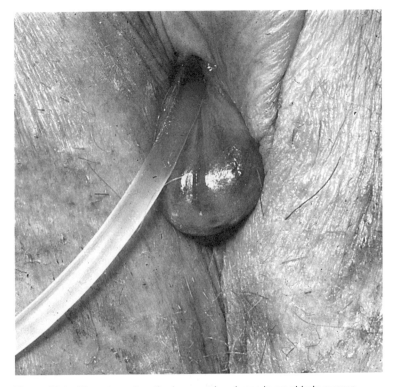

Figure 12.2   Thrombosed urethral mucosal prolapse in an elderly woman.

urinary cytology and intravenous urography. Urinary tract infections can cause hematuria and are considered at length in Chapter 11. However, patients with urinary tract infection may have persistent hematuria from another source, and need to be reevaluated after antibiotic treatment. Urinary tract stones and tumors which invade the bladder wall can be the locus of a persistent or recurrent infection. Urinary tract infection must be excluded before any sensory bladder disorder is diagnosed. A urethral discharge may be associated with either dysuria or urethral pain, and almost always represents some kind of infection. Vulvar pain often mimics dysuria and can be associated with irritative voiding symptoms. Vulvar pain may be associated with atrophic vulvitis, inflammatory vulvitis secondary to chemicals (most often soap, bubble baths, or fabric softeners), urethral caruncle or prolapse, and infectious vulvitis (most commonly monilial or herpetic). Vulvodynia is a symptom complex of chronic pain in the vulvar region described as burning, stinging, or vulvar ''rawness,'' which often requires meticulous evaluation by a specialist to obtain improvement. Finally, a urethral mass developing from a diverticulum or carcinoma may produce sensory disorders.

Specific Conditions and Their Management
Cystitis

Cystitis means inflammation of the bladder. It can be caused by infectious agents, radiation exposure, chemicals, or nonspecific etiologies. Because cystitis is so common, it should always be excluded in patients with irritative voiding symptoms or sensory disorders. The management of *infectious cystitis* is covered in Chapter 11. Radiation changes may lead to reduced bladder capacity and low compliance many years after the exposure. Certain drugs have pronounced effects on the bladder. For example, cyclophosphamide is well known to produce *hemorrhagic cystitis* in patients receiving chemotherapy for malignant disease. Cystoscopy may be necessary to exclude tumor recurrence in these patients. *Chemical cystitis* may mimic infectious cystitis both in terms of presenting symptoms and the appearance of the bladder at cystoscopy. A careful history should be taken and the use of irritating agents such as bubble bath, perineal deodorants or perfumes, and perfumed or colored toilet paper should be excluded. There is anecdotal evidence that certain foods may be concentrated in the urine and provoke an inflammatory reaction in the bladder. Patients suspected of having this problem should be helped to dilute their urine and avoid these substances. The Interstitial Cystitis Foundation has made dietary recommendations for patients with this problem (Table 12.1). *Nonspecific cystitis*, including the painful bladder syndromes, is covered in the third section of this chapter, ''Management of Nonspecific Conditions.''

Acute Urethritis (Including Sexually Transmitted Diseases)

Acute urethritis is an acute inflammation of the urethra, usually associated with dysuria, frequency, and urgency. The infectious agents are often transmitted sexually and include gonorrhea, chlamydia, herpes, trichomonas, and the human papilloma virus. Appropriate cultures should be taken and the patient and her sexual partner treated. The use of condoms should be encouraged. Herpetic lesions may respond to acyclovir, but if acute urinary retention is present, placement of a suprapubic catheter until the acute infection resolves is extremely helpful. This is easily done under local anesthesia using one of the commercially available catheters, such as the Bonanno catheter. The proper treatment of human papillomavirus remains controversial. Some practitioners recommend laser treatment of the urethra, but this has not been well studied and can cause significant complications. Noninfectious sources of urethral inflammation include the chemical irritants mentioned above. In our experience chemical irritants produce urethritis more often than they cause cystitis.

Malignancy

Transitional cell carcinoma of the bladder is a relatively common neoplasm. It is far more common in males than females, with a worldwide male:female ratio of about 3:1. It is rare in the first two decades of life and is most commonly seen in patients over the age of 50. Other risk factors include smoking, prolonged exposure to certain drugs (phenacetin, cyclophosphamide), and occupational exposure to a wide variety of chemicals, particularly those used in the manufac-

TABLE 12.1.   Foods to be Avoided in Painful Bladder Syndrome

1. Foods with acidic properties:
    All alcoholic beverages
    Most fruits (apples and cherries okay if cooked)
    Some vegetables, especially tomatoes
    Vinegar
    Curry
    Coffee and tea ("sun tea" is okay because tannic acid is not released)
2. Foods with high tyrosine, tryptophan, and aspartate levels:
    Vegetables, including avocados, eggplant, beans, and onions
    Cheese (processed cheeses including ricotta, cream cheese, and cottage
      cheese are acceptable)
    Beer and brewer's yeast
    Fruits, including bananas, raisins, pineapples
    Yogurt
    Chocolate
    Pepperoni and salami
3. Foods with possible toxic effects on the bladder:
    Eggs
    Milk
    Food colorings and flavorings
    Artificial sweeteners
    Wheat
    Chocolate
    Tomatoes
    Cola drinks
    Citrus fruits
    Some nuts

TABLE 12.2.   Staging of Bladder Cancer

Stage 0:   Carcinoma-in situ
Stage A: Tumor confined to the urothelium
Stage B: Infiltrating tumor which is confined to the muscularis
  B-1: Superficial invasion
  B-2: Deep invasion
Stage C: Tumor penetrating the muscularis

ture of chemical dyes or rubber products (see Table 3.16). Presenting symptoms include bladder pain, frequency, urgency, and dysuria. The presence of gross or microscopic hematuria, the age of the patient, and an acute onset of symptoms are helpful in identifying these patients. Bleeding at the *end* of voiding (terminal hematuria) should especially heighten the clinician's suspicion of malignancy. Urine cytology is useful in screening for malignant disease in patients with irritative bladder symptoms, particularly if some of these risk factors are present. If an IVP and cystoscopically-directed biopsies are negative, the patient with persistent microscopic hematuria should still be followed yearly with repeat urinary cytology and urinalysis. Periodic intravenous urography is also recommended. Patients with gross hematuria in whom the suspicion of malignancy is present should have an abdominal-pelvic CT scan even if they have had a negative IVP and cystoscopy. Although it is appropriate for the gynecologist to initiate the evaluation of patients in whom intravesical malignancy is suspected, these patients should undergo cystoscopy and biopsy by the urologist who will continue to take care of them. Carcinoma-in situ is frequently diagnosed only by random bladder biopsies because the urothelium may appear to be normal during gross inspection at cystoscopy. Liberal use of urinary cytology should be made in patients at risk for bladder cancer in order to pick up those who need further evaluation and biopsy. This is particularly important when following patients after treatment for a urinary tract malignancy. The staging of carcinoma of the bladder is given in Table 12.2.

Vulvovaginal Conditions

Because urine passes over the vulva during micturition, vulvar irritation leads to burning on urination. Vulvar burning with voiding is not really "dysuria," but may be reported by the patient as such. Acute vulvitis is often due to monilia, especially if the patient is a diabetic or has recently been treated with antibiotics. Chemical vulvitis is also common, usually from harsh deodorant soaps. Estrogen deficiency in postmenopausal women often leads to a chronic vulvitis which responds dramatically to hormone replacement. Vaginal discharge from monilia, trichomonas, or bacterial vaginosis may also produce vulvitis. Treatment of these conditions is directed at the vaginal source of the discharge.

Vulvodynia is chronic vulvar burning, sometimes characterized by the patient as "rawness," stinging, burning, or irritation. Itching is not a symptom of vulvodynia, but is reserved for pruritus vulvae. McKay has suggested that vulvodynia can be separated into five major diagnostic categories, each typically associated with a different anatomical location: (*a*) dermatoses in the labia majora; (*b*) papillomatosis in the labia minora; (*c*) vestibulis in the vulvar vestibule; (*d*) candida and cyclic vulvitis in the vagina; and (*e*) essential vulvodynia seen in normal skin with dysesthesia. The differential diagnosis of vulvodynia and pruritus vulvae is given in Table 12.3. Vulvar dermatoses, the most common of which is vulvar candidiasis, generally respond to specific treatment. Papillomatosis refers to the presence of multiple small cutaneous papillae, usually on the inner surface of the labia minora around the posterior vaginal introitus. The relationship of these findings to human papillomavirus infection is controversial, but it

TABLE 12.3. Differential Diagnosis of Vulvodynia and Pruritus Vulvae

Location	Presentation	Diagnosis
Labia majora	White hyperkeratotic or atrophic, friable	Lichen sclerosis
	Lichenified, dermatitic, often excoriated with pigmentary changes	Contact/irritant dermatitis or Lichen simplex chronicus
	Lilac plaques	Lichen planus
	Pink plaques, occasional scaling or fissuring	Psoriasis/tinea/seborrhea
	Dermatitic, swollen, satellite pustules	Candida
	Erythema	Steroid withdrawal dermatitis
	Verrucous or smooth, sessile papules	Condylomata acuminata
	Condylomatous, may ulcerate	Squamous cell carcinoma
Labia minora	Yellowish plaques— normal variant	Sebaceous hyperplasia
	Acetowhite papillae, mosaic vessel pattern	Papillomatosis
Vulvar vestibule	Dyspareunia; red, tender gland openings	Vestibulitis
Vagina	Discharge, KOH or culture positive	Candidiasis
	Erosive vaginitis	Bullous lichen planus or lichen sclerosis, autoimmune bullous diseases
	Recurrent symptoms, vary with menses	Cyclic vulvitis
Diffuse	Unremitting burning, older patient	Essential vulvodynia
	Radiation of pain down one or both legs	Pudendal neuralgia

a From McKay, Seminars in Dermatology, 1989; 8:40–47, with permission.

may represent subclinical HPV infection. Vulvar vestibulitis is a diagnosis usually associated with dyspareunia with penetration, erythema, and point tenderness of the vestibular glands. An acute inflammation of this area may be caused by monilial infections and resolves with treatment, but chronic vestibulitis may last for months or years. Surgical excision of this area may produce improvement in up to two-thirds of patients, but this should be considered only after a thorough investigation of other causes for symptoms. Cyclic monilial vaginitis should be suspected when the patient gives a history of symptom-free days or regular periodic flare-ups of the disease. A 6-week treatment with a topical and/or systemic anticandidal medication such as ketoconazole often brings relief, and patients may then be maintained on this medication in low tapered doses given every other day or every few days. Diffuse vulvar burning can be due to essential vulvodynia or to pudendal neuralgia which may respond to pudendal nerve blockade. Patients with essential vulvodynia have no obvious physical findings after careful examination but continue to complain of constant, nonradiating, unremitting, vulvar burning. These patients sometimes respond to treatment with tricyclic antidepressants such as amitryptiline, which is used to treat many kinds of peripheral neuritis. Amitryptiline may be started in low doses of 10 mg po at bedtime and increased gradually to 50–80 mg per day.

Bladder Stones

Foreign bodies may cause irritation of the urothelium and produce symptoms of frequency, urgency, and bladder pain. A stone at the bladder neck may occasionally produce a ball-valve type of obstruction. Patients with bladder stones may have a history of flank pain associated with passage of a ureteral calculi or a previous stone, but stones may also form spontaneously in the lower, as well as the upper, urinary tract. Hematuria may be present, but up to 15% of patients with urinary calculi do not have this symptom. An IVP and/or cystoscopy usually confirms the suspected diagnosis. A bladder calculus can usually be removed by ultrasonic or electrohydraulic lithotripsy during cystoscopy. Ninety percent of calculi are radiopaque and may be seen on a plain radiograph of the abdomen (KUB).

Diverticula of the Urethra and Bladder

Urethral diverticula are said to be present in up to 5% of the female population. The incidence is probably higher among those women with lower urinary tract symptoms. Bladder diverticula produce symptoms less commonly, unless they do not empty and retain residual urine or contain stones or tumors. The etiology of diverticula is uncertain. Bladder diverticula are felt to be the result of high bladder pressure, usually due to outflow obstruction, exerted on an area of relative weakness in the bladder wall. Urethral diverticula seem to be acquired due to repeated infection of the periurethral glands or urethral trauma.

Bladder diverticula are often asymptomatic, but may be implicated in recurrent urinary tract infections because they retain stagnant residual urine. Plain films are usually not helpful in diagnosing bladder diverticula, which are frequently picked up during intravenous urography. In a series of 142 double-contrast cystograms (dilute barium and gas), Lang found diverticula containing tumors in 3.5% and calculi in 26% of the cystograms. When found, bladder diverticula should be carefully examined with the cystoscope to exclude the presence of calculi and neoplasms. Excision of a bladder diverticulum should be reserved for those harboring calculi or tumors, or for patients with recurrent urinary tract infections who have had a complete evaluation and remain unresponsive to chronic suppressive therapy. Problematic vesical diverticula are best handled by urologists.

Urethral diverticula frequently produce symptoms of postvoid dribbling, dysuria, frequency, urgency, dyspareunia, and a painful urethral mass. These diverticula may arise from infection of the periurethral glands with subsequent obstruction of the neck of the gland. Gonorrhea is probably the most common organism which causes this type of urethral inflammation. Urethral diverticula are usually found in the distal third of the vaginal side of the urethra, where they may cause dysuria, stranguria, or incontinence, depending upon their position. Approximately half of all diverticula cannot be palpated or seen with a urethroscope. If a diverticulum is suspected but not confirmed on examination, it may often be seen during voiding cystourethrography. A double-balloon catheter may also be used to demonstrate a diverticulum by filling the space between the balloons with radiopaque dye under pressure (Fig. 10.2). Manually "milking" the urethra will often empty a urethral diverticulum, producing an efflux of urine or pus from the urethra. The patient with postvoid dribbling due to pooling of urine within a urethral diverticulum can solve her problem simply by stripping the urethra with her finger after voiding.

A urethral diverticulum should be excised if the mass is abscessed, if there is a question of malignancy, if it is contributing to recurrent urinary tract infection, or if the mass is painful. This procedure should not be undertaken lightly. If the mass is in the proximal urethra, excision may lead to incontinence. Incomplete healing of an excised diverticulum is one of the most common causes of urethrovaginal fistula formation. A urethral diverticulum is not always a small "bump" on the vaginal side of the urethra; they are sometimes complex, tortuous affairs which can corkscrew around the entire urethra or communicate with multiple other diverticula which are not obvious on physical examination. A cavalier approach to a "simple" operation can quickly turn into a nightmare if appropriate preoperative investigations have not been performed.

Urethral diverticula are generally excised vaginally. Placing a small Fogarty embolectomy catheter or a pediatric Foley catheter into the lumen of the diverticulum may facilitate the dissection. Some clinicians like to inject methylene blue dye through the lumen of the catheter to outline the diverticular sac. The urethral mucosa and smooth muscle around the diverticulum should be disturbed as little as possible during surgery, but failure to excise the neck of the diverticulum may result in its recurrence. The urethral mucosa, fascia, and muscularis should be closed in multiple layers using fine suture, and care should be taken to avoid overlapping suture lines if possible. Marsupialization of a distal diverticulum by the Spence procedure results in a wide urethral meatotomy but does not usually produce urinary incontinence unless the incision extends into the middle or proximal third of the urethra. Because marsupialization can resolve the symptoms without disturbing the rest of the urethra, this may be used as the therapy of choice for a distal diverticulum.

Urethral diverticula may be especially difficult to manage during pregnancy. Surgery should be avoided in pregnant patients since the pressure of a vaginal delivery is likely to disrupt a recent repair. Patients with symptomatic urethral diverticula during pregnancy should be placed on prophylactic antibiotics and taught to express the contents of the mass manually if possible. External drainage may occasionally be required. After pregnancy, many symptomatic diverticula will regress in size and become asymptomatic. Asymptomatic urethral diverticula should be left alone and merely observed, both in pregnant and nonpregnant patients. Treatment should be reserved for those that become symptomatic.

Pregnancy   Frequency and urgency beginning in the first trimester of pregnancy are well-known and probably related to rapidly expanding plasma volume and increasing production of progesterone. Once established, frequency and urgency persist throughout pregnancy, often worsening in the third trimester as the enlarging uterus and the weight of the fetus compress the bladder and reduce its functional capacity. Bladder pain and dysuria are not associated with pregnancy per se and suggest infectious cystitis. Urinary tract infection in the pregnant patient warrants prompt treatment because the development of pyelonephritis is an obstetrical emergency which is associated with premature labor and poor outcome. Urinary tract infection in pregnancy may present without dysuria but only as an increase in frequency and urgency. The clinical level of suspicion must remain high. In addition to the other causes, hematuria in pregnancy may suggest abnormal placentation with erosion into the bladder. Obstetricians should insist on a prompt and thorough evaluation of hematuria in a pregnant woman, just as they would in the nonpregnant patient, and should not allow the investigations to be delayed until "after delivery" by a reluctant urologist.

Detrusor Instability

Detrusor instability sometimes produces frequency and urgency in the absence of urge incontinence. In general, however, patients with this pattern have hypersensitive bladders which will respond to bladder drill and mild bladder antispasmodics such as phenazopyridine (Pyridium), hyoscyamine (Levsinex, Cystospaz), or combination-type preparations such as Urised (methenamine, methylene blue, phenyl salicylate, benzoic acid, atropine sulfate, and hyoscyamine). Bladder pain and dysuria are not commonly associated with detrusor instability, and should point toward another diagnosis. Cystometry is often helpful in categorizing these problems further. Management of the unstable bladder is discussed in Chapter 8.

Miscellaneous Problems: Estrogen Deficiency, Mass Compression, Endometriosis

Estrogen deficiency in the peri- and postmenopausal woman is a well recognized etiology of the urge syndrome. The vagina, urethra, and trigone of the bladder are all derived from the endoderm of the urogenital sinus and are estrogen-dependent tissues. Cytologic changes in the urinary tract mimic the changes seen in vaginal cytology throughout the menstrual cycle. The thinning of the urothelium seen in estrogen deficient women may be the source of the increased sensitivity to filling seen in some of these patients. Hormone replacement therapy is becoming the rule rather than the exception for postmenopausal women in the United States, and this treatment has been shown to reduce frequency and urgency in women with urogenital atrophy. Estrogen is also the treatment of choice for urethral caruncle, a common cause of dysuria in the elderly female (Fig. 12.1). Prolapse of the urethral mucosa through the external urethral orifice is unlikely to respond to estrogen therapy alone and may require excision (Fig. 12.2). Estrogen should be used to prevent recurrence of the prolapse once it has been removed.

Urinary frequency and urgency may be the presenting symptoms of a pelvic mass which reduces bladder capacity by external compression. Treatment should be aimed at removal of the mass. Fibroid tumors of the uterus are seen in 15% of white women over 35 years of age and in 30% of black women in the same age group. Fibroids are rarely responsible for frequency and urgency, and there is rarely justification for performing a hysterectomy on the basis of urinary tract symptoms alone. If a large fibroid uterus is present, particularly if there is a low lying anterior fibroid present, some patients may have bladder discomfort on this basis, but the hysterectomy in these patients is justified on the basis of their uterine pathology (the fibroids), not their urinary tract symptoms. Urinary tract symptoms associated with a uterus which would not otherwise be removed (such as an asymptomatic leiomyomatous uterus less than ''12 weeks'' size) are unlikely to be due to uterine pathology and are not indications for hysterectomy. Pregnancy should be excluded in the patient with frequency and urgency and an enlarged uterus.

Endometriosis may occur in the bladder and commonly presents with frequency and urgency. Cyclic hematuria may be present in the patient with vesical endometriosis, a symptom which can also be seen in patients with a uterovesical fistula. The diagnosis of endometriosis in the bladder can be made by seeing characteristic areas on cystoscopy, and the bladder biopsy must show endometrial-like stroma juxtaposed with glands and evidence of bleeding. It is, however, uncommon for a patient with endometriosis to present with urinary symptoms alone, and many women with extensive pelvic endometriosis are completely asymptomatic.

Management of Nonspecific Conditions
General Therapeutic Considerations

Personal choices, such as when to eat and when to sleep, are cherished freedoms of adulthood. However, when lower urinary tract symptoms begin to affect one's daily activities, instruction in fluid management and voiding habits is indicated. Patients can always take the option of ''cheating'' on therapeutic strategies on certain days, trading temporary convenience for a transient worsening of their symptoms.

Fluid Management

Although many patients have experimented with various forms of fluid management in an effort to control urinary tract symptoms, their efforts are not always grounded in a thorough understanding of bladder physiology. Some patients reduce their fluid intake to dangerously low levels of 500 ml or less per day on the assumption that the less urine they produce, the better off they will be. For patients with hypersensitive bladders, the highly concentrated urine thus produced may be far more irritating to their bladders than a larger volume of more dilute urine. Other patients will increase their intake to 4000 or 5000 ml daily based upon the logic that if this helps bladder infections, it may help other bladder symptoms too. The end result may be a dramatic increase in frequency, urgency, and incontinence.

Fluid management alone may resolve symptoms completely in some patients, and usually helps the majority of patients to control their symptoms. It is amazing how many patients with severe lower urinary tract symptoms *have not* attempted any formal fluid management. Fluid management is free, has no side effects, and gives the patient some control over her own symptoms.

Fluid management should not be started until the patient has kept a frequency/volume chart (Chapter 3). Sending the patient home with a plastic urinary "hat" that fits over the toilet bowl rim will greatly facilitate the collection of voided volumes. She should faithfully record the time and amount of every void for several days. Some physicians also ask the patient to record her fluid intake, but this can be gauged with some accuracy by looking at the voided volumes. Recording fluid intake may reveal that the patient drinks excessively at night or before bedtime. Two representative days of charting often provide adequate information and this schedule is helpful for working women who cannot keep a bladder chart at work.

Look for the following information when reviewing a patient's bladder chart:

1. Total fluid intake should range from 1500–2000 ml, unless there is a medical reason to alter it.

2. Volumes should be distributed throughout the day. If the patient drinks 1000 ml at lunch time, she should expect to have urinary frequency in the afternoon. Mealtime fluids should be limited to 300 ml and other fluids should be distributed equally between meals.

3. Fluid intake within 2 or 3 hours of bedtime should be minimal. If nocturia is present, patients should not drink before returning to bed after they have been to the bathroom at night.

4. Caffeine and alcohol may have an irritative effect on the bladder as well as induce a diuresis. Drinking alcohol before bedtime may lead to altered sleep patterns, nocturia, and enuresis.

Instructions for patients on fluid management are outlined in Table 12.4. A written instruction sheet of this type should be provided for patients.

Diuretic Timing

Patients who take diuretics and experience nocturia should make sure they take their medication in the morning hours. If it is necessary to take a diuretic twice a day, make sure the drug is taken in the early evening. Patients who experience severe frequency after taking a diuretic may find it useful to delay shopping and other activities outside the home until the afternoon.

Fluid Mobilization Management

Dependent edema often produces nocturia in some elderly patients, in patients with vascular insufficiency, and in patients who have had a pelvic lymphadenectomy. Physical examination will confirm the edema, and a frequency/volume bladder chart (with intake recorded) will confirm the nocturia. Patients with this problem should be encouraged to elevate the lower limbs periodically above the level of the heart in the afternoon and evening, to help mobilize fluids during their waking hours. A morning diuretic is sometimes useful but exchanges nocturia for daytime frequency. Specially fitted (Jobst) compression stockings may be useful in controlling the edema. Care should always be taken to make sure that patients with significant edema—particularly the elderly—are not in congestive heart failure, which requires treatment.

Bladder and Bowel Habits

Although every child is toilet trained to control detrusor contractions and to void voluntarily at the appropriate time and place, good bladder habits are taught

TABLE 12.4. Instructions to Patients in Fluid Management

Normal fluid intake is between 1500 and 2000 ml (50–70 ounces) per day, excluding what is taken in as food. Special circumstances, such as fever or hot environmental temperatures, will increase the amount of fluid you need. Drinking more than this amount may make you urinate more often and this is not necessarily abnormal. You may choose to drink more liquids, as may be required by certain diets, but if you do you will urinate more frequently.

The usual first desire to void occurs at a bladder volume of at least 150 ml (5 ounces). You do *not* have to go to the bathroom when you feel this first urge! Usually you can suppress this urge or "hold on" until a larger volume of urine is held in the bladder (200–300 ml or up to 10 ounces). Unless you have been drinking large amounts of liquid or you have a bladder infection, you should be able to wait to go to the bathroom for at least 2 hours. If you are having trouble delaying this urge to go, then make sure you space what you drink evenly throughout the day.

You should not drink liquids before going to bed! Your bladder will usually hold 400–600 ml (12–20 ounces) overnight. If you drink before going to bed you may make more urine than your bladder can hold until morning. If you drink during the night when you wake up, you can also make this problem worse. If you wake up at night for other reasons and do not normally need to void at night, it is best not to empty your bladder if you can help it. Try not to build bad bladder habits!

as poorly as good bowel habits. Young girls should be taught to wipe from front to back to avoid infection by contaminating the urethra with bowel flora. Other customs may result in less beneficial results, including fastidious placement of toilet paper on the toilet seat, voiding in a crouching position to avoid contact with the toilet seat (over 70% of women in one British study), and voiding prior to leaving home whether one needs to or not. Women may think that the first desire to void should be answered by voiding immediately, without thought as to the appropriateness of the bladder volume. This can predispose them to a vicious cycle of frequency and urgency. Likewise, the development of a bladder "holding pattern," where girls and women refuse to void except at home, can lead to overdistension of the bladder, voiding dysfunction, and even upper tract deterioration.

Bowel habits are likewise poorly taught. A gastrocolic reflex usually occurs 1/2 hour after eating. In combination with hot morning caffeine, a morning bowel movement is an ideal habit. Instead, women often suppress any natural urgency to defecate while getting the family ready for the day and/or going to work. Later, the urge having been lost, considerable strain may now be used to accomplish the task. Dysfunctional bowel habits are a source of considerable discomfort and morbidity for the female population of this country.

Bladder Drill

One of the most effective management techniques for patients with sensory disorders is bladder drill or bladder retraining. Childhood toilet training teaches young children to suppress the micturition reflex. This suppression of detrusor activity is the foundation for later bladder habits. Adults have often developed bad bladder habits, allowing detrusor contractions to be triggered by environmental influences such as coming into the front door with a full bladder (key-in-lock incontinence), voiding three times in a 10 minute period before leaving the house to "make sure the bladder is empty," or by voiding immediately whenever the slightest urgency occurs. The relearning process of adult bladder drill may therefore be more complex than the initial childhood lessons, but no less important.

Bladder drill has several basic principles: assignment of a specific time interval between voiding, avoidance of stimuli which may provoke the bladder into contracting (especially towards the end of the desired time interval), and progressive increases in the time intervals between voiding. Instructions to patients have been outlined in Chapter 8. Written instructions to patients of this kind are extremely helpful as part of a bladder drill program. The initial time interval for voiding should be assigned based on the information contained in the patient's frequency/volume chart. If the patient voids every 1–2 hours, set an initial goal of voiding every 1 hour and 15 minutes. The initial timed voiding interval must be achievable by the patient without great effort so that a solid starting point is established on which to build, *but under no circumstances should the patient go to the bathroom prior to the set time interval.* It is better to leak into a pad than to give in to the sensation of urgency. Provocative stimuli such as dishwashing, showering, arriving home, bathing children, etc., should be reserved for the earlier portion of the time interval, and avoided as much as possible as the goal approaches, since urgency is more difficult to control with a full bladder. This requires the patient to manage fluids strictly and to time her activities to coincide with her time goal. Rigorous adherence to this schedule may be difficult to achieve at work. Some patients will have more success initiating bladder drill during time off work, since the first several days with a new time interval are the most difficult to manage. It may be best to use weekends or days off to increase the time intervals between voiding. The interval should be increased by 15 minutes each week. If the previous goal was still difficult to reach by the end of the week, starting a new time interval should be delayed for another week. The final goal depends on patient wishes and fluid intake. Most patients should be able to achieve a voiding interval of between 2–3 hours.

Although bladder drill requires rigorous ''homework'' on the part of the patient, the technique benefits most patients. This technique *works* and can produce dramatic success breaking the disabling cycle of urgency and frequency which controls many patient's lives. Enthusiasm on the part of the instructor is extremely important, and a concerned and supportive nurse who is available for weekly telephone consultation will improve patient compliance. Bladder drill should be initiated for all patients with hypersensitive bladders, whether medical therapy is to be used concomitantly or not. Timed voiding regimens where the patient urinates at specific time intervals will also help many other patients with incontinence, voiding difficulty, or lack of normal bladder sensation. These techniques are particularly useful in the geriatric population.

Dietary Considerations

Certain foods seem to exacerbate urinary symptoms in certain patients. Dilution of the urine seems to help some patients, while others may benefit from excluding some foods entirely. A list of foods which have been reported to cause problems is given in Table 12.1. One note of caution: fanatical adherence to such diets have sometimes resulted in scurvy. Foods should be discontinued one group at a time. If symptoms remain unchanged, the food group may be reinstated.

Vulvar Hygiene

Patients with lower urinary tract symptoms should be taught to avoid perfumes and deodorant soaps in the vulvar area. If infectious vulvitis is present, it should receive prompt medical attention. Urine passing over an atrophic or inflamed vulva can irritate it further, and a glass of cool or tepid water poured over the vulva after voiding while the patient is still sitting on the toilet may give some relief. In hot or humid weather (and especially with obese patients) the vulva should be allowed to dry thoroughly after bathing. The patient should lie on the bed with her legs apart and use a hair dryer set on ''cool'' to dry the vulva. Cornstarch should be used instead of talcum powder in the vulvar region if the patient feels she needs a drying agent of some kind. Zinc oxide provides a barrier to protect irritated skin from urine, just as it does for babies with diaper rash. A variety of other skin barrier creams are also available. Wearing cotton crotch underwear and avoiding tight trousers or panty hose is also important. Many patients with incontinence must wear a pad at all times, and frequent changing may be economically unfeasible. Since a dry pad is less irritating, some patients will wear a panty liner inside a larger pad, and change the inner one more often. Other newer (but more expensive) pads have a gel lining which locks moisture in, keeping the surface dry. Instructions for patients in general vulvar hygiene are given in Table 12.5.

Painful Bladder Syndrome and Interstitial Cystitis

The diagnosis of painful bladder syndrome is based on symptoms of bladder pain, urinary frequency, urgency and sometimes nocturia occurring in the absence of urologic infection or other relevant pathology. The pain typically in-

TABLE 12.5. Practical Hints for Patients on Vulvar Care

The skin area around the outside of the vagina in women is called the "vulva." This area includes the skin around the urethra and the vaginal "lips." Many women experience burning in this area. This is often due to infection: A bladder infection can cause burning as urine passes through the urethra, and a yeast infection of the vulva can also cause burning as urine passes over the inflamed skin. Problems with urinary leakage can also make this area red, raw, and sore.

After an examination and possible treatment for an infection, you and your doctor may decide that you have a *chemical irritation* of the vulva. Many products in common use can irritate the sensitive skin in this area. Here are some practical things to do if this is a problem for you.

1. **Avoid colored toilet paper, douches or "feminine deodorant sprays," and tampons or absorbent pads with deodorants or scents.** Some tampons and pads contain special chemicals such as formaldehyde, and may need to be discontinued entirely.

2. **Be careful what soap you use on the vulva.** Soaps are a common source of irritation for the vulva. Avoid soaps whose names sound manly, invigorating, or bracing. Avoid any soap with a deodorant. Look for unscented soaps which emphasize hypoallergenic properties. A "pure" soap may be harsh and drying to some skin. Make sure soaps are rinsed completely from the vulva. A hand-held sprayer hose in the shower or bath can help rinse this area completely. Laundry detergent may also not be rinsed completely from underwear. Take a clean pair of underwear and rinse it vigorously in a tub of clear water: If a few bubbles are visible, you may need to rinse your underwear with a second cycle in the washing machine or by hand. Avoid using fabric softeners on your underwear, since they may also cause irritation to sensitive skin.

3. **Keep the vulva clean and dry.** Wear only cotton crotch underwear. Wear loose-fitting skirts instead of tight slacks. In very hot conditions, it may be helpful to wear no underwear at all. Avoid the use of talcum powder as a drying agent, particular scented talcum powder. If you feel you must use a drying agent, use only pure cornstarch from the grocery store. Sleep without underwear. Avoid wearing pantyhose. After bathing, make sure the vulva is dry before dressing. Some women find it helpful to lie on the bed and dry this area with a hand-held hair dryer on a cool setting. Since urine can burn an inflamed vulva, you may want to rinse this area after urination by pouring a glass of cool water over it. This can be done in the bathtub or while sitting on the toilet.

4. **If your vulva is inflamed, your doctor may prescribe medications or other treatments.** One effective treatment is to protect the vulva from further irritation with zinc oxide (often used to treat diaper rash in babies) or solid vegetable shortening after bathing. A special solution, called Burrow's solution, is available through most pharmacists, usually as a powder to prepare at home. The tablet or packet is usually diluted in a pint of cool water at a dilution of 1:40 and kept cool in the refrigerator. Soak a washcloth or gauze dressing and apply it to the affected area for 30 minutes. If the dressing becomes dry during this time, more solution can easily be added.

creases with bladder filling and is often relieved by emptying. Occasionally the pain is worse at the end of voiding. The pain is located suprapubically and dyspareunia is often present, two findings which may lead the patient to seek gynecologic evaluation.

The diagnosis of *interstitial cystitis* is given to patients with painful bladder symptoms who have typical findings at cystoscopy under anesthesia (Table 12.6). Since bladder filling is often quite painful in these patients, cystoscopy must be carried out under general or spinal anesthesia to reach the true *structural* bladder capacity unhindered by sensory input. Bladder filling during cystoscopy should be carried out by passive gravity filling under a pressure head of about 80 cm H_2O. This may be achieved by elevating the fluid bag on a high IV pole. The bladder capacity under anesthesia is generally reduced (less than 350–400 ml). When capacity is reached, the bladder should be left distended for a minute or so, and then drained. The terminal fluid is usually bloody or blood tinged in patients with interstitial cystitis. The bladder is then refilled. On the second cystoscopy, subepithelial petechial hemorrhages, glomerulations, and "cracking" of the urothelium will be seen. Ulcers and scarring of the bladder lining

TABLE 12.6.   Diagnosis of Interstitial Cystitis

1. Bladder pain
     Frequency, urgency, often nocturia
     Dysuria and incontinence are rare
2. Exclude other conditions:
     Bacteriuria (including fastidious organisms)
     Carcinoma in situ
     Mucosal dysplasia
     Radiation cystitis
     Tuberculous cystitis
     Prostatic syndromes (in males)
     Other gynecologic pathology
3. Urodynamic evaluation in selected patients
4. Cystoscopic findings under anesthesia
     Normal urethral lumen
     Blood tinged fluid at the end of the first bladder filling
     Petechiae and glomerulations seen during the second bladder filling
       "Early" interstitial cystitis
         Structural bladder capacity >400 ml
         No ulcers or scars
       "Classic" interstitial cystitis
         Structural bladder capacity <400 ml
         Ulcers and scars present
     Biopsy should be taken to exclude specific diseases such as carcinoma in situ

will often be seen in patients with late-stage interstitial cystitis. Many of these same findings can be caused by trauma from a careless cystoscopy, carcinoma in situ, radiation exposure, or acute infection. Biopsies taken from the areas of glomerulation are useful to rule out other pathology. If special stains are used, approximately 30%–50% of such biopsies will show increased numbers of mast cells (more than 20 cells/mm^2 of detrusor muscle tissue), but this finding is neither specific to nor diagnostic of interstitial cystitis.

There are over 100,000 diagnosed cases of ''classic'' interstitial cystitis in the United States; perhaps four to five times as many cases remain undiagnosed. In addition, there are probably over 1 million patients with the painful bladder syndrome (same symptoms, normal cystoscopy). Women with these conditions outnumber men by a ratio of 10:1, and the interval from the onset of disease to diagnosis is usually 3–7 years. Patients are frequently frustrated by the lack of a definitive diagnosis, and bounce from one physician to another looking for an answer. The effect of constant bladder pain on daily life is generally profound. A national survey, presented as part of an NIH consensus conference on interstitial cystitis, found that 40% of patients with interstitial cystitis were unable to work because of their disease, 58% were unable to have intercourse, 55% had considered suicide at some time in the course of their disease, and 12% had actually attempted suicide. In one large U.S. study, the quality of life for women with interstitial cystitis was found to be substantially lower than that of women with end-stage renal disease.

The etiology of painful bladder syndrome and interstitial cystitis is unknown and probably represents multiple causes presenting with the same symptoms. Possible etiologies include allergic phenomena, autoimmune processes, disruption of the glycosaminoglycan protective layer of the bladder urothelium, undetected infection with fastidious organisms, and reflex sympathetic dystrophy of the bladder.

The 1987 NIH consensus conference concluded that painful bladder syndrome includes multiple disease processes of unknown etiology and pathogenesis, and is therefore without rational therapy at present. Therapy is directed at symptom relief and referral to a center with extensive experience in the evaluation and treatment of chronic pain is often very useful. Treatment options include avoidance of possible bladder toxins (Table 12.1), intravesical instillation of

TABLE 12.7.   Instructions for Intravesical Instillation of DMSO in Patients with Painful Bladder Syndrome

General Considerations: Dimethyl sulfoxide (DMSO) is a widely available industrial solvent generated as a by-product of the pulp industry. In addition to its industrial uses, it has been approved by the Food and Drug Administration for instillation into the bladder as a treatment for interstitial cystitis. It produces a strong smell and garlic-like organic aftertaste which reminds many patients of "rotting oysters." The patient will be able to taste this in her mouth within minutes of DMSO instillation into her bladder. The nursing staff will appreciate it greatly if DMSO and the tubes or bottles used in instilling the solution are confined to a disposable drape. Any DMSO spilled on the carpet or examining room table will be detectable for the remainder of the day!

1. The patient should empty her bladder before instillation is undertaken.

2. A 50% solution of DMSO should be prepared. This can be done in either of two ways: 1) 25 ml of sterile water can be added to 25 ml of reagent grade DMSO (available through most laboratory supply sources); or 2) DMSO can be obtained preprepared as a prescription drug (RIMSO–50) in a sterile 50% solution. The patient can fill the prescription herself and bring to the office, or the drug can be obtained from most large hospital pharmacies. Some practitioners add 100 mg of hydrocortisone sodium succinate (Solucortef) or 10 mg of triamcinolone acetonide suspension (Kenalog) to the solution when it is prepared. Others have recommended the addition of 5000 units of heparin.

3. A red rubber catheter should be connected to a 60 ml catheter syringe (with the plunger removed) and inserted into the bladder using sterile technique. Once the catheter has been inserted, 50 ml of the 50% solution of DMSO should be poured into the bladder, taking care to avoid spillage. The catheter should then be removed. The perineum can be wiped dry with a tissue if spillage occurs.

4. The patient should hold the solution in her bladder for 20–30 minutes, and then void it out into the toilet. The patient must understand that she needs to keep the solution in her bladder for this length of time. Premature voiding will lead to inadequate exposure to the DMSO. Patients with very sensitive bladders may be able to retain the solution in the bladder better if a 1% solution of lidocaine has been injected into the bladder pillars bilaterally.

5. Instillations should be done every 2 weeks for 6 sessions. Many patients do not respond until after the third or fourth instillation.

DMSO (Table 12.7), bladder distension (both office distension under bladder pillar blockade with 2% lidocaine and distension under general anesthesia), inhibition of inflammatory mediators using H_1 and H_2 blockers (diphenhydramine hydrochloride 25–50 mg po TID with cimetidine 300 mg po TID); and amitriptyline, which is often used in the treatment of peripheral neuritis. Amitriptyline should be started at low doses of 10 mg po QHS and gradually increased by 10 mg QHS per week until dosage levels of 70–80 mg per night have been achieved. Starting with larger doses can cause overpowering side effects and result in poor patient compliance. Intermittent epidural blocks and treatment with transcutaneous nerve stimulators are other useful modalities of treatment for chronic pain processes, including interstitial cystitis. Other medical therapies include oral sodium pentosanpolysulfate (Elmiron), which theoretically replenishes the glycosaminoglycan layer of the bladder. Elmiron has not yet been approved for treatment purposes in the United States. Heparin is a synthetic glycosaminoglycan which can inhibit mast cell degranulation. It has produced mixed treatment results in the studies which have been done to date. It is usually administered as 5000 units, given subcutaneously, two or three times per day for 1 week. Intravesical instillation of 0.4% oxychlorosene sodium (clorpactin) appears to alleviate pain through oxidation of the bladder lining. It must be given under anesthesia. Anesthesia is also necessary for intravesical instillation of a 0.01% solution of silver nitrate, and for use of the neodymium-YAG laser. In some hands the laser has produced long-term benefits, but significant bowel and bladder injuries have also been reported. More radical ''end-stage'' therapies include denervation cystolysis, and supratrigonal cystectomy with substitution/augmentation cystoplasy for patients with shrunken, fibrotic, painful bladders. Cystectomy and urinary diversion can be used for the worst cases. Narcotics

Nocturia

should not be used in these patients because of the chronic nature of their complaints and the high potential which exists for drug abuse and addiction.

Evening fluid management, fluid mobilization management, and diuretic timing will greatly improve nocturia in many patients. With the use of bladder drill, improvement in nocturia usually lags behind improvement in daytime frequency, but will improve as the patient learns consciously and then unconsciously to suppress detrusor contractions. Desmopressin (DDAVP) is a synthetic antidiuretic hormone (ADH) analog which decreases urine production by increasing renal tubular resorption. Given as 10–20 micrograms intranasally at bedtime, the drug reduces urine output dramatically for the next 4–6 hours. Desmopressin has been shown to be safe and effective, and can produce striking results in the treatment of refractory nocturia and nocturnal enuresis. The drug cannot be used safely more than once per day. Patients using desmopression should be monitored for the development of hyponatremia and water intoxication, which can occur if the drug is abused and fluid intake is excessive.

Sensory Urgency

''Sensory urgency'' is a urodynamic diagnosis. It is given to patients with frequency, urgency, and sometimes with symptoms of urge incontinence who do not develop uninhibited contractions during provocative cystometry. Patients with urgency due to documented detrusor contractions are said to have ''motor urgency.'' Patients with urgency and frequency alone—without incontinence—rarely have detrusor instability. Some patients with sensory urgency may actually develop detrusor contractions which account for their symptoms outside the urodynamics laboratory, but they appear to differ from patients with urodynamically proven detrusor instability in that they seem to have better detrusor control. This probably makes patients with ''sensory urgency'' the best candidates for treatment with bladder drill. Anticholinergic drugs may be reserved for patients with sensory urgency who fail to improve significantly on bladder drill alone.

Conservative therapy for these patients may be initiated without formal cystometry. In these cases we make an artificial distinction between patients with frequency and urgency only (diagnosed as ''sensory urgency'' and treated initially with bladder drill) and those patients with frequency, urgency, *and urge incontinence* (presumptively diagnosed as ''detrusor instability'' and treated initially with medications, often in combination with bladder drill). There will be considerable overlap between these two groups. Failure of the initial therapy is an indication for urodynamic testing to help clarify the diagnosis.

Urethral Syndrome

The urethral syndrome is actually a symptom complex of dysuria associated with frequency, urgency, bladder pain, and voiding difficulty. Urethral syndrome has been called a ''wastebasket'' diagnosis given to patients in whom other diagnoses have been excluded. The prevalence of urethral syndrome is unknown, but probably is high: 40% of women in one study with suspected urinary tract infection who presented with dysuria, frequency, and urgency were found to have sterile urine on culture. There are many hypotheses regarding the etiology of urethral syndrome: infection with fastidious organisms which evade identification by standard culture techniques; urethral obstruction; neurologic disorders such as peripheral neuralgia; external urethral sphincter spasm; trauma; psychologic problems; and estrogen deficiency. Many of these theories are guesses based upon anecdotal success stories using various empiric therapies. For example, despite the absence of evidence for urethral obstruction, some patients seem to benefit from urethral dilation.

To make the diagnosis of urethral syndrome, the patient should relate a history of symptoms of dysuria and urethral pain, often accompanied by frequency, urgency, suprapubic discomfort, and voiding difficulty. A close relationship of symptoms to sexual activity suggests recurrent infection or irritation of the urethra due to various contraceptive substances. These patients may be helped by prophylactic antibiotics postcoitally and a change of contraceptive method. Chemical irritants, such as soap and bubble bath, must be excluded as causative factors. Incontinence or urge syndromes presenting without dysuria suggest other diagnoses. On examination of the patient, a urethral mass or discharge are suspicious for a diverticulum or an infection. A urine culture for fastidious organisms (which should be *labeled* as such) and a urethral culture for chlamydia, should both be negative. A frequency/volume chart is useful in documenting the frequency, and cystometry may be performed if detrusor instability is suspected. Urethroscopy should exclude anatomic abnormalities, and is usually painful but otherwise negative. Urine cytology should be negative.

Treatment for the urethral syndrome is usually symptom specific. As with any chronic pain condition, a plan should be developed consisting of initial therapies, subsequent therapies, and the expected time course for such management. The initial therapy should address the most prominent symptom, and subsequent therapy should utilize the least invasive options first. There is no reason why several noninvasive therapies cannot be used simultaneously, but if the patient improves under these conditions the intervention which caused the change in symptoms may not be immediately identifiable. The following therapies are often useful in managing the ''urethral syndrome.''

1. A trial of antibiotics is usually offered to the patient and her partner. This may consist of a 3-week course of tetracycline or doxycycline on the assumption that a chlamydial infection is present. Chlamydia is often difficult to culture and these drugs are effective in such infections. Patients may also be treated with chronic suppressive antibiotic therapy using Macrodantin 50–100 mg po QHS or trimethoprim 100–200 mg po QHS for 1–3 months, based on the assumption that a low-grade chronic infection may be present.

2. If the patient's symptoms are predominantly frequency and urgency with dysuria, and present in association with menopausal or postpartum atrophy, estrogen therapy may be offered. This may be given systemically or locally.

3. Urethral spasm associated with voiding difficulty may respond to diazepam 5–10 mg po TID, or prazosin 2 mg po BID, with variable results. Electrical stimulation and biofeedback hold some promise for the future, but are currently research techniques for treating the urethral syndrome.

4. Urethral dilation may be offered, especially if dysuria and voiding difficulties predominate. Although the mechanism of presumed obstruction is uncertain, it may be the result of previous infection or irritation. Equally unclear is why so many patients seem to respond to urethral dilation. Using anesthetic jelly, progressive dilation should be performed up to 36 Fr, usually in a single clinical session. This procedure can be extremely painful, and some patients may require dilation under anesthesia. One study showed that simple cystoscopy was as effective as urethral dilation in treating these patients. Anecdotal reports suggest that periurethral injection of steroids such as triamcinolone in small amounts may be helpful in some patients. Some clinicians recommend massage of the anterior vaginal wall at the time of dilation to facilitate emptying of small urethral diverticula into the expanded urethral lumen. Antibiotics should be given for a few days after urethral dilation and phenazopyridine (Pyridium, 200 mg po TID) or Urised (2 tablets po QID) will make the patient much more comfortable.

It should not be forgotten that multiple urethral dilations can cause pain, fibrosis, and scarring, and make the patient's complaints worse. If an initial urethral dilation has not produced benefits, the clinician should give serious consideration to trying other therapy rather than pursuing a potentially damaging and relatively unproven form of treatment.

SUGGESTED READING

Baskin LS, Tanagho EA. Pelvic pain without pelvic organs. J Urol 1992; 147:683–86.

Bodner D. The urethral syndrome. Urol Clin NA 1988; 15: 699–704.

Carson C, Osborne D, Segura J. Psychogenic characteristics of patients with female urethral syndrome. J Clin Psychol 1979; 35:312–16.

Friedrich EG Jr. Vulvar vestibulitis syndrome. J Reprod Med 1987; 32:110–14.

Gallagher D, Montgomerie J, North J. Acute infections of the urinary tract and the urethral syndrome in general practice. Br Med J 1965; 1:622–24.

George NJR, Gosling JR (Eds). Sensory Disorders of the Bladder and Urethra. New York: Springer-Verlag, 1983.

Gillenwater J. Summary of the National Institute of Arthritis,

Diabetes, Digestive, and Kidney Diseases Workshop on Interstitial Cystitis. J Urol 1988; 155:495–500.

Growdon WA, Fu YS, Lebherz TS, et al. Pruritic vulvar squamous papillomatosis: Evidence for human papillomavirus etiology. Obstet Gynecol 1985; 66:564–68.

Hanno PM, Staskin DR, Krane RJ, and Wein AJ (Eds). Interstitial Cystitis. New York: Springer-Verlag, 1990.

Holm-Bentzen M, Jacobsen F, Nerstrom B, et al. Painful bladder disease: Clinical and pathoanatomical differences in 115 patients. J Urol 1987; 138:500–02.

Kaplan W, Firlit C, Schoenberg H. The female urethral syndrome: External sphincter spasm as etiology. J Urol 1980; 124:48–51.

Klarskov P, Gerstenberg T, Hald T. Bladder training and terodiline in females with idiopathic urge incontinence and stable detrusor function. Scand J Urol Nephrol 1986; 20:41–46.

Lang EK. The roentgenographic assessment of bladder tumors. Cancer 1969; 23:717–24

Lynch PJ. Vulvodynia: A syndrome of unexplained vulvar pain, psychologic disability, and sexual dysfunction. J Reprod Med 1986; 31:773–80.

McKay M. Vulvodynia: A multifactorial problem. Arch Dermatol 1989; 125:256–62.

McKay M. Vulvodynia and pruritus vulvae. Seminars in Dermatology 1989; 8:40–47.

McKay M, Frankman O, Horowitz BJ, et al. Vulvar vestibulitis and vestibular papillomatosis: Report of the ISSVD committee on vulvodynia. J Reprod Med 1991; 36: 413–15.

Macaulay A, Stanton S, Stern S, Holmes D. Micturition and the mind: Psychological factors in the aetiology and treatment of urinary disorders in women. Br Med J 1987; 294: 540–43.

Parsons L, Mulholland G. Successful therapy of interstitial cystitis with pentosanpolysulfate. J Urol 1987; 138: 513–16.

Perez-Marrero R, Emerson L, Feltis J. A controlled study of DMSO in interstitial cystitis. J Urol 1988; 140:36–39.

Sobel J. Recurrent vulvovaginal candidiasis: a prospective study of the efficacy of maintenance ketoconazole therapy. New Eng J Med 1986; 315:1455–58.

Utz D, Zincke H. The masquerade of bladder cancer in situ as interstitial cystitis. J Urol 1974; 111:160–61.

Webster GD, Galloway NTM. Surgical treatment of interstitial cystitis: Indications, techniques, and results. Urology (Suppl) 1987; 29(4):34–39.

Zingg EJ, Wallace DMA (Eds). Bladder Cancer. New York: Springer-Verlag, 1985.

13

Bladder Emptying Problems

General Considerations and Patient Triage

Bladder emptying problems are common in men because benign prostatic hypertrophy often leads to obstructed voiding. In contrast, obstructed voiding is uncommon in women unless they have had bladder neck suspension operations or other pelvic surgery. Gynecologists tend to be more familiar with disorders such as urge and stress incontinence which are troublesome but rarely life-threatening conditions. Abnormal emptying, on the other hand, can lead to serious damage to the upper urinary tract. Voiding disorders which result in chronic residual urine may promote chronic infection, while the high intravesical pressure sometimes associated with bladder outlet obstruction may lead to hydronephrosis and kidney damage. Some voiding disorders are predictable and others are certainly preventable. The evaluation and management of voiding disorders takes experience and training, and often requires consultation with a specialist. Once a treatment plan has been initiated it can usually be continued by the primary physician. Gynecologists are gaining increasing experience with the routine use of clean intermittent self-catheterization, which greatly facilitates the management of chronic emptying problems. The general gynecologist should strive to recognize voiding dysfunction so that further evaluation is not delayed. In many instances, anticipation or early recognition of voiding difficulty may prevent the development of severe voiding dysfunction and its possible consequences.

The term *voiding difficulty* is generally used to refer to problems with bladder emptying. Emptying problems can be broken down further into *voiding dysfunction,* which means that the patient either cannot generate an appropriate detrusor contraction, cannot relax the pelvic floor and external urethral sphincter appropriately, or has various combinations of the two, and *obstructed voiding,* which means that the patient voids by generating high detrusor pressures but a low urinary flow. Bladder emptying problems manifest themselves in one of two ways: inability to empty the bladder completely, or emptying in an abnormal fashion. Some patients have both of these problems simultaneously.

Significant Residual Urine

There is no consensus as to what absolute volume constitutes a pathologic residual urine. For the purposes of postoperative catheter management, clinicians use postvoid residuals as low as 30 ml and as high as 150 ml as acceptable volumes which no longer require catheterization. In patients with atonic bladders who are entirely dependent upon intermittent catheterization for emptying, residual volumes of 400–600 ml may be tolerated as long as the bladder is emptied several times during the day. The residual must always be interpreted in light of the volume voided: A 50 ml residual is insignificant if the voided volume is 400 ml, while the same residual becomes significant if the voided volume is 25 ml.

Although there is no agreement on what constitutes a "significant residual," more than 100 ml on several occasions warrants close monitoring, especially in elderly patients. Patients with *asymptomatic* residuals of up to 200 ml or 300 ml may be followed, but must be watched closely for overdistension of the bladder, the development of upper tract damage, recurrent infection, or incontinence. Patients with residual urine volumes this large are likely to have a reduced functional bladder capacity and will probably become symptomatic over time. Falsely elevated residual urine measurements are sometimes obtained from patients who feel pressured to "produce" in the clinic or the urodynamics laboratory; due to anxiety or tension they may void less than 150 ml. Patients who are discovered to have an elevated residual urine should have the measurement repeated on another day after emptying a comfortably full bladder.

Abnormal Voiding Patterns: "No Go," "Go Slow," "Stop and Go"

Female patients are not accustomed to discussing voiding symptoms. For this reason they must be asked specific questions by the physician who takes their history. Voiding problems are difficult to evaluate without urodynamic studies, yet the very nature of a urodynamics laboratory may produce situational voiding dysfunction from patient embarrassment and urethral instrumentation. In many laboratories women are made to void in a standing position in front of a fluoroscopy unit, with catheters in place and with a crowd of physicians, nurses, and radiology personnel looking on. This may lead to "iatrogenic voiding difficulty." Urodynamic studies must always be correlated with the symptoms experienced by the patient at home, and every effort should be made to provide the most comfortable environment for micturition. Laboratory personnel should be kept to a minimum, and these individuals may need to leave the room briefly to allow the patient to void in private. The clinician should be extremely cautious about making the diagnosis of voiding dysfunction based on one isolated abnormal study.

Approximately one-third of women void by a combination of urethral relaxation and detrusor contraction, one-third by urethral relaxation alone, and one-third void by a combination of straining (Valsalva) and detrusor contraction. There are several patterns of abnormal voiding in women:

"No go," or hesitancy (difficulty in initiating the urine stream), is often related to an inability to relax the pelvic floor or to initiate the micturition reflex. A "shy bladder" is common in teenage girls attempting to void in a public rest room, but would be unusual in most adult women voiding in the privacy of their own homes. It can be normal, however, for the first morning void to be associated with mild hesitancy if the bladder is overly full.

"Go slow," a poor but uninterrupted urinary stream, is suspicious for outlet obstruction or voiding with a low detrusor pressure. Alterations in the position or configuration of the urethra after surgery will sometimes produce spraying or redirection of the urine stream. This situation is a nuisance for the patient but has no real remedy except for having her change her position while voiding or submitting to a takedown of her anti-incontinence procedure.

"Stop and Go," an interrupted stream, has multiple etiologies, including failure to maintain a sustained detrusor contraction (mediated by the pontine micturition center), failure to coordinate the detrusor contraction with simultaneous urethral relaxation, active sphincteric contraction in association with a detrusor contraction (detrusor-sphincter-dyssynergia), outflow obstruction, and the use of excessive straining which requires interruption of voiding to take another breath.

This chapter will discuss how to separate these entities and how to treat each one.

Diagnosis of Voiding Difficulty

Patients with difficulty voiding complain of either abnormal voiding patterns or of symptoms which are subsequently found to be due to voiding abnormalities. Examples of this include frequency caused by a small functional bladder capacity where most of the anatomic bladder space is filled with residual urine, or recurrent urinary tract infections. Patients who complain of "incomplete emptying" often have frequency and urgency rather than an emptying disorder. A patient does not always know that she has an increased residual urine after voiding. Because these symptoms may be related to a number of urinary tract complaints, exclusion of a large residual urine is one of the most important steps in the evaluation of any woman with lower urinary tract symptoms. Voiding abnormality may occur even though the bladder empties completely: an example would be patients who experience spraying of urine after anti-incontinence surgery. The patient who empties completely but who must sit and strain and struggle for 20 minutes to void 300 ml has significant voiding dysfunction irrespective of how much urine is left in her bladder. On the other hand, one significant postvoid residual by itself does not make the diagnosis of voiding dysfunction (see below).

Uroflowmetry is a useful way of screening for abnormal voiding patterns (see Chapter 4, "Practical Urodynamics"). The peak flow rate in patients with voiding difficulty is often reduced, but it is possible to produce an artificially high peak flow by straining. The pattern of urine flow is often interrupted in these patients, either due to straining, inadequate urethral relaxation, or poor coordination between the bladder and urethra. The total voiding time is often prolonged with gaps between episodes of urine flow. This produces a low mean flow rate, which is probably a more accurate measurement of urine flow than the peak flow rate. Since voiding patterns are highly dependent upon the volume voided, interpretation of uroflowmetry must be done cautiously in patients who void less than 150 ml. Rather than looking at an arbitrary standard for diagnosing voiding problems (such as a peak flow rate of 15 ml/sec), it makes more sense to use a nomogram to analyze voiding patterns in terms of centile rank in a comparable population (see Chapter 4). This allows some compensation to be made for the variation in voiding which will normally occur based on the volume of urine passed. Patients whose voiding studies are persistently in the bottom 5%–10% of the population nomogram are probably at increased risk for the development of clinically significant voiding problems.

The most complete evaluation of voiding is obtained by performing pressure-flow voiding studies under fluoroscopic observation with simultaneous pelvic floor electromyography. This allows simultaneous measurement of pressure, urine flow, and pelvic muscle activity. Simultaneous fluoroscopy (voiding video-cystourethrography) permits visualization of the actual flow of urine through the urethra. This can then be correlated with the other measured parameters. Urodynamic testing of this type is helpful in identifying specific mechanisms of dysfunction and in suggesting treatment options, but it cannot reliably indicate whether the condition is transient or chronic.

Voiding difficulty may be transient or chronic. Transient voiding problems may be associated with medication, overdistension of the bladder, "psychogenic" causes, urethral pain associated with infection or surgery, etc. Chronic voiding trouble may be associated with neuropathology, pelvic denervation injury, bladder outlet obstruction, or the development of dysfunctional voiding patterns stemming from bad bladder habits which are often acquired as the result of misguided parental influences during childhood, or as a result of time constraints in a profession (e.g., "nurse's bladder"). Transient voiding difficulty should be suspected when the problem has started recently, particularly if it has developed in association with surgery or a change of medication, or if symptoms such as dysuria or frequency have started at the same time. All too often patients are referred for a complex evaluation of voiding disorders or incontinence which are actually side effects of medication. Table 13.1 lists medications likely to produce voiding difficulty. However, the recent onset of symptoms does not preclude the possibility that the problem will eventually become chronic due to a precipitating cause such as a cerebrovascular accident. Work-up of voiding abnormalities should always include a review of neurologic symptoms, medications, and other medical conditions. The history may also be obscured by other medical crises: The postoperative patient in the recovery room or the victim of a recent stroke may both have experienced overdistension which produces transient bladder denervation. This kind of voiding dysfunction (in isolation) would be expected to improve with time.

The evaluation of chronic voiding difficulty should include assessment of neurologic function and the search for potentially reversible causes of voiding dysfunction. The management goals in chronic cases are first, to prevent upper

TABLE 13.1.   Medications Which can Cause Voiding Difficulty or Urinary Retention

1. Drugs with anticholinergic effects:
   a) Overdosage of medications used for the treatment of urge incontinence: Propantheline; oxybutynin; flavoxate; imipramine
   b) Over-the-counter antihistamines and decongestants
   c) Antidepressants such as imipramine
   d) Antispasmodics: Dicyclomine; Donnatol (phenobarbital, hyoscyamine, atropine, scopolamine)
   e) Antipsychotics: Haloperidol; thioridazine
   f) Anti-Parkinson agents: Benztropine mesylate; trihexyphenidyl
   g) Opiates
2. α-Adrenergic agents:
   Pseudoephedrine and ephedrine (in many over-the-counter cold remedies and diet pills)
   Phenylpropanolamine (cold remedies)
3. Calcium channel blockers (reduce smooth muscle contractility)

TABLE 13.2.   Risk Factors for Postoperative Voiding Difficulty in Women

1. Straining to void, poor flow, or difficulty initiating urinary stream before surgery
2. History of previous voiding dysfunction after childbirth (except in the first 24 hours after epidural anesthesia) or other surgery
3. History of acute urinary retention requiring catheterization
4. Significant postvoid residual urine prior to surgery
5. Abnormal urodynamic findings
   (Note: These must be interpreted in relation to volume voided)
   a) Preoperative flow rate less than 15 ml/sec (without strain)
   b) Prolonged flow time (greater than 30 seconds)
   c) Maximum detrusor pressure during voiding of less than 20 cm H_2O
   d) Isometric "stop flow" test with an increase in detrusor pressure of less than 10 cm H_2O
6. Surgical procedures which interfere with normal voiding by producing
   a) Relative bladder neck obstruction (many anti-incontinence operations)
   b) Spasm of the muscles of the pelvic floor (many operations to correct pelvic relaxation)

Prediction of Postoperative Voiding Difficulty

tract damage, and second, to reduce undesired symptoms such as frequency and incontinence by facilitating bladder emptying.

One mechanism by which bladder neck suspension surgery improves incontinence is through the creation of relative outflow obstruction or urethral kinking. Although this improves urine storage, the bladder's ability to empty may be compromised. The average length of time for which catheter drainage is needed after bladder neck suspension surgery ranges from a few days to several weeks. Catheter drainage time is generally longer after sling procedures and shorter after paravaginal operations. Comparing studies with one another is difficult because of the variable criteria used to determine when the catheter should be removed. If the likelihood of developing postoperative voiding problems could be predicted before surgery, patients could be counseled about it and taught techniques such as clean intermittent self-catheterization prior to surgery, or the proposed operation could be modified to reduce the likelihood of voiding dysfunction or outflow obstruction. In some cases, surgery might be canceled altogether.

Who is at risk for postoperative voiding difficulty? A list of risk factors is given in Table 13.2. Patients who habitually strain during voiding are at increased risk, since these patients may not be generating an adequate detrusor pressure during micturition. Up to one-third of women may void by urethral relaxation alone without a detrusor contraction. Many women in this group may not be able to increase intravesical pressure enough to void postoperatively against the relative obstruction created by bladder neck surgery. Some women, however, will be able to generate a sufficient detrusor contraction postoperatively, even though they did not do this routinely before their operation. Attempts have been made to correlate preoperative urine flow rates with postoperative voiding trouble. According to several studies, patients with preoperative peak flow rates of less than 15 ml/sec are at increased risk of developing this problem; however, uroflowmetry alone is a relatively unreliable test. Many patients can achieve high peak flow rates by straining. Maximum detrusor pressure during voiding has also been used to predict postoperative voiding problems, and it appears that patients who generate subtracted detrusor pressures of less than 20 cm H_2O are at increased risk of developing emptying problems after surgery. The patient who voids by urethral relaxation alone may be perfectly capable to generating a detrusor contraction when she is forced to do so, and the ''stop flow'' or isometric detrusor pressure (Piso) test can be used to identify these patients. In this test, the patient is asked to stop her urine flow suddenly during the voiding phase of subtracted cystometry (Fig. 4.22). The patient accomplishes this by contracting the striated urethral sphincter and the pelvic floor. The sudden occlusion of the urethra should produce a rapid rise in detrusor pressure because the detrusor is still contracting against a closed outlet. The pressure rise which then develops is used as a measurement of inherent detrusor strength. This may reflect how much pressure the detrusor is capable of generating against the relative outflow obstruction created by bladder neck surgery. Isometric detrusor pressure increases of less than 20 cm H_2O have been correlated with postoperative voiding dysfunction. Concern that a patient may be at risk for postoperative voiding problems is an indication for urodynamic testing, and counseling any patient of this risk is an important part of the pre-operative discussion.

Management Techniques for Bladder Emptying Problems

Continuous Transurethral Drainage

Continuous transurethral bladder drainage is often used by default because the catheter can be inserted by nursing personnel. Continuous transurethral drainage has three advantages and many disadvantages. Placement of a transurethral Foley catheter does drain the bladder adequately, is widely available, and requires minimal skill. However, because it blocks the urethra, patients are unable to void with the catheter in place and it must therefore be removed to evaluate voiding function. As a result, the catheter is often removed and replaced several times in trying to see if it is still needed. Urethral catheters are uncomfortable and interfere with both ambulation and coitus. Chronic use of a urethral catheter is also associated with a higher incidence of urinary tract infection than the other methods discussed below. If used chronically, particularly with a large balloon, urethral catheters may destroy the bladder neck. Transurethral drainage should be reserved for acute situations and limited periods of time while a better management plan is being developed.

Suprapubic Catheter Drainage

Suprapubic catheters allow the patient to attempt to void when the catheter is clamped but preserves the option of maintaining continuous drainage. These catheters are usually placed during surgery, although some, such as the Bonanno catheter, can be inserted under local anesthesia if the patient's bladder is full (400 ml). During surgery, catheters may be placed before the procedure is started (such as before beginning a vaginal hysterectomy and repairs), after the abdomen is closed, or during the case by direct cystotomy through the bladder dome.

The most popular commercially available suprapubic catheters are: (a) the Bonanno, which is easy to place but is somewhat prone to kinking due to its narrow gauge (Fig. 13.1); (b) the Stamey, a Malecot-style catheter which is slightly more difficult to place but wider and less likely to block if there is bleeding or catheter kinking (Fig. 13.2); and (c) the Cystocath (Dow), which is relatively expensive and utilizes a fussy paste and plastic plate system of attachment (Fig. 13.3).

A regular Foley catheter may also be used, placed either by direct cystotomy during surgery, or by passing a tonsil forceps through the urethra, up through the bladder and abdominal fascia, and then out through a stab incision in the

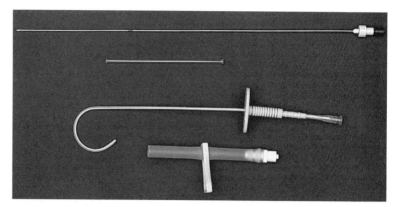

Figure 13.1   Bonanno suprapubic catheter showing the sharp needle trocar which threads through the catheter to facilitate placement, the catheter itself (which has a self-retaining "J" shape once the trocar is removed), and the connector for attaching the tubing for the catheter bag.

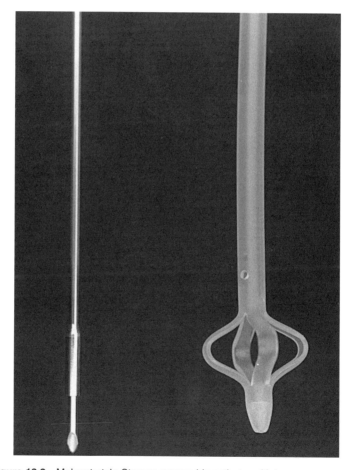

Figure 13.2   Malecot-style Stamey suprapubic catheter with trocar.

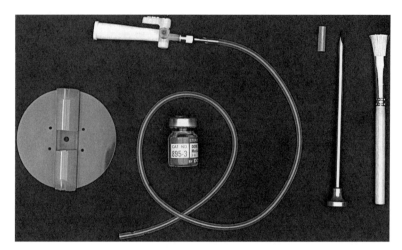

Figure 13.3   The Cystocath suprapubic catheter, including trocar, catheter tubing, valve, and adhesive catheter-fixation device.

suprapubic skin. The end of the catheter is then grasped, drawn back through the bladder and out the urethra (to determine its position), the forceps released, and the catheter gently drawn up into an intravesical position and the balloon inflated (Fig. 13.4) The catheter should then be sutured to the skin with permanent suture so it cannot become dislodged inadvertently.

Suprapubic catheters are less prone to infection than urethral catheters and are tolerated better by patients; nevertheless, the catheter may still be irritating and does require a bag. Blockage, kinking, or extravesical positioning of the catheter are common problems. Although many of the commercially prepared catheters have flanges, pigtails, or other devices to hold them in place, it is a good idea to suture them to the skin at their insertion site for extra security. The catheter should then be carefully taped with silk tape so that it does not become kinked. Nondraining catheters should be flushed copiously with several hundred ml of sterile water or saline with a 60 ml syringe. If the instilled fluid cannot be withdrawn into the syringe, the catheter is probably in a extravesical position and should be removed. Once voiding has been reestablished, the catheter can be removed on an outpatient basis. The bladder must be empty when this is done or a geyser of urine will erupt from the suprapubic catheter site. After the catheter has been removed, the insertion site will leak small amounts of urine for a few hours. This leakage can be easily managed with several gauze sponges; if it persists or is excessive, urinary retention should be suspected.

Chronic suprapubic catheterization can be used in some patients for whom intermittent catheterization is unacceptable or impractical (Table 13.3). After 6–8 weeks the catheter tract epithelializes and the catheter may be changed easily in the office every 6 weeks. Excessive mucus production in response to the indwelling catheter may encrust and block the catheter lumen. Acidifying the urine by having the patient ingest 3 g of vitamin C every 8 hours will help prevent this.

Clean Intermittent Self-Catheterization (CISC)

In the early 1970's, Jack Lapides introduced the idea of intermittent self-catheterization performed by patients as a *clean*, rather than a *sterile,* procedure. He argued that overdistension and high intravesical pressures were the key factors in the development of urinary tract infection, and that the introduction of a few host organisms by self-catheterization was unlikely to produce infection as long as the bladder was emptied regularly.

Self-catheterization is simple. The technique can be used by most patients, including children and the elderly. Individuals who are unable to use their hands or who are mentally incompetent are not good candidates for CISC unless they

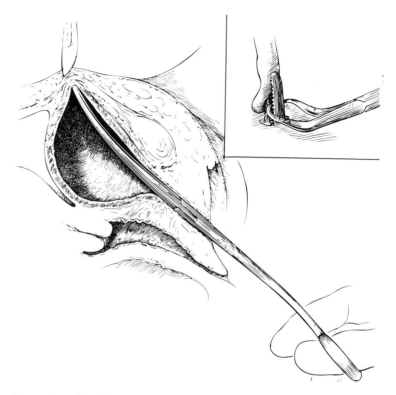

Figure 13.4 Introduction of a suprapubic catheter from below at the time of vaginal surgery. A long instrument such as a uterine dressing forceps is passed through the urethra into the bladder, which has been filled with 300 ml of sterile water or saline. The forceps is forced through the bladder dome until its tip can be palpated under the skin. A 1 cm incision is made and the end of forceps is pushed through the skin. A towel clip or other instrument is sometimes needed to separate the tips of the forceps so that the end of a Foley catheter may be grasped with the clamp and pulled down into the bladder (*Inset*). Once inside the bladder, the catheter balloon is inflated and the forceps is removed. The suprapubic catheter is then anchored to the skin with a stitch of permanent suture. (From Nichols and Randall, Vaginal Surgery, 3rd ed. Baltimore: Williams and Wilkins, 1989, with permission.)

have consistent care from their families or nursing personnel. The technique can be used in nursing homes, although the probability of nosocomial infection is increased. Patients should be given simple written instructions (Table 13.4), but they *must* be taught the technique one-on-one by an enthusiastic nurse or other health care worker, using a 14 Fr female self-catheter (Fig. 13.5).

Self-catheterization is as easy to learn as how to insert a tampon. Patients can be reassured that they are doing it correctly because urine comes out when the catheter goes in! Women can easily use a small short, moderately rigid catheter to perform self-catheterization. Telling patients to use a long floppy red rubber catheter is much more difficult. Men may need the extra length provided by these catheters, but women do not. If voiding problems are anticipated after surgery, CISC should be taught to patients preoperatively. The patient will be more comfortable if she knows what to expect and has had time to practice at her own pace, rather than being forced to learn in a hospital room while contending with a painful surgical incision. Some surgeons utilize this technique routinely for their postoperative patients, usually after an initial few days of continuous transurethral bladder drainage.

Intermittent self-catheterization allows attempted voiding without the irritation of an intravesical catheter or the need for a bag. Voiding should be attempted

TABLE 13.3.   Caring for Suprapubic Catheters

I. During the first 48 hours aftery surgery
   1. If hematuria is present, a larger diameter catheter (Stamey or Foley) is pre-ferred. The catheter should be left open to free drainage until the hematuria disappears.
   2. Although many catheters are sutured to the skin, narrow gauge suprapubic catheters, such as the Bonanno, should be taped in two positions to add security and to prevent kinking of the catheters.
   3. If the catheter does not appear to be draining, examine the catheter to make sure it has not become kinked. This is a common problem and it may occur beneath tape or at the site where the catheter emerges from the skin. Nursing personnel may be less aware of this possibility than the surgeon who placed the catheter. Considerable time can be saved and much overdistension of the bladder prevented by checking the catheter yourself.
   4. If the catheter is not draining but is not kinked, it may have become blocked by blood or debris, or have migrated out of the bladder. This can be checked by flushing the catheter with sterile water or saline injected through a 60 ml syringe connected directly to the catheter. Any blockage should be cleared by flushing the catheter. The fluid that has been injected (100–150 ml) should be recovered if the catheter is still in the bladder. If the catheter has migrated into the space of Retzius or the subfascial space, this will not occur. When catheter migration of this kind occurs, transurethral catheterization should be instituted. This may be accomplished by placing an indwelling Foley or by beginning intermittent catheterization.
   5. If the catheter does not seem to be draining, yet is not kinked and does not appear to have migrated out of the bladder, a renal or ureteric etiology for decreased urinary outout should be considered.

II. Long-term catheter care
   1. If the decision to use a chronic suprapubic catheter has been made, scrupulous care should be taken to ensure downward drainage into the catheter bag occurs at all times and that aseptic technique is used when changing catheter tubing.
   2. Once the catheter site has matured (usually in 6–8 weeks), a 14 Fr Foley catheter can easily be changed each month by a visiting nurse. To change the catheter its balloon should be deflated and the catheter pulled out through the suprapubic puncture site. When the tract has epithelialized, a new catheter can simply be inserted into the opening and advanced into the bladder. Urine can then be aspirated from the tube to check for proper placement, and the new balloon inflated. No suture is used to hold the catheter in place, but a catheter attachment device (usually of Velcro) should be used to hold the catheter in place along the upper thigh. The catheter entry site should be kept clean and dry. Cleaning this site periodically using a Q-tip and hydrogen peroxide is often useful.
   3. The major problem with these catheters is clogging due to encrustation of the catheter as a result of chronic irritation of the bladder lining. High doses of vitamin C (3 g by mouth 3 times per day) can help acidify the urine and reduce this problem. Routine irrigation of chronic suprapubic catheters with antiseptic solutions does not seem to be beneficial.
   4. Suppressive antibiotics should *not* be used, since they will only breed resistant organisms.

every 2–3 hours in acute cases, and catheterization should be performed, at minimum, the first thing in the morning and the last thing at night. The patient should attempt to void prior to catheterizations. The need for additional catheterizations during the day depends upon fluid intake, voided volumes, and the amount of the postvoid residual. Consistent residuals of 500 ml require more frequent catheterization; if the residuals are substantially smaller, for example 75 ml, the patient may catheterize less often.

Patients who are unable to void at all generally catheterize themselves every 3–4 hours and keep their catheterized urine volumes around 350 ml at each catheterization. Since 50% of patients on CISC have urine colonized by bacteria at the end of 1 year, only *symptomatic* infections should be treated. Treating "positive" urine cultures in self-catheterization patients who do not have symptoms is a waste of antibiotics. Persistent use of antibiotics will only encourage the

TABLE 13.4. Patient Instructions for Clean, Intermittent Self-Catheterization

Many patients think that only doctors or nurses can insert catheters into the bladder, but many people with bladder emptying problems catheterize themselves to make sure the bladder empties completely.

Learning to catheterize yourself is as simple as inserting a tampon! The first time you learned to put in a tampon it was difficult because you were uncertain about the vaginal opening and the anatomy of the vagina. Once you become familiar with this, it was easy to do. The same thing is true with self-catheterization, and you will soon be doing it with ease!

1. Always wash your hands with soap and water before beginning. You may also want to wash around the urethra with soap and water before starting. This is all that is needed. You do *not* need to clean the area with special solutions or disinfectants before catheterizing.

2. A special female catheter is the easiest to insert. One end of the catheter is smooth with small holes: This is the end which is put into the bladder, so try not to touch it so that it stays clean. Hold the catheter at the other end; this end will not be put in the bladder, so keeping this end very clean is not as important. The catheter should be stiff enough for you to hold it like this. If your catheter is too floppy and you have to hold it very close to the "business end" of the tube, ask your doctor to order some "female self-catheters."

3. Sit *backwards* on the toilet so you can get to the area between your legs more easily. If you are right-handed, spread the vaginal "lips" with your (clean) left hand. Hold the catheter at the far end and insert the near end (with holes) into the urethra. Once the catheter is in the urethra, push it in another inch to make sure you are in the right place.

4. How do you know you are in the right place? Urine comes out! With practice, finding the opening to the urethra is easy, but you may want to use a mirror at first to help you get it right. The most common mistake is putting the catheter into the vagina. If this happens, wash the catheter off and try again. Don't be afraid to touch yourself! Put the middle finger of your left ("spreading") hand into your vagina. The opening of the urethra should be just above (closer to your navel) the vaginal finger. Later on, you may find it easier to pass the catheter while standing up with one leg on a step or on the edge of the toilet bowl, and aim the urine stream into the toilet. This takes a little practice, but many women find it easier than sitting down.

5. The catheter does not need to be sterilized or boiled. Keep a glass of water with some dishwashing liquid in it next to the bathroom sink. The catheter should be stored "business end" down. When you are ready to use the catheter, hold it by the opposite end and rinse off all the soap in running water. After use, rinse the catheter again and put it back in the glass. The soapy water in the glass should be changed every day.

6. When you are away from home, take your catheter with you in a clean plastic container such as those used for toothbrushes. A plastic bag will also work, but is not quite as sturdy.

7. If you take care of your catheters each one will last several weeks. *You do not have to use a new catheter each time you catheterize yourself.* Start using a new one when the plastic on the old one starts looking dark or is beginning to feel uncomfortable.

8. You and your doctor will discuss how often you need to catheterize yourself. You will need to do this at least once each day. If you cannot pass any urine at all on your own, you may need to catheterize yourself 4–6 times each day.

9. After you have been catheterizing yourself for a while, you will probably have some bacteria growing in your urine, but you should only take antibiotics if you have *symptoms* of an infection. For this reason, always tell healthcare workers that you are catheterizing yourself—having bacteria in a sample of your urine does *not* necessarily mean that you have an infection.

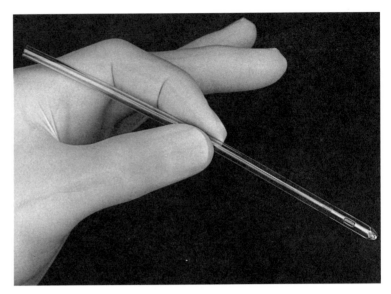

Figure 13.5 14 Fr plastic catheter for clean intermittent self-catheterization in women.

development of resistant bacteria, which may then cause more serious problems. Antimicrobial prophylaxis should be reserved for women who have just started their catheterization program, and for those who continue to have frequent bouts of symptomatic cystitis despite corrections in technique. Patients on long-term self-catheterization should have access to antibiotics at home and should be able to self-medicate for 2–3 days when they begin to notice symptoms of infection. Intermittent treatment of this kind is less likely to produce resistant organisms than chronic antibiotic suppression.

Techniques for Bladder Emptying (Credé, Valsalva, Double-Voiding, etc.)

Bladder emptying can often be improved by the use of specific techniques. Although some patients have discovered these techniques on their own, others have not tried them.

Double Voiding. This technique is well suited to those women who empty incompletely. After voiding, the patients stands and may walk around for a few minutes, but then sits and voids again. Running water or flushing the toilet may help trigger a second detrusor contraction in these patients.

Credé. This maneuver improves bladder emptying through the application of external pressure. The patient should place a hand in the suprapubic region and push downward with voiding. This technique is particularly useful for women with acontractile bladders, and is often employed by patients with neurologic bladder dysfunction.

Valsalva. Many women empty their bladders by abdominal straining. However, because straining may exacerbate genital prolapse, rectal prolapse, and hemorrhoids, it should be used only by those women who have not improved their voiding with other techniques.

Additional Tricks. Leaning forward or standing over the toilet may improve voiding for some women, especially if their voiding difficulty is related to postoperative anatomic changes. Patients who have had sling surgery for stress incontinence often report having to utilize some form of altered posture in order to improve their voiding, probably by decreasing the tension on the supportive suburethral strap. Often the patient will need to sit forward and reposition the buttocks more posteriorly on the toilet seat, again changing the angle of the pelvis. Tapping on the bladder with a finger can be used by some patients with autonomic neurologic dysfunction to trigger a reflex detrusor contraction. Occasionally patients report that gently stroking or ''tickling'' the lower back is effective in helping them urinate; presumably this also helps trigger the micturition reflex. Others have found that voiding is improved by pressing toilet paper against the perineum. Finally, patients with voiding dysfunction should always take the time to void in a private place where they can feel comfortable and will not be interrupted. Proper leg and foot support is helpful in obtaining maximal pelvic muscle relaxation, and patients with short legs may find the use of a small stepstool helpful in improving their voiding function.

Pharmacologic Agents

Clinicians are often tempted to "do something" when acute voiding problems occur. Often the best plan is to provide adequate bladder drainage and to reassure patients that the condition will improve with time. Although there is anecdotal evidence that medical therapy for voiding dysfunction is effective, clinical studies have not substantiated the usefulness of most drugs commonly used for these conditions. If the urge to prescribe a medication cannot be overcome, here are the options:

α-Blockers (Prazosin, Phenoxybenzamine). α-Adrenergic antagonists relax the urethra and bladder neck, and in several studies have been shown to be more effective than placebos. The most commonly used drugs are phenoxybenzamine (10 mg po TID/QID) and prazosin (1–2 mg BID/TID). Patients who are started on prazosin (Minipress) should be observed for 60–90 minutes after the initial administration of the drug, because of the possibility of syncope, tachycardia, and hypotension. Because of this first dose effect, prazosin is best started at bedtime.

Cholinergic-agonists. Acetylcholine-like agents, of which bethanechol chloride (Urecholine) is the most common, have been used to attempt to stimulate detrusor contractions in patients with voiding dysfunction. Because it produces a general stimulation of muscarinic receptors, this drug also produces typical cholinergic side effects such as flushing, tearing, and bowel contractions. The drug may be given parenterally or orally. When given subcutaneously, the usual starting dose is 5 mg three or four times per day. As an oral drug, the usual starting dose is 10 mg three or four times per day, gradually rising to as much as 50 mg three or four times per day. The drug is contraindicated in patients with asthma, hyperthyroidism, peptic ulcer disease, epilepsy, Parkinson's disease, or coronary artery disease. Although this drug produces contractions in bladder muscle strips in a pharmacologic laboratory, the drug does not appear to enhance detrusor activity in a clinically significant way. Most studies done with the drug have been uncontrolled. In the one controlled study of postpartum women the drug was not helpful in the treatment of urinary retention.

Prostaglandins. In theory, prostaglandins are useful in producing detrusor activity due to their ability to stimulate smooth muscle contractions. Prostaglandin $F_2\alpha$ has shown some benefit compared to controls in one study, while prostaglandin E_2 has shown less favorable results. In general, the clinical use of these drugs for promoting bladder emptying has been disappointing.

Diazepam. Relaxation of the pelvic floor is necessary for normal voiding. In some cases of acute urinary retention, muscle relaxants may help improve voiding function. Diazepam may be given in doses of 2 mg po TID to help accomplish this. In some cases, higher doses may be needed. Unfortunately, the relaxation produced by this drug is not specific to the urethral sphincter and pelvic floor, and patients commonly experience side effects such as drowsiness, ataxia, and fatigue. Diazepam also has a high potential for abuse and must be prescribed cautiously.

Biofeedback

Biofeedback using EMG of the striated urethral musculature or pelvic floor will help increase patient awareness of urethral contraction and relaxation, and may benefit patients who have detrusor-sphincter-dyssynergia or dysfunctional voiding due to an inability to relax the urethral sphincter or pelvic floor. Most practitioners will not have either the experience or equipment necessary to do this and will need to refer patients to centers with an interest in treating these disorders in order to obtain this type of treatment.

Surgical Management of Voiding Dysfunction

Urethral dilation to size 36 Fr or beyond has often been used in managing voiding dysfunction. The results are variable and have not been well studied. Excessive dilation can cause fibrosis and scarring and lead to further problems. Internal urethrotomy and bladder neck incision have been used occasionally, but have a high potential for significant complications which may be worse than the original problem. These procedures are less popular now than in the past.

Management of postoperative obstruction should begin with reassurance, drainage, and time. If the patient is still having problems after several months, taking down the obstructive procedure should be considered. The diagnosis of outflow obstruction is made on the basis of high detrusor pressure and low urinary flow during urodynamic studies, and these should be obtained prior to embarking on another operation. Takedown of a previous surgical repair because of postoperative voiding difficulty may not improve voiding unless outflow obstruction is present. In cases where voiding trouble exists but outflow obstruction is not present, the patient should generally be managed conservatively. Although some patients remain continent after taking down previous suspensory procedures, the possibility of developing recurrent stress incontinence should be recognized. A second, less obstructive, procedure such as a paravaginal repair or vagino-obturator shelf operation, may be performed at the same time as the takedown, attempting to maintain a balance between continence and the ability to void normally.

Specific Problems
Voiding Difficulty after Pelvic Floor Surgery

Surgical procedures involving the pelvic floor may produce transient voiding difficulty which may last several days to several weeks. In addition to the causes listed below, narcotics and postoperative ileus may also exacerbate voiding problems. Patients with difficulty urinating after surgery should understand that the time to recovery is quite variable. It is impossible to predict the duration of these symptoms. If problems do arise, patient acceptance of this situation is improved if there has been a candid preoperative discussion of the possibility (or probability) of such an occurrence. If the patient can empty partially, supplementary voiding techniques may be useful (see below). These techniques, when combined with self-catheterization once or twice a day, may enable her to avoid the need for continuous catheter drainage.

After Anterior Vaginal Repair. After anterior colporrhaphy or Kelly plication, edema in the periurethral tissues may produce transient voiding difficulty. These operations may also alter the anatomy of the urethra and bladder neck, producing urethral kinking which can lead to partial outlet obstruction. Care should be taken to provide adequate postoperative bladder drainage in these patients so that they do not become overdistended. If a catheter was not placed during the surgery, regular interval drainage should be used to avoid bladder injury. Some surgeons report little urinary retention after anterior vaginal wall procedures, while others note that this happens frequently. These surgeons often place a suprapubic catheter as part of their postoperative regimen until normal voiding returns. Patients who have a history of previous postpartum or postoperative retention, or those who strain to void, will benefit particularly from this approach. If continuous drainage is not used after anterior vaginal surgery, all patients should be watched carefully for voiding trouble and toileted regularly.

After Posterior Colporrhaphy. Many surgeons are surprised that voiding dysfunction is often associated with posterior colporrhaphy. Stimulation of the levator ani muscles effectively inhibits detrusor contractility, and pain in the pelvic floor often makes it difficult for the patient to relax these muscles sufficiently to permit the free flow of urine through the urethra. Stool impaction, by itself, can also cause voiding dysfunction through a similar stimulation of the levator muscles. This can be seen in normal individuals, where voiding will cease transiently as a bowel movement traverses the pelvic floor and is evacuated. If excessive abdominal straining is used, the patient may empty both her bowels and bladder simultaneously. The pain and edema created in the posterior pelvic floor by a posterior colpoperineorrhaphy is a powerful inhibitor of pelvic muscle relaxation. Voiding dysfunction may persist for several days until the pain and edema resolve. Placement of a suprapubic catheter at the time of surgery is often wise, particularly in patients who strain to void or have a history of previous postoperative voiding difficulty.

Bladder Drainage after Surgery for Incontinence

The average time that catheterization is needed after anti-incontinence surgery varies greatly with the procedure performed, the surgeon, the patient, and the criteria used to determine when bladder function has returned to normal. The paravaginal repair operation appears to produce less postoperative voiding difficulty than other retropubic operations such as the Burch or Marshall-Marchetti procedures, but to date no urodynamic data have been produced to document this fact, and no comparative studies of postoperative voiding function have been undertaken. Sling procedures and operations which overelevate the bladder neck often result in prolonged voiding difficulty due to the creation of varying degrees of outlet obstruction. The reported average length of catheterization after a Burch procedure ranges from 4 days to more than 12 days.

The regimens used in voiding trials and the various criteria used to determine when no significant residual urine is left vary greatly. Some surgeons wait until the patient is discharged to begin voiding trials, although most patients are asked to attempt voiding once they are ambulatory and bowel function is returning. Periodic clamping of a transurethral Foley catheter to allow the bladder to "regain its tone" does little to enhance the return of normal bladder function. Neither is there much evidence that medications such as bethanechol chloride (Urecholine) are clinically effective in restoring normal voiding. Some surgeons ask their patients to try to void on a regular schedule and check the residual urine after each attempt at voiding; others feel that patients are less anxious, and nurses are less taxed, if a postvoid residual is checked only in the morning and late afternoon, or any time the patient feels uncomfortable. The best regimen is the one that both the surgeon and the nursing staff are familiar with, and the one that reassures the patient that voiding difficulty is expected but that bladder function will return over time.

Overdistension of the bladder *must* be avoided, since it is both painful and will prolong the need for catheterization. There is no evidence that scheduled voiding every 2 hours will necessarily return bladder function to normal more rapidly, but it may be more effective in avoiding accidental overdistension programs where bladder emptying is encouraged at much longer intervals. Regimens for the use of suprapubic catheters after bladder neck surgery for incontinence are given in Table 13.5.

Postpartum Voiding Difficulty

Two conditions common to postpartum women may produce transient voiding difficulty: perineal pain and edema which prevent effective relaxation of the pelvic floor during voiding, and bladder overdistension from the use of epidural anesthetics or narcotics. Adequate intrapartum and postpartum bladder drainage will help minimize these problems. Allowing a sedated postpartum woman to sleep for hours while a brisk diuresis overdistends her bladder is no kindness. If regular toileting is impractical for such patients, a temporary urethral catheter may be placed. If extensive surgical repair of vaginal or perineal lacerations was necessary or if significant periurethral lacerations occurred at delivery, placement of an indwelling catheter for 24 hours should be considered. Epidural anesthesia is known to be associated with bladder dysfunction, and a transurethral Foley catheter should be placed at delivery in all women with epidural anesthesia and removed 12–24 hours after discontinuation of the anesthesia.

Emptying Problems after Radical Hysterectomy or Extensive Pelvic Surgery

Dissection of the cardinal ligaments during radical hysterectomy disrupts the autonomic innervation of the bladder and generally leads to transient voiding dysfunction. The degree and duration of the dysfunction which develops appears to be directly related to the extent of the dissection, and this is compounded if the patient receives radiation therapy. Because of this, patients undergoing radical hysterectomy *must* have adequate postoperative bladder drainage. After surgery, the catheter should be left to free drainage for 7–14 days before a trial of voiding is begun. This can be accomplished by placement of a suprapubic catheter which

TABLE 13.5. "Clamp and Release" Regimens for Postoperative Suprapubic Catheters

Suprapubic catheters are more comfortable for patients than urethral catheters. They allow the patient to attempt to void on her own and also allow a convenient way of measuring the postvoid residual urine. The object of catheter clamping is to find out when the patient is voiding well enough on her own so that the suprapubic catheter may be removed. Unless the suprapubic catheter is clamped for a period of time, enough urine will not accumulate in the bladder to permit voiding.

There are two basic regimens for clamping suprapubic catheters: Checking a residual urine volume after every void or attempted void, or checking the residual only once or twice throughout the day or when the patient complains of discomfort. Both regimens leave the catheter open to free drainage overnight to facilitate sleeping.

The suprapubic catheter should be clamped when the patient is ready to begin an attempt at voiding. Generally this can be done on the morning of the second postoperative day, unless the urine is still bloody or there is some other medical reason to delay a voiding trial. There is no reason to wait routinely for 4 days before allowing the patient to void. This only delays the process and prolongs the patient's hospital stay.

Regimen No. 1: Check Postvoid Residuals after Every Void

The suprapubic catheter should be clamped when the patient wakes up in the morning. She should try to void every 2 to 3 hours thereafter, sooner if she is uncomfortable or feels the urge to go. The voided volume should be recorded after every void, and the catheter should then be opened and allowed to drain for 15 minutes. The volume which drains out should be recorded as the residual urine volume and the catheter should then be reclamped. The catheter bag should be low enough to permit the catheter to drain easily during the 15 minutes in which it is opened after each void. The residual volume should be recorded whether the patient is able to void or not. After the last attempt at voiding in the evening, the residual urine should be recorded after 15 minutes and the catheter left to open drainage overnight. The patient should be allowed to unclamp the catheter at any time if she is unable to void or is in pain.

Advantages: The bladder should never become over-distended.

Disadvantages: Some patients become obsessive about voids and residuals, to the detriment of normal urination.

Regimen No. 2: Check Postvoid Residuals at Intervals During the Day

The suprapubic catheter should be clamped when the patient wakes up in the morning. She should try to void every 2 to 3 hours thereafter; sooner if she is uncomfortable or feels the urge to go. All voided volumes should be recorded. The residual should be checked after the first void in the morning, after the last void in the evening, and anytime the patient feels uncomfortable. If the patient is unable to void at all, the catheter should be opened for 15 minutes every 4 to 6 hours and the residual should be recorded. The interval between opening the catheter can be changed based on the residual urine volume which is obtained: The residual urine volume should be kept under 500 ml. After the last attempt at voiding in the evening, the residual urine should be recorded after 15 minutes and the catheter left to open drainage overnight. The patient should be allowed to unclamp the catheter at any time if she is unable to void or is in pain.

Advantages: The patient may attempt voiding more often during the day because the bladder is not emptied regularly. It is often easier for patients to check their residual urine volumes only occasionally.

Disadvantages: A less rigid protocol of this nature requires superb nursing supervision. This is easier to do in an "open ward" setting where all patients can be seen a one time, than situations where the patients are all in private rooms. It is easy for the bladder to become overdistended if the patient is not supervised closely.

is left open for 1–2 weeks before starting a "clamp and release" regimen until voiding returns. Alternatively, patients may be taught clean intermittent self-catheterization. Many patients who undergo a radical hysterectomy will need long-term self-catheterization, and some will need to continue this for life. Preoperative baseline urodynamic studies and periodic re-evaluation of these patients will improve their care. The goal is to avoid upper tract damage and to allow the patient the most normal lifestyle possible. If some detrusor contractility is present and the patient is able to empty partially, although not completely, she may be helped by the use of the voiding techniques mentioned above.

Bladder Distension Injury

Overdistension of the bladder may produce transient voiding dysfunction from stretch injury to the bladder wall and its sensory fibers. The amount of distension that is needed to produce injury of this type varies greatly according to the individual and the circumstances. In normal patients, injury of this type would be unusual at volumes under 1,000 ml. Nonetheless, such injuries do occur, particularly in stroke victims, postpartum women, and postoperative patients. The pain associated with bladder distension in a postoperative or postpartum patient may be dismissed improperly as "routine" pain and treated with analgesia. Indwelling catheters may become kinked or blocked, and should be checked regularly to prevent distension injury. If overdistension occurs and the patient is unable to void, a transurethral catheter should be left in place for at least 24 hours to decompress the bladder prior to a trial of voiding. Although these injuries usually resolve in a few days, they are preventable and should not occur.

Acute Inflammation or Infection

Acute inflammation or urinary tract infection may lead to difficulty voiding due to pain. Treatment of the underlying condition will resolve this, but may take some time. Occasionally a urethral or even a suprapubic catheter must be placed to facilitate drainage. Patients with acute genital herpes are the most likely to require treatment of this kind. Phenazopyridine (Pyridium) or Urised tablets often offer sufficient relief for patients with voiding dysfunction due to acute urinary tract infection. Patients with acute herpetic infections can be made more comfortable by the use of topical anesthetic sprays or voiding while sitting in a bathtub full of warm water. Normal voiding usually returns promptly when the attack clears.

Neurologic Causes of Voiding Difficulty

Women with neurologic disorders may have voiding dysfunction due to detrusor-sphincter-dyssynergia or detrusor acontractility, in addition to incontinence produced by detrusor hyperreflexia. Multiple sclerosis, Parkinson's disease, congenital abnormalities such as myelodysplasia, spinal cord injury, and stroke, are the most common neurologic conditions leading to voiding abnormalities. Close neurologic consultation is mandatory in the care of these patients. Urodynamic testing with EMG will help pinpoint the cause of the patient's bladder dysfunction. Because these patients are at risk of upper tract deterioration, they are best treated by those with extensive experience in neuro-urology.

Dysfunctional Voiding

"Dysfunctional voiding" includes a variety of complaints pertaining to patients' voiding patterns. A few patients may complain of "spraying" of the urine stream after anti-incontinence surgery. Unless there is a symptomatic residual urine or some other problem, the condition is rarely severe enough to warrant reoperation. Spraying results in a wet toilet and a wet patient. This may be resolved with the use of a clean plastic tube about the caliber of an empty toilet paper roll to direct the stream into the toilet. The tube should be pressed tightly against the perineum centered over the urethra. These tubes are readily available, such as 50 ml Falcon tubes (with the end removed) which are used in most medical laboratories. A large plastic hair roller will serve a similar purpose. Some patients are unable to relax the urethral sphincter and pelvic floor during voiding and may benefit from biofeedback training using EMG to help them learn to relax these muscles. Muscle relaxants, such as diazepam, or α-blockers, such as prazosin, may be useful for short-term trials. Many women are unable to void unless their feet are properly supported. Keeping a small stepstool in

Detrusor Hyperactivity with Impaired Contractility Genital Prolapse

the bathroom may help improve voiding in some women, particularly those who are exceptionally short of stature.

DHIC refers to an overactive detrusor which causes incontinence but fails to empty the bladder completely. This is an important cause of emptying problems in the elderly and is discussed in Chapters 9 and 15.

A large cystocele may collect urine at a level below the urethra; urine must then travel uphill to be expelled. In some large (second and third degree) cystoceles and cystourethroceles, the urethra may kink and become transiently obstructed, compromising voiding. Many patients need to reduce the cystocele in order to void. Surgical correction of the prolapse may cure the voiding problem, but the surgeon cannot be certain that there is not another coexistent voiding problem and therefore should not promise a resolution of voiding difficulties after surgery. Vaginal vault prolapse and large enteroceles can also cause voiding dysfunction, but voiding dysfunction due to isolated urethroceles is uncommon. First degree cystoceles (descent toward, but not to, the introitus) are unlikely to cause significant voiding difficulty. Some patients relate a history of stress incontinence which improved with worsening of their prolapse. These patients may have become dry due to the development of functional outlet obstruction. Surgery may cure the prolapse but cause the incontinence to worsen by removing this outlet obstruction. Patients of this kind should be carefully examined with a full bladder and the prolapse reduced by a pessary, a Sims speculum, or a ring forceps while performing a cough stress test to check for this possibility.

Acute Urinary Retention

Acute urinary retention refers to a sudden inability to void leading to overdistension of the bladder. The condition is painful and requires catheterization for relief. Although this is seen most commonly in postpartum or postoperative patients, or as a side effect of medication in a susceptible patient, other pathology may also lead to this condition. Among the other causes that may be cited are pelvic tumors, herniated vertebral discs, Guillain-Barré syndrome, and a variety of other neurologic conditions, many of which are potentially life-threatening. Immediate management of these patients requires bladder decompression with either an indwelling catheter or intermittent catheterization while investigations are undertaken to determine the etiology of the condition.

"Psychogenic" Urinary Retention

"Hysteria" is often regarded as a common cause of acute urinary retention in women. Although emptying problems in men have many recognized etiologies, the most common being prostatic hypertrophy, it is interesting that much of the literature on female voiding disorders is devoted to discussions of psychogenic urinary retention "related to a hysterical character disorder." There are many real etiologies for urinary retention in women, and *all* of these must be ruled out by a meticulous evaluation before consideration is given to a possible psychogenic etiology. Although many female patients who present with acute retention will have a history of being sexually abused, "psychosomatic urinary retention" is a diagnosis of exclusion.

Bladder Outlet Obstruction in Women

True bladder neck obstruction is unusual in women, and when it occurs it is most commonly the result of anatomic overelevation of the bladder neck following anti-incontinence surgery. Other possible anatomic causes include extrinsic compression from fibroid tumors or a prolapse, intraurethral stenosis or obstruction from a diverticulum, fibrosis or a neoplasm. Primary bladder neck obstruction has been said to occur due to hypertrophy of the smooth muscle and collagen surrounding the urethra, or from increased α-adrenergic receptors within the bladder neck. Functional bladder outlet obstruction may occur from inappropriate urethral contraction, such as in detrusor-sphincter-dyssynergia. The patient should be examined to assess the extent of bladder neck elevation and to look for any extrinsic mass that might be obstructing the urethra. A large postvoid residual may be present, especially if the obstruction is long-standing.

Bladder outlet obstruction is diagnosed during urodynamic testing by the presence of high pressure and low flow. Simple uroflowmetry typically shows low peak flow rates (less than 15 ml/sec), and the pattern is often interrupted. Because this voiding pattern may be associated with an underactive detrusor, subtracted cystometry should be performed in patients suspected of having outflow obstruction. The pressure-flow study should reveal high detrusor pressures during voiding (over 50 cm H$_2$O) with a simultaneous low flow rate (less than 15 ml/sec). Videocystourethrography is very useful in evaluating outlet obstruction. When performed in association with subtracted cystometry, this technique allows measurement of bladder and urethral pressures while the passage of fluid is visualized by fluoroscopy. This may be used to localize the site of obstruction. EMG is an important part of the evaluation of voiding disorders because it can detect inappropriate contraction of the sphincter during attempted voiding. Cystourethroscopy will occasionally reveal intraurethral stenosis, fibrosis, or extreme angulation of the urethra, but these may sometimes be detected by careful physical examination as well.

Treatment is aimed at the specific etiology of the obstruction once it has been identified. Bladder outlet obstruction due to anti-incontinence surgery should be *prevented* by avoiding overcorrection at the time of surgery. Patients with postoperative obstruction may be helped by a takedown operation and resuspension of the bladder neck at a lower level, such as by replacing a Burch or MMK operation with a paravaginal repair. In some cases, periurethral scarring may still elevate and occlude the urethra after resuspension. In other cases, incontinence may return after the takedown operation. Urethral dilation should be reserved for documented distal urethral stenosis; repetitive dilation is a common *cause* of proximal urethral stenosis and is generally overused in the treatment of voiding problems. Functional obstruction due to urethral spasm or poor pelvic muscle relaxation may respond to a combination of bladder retraining, biofeedback, and diazepam or prazosin to relax the urethral musculature. Surgical incision or resection of the bladder neck has little place in the treatment of female voiding disorders and can lead to total incontinence.

SUGGESTED READING

Andersson KE, Ek A, Hedlund H, Mattiasson A. Effects of prazosin on isolated human urethra and in patients with lower motor neuron lesions. Invest Urol 1981; 19:39–42.

Andersson K. Current concepts in the treatment of disorders of micturition. Drugs 1988; 35:477–94.

Bass J, Leach G. Bladder outlet obstruction in women. Prob Urology 1991; 5:141–53.

Beck RP, Warren KG, Whitman P. Urodynamic studies in female patients with multiple sclerosis. Am J Obstet Gynecol 1981; 139:273–76.

Bennett D, Diokno A. Clean intermittent self-catheterization in the elderly. Urology 1984; 24:43–45.

Bendtsen AL, Andersen JR, Andersen JT. Infrequent voiders syndrome (nurses bladder): Prevalence among nurses and assistant nurses in a surgical ward. Scand J Urol Nephrol 1991; 25:201–04.

Bhatia N, Bergman A. Urodynamic predictability of voiding following incontinence surgery. Obstet Gynecol 1984; 63: 85–91.

Blaivas JG, Labib KB. Acute urinary retention in women: Complete urodynamic evaluation. Urology 1977; 10: 383–89.

Doran J, Roberts M. Acute urinary retention in women. Br J Urol 1976; 47:793–96.

Bonannao PJ. Bladder drainage with the suprapubic catheter needle. Obstet Gynecol 1970; 35:807–13.

Bradley W, Bockswold G, Timm G. Neurology of micturition. J Urol 1976; 115:481–87.

Caplan LR, Kleeman FJ, Berg S. Urinary retention probably secondary to herpes genitalis. N Eng J Med 1977; 297: 920–21.

Clarke-Pearson DL, Soisson AP, Wall LL. Surgical treatment of early-stage cervical cancer. In Greer BE, Berek JS (Eds). Gynecologic Oncology: Treatment Rationale and Techniques. New York: Elsevier, 1991:187–205.

Constantinou C, Djurhuus J, Silverman D, Towns A, Wong L, Govan D. Isometric detrusor pressure during bladder filling and its dependency on bladder volume and interruption to flow in control subjects. J Urol 1984; 131:86–90.

Delaere K, Thomas C, Moonen T, Debruyne F. The value of prostaglandin E$_2$ and F$_2$-α in women with abnormalities of bladder emptying. Br J Urol 1981; 53:306–09.

Diokno AC, Sonda LP, Hollander JB, Lapides J. Fate of patients started on clean intermittent self-catheterization therapy 10 years ago. J Urol 1983; 129:1120-22

Finkbeiner A. Is bethanechol chloride clinically effective in promoting bladder emptying? J Urol 1985; 134:443–49.

Fishman I, Shabsigh R, Kaplan A. Lower urinary tract dysfunction after radical hysterectomy for carcinoma of the cervix. Urol 1986; 28:462–68.

Frymire LJ. Comparison of suprapubic versus Foley drains. Obstet Gynecol 1971; 38:239–44.

Givens C, Wenzel R. Catheter-associated urinary tract infections in surgical patients: A controlled study on the excess morbidity and costs. J Urol 1980; 124:646–48.

Graham C. Making a catheterization program work in patients with functional limitations. Prob Urol 1989; 3: 54–71.

Kunin C, Chin Q, Chambers S. Indwelling urinary catheters in the elderly: Relation of "catheter life" to formation of encrustation in patients with and without blocked catheters. Am J Med 1987; 82:405–11.

Lapides J, Diokno A, Silber S, Lowe B. Clean intermittent self-catheterization in the treatment of urinary tract disease. J Urol 1972; 107:458–61.

Lapides J, Diokno AC, Lowe BS, Kalish MD. Follow-up

on unsterile, intermittent self-catheterization. J Urol 1974; 111:184–87.

Lose G, Lindholm P. Prophylactic phenoxybenzamine in the prevention of postoperative retention of urine after vaginal repair: A prospective randomized double-blinded trial. Int J Gynecol Obstet 1985; 23:315–20.

Lose G, Jorgensen L, Mortensen S, Molsted-Pedersen L, Kristensen J. Voiding difficulties after colposuspension. Obstet Gynecol 1987; 69:33–37.

McGuire EJ, Savastano JA. Long-term follow-up of spinal cord injury patients managed by intermittent catheterization. J Urol 1983; 129:775–76.

Massey J, Abrams P. Obstructed voiding in the female. Br J Urol 1988; 61:36–39.

Mundy A. An anatomical explanation for bladder dysfunction following rectal and uterine surgery. Br J Urol 1982; 54:501–04.

Norton P, Stanton S. Isometric detrusor test as a predictor of postoperative voiding difficulties. Neurourol Urodynam 1988; 7:287–88.

Norton P, Peattie A, Stanton S. Estimation of urinary residual by palpation. Neurourol Urodynam 1989; 8:330–32.

Parikh A, Chapple CR, Hampson SJ. Suprapubic catheterisation and bowel injury. Br J Urol 1992; 70:212–13.

Parkin DE. Lower urinary tract complications of the treatment of cervical carcinoma. Obstet Gynecol Surv 1989; 44:523–29.

Prasad M, Abcarian H. Urinary retention following operations for benign anorectal diseases. Dis Colon Rectum 1976; 21:490–92.

Preminger GM, et al. Acute urinary retention in female patients: Diagnosis and treatment. J Urol 1983; 130:112–13.

Raz S, Smith R. External sphincter spasticity syndrome in female patients. J Urol 120(1976); 115:443–46.

Richardson D, Bent A, Ostergard D. The effect of uterovaginal prolapse on urethrovesical pressure dynamics. Am J Obstet Gynecol (1983); 146:901–05.

Riehle R, Williams J. Transient neuropathic bladder following herpes simplex genitalia. J Urol (1979); 122:263–64.

Shapiro J, Hoffman J, Jersky J. A comparison of suprapubic and transurethral drainage for postoperative urinary retention in general surgical patients. Acta Chir Scand 1982; 148:323–27.

Singer A, Bartlett J, Abbe R, Gavrell G, Quinn A, Leidich R. Postoperative urinary retention. Postgrad Med 1987; 81:154–56.

Stanton S, Cardozo L, Chaudhury N. Spontaneous voiding after surgery for urinary incontinence. Br J Obstet Gynaec 1978; 85:149–52.

Tanagho E, Miller E. Initiation of voiding. Br J Urol 1970; 42:175–80.

Twombley G, Landers D. The innervation of the bladder with reference to radical hysterectomy. Am J Obstet Gynecol 1956; 71:1291–1300

Van Nagell J Jr, Penny R Jr, Roddick J Jr. Suprapubic bladder drainage following radical hysterectomy. Am J Obstet Gynecol 1972; 113:849–50.

Webster G, Kreder K. Voiding dysfunction following cystourethropexy: Its evaluation and management. J Urol 1990; 144:670–73.

Wein A. Physiology of micturition. Clin Geriatr Med 1987; 2:689–99.

Wennergren HM, Oberg BE, Sandstedt P. The importance of leg support for relaxation of the pelvic floor muscles: A surface electromyograph study in healthy girls. Scand J Urol Nephrol 1991; 25:205–13.

Zimmern PE, Hadley RE, Leach GR, Raz S. Female urethral obstruction after Marshall-Marchetti-Krantz operation. J Urol 1987; 138:517–20.

14

Prolapse and the Lower Urinary Tract

Gynecologists are involved in the care of patients with genital prolapse and lower urinary tract disorders because of the intimate interrelationship of these two organ systems. The term "genitourinary" is a manifestation of this interrelationship, and explains why both urologists and gynecologists are genitourinary surgeons. The close relationship between the genital and urinary tracts derives not only from their common embryologic origins, but also from their anatomic proximity and physiologic interdependence. It is impossible to divide the problems of one system from the other. Consider, for example, the paradoxical relationship between stress incontinence and urinary retention in patients with cystoceles. How can poor support of the bladder and urethra give rise to urinary incontinence in some individuals, but voiding difficulty in others? This chapter discusses the relationship between genital prolapse and lower urinary tract dysfunction.

Elements of both structure and function are involved in this relationship. Prolapse is primarily a *structural* problem, while continence and voiding are *functional* issues. Patients with stress incontinence have altered physiologic function, but this is generally the result of structural alterations in urethrovesical support. The same is true for patients with large cystourethroceles who develop voiding disorders. In these patients structural defects have resulted in urethral kinking and the development of functional outlet obstruction. This typically results in an intermittent urinary stream because straining to empty the bladder forces the cystocele against the urethra, slowing or stopping the flow completely (Fig. 14.1).

From what has been covered elsewhere in this book, however, it should be clear that *both* stress incontinence and voiding difficulty may be due to causes other than defective anatomic support. The link between structure and function is very important in genitourinary disorders, but it is not absolute. Patients who have stress incontinence associated with urethral hypermobility generally obtain a good surgical result from operations which correct the anatomic defect and stabilize urethral support. Similarly, patients who have voiding difficulty, large residual urine, and an associated *large* cystourethrocele can usually expect their voiding to improve after surgery. A *small* cystocele is unlikely to be the cause of voiding dysfunction, and correction of a minimal defect is unlikely to improve bladder emptying. These patients may have another cause for their problems, such as denervation of the lower urinary tract from a neurologic disease like multiple sclerosis.

Vaginal birth is probably the single most significant factor in the development of both prolapse and incontinence in women. Tissue trauma from the passage of the large human head through the female pelvis is probably the common pathway linking these conditions with each other. Avulsion of connective tissue from its normal attachments, neuromuscular damage, and alterations in the geometry of the pelvis are probably all important in the genesis of these problems. This can only be understood if prolapse and incontinence are considered together.

The goal of this chapter is to help the reader understand how to evaluate and

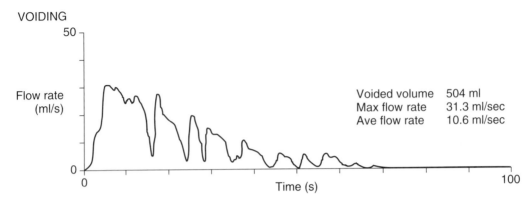

Figure 14.1   Urine flow study in a patient with a large cystocele, resulting in an interrupted flow pattern.

manage lower urinary tract problems associated with prolapse. Urinary tract symptoms clearly occur in women who do not have prolapse, as well as women who do. It is, therefore, important to decide whether these symptoms are caused by prolapse in women who have defective pelvic support, or whether they are coincidental unrelated findings. The material presented here should help clinicians sort out the different problems of patients in this situation, such as a woman with a cystourethrocele and symptoms of urgency and frequency whose urinary symptoms originate from causes other than her prolapse (such as a bladder tumor).

The following list of questions summarizes the problems that arise from the close relationship of the urinary and genital tracts in women:

- How do you decide when prolapse is causing a patient's bladder symptoms and urinary tract dysfunction?
- How should you evaluate incomplete emptying occurring in a patient with a cystourethrocele to see if it will resolve after reconstructive surgery?
- How can patients be evaluated to see if they will develop stress incontinence after surgery to correct a prolapse?
- How can patients with stress incontinence be evaluated to see if they will develop a prolapse after the urethra is resuspended?
- How do operations for stress incontinence influence pelvic support?

Before these issues can be addressed, the various types of prolapse must be understood, including how they may be detected on physical examination and the kinds of symptoms they may cause.

Classification of Prolapse
Types of Prolapse

Patients with prolapse have defective pelvic support, allowing the vagina, uterus, and their adjacent organs to descend below their normal positions. Traditionally, prolapse has been named according to the organ lying next to that part of the vagina which has prolapsed, i.e., when the anterior vaginal wall prolapses, it is called a cystocele. While this is a convenient descriptive system, the term cystocele may imply that there is something wrong with the bladder or that a defect in the bladder wall has caused a herniation. This is not true. Prolapse is actually a problem of vaginal and uterine support, not an abnormality of the bladder or rectum. Descent of the bladder, rectum, or uterus does not have much to do with the organs themselves, but has a lot to do with their connections to the pelvic sidewalls. It is defective support of the anterior vaginal wall and pubocervical fascia that allows the bladder to prolapse, not some defect in the bladder itself.

Prolapse is divided into 5 types: urethrocele, cystocele, uterine prolapse, enterocele, and rectocele (Fig. 14.2). These occur in various combinations and different degrees of severity. They will be defined, described, and illustrated in this chapter.

Urethrocele, Cystocele, and Cystourethrocele

The urethra is approximately 4 cm long and is fused to the lower 4 cm of the vagina. Descent of this portion of the vagina is called a *urethrocele.* Loss of support in this region is most often associated with stress incontinence. When the urethra and bladder are in their normal anatomic relationships, this portion of the anterior vagina is angulated anteriorly. This is easy to see during a pelvic examination if the blade of a speculum is used to retract the posterior vagina out of the way. The bladder lies adjacent to the anterior vagina above the urethrovesical junction. Loss of support in this region is called a *cystocele.* The term *cystourethrocele* is used when support of the anterior vagina is defective in both areas. Isolated urethroceles are rare.

Uterine Prolapse

Uterine prolapse is usually classified by describing the degree of descent of the uterine cervix when the patient strains. Normally the cervix is located in the upper third of the vagina. It may descend to within a few centimeters of the hymenal ring in multiparous women without causing any symptoms or changes in physiology. The cervix can often be pulled below this point in normal parous women if enough traction is applied to it. Just because the cervix can be pulled out of its normal position does not mean the patient has a clinical prolapse! This is an unnatural way of detecting prolapse and does not make a diagnosis unless the cervix extends well below the hymenal ring with traction. Once the diagnosis of prolapse has been made, however, the application of traction of this kind can help evaluate the maximum degree of cervical descent. Traction may also help the clinician detect potential prolapse that may worsen after surgery to correct stress incontinence.

Enterocele

The peritoneal fold, called the cul de-sac or pouch of Douglas, extends approximately 3 cm below the junction of the posterior vaginal wall and the uterine cervix. This is the area in which an enterocele develops. A true enterocele is often referred to as a *pulsion enterocele* because it is filled with bowel and is distended by abdominal pressure. Enteroceles of this type present as a protruding mass in the upper part of the posterior vaginal wall. The second type of enterocele is called a *traction enterocele,* because the peritoneum of the cul-de-sac is pulled into an abnormally low position by prolapse of the cervix. Since it is not filled with bowel, this is not a true enterocele. It is only a manifestation of loss of uterine support. Once the uterus has been removed, however, a true enterocele may develop if the peritoneum is not closed and the vagina is not supported adequately.

Rectocele

An anterior protrusion of the rectal wall into the vaginal canal is called a rectocele. This develops because the rectovaginal fascia no longer restrains the rectum in its normal position. A rectocele produces symptoms when it forms a pocket which traps stool. Patients in whom this occurs may complain of ''constipation,'' but it must be emphasized that most constipation in women is due to causes other than rectoceles. The anterior rectal wall is normally quite mobile, and this is often confused with a true rectocele. If the perineal body is deficient, there may also appear to be a rectocele because the normal angulation of the rectum has been exposed, rather than there being any true alteration in rectal support.

Procidentia

The most severe form of prolapse occurs when the vagina and uterus extend completely outside the body. The term *procidentia* is used for this condition (Fig. 14.3). Management of this condition can be quite challenging.

Assessing the Degree of Prolapse

A number of clinical classification systems have been developed to describe the severity of prolapse. While each system clearly describes the criteria used to grade a prolapse, unless another physician knows which system is being used he does not know what degree of prolapse is really present without examining the patient himself. Until a formal system for the classification of prolapse has been agreed upon by gynecologists and comes into general use, the clearest method is probably descriptive (Table 14.1). The prolapse may be described

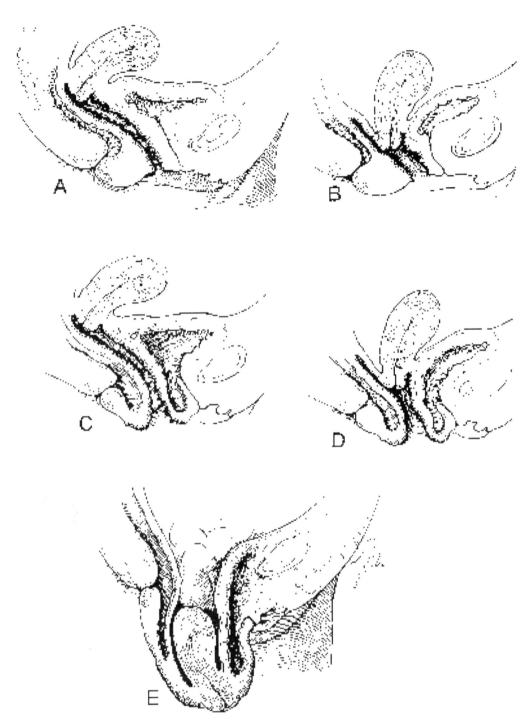

Figure 14.2 Various types of prolapse: *A* normal support, *B* pure uterine prolapse, *C* cystocele and rectocele with normal uterine support, *D* cystocele and rectocele with uterine prolapse, *E* complete uterine procidentia with cystocele, rectocele, and enterocele. (From Nichols and Randall, Vaginal Surgery, 3rd ed. Baltimore: Williams and Wilkins, 1989, with permission.)

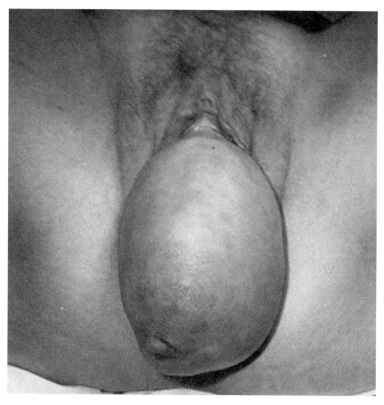

Figure 14.3   Procidentia. The entire vagina is everted and the entire uterus lies below the pelvic floor.

TABLE 14.1.   Grading of Urogenital Prolapse and its Implications

Position of the Bulge During Maximum Straining (Measured in centimeters)	Clinical Significance
Above hymenal ring	Occult: Probably not significant
At the hymenal ring	Borderline
Below the hymenal ring	Clinically significant

simply by noting the position of the cervix (or "bulge" in question) in relation to the plane of the hymenal ring. The position that the bulge reaches during maximal straining can then be estimated in centimeters above or below this point of reference. For example, a uterine prolapse could be described by saying that the cervix descended 2 cm below the hymenal ring during straining. A similar assessment of a cystourethrocele could be made by noting the location of the urethrovesical junction and the relative positions of the bladder and urethra (e.g., "A cystocele was present extending 1 cm below the hymen and the urethra was supported normally."). In the case of a prolapse that breaks the plane of the hymen, estimating the diameter of the bulge helps establish the size of the prolapse further (e.g., "The cystourethrocele dilates the hymenal ring to a diameter of 5 cm.").

Examining Patients to Detect Prolapse

The evaluation of patients with lower urinary tract problems should include a thorough examination intended to detect occult as well as overt prolapse. This

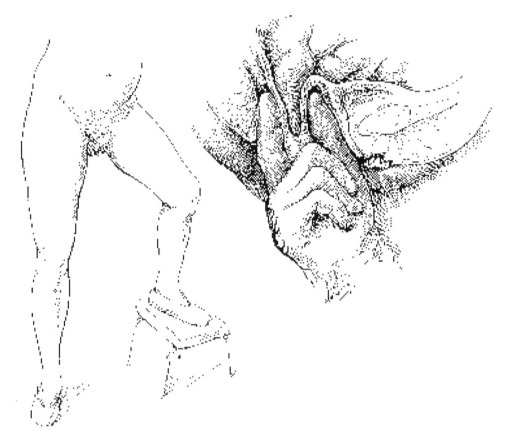

Figure 14.4 Standing examination of the patient to detect prolapse and enterocele formation. (From Nichols and Randall, Vaginal Surgery, 3rd ed. Baltimore: Williams and Wilkins, 1989, with permission.)

should be an area in which gynecologists excel. Women with stress incontinence may also have poor uterine support or thin rectovaginal septa that have gone unnoticed. These findings may not be obvious if an examination is performed only in the lithotomy position using an ordinary bivalve speculum.

How to Examine Patients with Prolapse.   The diagnosis of genital prolapse is made on physical examination. The basic aspects of this evaluation have been covered in Chapter 3; however, there are two fundamental points which must be made regarding the examination of patients with prolapse: (*a*) The examination must be made with the patient straining forcefully enough to demonstrate the prolapse at its largest extent, and (*b*) the clinician must examine each element of support independently. These are critical points. The various components of a prolapse can only be assessed when the prolapse is seen at its fullest extent. If the entire extent of the prolapse is not observed, important elements may be overlooked. For example, a large cystocele may be seen initially when the patient strains but her concurrent prolapse of the vaginal apex and the associated enterocele may only be seen with prolonged straining. To make sure all aspects of the prolapse are evaluated, ask the patient how large her prolapse is when it is largest, and persist in the examination until that size is observed. Once the full prolapse is visible, its component parts can be evaluated. Clinical examination should then focus on the specific support defects that are present, the severity of the prolapse, and an evaluation of the cause of the prolapse. Because prolapse is worse when the patient is erect, this means that these patients should generally have a *standing* pelvic examination as well as the more traditional examination in the dorsal lithotomy position (Fig. 14.4).

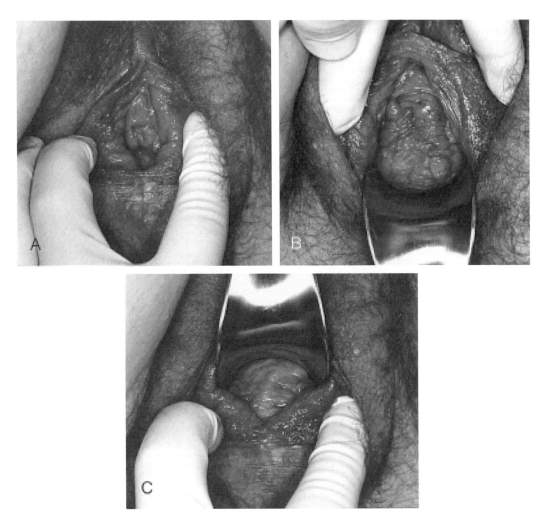

Figure 14.5 Examination of individual portions of the vagina. *A* Cursory inspection of the vagina when the patient strains demonstrates minimal prolapse. *B* Examination of the anterior vagina while retracting the posterior vaginal wall reveals a moderate cystocele. *C* Examination of the posterior vagina while retracting the anterior vaginal wall reveals a moderate rectocele.

Evaluate the Support of Each Aspect of the Vagina Individually. Once the prolapse is developed maximally, identify how much of the anterior vaginal wall, the cervix, and the posterior wall have prolapsed downward. The anterior and posterior walls of the vagina should each be examined separately by retracting the opposite wall with the posterior half of a vaginal speculum (Fig. 14.5 *A–C*). This is important because, for example, a large cystocele may hold a potential rectocele in place and hide it from a cursory view. If this is not recognized before surgery, the rectocele may not be repaired and may become symptomatic postoperatively.

The urethra and vaginal wall are fused together. The state of urethral support can be determined by examining the lower third of the anterior vaginal wall below the urethrovaginal crease (Fig. 14.6). The vaginal wall in this area should be above the hymenal ring during straining. This area is mobile in all women, and may move significantly in continent multiparous patients. Descent below the hymenal ring is definitely abnormal.

Above the urethrovesical crease, the anterior vaginal wall usually lies in a

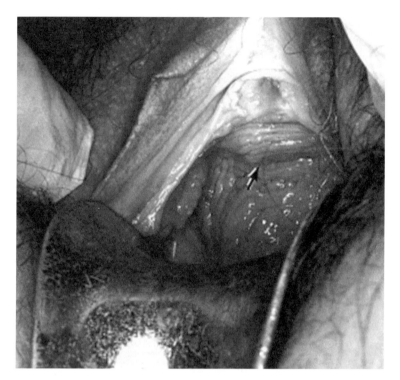

Figure 14.6 Examination of the normal anterior vaginal wall showing the crease which indicates the normal angle between the urethra and the vagina (*arrow*).

flat plane at about 45° from the horizontal. Any descent of the anterior vaginal wall below the level of the hymenal ring in this area is significant. This descent can be caused by three things: (*a*) separation of the paravaginal attachment of the pubocervical fascia from the white line, (*b*) detachment of the vagina from the cervix, and (*c*) tearing of the pubocervical fascia resulting in herniation of the bladder through this layer of tissue.

The pubocervical fascia is normally attached laterally to the pelvic wall at the white line. This can be recognized during pelvic examination as the area where the superior lateral sulcus of the vagina meets the vaginal sidewall (Fig. 14.7). If this attachment breaks, the lateral crease falls below its normal line of attachment to the pelvic sidewall. This line of attachment normally runs between the inferior edge of the pubic symphysis and the ischial spine. In patients with normal support the anterior vaginal wall retains its rugal folds and is not stretched as it is in other patients. This condition is referred to as a displacement cystourethrocele (Fig. 14.8). Many individuals with a displacement cystourethrocele will also have an avulsion of the pubocervical fascia from the cervix. This condition can be recognized by loss of the anterior fornix between the cervix and vagina.

These defects have clinical importance. For example, traditional anterior colporrhaphy works better for correcting a central defect in the fascia (distension cystourethrocele) than for correcting a defect arising from a detachment of the fascia from the pelvic side wall (displacement cystocele, Figure 14.9). If there is a paravaginal detachment of the pubocervical fascia which results in a displacement cystourethrocele, an anterior colporrhaphy will only gather the pubocervical fascia in the midline. It will do nothing to elevate the lateral borders of this fascia where the defect lies. Similarly, if the pubocervical fascia has been detached from the cervix, this fascia should be retrieved at the time of vaginal hysterectomy and included in the vaginal closure. This will elevate the anterior

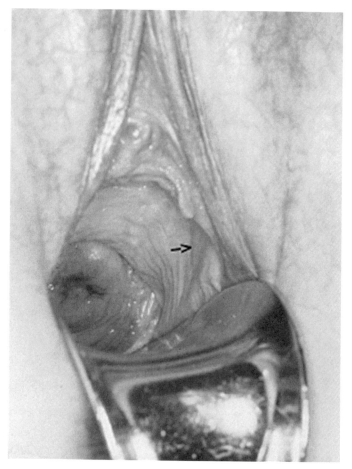

Figure 14.7 Attachment of the anterior vaginal wall to the pelvic sidewall at the lateral vaginal sulcus.

vaginal wall by connecting the upper edge of the pubocervical fascia to the cardinal and uterosacral ligaments.

The severity of uterine prolapse is determined by the location of the cervix. The position of the cervix relative to the hymenal ring should be noted while the prolapse is at its largest. If the cervix is not visible due to a cystocele or rectocele, then its location may be determined by palpation when the patient is straining. If the cervix descends to within a centimeter of the hymenal ring there is significant loss of support. If plans have not been made to remove the uterus at the time of incontinence surgery, uterine support should be tested further before assuming that it is normal. This can be done by applying traction to the cervix with a tenaculum. This may reveal an occult prolapse extending below the hymenal ring. As has been mentioned, unless the cervix extends below the hymen with traction, descent is still within physiologic limits.

In addition to seeing how far the cervix descends, its length should be determined. Cervical elongation frequently occurs in patients with prolapse even though the uterine corpus is in a normal location and may result in a cervix which is 10–12 cm long. Knowing this fact preoperatively will allow the surgeon to proceed quickly with a vaginal hysterectomy, rather than hoping with every pedicle that the uterine arteries will soon appear. It is also important to recognize that the upper portions of the cardinal ligaments are in a normal location in patients with cervical elongation. These structures can be attached to the vaginal

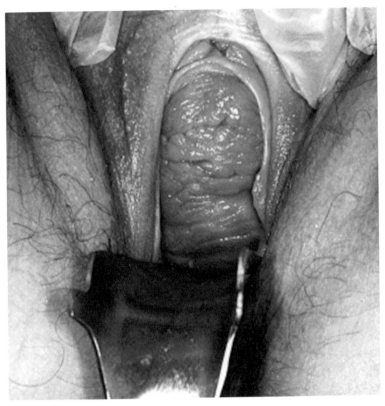

Figure 14.8 Displacement cystocele with obliteration of the urethrovesical crease in the vagina.

apex at the end of the hysterectomy to help resuspend the vagina. If the cervix is not elongated, then the strength of the entire cardinal/uterosacral ligament complex may be suspect. Special efforts should be made in these patients to perform a thorough McCall-type culdeplasty to elevate the vaginal apex.

Defects of support in the posterior vagina are understood less well than any other form of prolapse. The evaluation and correction of these defects challenge even the most experienced gynecologic surgeons. Distinguishing a high rectocele from an enterocele is often quite difficult. Since dyspareunia can follow a repair operation, correction of asymptomatic posterior wall defects is not without risk. On the other hand, the development of a rectocele or enterocele after vaginal hysterectomy and anterior colporrhaphy, or surgery for incontinence, is also undesirable. The support of the posterior vaginal wall must therefore be considered carefully.

Three questions should be asked when examining the posterior vagina: (*a*) Is it normally supported? If not, (*b*) is a true rectocele present or is it a pseudorectocele?, and (*c*) Is an enterocele present? When the posterior vaginal wall descends below the hymenal ring, there is significant prolapse. This can be caused by either a rectocele, an enterocele, or both. There are also occasions in which the posterior wall seems to bulge into the vagina when in fact it is well supported. This often occurs not because the rectal wall is poorly supported, but because the perineal body is deficient. Nichols has referred to this as a *pseudorectocele.* It can easily be differentiated from a true rectocele because the contour of the anterior rectal wall is normal on rectal examination (Fig. 14.10 *A* and *B*).

The hallmark of a typical rectocele is the formation of a vaginal pocket which bulges outward beyond the axis of the anal canal. This finding not only makes

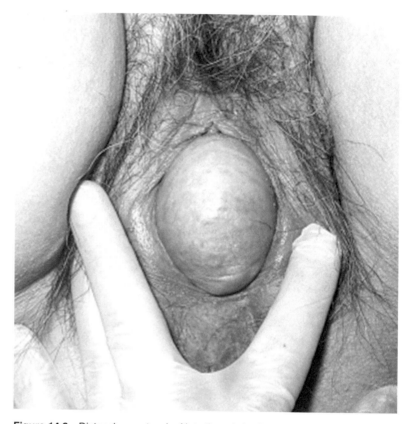

Figure 14.9 Distension cystocele. Note the relative lack of rugal folds.

the diagnosis, but also illustrates the mechanism by which rectoceles produce symptoms. Even though the anterior rectal wall may be more mobile than normal, as long as it has a smooth contour stool will pass out through the anus. However, when the patient strains, and a pocket develops in the lumen, stool becomes trapped, and difficulty evacuating can occur. This often requires the patient to push on the perineal body or to "splint" the rectum by putting two fingers in the vagina to help push stool out. Generally, patients must be asked specifically if they do this, as they are often too embarrassed to mention the subject on their own.

A protrusion of the upper part of the posterior vaginal wall can either be caused by an enterocele or a high rectocele (Fig. 14.11). These conditions are distinguished most easily by performing a rectovaginal examination while the patient is standing (Fig. 14.4). The index finger is placed in the rectum and the thumb is placed in the vagina. The examiner then attempts to palpate small bowel between them. Finding this confirms that an enterocele is present. If this is not found, the bulge is probably due to a sacculation of the rectal wall, indicating the presence of a high rectocele. This distinction is critical because an undetected enterocele may persist after surgery and lead ultimately to failure of the surgical repair. The differentiation between an enterocele and rectocele should be made with the patient awake, before surgery, because bowel is present in the enterocele sac only when the patient strains. Seeing the enterocele develop and palpating the bowel in its sac is rarely possible in the operating room with the patient supine, asleep, and paralyzed by muscle relaxants.

Prolapse after Hysterectomy

In patients who have had a previous hysterectomy and subsequently present with prolapse, special attention must be devoted to examining the vaginal apex

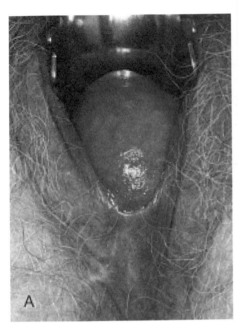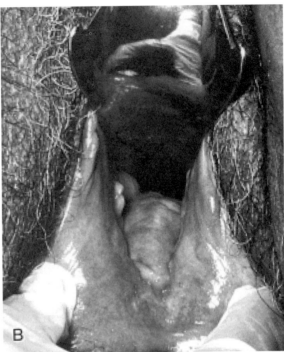

Figure 14.10 Rectocele and pseudorectocele. *A* True rectocele with extension of the prolapse below the hymenal ring. *B* Pseudorectocele caused by exposure of the lower rectum due to separation of the perineal body. Note that the bulge does not extend below the hymenal ring. On palpation, the anterior rectal wall is normal.

to see if it is prolapsing. When the uterus is in place, the position of the cervix serves as a marker for poor support of the upper vagina. However, descent of the vaginal apex is often missed in cases of posthysterectomy vaginal prolapse. If the vaginal vault is not suspended in these patients, and if only an anterior/posterior colporrhaphy is performed, the operation will fail to cure the problem and the prolapse will invariably recur, often quite rapidly.

Examination of the patient who has had a prior hysterectomy should include a specific effort to determine the location of the vaginal apex when the prolapse is at its largest. The apex may be identified by the scar that exists where the cervix was removed (Fig. 14.12). If the apex descends to the lower third of the vagina on straining, this is significant and the vagina should be resuspended at the time of surgical repair. Another technique which allows evaluation of the degree of apical descent is to place the full length of posterior half of a speculum into the vagina to elevate the vaginal apex into a normal position (Fig. 14.13 *A–C*). If the bulge is eliminated when the half speculum is placed both anteriorly and then posteriorly, then elevation of the apex has corrected the problem, not support of the anterior or posterior vaginal wall. These patients need an operation to support the vaginal apex.

Relationship Between Prolapse and Symptoms

All types of prolapse have several symptoms in common. Once the vagina has prolapsed below the introitus, it is the only structural layer separating the high pressure inside the abdomen from the much lower atmospheric pressure. The downward force created by this pressure differential puts enormous tension on the supporting ligaments and fascia. This results in a dragging feeling noticed where the tissues connect to the pelvic sidewall (usually described as pressure in the groin) and a sacral backache caused by traction on the uterosacral ligaments. This discomfort typically resolves when the patient lies down and the

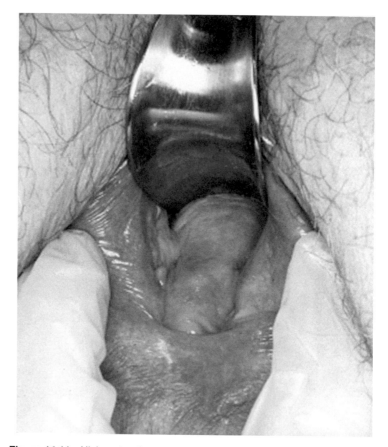

Figure 14.11   High rectocele versus enterocele. Notice the "double bump" with the upper portion of the bulge representing either a high rectocele or an overriding enterocele. This can only be resolved by palpating the rectovaginal septum to see if bowel or omentum can be detected in the bulge.

downward pressure is reduced. Exposure of the moist vaginal walls may lead to a sensation of perineal wetness that the patient may confuse with urinary incontinence. It may also lead to cornification and ulceration of the vaginal wall. Most patients describe an underlying sense of pelvic insecurity that is difficult for them to articulate precisely. Although patients may have difficulty expressing this in any way other than saying "something is just not right," this is a consistent finding and should not be ignored, particularly in patients who have had a prior hysterectomy.

Symptoms of Anterior Wall Prolapse

The two primary symptoms of anterior vaginal wall prolapse are paradoxical. Loss of support can lead both to stress incontinence and to voiding difficulty. Symptoms of incomplete bladder emptying are probably most common in women who void by straining. If she is able to generate a sustained detrusor contraction, then there really is no reason why a woman with a cystocele should not empty her bladder completely. It should not be surprising, therefore, that many women with significant cystoceles have no significant postvoid residual urine. A woman who strains to void, however, increases her abdominal pressure in order to force urine out of the bladder. This increasing abdominal pressure distends the cystocele, which gets bigger and bigger, and results in functional outlet obstruction as the urethra is compressed by a "flap valve" effect. Patients who experience this phenomenon may complain of prolonged voiding and an intermittent urinary stream that stops and starts during urination (Fig. 14.1).

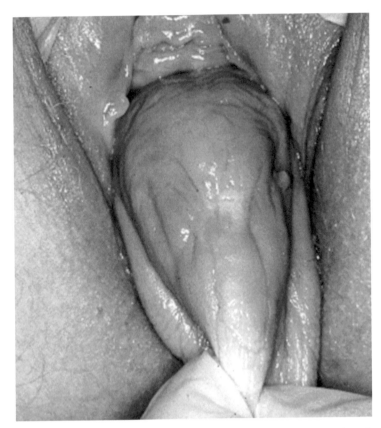

Figure 14.12 Posthysterectomy vaginal vault prolapse. Note the scar where the cervix was removed at the time of prior hysterectomy.

In addition to these functional symptoms, many patients with a cystourethrocele complain of urinary urgency and frequency. This probably arises from stretching of the bladder base as it prolapses through the vaginal introitus. These symptoms are often less pronounced at night when the patient is supine.

Patients have varying degrees of loss of support beneath the bladder and urethra, and their symptoms will vary along a continuum, ranging from urinary incontinence to complete urinary retention. It is important to correlate the patient's symptoms with her physical findings in order to address these problems intelligently.

Symptoms Associated with Prolapse of the Uterus or Vaginal Apex

There are few symptoms related specifically to prolapse of the uterus, the vaginal apex, or to the formation of an enterocele. These patients usually complain of the generalized symptoms of prolapse mentioned above, particularly the protrusion of an uncomfortable bulge. Some have urgency and frequency, probably related to the pressure of the prolapse on the bladder base, but this is variable. It should not be forgotten that patients may also have urinary stones, detrusor instability, or other problems in addition to their prolapse! Although uncommon, an occasional patient with a large thin enterocele will have a sense of impending rupture. This should not be ignored. Vaginal evisceration from a ruptured enterocele is a surgical emergency.

Symptoms of Rectocele

The cardinal symptom of a rectocele is difficulty in emptying the rectum. As a woman bears down to evacuate the rectum, stool is pushed into the rectocele, and the harder she strains, the bigger the rectocele becomes. "Constipation" is common in older women and may be due to a variety of causes, most of which have nothing to do with prolapse. It is important to understand what the patient means by "constipation." Infrequent bowel movements due to poor colonic

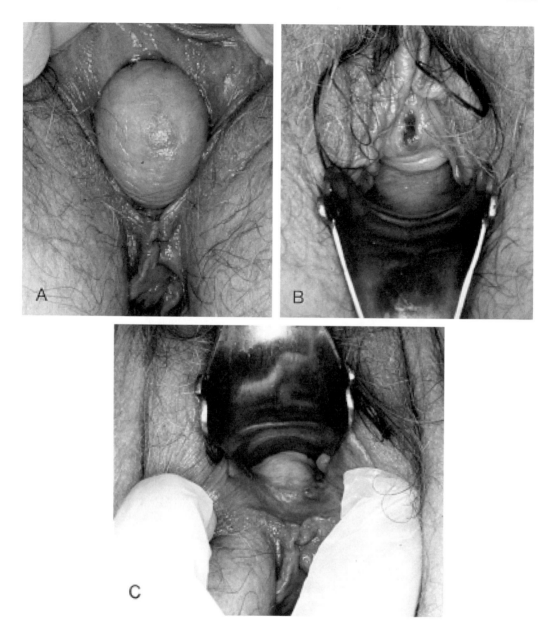

Figure 14.13 Examination of a prolapse whose nature is unclear. *A*. Without more careful examination, the components of this prolapse are uncertain. When a speculum is placed posteriorly (*B*) and anteriorly (*C*) to inspect each vaginal wall separately, the prolapse goes away. This indicates that the patient has a prolapse of the vaginal apex which has been elevated by the speculum in each instance.

motility are different from those due to hard dry feces from inadequate dietary fiber. Difficulty in passing a stool of otherwise normal consistency and texture is different still. Many women have found that if they press between the vagina and rectum to elevate the rectocele, this maneuver helps with defecation. If this history is elicited from a patient, it tends to support the idea that her rectocele is part of her problem with defecation. Small pencil size stools may be associated with rectal stricture due to carcinoma or some other process. This should not be forgotten when evaluating women with rectal complaints.

Effects of Prolapse on the Lower Urinary Tract
Equivocal Prolapse and Lower Urinary Tract Symptoms: Will an Operation Help?

Having determined the patient's symptoms and the presence and severity of any prolapse, the relationship between support and symptoms must be considered. A woman who presents with a small cystourethrocele or minor uterine prolapse in association with lower urinary tract complaints should know prior to surgery whether or not an operation for the prolapse will alleviate her urinary symptoms. When the prolapse is so large that it requires surgery irrespective of the presence of lower urinary tract symptoms, the impact of surgery on the urinary tract must still be evaluated. In women with mild prolapse, the decisive factor in planning surgery is often whether her symptoms are caused by the prolapse or are simply the result of a coexisting condition. Symptoms of urgency, frequency, and voiding difficulty are all symptoms that may be caused by prolapse, but they may also be caused by other factors such as cystitis, estrogen deficiency, or neurologic disease. In women whose prolapse lies above the level of the hymenal ring, the relationship between her symptoms and prolapse should be assessed carefully.

The first way to assess whether symptoms are due to the patient's prolapse is to ask her what happens to her symptoms when she lies down. Since the pressure on the prolapse is greatest in the erect position, symptoms that are related to prolapse should resolve when the patient lies down. Symptoms of prolapse will usually subside after a few minutes or an hour. If the patient has not noticed a relationship of this kind, it may be worthwhile to see her again in a few weeks after instructing her to watch for this. Patients who have persistent symptoms at night should be presumed to have another cause for their symptoms and should be evaluated carefully to find another etiology before surgery is performed for symptom relief.

Urinary tract symptoms are much less dependent upon position, even though frequency and urgency are usually less when patients are supine. Some women with significant prolapse and stress incontinence leak more when they cough while supine, since their prolapse may plug up the urogenital hiatus when they are standing and prevent the escape of urine. Some women with massive prolapse may have to lie down in the bathtub and reduce their prolapse in order to void. Estrogen deficiency may cause irritative bladder symptoms and this can be treated with vaginal estrogen cream. Urinalysis and culture (where appropriate) should be obtained to rule out the possibility of a urinary tract infection. The patient with uninfected urine who does not respond to estrogen cream may benefit from a trial using a pessary to confirm that prolapse is the cause of her symptoms. Although a pessary may press on the bladder and cause symptoms on its own, relief of symptoms by a pessary suggests that surgery may be helpful.

Voiding Difficulty

One of the most common reasons given for repair of a cystourethrocele is the presence of an elevated postvoid residual urine volume and recurrent urinary tract infections. In normal voiding, the bladder empties by a combination of urethral relaxation and detrusor contraction. Since normal bladder emptying occurs through a sustained contraction of the bladder musculature which forces the urine out through the urethra, the bladder should be able to empty itself completely even if urine must be forced "uphill." The patient with a cystocele should still empty her bladder completely in spite of her prolapse. The patient who has recurrent urinary tract infections and a normal postvoid residual should receive the same evaluation as anyone else in spite of her cystocele.

In patients with a large prolapse, the bladder lies further from the sacrum than it does in normal women. It is plausible that the nerves which run from the sacral foramina to the bladder base may suffer stretch injury under these circumstances, much as patients with severe perineal descent have been shown to develop anal sphincter denervation from chronic straining at stool. Under these circumstances, elevated residual urine may be due to neurologic damage. Many women void by combining straining with urethral relaxation. The presence of a large cystocele in these individuals may make voiding difficult because increases in abdominal pressure simply increase the distension of the cystocele and compress the urethra closed. In these individuals cystocele repair has the potential to improve their voiding by eliminating the obstructing bulge and making bladder emptying more efficient. Similar symptoms may also be seen in patients with complete vaginal vault eversion after hysterectomy or massive rectoceles, but even the most expert surgical repair cannot restore damaged nerves. In fact, anterior colporrhaphy probably increases denervation injury since the parasympathetic ganglia which innervate the bladder lie in the vesicovaginal space. Damage to these ganglia may be responsible for some of the delayed return of voiding that occurs after anterior colporrhaphy.

The Large Prolapse

When a large prolapse is present it will require treatment whether or not lower urinary tract symptoms are present. Significant urinary tract symptoms must still be evaluated when they are present. If they are not present, the clinician must still make sure that the urinary tract is not affected by the patient's prolapse. Preoperative evaluation of these patients should include:

—Screening for urinary tract infection and checking the urinary sediment to make sure it is normal. This can be done by microscopic urinalysis and appropriate culture.
—Careful examination to make sure that the patient's prolapse is not protecting her from having stress incontinence by providing additional urethral closure.
—Evaluating the possibility that the prolapse is causing ureteral obstruction and renal damage.

Prolapse and Occult Stress Incontinence

It has been observed for many years that stress incontinence may suddenly appear in women following prolapse surgery. If the prolapse is reduced by surgical repair, the underlying defect in the continence mechanism may suddenly be revealed. A cystocele may improve urethral closure by two potential mechanisms: (*a*) The protruding bladder may push against the urethra improving its closure during a cough, or (*b*) it may act as a "shock absorber" by damping sudden increases in bladder pressure. In this case urine could be pushed into the cystocele by a cough or sneeze rather than spurting out of the urethra. No matter what the mechanism may be, the possibility that stress incontinence may develop after prolapse repair must be anticipated.

There is no way short of doing the operation to create the exact anatomic situation that will exist after surgery, but it is possible to approximate the postoperative state to see if stress incontinence will develop. This may be done by elevating the anterior vagina into its expected postoperative position with the posterior blade of a Grave's speculum, a rolled gauze sponge held on a ring forceps, or a similar instrument. If the uterus is still present, the blade should be placed in the anterior vaginal fornix and used to elevate the uterus until the anterior vaginal wall is in the position that is expected after surgery. If stress incontinence occurs when the patient coughs with a moderately full bladder, then corrective steps must be taken at surgery to prevent postoperative incontinence. On the other hand, if reduction of the prolapse does not lead to incontinence, then development of this problem after surgery is much less likely.

Some authors use a vaginal pessary instead of a speculum to reduce the prolapse while testing for stress incontinence. This allows the patient to walk around and perform other activities under observation to see if incontinence occurs; however, a pessary can also obstruct the urethra, producing a false sense of security. Direct elevation of the anterior vaginal wall during the examination allows the clinician to have much greater control over the anatomy that is being evaluated. This would, therefore, appear to be a better test. Care must be taken not to press on the bladder base when this test is done. Even normal women may leak if their bladders are pushed forcefully from below. The goal of this examination should be to recreate the expected postoperative anatomical relationships as nearly as possible and nothing more.

The type of surgery that is done to prevent the development of stress incontinence in these cases will depend upon the surgeon's skill and preference. If the prolapse operation is to be done vaginally, then a needle suspension (e.g., Pereyra, Stamey) will often provide adequate urethral support. Good results in such cases have been reported by some authors using a strictly vaginal approach in which the tissues near the pubic symphysis are plicated under the urethra. It should be emphasized that this is *not* a simple anterior colporrhaphy. It requires specific placement of deep sutures at the vesical neck, which are sometimes driven into the periosteum of the pubic symphysis. Of all the techniques utilized for the cure of stress incontinence, this one is the most dependent upon the quality of the tissues present and the skill of the surgeon. Failures result both from poor local tissue and from deviations, however minor they may seem, from the techniques utilized and described by master vaginal surgeons. Paravaginal repair will alleviate both the cystourethrocele and the stress incontinence by reattaching the ruptured endopelvic fascia to its normal location along the arcus tendineus fasciae pelvis. Although it is possible to perform this operation vaginally, the only good published results to date have been achieved using a transabdominal approach. Other retropubic bladder neck suspension operations such as the ''MMK'' and Burch colposuspension should also be effective in preventing stress incontinence. Of these two operations, the Burch procedure is the better choice if a cystocele is present.

The authors make the following recommendations: In patients with minimal occult stress incontinence and good local tissues, the surgeon who is confident in his ability to achieve adequate support may use an anterior colporrhaphy, with appropriate attention to plication of the suburethral tissues. Surgeons experienced in the use of needle suspension operations may perform their operation of choice in connection with the repair. However, if the incontinence seems severe when the prolapse is reduced or if the local tissues are weak, then some form of retropubic bladder neck suspension would seem to be the best choice. A small number of patients with intrinsic sphincteric weakness will require a sling procedure.

Prolapse and Ureteral Obstruction

A large prolapse can cause ureteral obstruction. This most often occurs in patients who have total uterine procidentia or complete posthysterectomy vaginal vault eversion. If ureteral obstruction is present renal function may deteriorate and this is a clear indication for surgical intervention. For this reason the blood urea nitrogen (BUN), creatinine, and serum electrolytes should be checked on patients before undergoing surgery for massive prolapse of this kind. If the BUN and creatinine are elevated, an intravenous urogram should be performed *with the patient standing and the prolapse protruding* to see if ureteral obstruction is responsible for the deterioration in her renal function (Fig. 14.14). Obviously, other factors such as hypertension or diabetes may be the cause of the patient's kidney damage, but if obstructive uropathy is resulting from the prolapse, surgical intervention should prevent further deterioration in renal function by relieving the high back-pressure which is responsible. If the IVP does not reveal an obstruction, then a further search for other causes of renal damage should be pursued.

Urinalysis in the Patient with Prolapse

Since prolapse may result in incomplete voiding, it is necessary to rule out urinary tract infection prior to surgery. Although a clean-catch midstream urine is usually satisfactory for urinalysis and urinary sediment examination in most women, patients with a large prolapse often collect contaminated specimens because the urine washes over the prolapse before it reaches the collection cup. If it is negative, a specimen of this kind is adequate; but if the results are questionable, then a catheterized urine sample should be obtained. Although the presence of a few epithelial cells in the specimen may explain the bacteria seen on microscopic examination, assuming this to be the case may result in a significant urinary tract infection being missed before surgery. This could lead to serious postoperative pyelonephritis. Red blood cells in the urinary sediment should be investigated further. The urinary urgency and frequency that often accompany prolapse can mask the urgency and frequency that develop due to a bladder neoplasm. If any doubt exists about the quality of the urine specimen from a patient with prolapse, a catheterized specimen should be obtained for analysis.

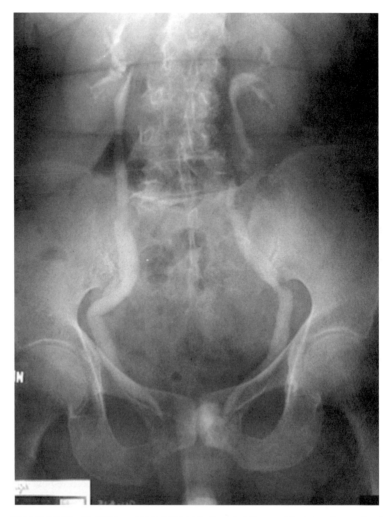

Figure 14.14   Excretory urogram taken in the standing position showing ureteral obstruction secondary to massive prolapse. Note the prolapsed bladder well below the pubic symphysis.

Effects of Surgery for Stress Incontinence on Prolapse

Many women with stress incontinence have genital prolapse and many patients with genital prolapse have stress incontinence. The fact that *not all* women who have one of these two conditions has the other suggests that each situation should be considered individually. Previous sections have emphasized the need to detect occult stress incontinence that may appear after prolapse repair. This section will discuss the problem of genital prolapse which appears after surgery for stress incontinence.

Patients who present with overt prolapse and stress incontinence do not pose any particular diagnostic problem, but those who seek help for stress incontinence may be unaware that they have defective pelvic support. All patients should be examined carefully for the presence (or absence) of prolapse. This is important for two reasons. First, women who have poor urethral support will often have poor support in other areas. Because routine pelvic examinations are generally performed in the dorsal lithotomy position, a prolapse may not be evident unless it is looked for specifically. Second, many urethral suspension procedures alter the vaginal axis. This may lead to the development of an enterocele, rectocele, or uterine or vaginal prolapse due to the altered vectors of force affecting these structures. Attention to the principles of examination outlined earlier in this chapter is critical for making the proper diagnosis. This includes performing a pelvic examination in the standing position. Although this is initially awkward, it is extremely worthwhile.

In addition to the search for overt prolapse, it is important to identify women who have suboptimal pelvic support even though they do not currently have a prolapse. These patients are at risk for developing prolapse after stress incontinence surgery. Because stress urinary incontinence is often associated with a cystourethrocele, other forms prolapse may develop once this has been reduced. Patients with cystoceles often have a gaping introitus that is filled by the prolapsed anterior vagina. When the protruding cystourethrocele has been eliminated, the opening in the lower vagina is still there. A rectocele, which may formerly have been held in place by the other prolapse, may now fill the unoccupied space in the vagina to become a clinical problem.

Hysterectomy and Surgery for Stress Incontinence

The relationship between hysterectomy and stress incontinence has long been controversial. The controversy centers around two questions: (*a*) Does simultaneous hysterectomy improve the outcome of surgery in women with stress incontinence? and (*b*) Is hysterectomy justified at the time of surgery for stress incontinence in a woman with no significant prolapse and no other gynecologic complaints?

Does Hysterectomy Improve the Outcome of Surgery For Stress incontinence?

Many clinicians have the impression that hysterectomy improves the outcome of surgery for stress incontinence. This idea has not been borne out by clinical studies. In the absence of uterine prolapse there is no reason why hysterectomy should influence the success of operations designed to cure stress incontinence. Many women with stress incontinence *do* have some degree of uterine prolapse, and if present this should usually be treated if childbearing has been completed. Removal of the uterus allows the surgeon to use the cardinal and uterosacral ligaments to reinforce the support of the vaginal apex and also to perform a culdeplasty to prevent subsequent enterocele formation. In addition, hysterectomy permits resuspension of the upper edge of the pubocervical fascia to the suspensory ligaments. This normal attachment has been lost in many women with a cystocele so that the anterior fornix is obliterated and it is no longer elevated. After the uterus has been removed, the margin of this fascia can be retrieved and attached to the cardinal and uterosacral ligaments, reestablishing the normal elevation of this fascia and reducing the cystourethrocele.

Preservation of Childbearing

Some young women may have such severe incontinence that they wish to have it treated surgically before they have completed childbearing. Ideally, surgery of this kind should be postponed until after the patient is finished with reproduction so that possible damage to the repair by subsequent pregnancy or delivery is avoided. However, situations occasionally arise in which the incontinence is so severe that immediate repair with retention of the uterus is warranted. A frank and open discussion should be held with the patient about the possibility of *pregnancy itself* causing incontinence, apart from any trauma sustained at delivery. If she proceeds to have a surgical repair, the possibility of cesarean delivery for future pregnancies should also be discussed, to avoid additional trauma to the pelvic floor. If the patient decides *not* to have surgery before her childbearing has been completed, she needs to understand that cesarean delivery will not cure her problem. She will probably need surgery irrespective of the route of future deliveries, but she should be re-evaluated after childbearing has been completed. Furthermore, if stress incontinence persists following a subsequent delivery, no surgery should be performed for at least 3 (and probably at least 6) months postpartum to allow her pelvic floor to stabilize following childbirth. There is no role whatsoever for a retropubic bladder neck suspension performed at the time of cesarean section in patients who have stress incontinence during pregnancy.

If a patient who wishes future childbearing decides to proceed with surgery for her stress incontinence, the question of uterine support must be addressed.

If the uterus has normal support then only a urethral suspension needs to be performed. Imperfect uterine support may be improved by shortening the utero-sacral ligaments and reattaching them to the back of the cervix. This is done by placing a permanent suture through each ligament approximately 3 cm from the cervix. Each suture is then brought back through the cervix midway between the two ligaments, shortening and tightening them. This should be done with the uterus elevated under tension after the ureters have been clearly identified on each side. This procedure not only narrows the cul-de-sac, but also elevates the cervix by bringing it closer to the sacrum. Although this mechanical change is not apparent when the patient is supine, it can be noticed when she stands up. Since the uterosacral ligaments originate above the cervix, these sutures also elevate the uterus.

An alternate way of achieving these goals is to perform a careful culdeplasty. The Halban culdeplasty is performed by placing a series of sutures in the sagittal plane, obliterating the cul-de-sac by closing it front-to-back, and sewing the rectum against the back of the vagina and cervix. The most lateral suture can be placed through the uterosacral ligament and driven into the back of the cervix to provide more elevation and further closure. The course of the ureter should be checked after the placement of the sutures to make sure that it has not been kinked. A Moschcowitz culdeplasty utilizes a series of concentric purse string sutures to obliterate the cul-de-sac. This not only prevents the formation of an enterocele, but can also add significant elevation if the uterosacral ligaments are incorporated in it.

Preservation of the Uterus after Childbearing

Some women may not wish to have a hysterectomy at the time of surgery for stress incontinence. This is an important issue and should be discussed thoroughly with the patient. Uterine support should be assessed to see if prolapse is definitely present or support is weak. If uterine support is good, then there is no reason to perform a hysterectomy at the time of surgery for stress incontinence. If definite prolapse is present and the cervix lies at or below the hymenal ring, the patient should know that this will probably worsen and she may develop a rapidly worsening prolapse after surgery if a hysterectomy is not performed. It is possible to plicate the uterosacral ligaments and improve the support of a uterus without removing it, but the patient needs to know that there is little information about the success of this type of surgery. If uterine support is somewhat lax, but no definite prolapse is present, then each case must be considered individually.

Elective Hysterectomy at the Time of Urethral Suspension

Some patients request hysterectomy at the time of surgery for stress urinary incontinence even though they have no specific gynecologic pathology. Removing the inconvenience of menstruation, reducing the possibility of ovarian cancer through oophorectomy, and eliminating the risk of endometrial and cervical malignancy are potential benefits for these patients. On the other hand, increased blood loss, ureteral injury, and postoperative pelvic infection are real complications of hysterectomy, and they must be considered seriously. It seems reasonable to perform a hysterectomy at the time of incontinence surgery if the patient desires this and accepts the increased risks of the procedure; however, insistence on *routine* performance of a hysterectomy in the absence of prolapse or gynecologic pathology cannot be justified.

Hysterectomy and Sensory Disorders

Some patients with sensory disorders of the bladder and urethra are advised to have a hysterectomy. The rationale for this advice is that the uterus is pushing on the bladder and producing urgency or bladder pain. This explanation is without scientific foundation. Anteversion and anteflexion are common normal uterine positions which have never been shown to produce sensory disorders of the bladder. Occasionally a very large fibroid uterus may cause some bladder discomfort, especially if a low-lying anterior fibroid is present. In such a case the uterine pathology itself provides sufficient indications for a hysterectomy. Similar symptoms in a patient with a uterus which would not otherwise be removed, such as an asymptomatic leiomyomatous uterus less than "12 weeks" in size, are unlikely to be due to uterine pathology. In general, hysterectomy is rarely justified for attempted relief of sensory disorders of the bladder.

Hysterectomy and the Development of Urinary Tract Symptoms

A brief final word is necessary regarding the potential role of hysterectomy in creating stress incontinence or other lower urinary tract symptoms. Allegations to this effect are found from time to time in the medical literature, but little data has been produced to support them. It is possible that hysterectomy can damage some elements important to pelvic support and that over time this may lead to the development of stress incontinence in some patients. What is more likely, however, is that some patients who have had a hysterectomy for symptomatic pelvic relaxation *without stress incontinence,* have gradually developed symptomatic urine loss as a manifestation of the underlying problem for which they had their original surgery. There are also some patients who are extremely troubled by gynecologic problems such as refractory dysmenorrhea, and who also have mild stress incontinence which does not trouble them. Once their menstrual difficulties have been eliminated by hysterectomy, they may start to notice the stress incontinence that they had before which was overshadowed by their other problem. Since hysterectomy is such an important life-event, many women may relate the onset of their troubles to their hysterectomy simply because they remember that they developed it in the "posthysterectomy period." Most studies have shown that the best indicator of urinary tract function after hysterectomy is the state of the urinary tract before the operation. Pre- and postoperative urodynamic studies have not detected significant changes in lower urinary tract function following simple hysterectomy. Radical hysterectomy, however, often causes major changes in bladder and urethral function due to injury to the autonomic nervous supply of the lower urinary tract during extensive dissection of the cardinal ligaments.

SUGGESTED READING

Baden WF, Walker T. Genesis of the vaginal profile. Clin Gynecol Obstet 1972; 15:1048–54.

Baskin LS, Tanagho EA. Pelvic pain without pelvic organs. J Urol 1992; 147:683–86.

Bartscht KD, DeLancey JOL. A technique to study the passive supports of the uterus. Obstet Gynecol 1988; 72:940–43.

Berglas B, Rubin IC. Study of the supportive structures of the uterus by levator myography. Surg Gynecol Obstet 1953; 97:677–92.

Bump RC, Fantl JA, Hurt WG. The mechanism of urinary incontinence in women with severe uterovaginal prolapse: Results of barrier studies. Obstet Gynecol 1988; 72:291–95.

DeLancey JOL. Anatomic aspects of vaginal eversion after hysterectomy. Am J Obstet Gynecol 1992; 166:1717–28.

Farquharson DIM, Varner RE, Orr JW, Shingleton HM, Hester S. Immediate and short-term effects of abdominal and vaginal hysterectomy on bladder function and symptomatology. J Obstet Gynaecol 1987; 7:279–84.

Fiani S, Kjaeldgaard A, Larsson B. Preoperative screening for latent stress incontinence in women with cystocele. Neurourol Urodynam 1985; 4:3–8.

Fothergill WE. On the pathology and the operative treatment of displacements of the pelvic viscera. J Obstet Gynaecol Br Emp 1908; 13:410–19.

Friedman EA, Littel WA. The conflict in nomenclature for descensus uteri. Am J Obstet Gynecol 1961; 81:817–20.

Grady M, Kozminski M, DeLancey JOL, Elkins T, McGuire EJ. Stress incontinence and cystoceles. J Urol 1991; 145:1211–13.

Hanley HG. The late urological complications of total hysterectomy. Br J Urol 1969; 41:682–84.

Hertogs K, Stanton SL. Mechanism of urinary continence after colposuspension: Barrier studies. Br J Obstet Gynecol 1985; 92:1184–88.

Jequier AM. Urinary symptoms and total hysterectomy. Br J Urol 1976; 48:437–41.

Kujansuu E, Teisala K, Punnonen R. Urethral closure function after total and subtotal hysterectomy measured by urethrocystometry. Gynecol Obstet Invest 1989; 27:105–06.

Langer R, Neuman M, Ron-El R, Golan A, Bukovsky I, Caspi E. The effect of total abdominal hysterectomy on bladder function in asymptomatic women. Obstet Gynecol 1989; 74:205–07.

McCall ML. Posterior culdeplasty: Surgical correction of enterocele during vaginal hysterectomy; a preliminary report. Obstet Gynecol 1957; 10:595–602.

McGuire EJ, Gardy M, Elkins T, DeLancey JOL. Treatment of incontinence with pelvic prolapse. Urol Clin NA 1991; 18:349–53.

Mengert WF. Mechanics of uterine support and position I: Factors influencing uterine support (an experimental study). Am J Obstet Gynecol 1936; 31:775–81.

Nichols DH, Randall CL. Significance of restoration of normal vaginal depth and axis. Obstet Gynecol 1970; 36:251–56.

Paramore RH. The supports in chief of the female pelvic viscera. J Obstet Gynaecol Br Emp 1908; 13:391–409.

Parys BT, Haylen BT, Hutton JL, Parsons KF. The effects of simple hysterectomy on vesicourethral function. Br J Urol 1989; 84:594–99.

Porges RF, Porges JC, Blinick G. Mechanisms of uterine support and the pathogenesis of uterine prolapse. Obstet Gynecol 1960; 15:711–26.

Richardson AC, Lyon JB, Williams NL. A new look at pelvic relaxation. Am J Obstet Gynecol 1976; 126:568–73.

Richardson DA, Bent AE, Ostergard DR. The effect of uterovaginal prolapse on urethrovesical pressure dynamics. Am J Obstet Gynecol 1983; 146:901–05.

Shull BL, Capen CV, Riggs MW, Kuehl TJ. Preoperative

and postoperative analysis of site-specific pelvic support defects in 81 women treated with sacrospinous ligament suspension and pelvic reconstruction. Am J Obstet Gynecol 1992; 166:1764–71.

Stanton SL, Norton C, Cardozo L. Clinical and urodynamic effects of anterior colporrhaphy and vaginal hysterectomy for prolapse with and without incontinence. Br J Obstet Gynaecol 1982; 89:459–63.

Symmonds RE, Jordan LT. Iatrogenic stress incontinence of urine. Am J Obstet Gynecol 1961; 82:1231–37.

Vervest HAM, van Venrooji GEPM, Barents JW, Haspels AA, Debruyne FMJ. Nonradical hysterectomy and the function of the lower urinary tract I: Urodynamic quantifi-

cation of changes in storage function. Acta Obstet Gynecol Scand 1989; 68:221–29.

Vervest HAM, van Venrooji GEPM, Barents JW, Haspels AA, Debruyne FMJ. Nonradical hysterectomy and the function of the lower urinary tract II: Urodynamic quantification of changes in evacuation function. Acta Obstet Gynecol Scand 1989; 68:231–35.

Wall LL, Hewitt JK. Urodynamic characteristics of women with complete posthysterectomy vaginal vault prolapse. Urology, In press.

Wiskind AK, Creighton SM, Stanton SL. The incidence of genital prolapse after the Burch colposuspension. Am J Obstet Gynecol 1992; 167:406–11.

15 Special Considerations in the Elderly

The American population is aging. The average 65-year old woman can expect to live another 24 years; a 75-year old woman can expect to live an additional 14 years; and, on average, an 85-year old woman will live another 8 years. Therefore, conditions which are more prevalent among the elderly will account for an increasing proportion of gynecologic practice.

Urinary incontinence is a common problem among the elderly. As many as one-third of women over 65 suffer from significant incontinence, a problem which may compromise their dreams of an active retirement. Among community dwelling older persons, an estimated 15%–30% suffer from significant incontinence. In perhaps one-quarter of these people the problem is severe. The prevalence of urinary incontinence in nursing homes is even higher; at least one-half of the 1.5 million Americans in nursing homes suffer from this problem. Significant morbidity is associated with this problem, including falls and fractures from slipping on slick bathroom floors, rashes and excoriation of the skin from chronic exposure to urine, and "idiopathic cellulitis." In nursing homes, many incontinent residents are managed by using indwelling catheters, a practice which is often unnecessary and carries with it an increased risk of significant infection and urosepsis. In addition to the medical problems associated with incontinence, the financial costs of this problem for both community-dwelling and institutionalized patients is staggering. In 1988, the National Institutes of Health estimated that the costs of managing urinary incontinence ran to at least $10.3 billion per year. As the percentage of Americans over 65 years of age increases, we can expect the expense of managing incontinence to rise even higher.

In spite of these problems, however, it is important to emphasize that two-thirds of elderly women do *not* have urinary incontinence. Although it is more common in the elderly than in the rest of the population, it is *not* a normal part of aging and should never be regarded as such. Many elderly people think that incontinence is an unavoidable and untreatable consequence of growing old, and bear this burden in resigned silence, avoiding physical and social activity. One accident on a neighbor's sofa can turn an otherwise vigorous woman into a virtual recluse. Fear of being placed in a nursing home or of having surgery may also lead to delay in seeking medical help. For the elderly woman who remembers that Aunt Tilly was forced to go into a nursing home after she became incontinent, the onset of her own incontinence may seem to herald the loss of her adulthood and sense of independence. Fear, embarrassment, and lack of knowledge cause many elderly women to fail to seek medical advice about their condition.

Unfortunately, many members of the medical profession share the common public misperceptions about urinary incontinence in the elderly. What changes actually *are* seen with aging in the lower urinary tract? How does the management of urinary incontinence differ in the elderly patient? Physicians sometimes believe that elderly patients do not benefit from many forms of treatment used for younger women. This is not true. Because urinary incontinence is rarely life-threatening, some physicians believe that it is merely a normal part of the aging process. Many health professionals therefore neglect the evaluation of incontinence in favor of "real diseases," which are more respectable and less aesthetically displeasing. Yet unlike many other medical conditions, urinary incontinence is usually treatable, with a tremendous resultant impact on the patient's quality of life and self-esteem. In many cases physicians are reluctant to consider surgery for this problem because the patient is "too old" and does not have a life expectancy long enough to justify elective surgery, or because the risks of operation are felt to be "more than they could stand," without a true appreciation of what might be involved. No one should be excluded from surgical cure of their problem on the basis of age alone. Many conservative treatment methods have also been viewed as inappropriate for elderly patients, for similarly unjustified reasons. Elderly women are often thought to be incapable of performing clean intermittent self-catheterization or to be poor candidates for doing pelvic muscle exercises. Many elderly women are thought to be "too many years postmenopausal" to justify hormone replacement therapy. None of these perceptions is true.

The following story is tragically illustrative of the problem. A woman in her 80's had had a pessary placed for treatment of genital prolapse, but as she gradually became senile she neglected to inform her family of its presence. After 10 years her family brought her in for a medical evaluation because she was "passing rocks from her vagina." The ring pessary had eroded into the bladder, creating a vesicovaginal fistula exactly the size of the pessary. This woman had been incontinent for 7 years before the calculi which had formed on the pessary began to break loose and come out of the vagina. Although her urinary incontinence was regarded as "normal," it took the passage of vaginal "rocks" to bring her to medical attention.

The Physiology of Aging

Normal physiologic changes in the lower urinary tract of elderly women make them more susceptible to the development of incontinence, not because incontinence is "normal," but because the balance between normal storage and emptying is more precarious. Because the elderly lack the normal physiologic reserve which is found in younger patients, minor factors such as a change in drug dosage can upset this balance and precipitate incontinence.

Intrinsic Factors

Many changes associated with normal aging have profound effects on the lower urinary tract. In women, adequate levels of estrogen are linked to the integrity of bone, a reduction in cardiovascular disease, a prolongation of their life span, and the maintenance of psychologic well-being. The intrinsic effects of aging on the lower urinary tract are related mainly to the loss of estrogen which occurs after menopause. Because the bladder and urethra are estrogen sensitive organs, decreased estrogen levels result in urogenital atrophy with thinning of the tissues in the vulva and vagina. In addition to these genital changes, the trigonal urothelium becomes thin and the normal coaptation of the urethral mucosa is lost. Connective tissue demonstrates decreased elasticity, increased cross-linking of collagen, and reduced total amounts of collagen. Urethral support may be lost as the amount of connective tissue decreases, striated muscle atrophies, and the volume of blood flow through the urethral vascular plexus falls off. Hypertrophy of the detrusor muscle may occur, resulting in trabeculation of the bladder and the development of diverticula. Loss of the normally protective glycosaminoglycan layer of the bladder may lead to an increased susceptibility to bacterial invasion and urinary tract infection. The neurologic effects of aging may lead to a reduction in the number of α-adrenergic receptors in the urethra and a gradual slowing of nerve conduction time. The combination of all these factors may result in decreased bladder capacity, increased sensitivity of the bladder and urethra, increased bladder neck mobility, and a decrease in the patient's ability to suppress or initiate a detrusor contraction.

Extrinsic Factors

Changes in other organ systems can also produce dramatic effects on the lower urinary tract. Among the extrinsic factors involved are inappropriate drug

TABLE 15.1.   Normal Urologic and Urodynamic Changes in Elderly Women

History
  Increased nighttime diuresis
  Nocturia 1–2 times per night
  Overall reduction in fluid intake
Physical examination
  Absent anal wink reflex in 25%
  Urogenital atrophy due to estrogen deprivation
Urodynamic findings
  Postvoid residual urine increased (50–100 ml)
  Decreased functional capacity due to increased residual urine
  Reduced cystometric capacity (below 400 ml)
  Earlier first desire to void (below 150 ml)
  Reduction in intrinsic urethral pressure
  Decreased urine flow rate during voiding

administration, changes in the patient's functional status, or disease processes in other organ systems. The elderly often produce proportionally more urine at night than do younger people. Kidney filtration decreases with age and this organ works to "catch up" on the night shift, producing a nighttime diuresis which may be exacerbated by problems such as venous stasis or congestive heart failure. When these effects are added to a decreased bladder capacity, nocturia increases. It is not abnormal for an otherwise healthy 80-year old woman to get up from sleep twice per night to void. Venous insufficiency may result in dependent edema. The fluids which are pooled in the legs during the day, re-enter the circulation at night when the patient is supine and increase her urine output. Chronic pulmonary conditions will exacerbate stress incontinence, particularly as the sphincteric mechanism ages. The neurologic compromise seen after stroke or in association with Parkinson's disease or various forms of dementia will contribute to a decreased awareness of bladder habits and an increase in detrusor overactivity. Diabetes is more prevalent in the elderly and represents a major reason for increased urinary output and increased peripheral neuropathy in this age group. Genital prolapse also tends to worsen with age and may affect bladder sensation and bladder emptying. Finally, decreased mobility may simply make it more difficult for patients to get to the toilet in time once the urge to urinate arises.

The combination of intrinsic and extrinsic factors produces a decrease in bladder capacity and urethral closure pressure, lower urinary flow rates, and decreased detrusor contractile power in the elderly (Table 15.1). Postvoid residual urine typically increases to 50–100 ml in the elderly. At the same time there appears to be a decrease in the ability of older people to suppress spontaneous detrusor contractions. Resnick has reported unstable detrusor contractions during cystometry in up to 20% of otherwise normal females between the ages of 60 and 70, not just those with urinary tract dysfunction. All of these changes make the lower urinary tract in the elderly patient more vulnerable to dysfunction from relatively minor insults. On the other hand, this also means that simple medical measures may correct this dysfunction by restoring the proper balance.

Etiology of Incontinence in the Elderly

Stress, Urge, and Mixed Incontinence

Although both young and elderly women may experience stress incontinence, urge incontinence, or mixed (stress and urge) incontinence, there are several important differences between these age groups. The prevalence of these conditions varies according to the patient population and the criteria used for making the diagnosis. Most studies have found that detrusor instability increases with age. This is probably a manifestation of gradually increasing neuropathology in the aging population. Stress incontinence is common in women over 65, being present in 30%–46% of patients depending on the techniques used to make the diagnosis. Chronic pulmonary diseases are more prevalent among the elderly and exacerbate problems with stress incontinence. Neurologic problems are also more common in an elderly population and may cause urinary incontinence due to detrusor overactivity. In an older population of nursing home patients with a mean age of 88.6 years, Resnick found detrusor instability/hyperreflexia to be the predominant cause of incontinence in 61%. Half of these patients had impaired detrusor contractility as well as detrusor overactivity. Patients with this problem experienced urge incontinence which only emptied their bladders partially. The same was true for voluntary voiding. The finding of increased residual urine volumes in incontinent patients with detrusor hyperactivity was surprising, since it had previously been assumed that an unsuppressed detrusor contraction resulted in complete bladder emptying. Genuine stress incontinence was found in 21% of Resnick's patients, but only 4% had mixed incontinence at the time of videourodynamic testing. Elderly patients with incontinence due to detrusor instability/hyperreflexia often have very little warning before urine loss occurs. Incontinence may present as sudden uncontrollable urine loss without prodromal urgency. At other times the patients are conscious of impending incontinence, but they simply cannot get to the toilet in time due to impaired mobility.

Incontinence Associated with Incomplete Emptying

Impaired detrusor contractility is a special problem in the elderly population. As previously mentioned, it had generally been assumed that an uncontrolled, uninhibited detrusor contraction resulted in complete or nearly complete bladder emptying. However, Resnick and Yalla found that in one-half of the 47 elderly women they investigated, both unsuppressed involuntary detrusor contractions as well as voluntary voiding resulted in incomplete emptying and a large residual urine. This syndrome has been termed "DHIC," or detrusor hyperactivity with impaired contractility. Although dementia, Parkinson's disease, and stroke all contribute to DHIC, the condition is often seen in elderly people who have no other evidence of neurologic compromise. Treatment of this condition is usually complicated because the pharmacologic treatment of detrusor instability/hyperreflexia is usually aimed at blocking detrusor contractility—a management plan that can make the situation worse in these patients if it increases the amount of residual urine that they carry. If patients with DHIC are able to self-catheterize, suppression of detrusor activity by drugs in combination with periodic self catheterization is a satisfactory solution to the problem. This can also be accomplished if there is ready access to good nursing care. Otherwise, these patients present a real management dilemma.

Reversible Causes of Incontinence

Due to the somewhat frail physiologic balance between storage and emptying which exists in the elderly, transient medical conditions can often lead to incontinence. Correction of these medical conditions often restores the proper homeostatic balance and eliminates the problem. This means that a thorough medical evaluation is the cornerstone of managing urinary incontinence in the elderly patient. Problems can often be solved without resort to sophisticated urodynamic testing, which may not always provide the "real" answer to what is going on in these patients. Resnick has devised the useful mnemonic "DIAPPERS" to categorize the reversible causes of urinary incontinence which are commonly found among the elderly (Table 15.2).

Delirium.   Delirium is disorientation. This may be "classic" disorientation to time and place, but delirium may also take more subtle forms. Patients with

TABLE 15.2.   Reversible Causes of Incontinence

Delirium
Infection
Atropic urethritis and vaginitis
Pharmacologic causes
Psychologic causes
Excess fluid excretion
Restricted mobility
Stool impaction

(After Resnick)

delirium may be acutely confused, but more often lack the ability to focus on sequenced tasks. These individuals may become incontinent because they do not perceive the need to void or because they do not perceive the need to maintain continence. A useful screening test for delirium is to make the patient attempt to perform a repetitive sequenced task, such as serial subtraction of seven, starting at 100. A diagnostic test such as this is important, because the delirious patient may appear relatively normal until forced to undertake a repetitive task of this nature. Diagnosing delirium is *important,* not just an academic exercise. The onset of delirium is associated with serious underlying medical problems, and carries a risk of increased morbidity and mortality.

Infection. An increased postvoid residual and changes in the bladder lining predispose elderly women to develop symptomatic urinary tract infection; however, the presenting symptoms of a urinary tract infection may be different in these patients. Many older women will present with urinary incontinence and bacteriuria without the dysuria which is so commonly associated with acute cystitis in younger women. Nonetheless, infections can cause bladder irritation which may lead to unsuppressible detrusor contractions. For this reason infection should always be investigated as a possible cause for incontinence, particularly in the older patient. Many elderly women without incontinence will also have asymptomatic bacteriuria if their urine is examined. Screening for this condition should be carried out early in any general evaluation of elderly women.

Atrophic Urethritis and Vaginitis. Estrogen deprivation commonly results in increased sensitivity of the lower genitourinary tract and is often responsible for irritative symptoms in postmenopausal women. Atrophic irritation of this kind can trigger detrusor instability in some patients, and loss of urethral coaptation can lower outlet resistance. This condition generally responds rapidly to local estrogen application over a few weeks (see below).

Pharmacologic Causes. Many medications used to treat urinary incontinence may actually exacerbate the problem if their use is not monitored carefully. Drugs which impair detrusor contractility may reduce voiding efficiency and lead to overflow incontinence by increasing the residual urine volume. The weakest antidepressants, such as trazodone (Deseryl), have greater anticholinergic effects than do the strongest antipsychotic medications. Sedative-hypnotics, including flurazepam (Dalmane), diazepam (Valium), and alcohol, reduce patients' awareness of bladder sensation. Alcohol also has a diuretic effect, and may produce problems in patients who drink at bedtime to help themselves sleep. Certain diuretics, such as furosemide (Lasix), ethacrynic acid (Edecrin), and bumetanide (Bumex), can produce incontinence by overwhelming the bladder's ability to handle the increased urine output. Many other medications have unexpected anticholinergic side effects. These include antispasmodics like Bentyl (dicyclomine) and Donnatol (atropine, phenobarbital, hyoscyamine, and scopolamine); anti-Parkinson medications (except Sinemet); antiarrhythmics such as Norpace (disopyramide); antihistamines (most of which are obtained in over-the-counter cold remedies); opiate preparations; antidiarrheal medications like Lomotil (diphenoxylate and atropine); and psychotropic drugs. All of these medications may lead to decreased voiding efficiency and increased residual urine, which may worsen incontinence in some patients. Antipsychotic medications, such as Haldol (haloperidol) and Navane (thiothixene), have Parkinsonian extrapyramidal side effects and may compromise patient mobility, while thioridazine (Mellaril) and thorazine inhibit detrusor contractility. Elavil (amitriptyline) has significant anticholinergic effects and may also cause orthostatic hypotension. Xanax (alprazolam) does not affect lower urinary tract function. Narcotics and calcium channel blockers (nifedipine, verapamil) may inhibit bladder contractility. α-Agonists (ephedrine, pseudoephedrine, phenylpropanolamine) will increase outflow resistance and may cause acute urinary retention. α-Blockers (prazosin, terazosin) will lower resistance in the bladder neck and urethra and may precipitate urinary incontinence in some patients.

Psychologic Causes.   Depression and behavioral disturbances decrease patient motivation and may lead to a decreased awareness of bladder sensation. These problems may be seen especially during life-crisis situations, such as the death of a spouse or a close friend.

Excess Fluid Excretion.   Excessive fluid intake and a variety of metabolic disorders (diabetes mellitus, hypercalcemia, diabetes insipidus) lead to excessive fluid excretion. Venous stasis in the lower extremities and congestive heart failure are very common in elderly women and are often associated with urinary incontinence because of their relationship to excess fluid excretion. Reabsorption of edema fluid at night while the patient is supine is a frequent cause of nocturia in the elderly. Edematous states may also be caused by decreased albumin and the use of nonsteroidal anti-inflammatory drugs or calcium channel blockers such as nifedipine.

Restricted Mobility.   Elderly patients may not be able to make it to the toilet in time because it takes them so long to *get* to the toilet! Impaired mobility is a correctable cause of incontinence which is often overlooked. Treatable causes of impaired mobility include disorientation in unfamiliar settings, neurologic conditions (spinal stenosis), mechanical problems (e.g., amputation), motivation (fear, depression), foot problems, drugs causing weakness or dizziness, deconditioning of the baroreceptors which control intravascular pressure (often due to prolonged bedrest), and visual impairment. If it is not possible to correct the patient's immobility, placing a commode within easy reach both day and night is often a good solution to this problem.

Another major cause of restricted mobility in the elderly is clothing. Many patients can make it to the toilet in time but leak urine because they cannot undress quickly enough once they are there. Visual impairment as well as lost manual dexterity due to arthritis are common reasons that this occurs. Patients should be encouraged to wear comfortable, loose fitting clothing that is easy to take off and put on. Find out how long it takes a patient to get dressed. Many elderly women wear elaborate combinations of intertwined corsets, girdles, belts, garters, slips, and stockings which take forever to remove and put on again. This kind of dressing should be discouraged in patients with bladder control problems. Correcting this problem may be all that some patients need in order to be dry.

Stool Impaction.   Distension of the rectum and pelvic floor by impacted stool may cause reflex inhibition of the parasympathetic innervation of the bladder and lead to urinary retention, voiding dysfunction, and incontinence. This problem can be treated easily with stool softeners, attention to proper diet, and disimpaction of the acutely impacted patient. Again, this simple cause for incontinence is often overlooked.

Other Problems Specific to the Elderly

Urethral caruncle and urethral prolapse (Fig. 12.2 *A* and *B*) result from estrogen deficiency and may produce symptoms of urgency, dysuria, and voiding difficulty in this age group. Voiding difficulty is not always associated with urinary incontinence, and a chronically elevated residual urine may result in recurrent urinary tract infection. Large cystoceles or other forms of prolapse may also result in voiding problems. Loss of estrogen may make the bladder more susceptible to urinary tract infection. Decreased fluid intake and abnormal metabolism of calcium and urate may produce stones. The acute onset of irritative voiding symptoms in elderly women should prompt the clinician to investigate the possibility of neoplasia, which is more common among older patients.

Evaluation of the Elderly Patient

History and Associated Medical Conditions

It is important to recognize that an enormous amount of embarrassment and distress generally accompanies urinary incontinence in the elderly. Imagine the feelings of an elderly grandmother who wets her pants in front of grandchildren. They will not understand this and may even make fun of her. Trying to discuss this problem with a physician or nurse may be just as traumatic for her. Medical personnel must learn to inquire about the presence of urinary tract complaints in these patients in a manner which relieves them of anxiety. Prefacing questions by mentioning the high prevalence of incontinence in women of a similar age group often eases patient fears about being ill, senile, or abnormal. Phrases such as "Many of my patients cannot make it to the bathroom in time and sometimes have an accident. Does this ever happen to you?" may be very helpful. Acknowledging their stress and embarrassment will also help put them at ease.

The medical history is extremely important in evaluating an elderly patient. Medications are far more likely to contribute to the development of incontinence in older patients than in younger ones. All medications should be reviewed with the patient, including over-the-counter drugs. Many patients do not realize that these are "real" medications with potentially serious side effects. Patients should be encouraged to bring all of their medications with them to their appointment. In taking the incontinence history, active questioning by the physician is necessary to round out the details because the elderly patient may fail to make important distinctions, such as the difference between urge and stress incontinence. The physician must also examine the elderly patient carefully for changes in mental status. Continence depends upon her ability to remember when she last voided and to perceive the benefits of dryness or of treatment. An evaluation of mobility is exceptionally important, as are questions about manual dexterity and the time it takes a patient to dress or undress. Observing the patient for signs of stroke is important since the patient herself may not have realized that this has occurred, or because she has purposely concealed it from her family and friends. If a stroke has occurred, this information will help to identify the etiology of her problem and the type of incontinence that is occurring. Anticholinergic medications should be used cautiously in stroke patients as they may precipitate urinary retention even when detrusor hyperreflexia is present. Anticholinergic drugs may also cause problems in patients with glaucoma, constipation, or severe diverticulosis. Inquiries should be made regarding lower extremity edema, since this may contribute to nocturnal diuresis and increased nocturia. The importance of fluid intake and the use of a frequency-volume bladder chart has been emphasized repeatedly throughout this book. Diabetes is an important cause of polyuria in the elderly.

Fecal incontinence is often associated with urinary incontinence, and patients are even more reluctant to talk about this than about loss of bladder control. Patients should be questioned actively about anal problems, and although most patients will discuss constipation easily enough, the presence of fecal incontinence is greatly distressing and rarely volunteered. If bladder sensation is absent or markedly decreased, this may be a sign of neuropathy which needs further investigation.

The goals of treatment should be reviewed with the patient and her family. In the absence of reversible or potentially dangerous conditions, treatment should first be directed towards the worst (most severe or bothersome) symptoms. The goal of treatment is not always complete cure at all costs, but preconceived limitations based on age should be avoided when discussing more radical treatments such as surgery.

Physical Findings in Elderly Patients

The physical examination of the elderly patient is different from that needed for a younger patient. Since conditions such as congestive heart failure, arthritis, orthostatic hypotension, and peripheral edema may contribute significantly to continence problems in the elderly, all such patients should be given a good general physical examination. Special attention should be given to gait, mobility, and manual dexterity. Because of the increased prevalence of breast cancer in the elderly, the breast exam should not be neglected and mammograms should be encouraged. It is striking how many elderly women have never had a screening mammogram. The increased incidence of stroke in these patients means that the neurologic screening examination is important and should not be neglected. The anal wink reflex may be absent in up to one-quarter of elderly women, but the bulbocavernosus reflex is almost always intact. A rectal examination should always be performed to check for fecal impaction and the presence of occult blood in the stool. Because increased abdominal pressure may lead to urinary incontinence, the gynecologic exam should be thorough, looking for a possible pelvic mass. The patient's estrogen status should be evaluated. Significant prolapse is often present. The clinician should attempt to demonstrate stress incontinence by having the patient cough with a full bladder. The limitations of the Bonney-Marshall test have previously been discussed, but this test may be even more misleading in the elderly population due to reductions in vaginal capacity and mobility. Since there is an increased prevalence of incomplete emptying in the older patient, the postvoid residual urine should be assessed on at least one occasion. If elevated, further investigation is warranted. The importance of occult urinary tract infection in the elderly should not be overlooked, particularly in patients with increased urinary residuals.

Urodynamic Testing in the Elderly

Not all test procedures need to be extensive or exhaustive. The frequency-volume bladder chart provides invaluable information on excessive fluid intake, inappropriate fluid restriction, the number of incontinent episodes, and the patient's pattern of frequency and nocturia. A plastic collection "hat" that fits over the toilet bowl rim is very useful in helping elderly patients collect and measure their urine volumes. Resnick estimates that the bladder chart yields the diagnosis in one-quarter of his population of elderly women with incontinence (personal communication). A chemical and metabolic laboratory survey may reveal the reason for increased urinary output or declining mental status. Urinary cytology should be obtained in patients with frequency and urgency of recent onset. Either gross or microscopic hematuria is worrisome, since malignancy or other significant urinary tract disease is present in over 20% of elderly women with this finding. Anal incontinence is often seen in elderly patients with urinary incontinence. Anorectal manometry is a quick and relatively inexpensive way of evaluating rectal sensation, baseline pressure, sphincter tone, and squeeze pressures, and can often provide information useful in the treatment of these patients. More sophisticated gastrointestinal studies such as colonic transit times or defecography can help assess the progress of stool through the large bowel and rectum.

Many elderly patients do not need formal urodynamic testing. Simple cystometry at the bedside may demonstrate unstable detrusor activity or stress incontinence in many cases. If pure stress incontinence is present or pure urge incontinence is found in the absence of a significant neurologic history, a trial of conservative management is completely appropriate. However, if the patient's symptoms are mixed or severe or if surgery is contemplated, more sophisticated urodynamic testing should be performed. Elderly patients should never be systematically excluded from urodynamic evaluation because of their age, frailty, or the fact that they are institutionalized. Resnick has clearly demonstrated that the only adverse sequelae of complex urodynamic testing in elderly patients is asymptomatic bacteriuria. Urodynamic studies are generally done most efficiently by two people working together. When elderly patients are involved, the assistance of another pair of hands is always welcome.

Hilton and Stanton have developed an algorithm for the evaluation of incontinence in the elderly using simple tests and bedside urodynamic studies which resulted in an adequate evaluation of 90% of geriatric and nursing home patients (Fig. 15.1). Patients who have undergone recent pelvic surgery, had recurrent urinary tract infections, suffer from marked genital prolapse, stress incontinence, significant voiding symptoms, or residual urine volumes greater than 100 ml should have complex urodynamic testing. Both Castelden and Resnick advocate formal urodynamic evaluation of most elderly patients because of the complexity of findings in this group. Of particular concern is the presence of impaired detrusor contractility in elderly women who also have detrusor overactivity (DHIC). The use of anticholinergic medication is complicated in these patients and may require simultaneous self-catheterization.

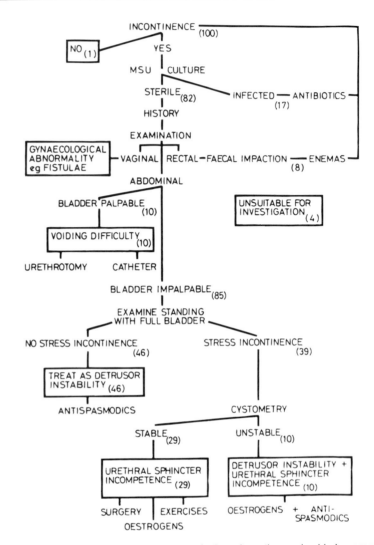

Figure 15.1 Algorithm for assessment of urinary incontinence in elderly women. The figures in parentheses are the numbers of patients who followed each route when the algorithm was applied to 100 patients retrospectively. = Midstream specimen of urine. (From Hilton and Stanton, Br Med J 1982; 282:942, with permission.)

Management of Urinary Incontinence in the Elderly

General Considerations

Age alone should not be the major reason for rejecting any given mode of therapy in an elderly patient. Discussion of the quality of life with the patient and her family, her expected level of activity, and priority of symptoms will help individualize the management of urinary incontinence. Surgery for stress incontinence should be considered against the background of the patient's general health and level of activity at any age, especially if conservative management has not been successful.

Elderly patients frequently have concurrent problems. Treatment of these contributing factors may improve their continence significantly. The following general suggestions may be helpful in managing elderly patients with incontinence. Because obstipation often exacerbates patients' urinary tract symptoms, they should be offered both bowel stimulants and stool softeners as necessary. Since nighttime diuresis often results in significant urine output during sleep with the patient waking to void every 2–3 hours, women with this problem should be instructed to elevate their legs in the evening, restrict their fluids for several hours before going to bed, and to use diuretics early in the day. A commode may be placed at the patient's bedside during the night and in a convenient living area during the day to provide easy patient access to toileting. Clothing should be made as simple as possible to allow quick and easy undressing (e.g., eliminate multiple layers of clothing, replace buttons with Velcro, etc.). The use of a walker may help the patient feel more secure in getting to the bathroom. Toilet seat adapters and the installation of siderails or sidebars will improve patient mobility and access to toilets even further. Modifications of this kind should not be made so that they compromise the patient's ability to sit on the toilet with her feet on the ground, since this has been shown to make voiding more difficult. Changing the patient's medication is often useful. Antidepressants with fewer anticholinergic effects (such as Prozac) should be used to replace those with more powerful antimuscarinic activity. Diuretics or α-blockers such as prazosin which are used for the treatment of hypertension can often be replaced by ACE inhibitors or other medications that do not compromise bladder function quite so much.

Genital prolapse often exacerbates incontinence in elderly women. If the pelvic relaxation is symptomatic, a pessary may relieve symptoms without resorting to surgery. The pessary should be chosen so that it does not compromise bowel or bladder emptying. Some trial and error may be necessary to find a pessary that works. Cube pessaries are attractive because they tend not to compress the bowel or bladder. However, since these pessaries are held in place by a mild suction effect, the cube may erode the vaginal mucosa if it is not removed and cleaned on a regular basis. Gelhorn pessaries and ring or ''doughnut'' pessaries may compress the bowel or bladder, and some patients may find that they have to remove or adjust them in order to void or defecate. This greatly compromises their usefulness, particularly in patients with limited manual dexterity. Even if a pessary is not used, patients with significant genital prolapse can be instructed to facilitate emptying by reducing their cystocele at the end of voiding or by compressing a rectocele with two fingers to help with defecation.

Estrogen Status

The use of estrogen replacement therapy should be considered in every postmenopausal woman. It is well known that estrogen use decreases the risk of cardiovascular disease and plays a crucial role in preventing the postmenopausal bone loss which may lead to debilitating osteoporosis. It is also well known that starting hormone replacement therapy will arrest the further development of osteoporotic bone loss even in the patient with significant disease, although it will do little to restore the bone that has already been lost. At present there is no clear evidence that estrogen use, by itself, increases the risk of a patient developing breast cancer.

In spite of these facts many physicians continue to hold the opinion that hormone therapy is ''not worthwhile'' in the geriatric population. This is not true, and the decision to institute hormone replacement therapy should be made on the basis of an individual's needs regardless of her age. The only *absolute* contraindications to hormone replacement therapy are the presence of active gallbladder or liver disease, hormonally dependent cancers (breast, endometrium), active thromboembolic disease or acute deep venous thrombophlebitis, and undiagnosed vaginal bleeding, which must be evaluated immediately to rule out the presence of genital cancer. Relative contraindications to hormone replacement therapy include a strong history of documented thromboembolic events, peripheral vascular disease, and migraine headaches. Patients who have had a stage I carcinoma of the endometrium completely treated by adequate hysterectomy may receive hormone replacement therapy. Women with a past history of node-negative breast cancer which has been in remission for a prolonged period of time are sometimes given hormone replacement therapy on an individual basis, depending on their symptoms. Because there are no data regarding the effects of such therapy on their malignancy, these patients must give informed consent and must understand that their risk for tumor recurrence, while probably small, is also probably increased if they take hormones. This risk may be justified in the presence of debilitating symptoms which can be corrected by hormone replacement. Physicians must continue to treat patients, not medico-legal risk factors.

Is estrogen efficacious in treating lower urinary tract disorders? Although the use of estrogen is best established in the treatment of urge syndromes, recent evidence confirms its usefulness in the treatment of stress incontinence. Our practice is to offer estrogen replacement therapy to all postmenopausal women with urinary incontinence or sensory disorders of the lower urinary tract unless there is a contraindication. Even patients who have been menopausal for many years may benefit from this form of treatment. Estrogen also improves the thickness and vascularity of the vaginal epithelium and endopelvic fascia, thus improving the handling of these tissues during surgery and their response during healing.

Hormone replacement therapy in the elderly woman with lower urinary tract complaints can be carried out through the application of vaginal estrogen cream. These creams are supplied in a tube with an applicator which is filled to a predetermined level and inserted into the vagina. The plunger on the end of the tube is then depressed, depositing the cream in place. The most commonly used creams are Premarin (conjugated equine estrogens), Estrace (17-β-estradiol), and Ogen (estropipate). Initial treatment of the geriatric patient with atrophic vaginitis generally involves the use of one full applicator of the cream at night for 2–4 weeks, then tapering the dose to a lower maintenance level using a full or half-applicator two or three times per week. The lowest level of estrogen that will control symptoms should be used. After adequate estrogenization has been achieved, many patients can be maintained on as little as 1/2 applicator of estrogen cream once per week. There is some systemic absorption of estrogens given vaginally, and patients may complain of breast tenderness. The reason that this may occur should be explained to the patient beforehand, to spare her unnecessary anxiety. Patients who have had a hysterectomy may use the cream continuously, but patients with a uterus in place require special consideration. Spotting which occurs during vaginal estrogen use must be investigated to rule out endometrial neoplasia. Elderly patients with a uterus who use vaginal estrogen creams for prolonged periods of time, may find it useful to use the cream only 3 out of every 4 weeks. Before prescribing vaginal estrogen creams, make sure that the elderly patient will use them! Many older women don't want to use anything "down there." The use of systemic estrogens may be preferable for such patients.

Using oral or transdermal estrogen is perfectly acceptable in the older patient providing no specific contraindications exist. If the patient has had a hysterectomy, systemic estrogens may be used on a continuous dosage regimen. If the patient still has a uterus, estrogen must be used in combination with a progestin to avoid the development of endometrial hyperplasia or, in rare cases, endometrial adenocarcinoma. The problem with the use of systemic estrogen and progestin is that it tends to produce vaginal bleeding, which may be disturbing to the woman who is well past menopause.

The lowest dose of estrogen which will control symptoms should be used. Typical equivalent daily starting doses of estrogen are 0.625 mg of Premarin or Ogen, or 1 mg of Estrace. The transdermal estrogen skin patch (Estraderm) is started as a single 0.05 mg skin patch changed two times per week. The location of the skin patch should be changed each time one is used. Patches should be applied to the lower abdomen, hips or thighs. They should *not* be applied directly to the breasts. The skin under the patch is often slightly reddened or discolored after the patch has been removed, but this should not cause concern.

The progestin used in combined regimens is usually medroxyprogesterone acetate (Provera, Cycrin) or, less commonly, norethindrone acetate (Aygestin, Norlutate). The progestin may be given continuously or in cyclic fashion. Most practitioners starting an elderly woman on systemic hormone replacement would probably begin with 0.625 mg of Premarin or 1 mg of Estrace every day, with

2.5 mg of Provera given every day as well. The reason for using a continuous daily dose of both drugs is that these patients already have an atrophic endometrium. By giving a continuous daily dose of progestin, endometrial hypertrophy can be prevented, and the problem of unwanted bleeding can often be avoided altogether. Because the development of spotting on this regimen is unpredictable, patients who develop such bleeding need close surveillance. It is not uncommon for unpredictable spotting to develop early in the course of such treatment, particularly in younger women, but to fade away over time as the progestin effect comes to dominate.

Cycled estrogen-progestin combinations are usually given as daily estrogen with a period of concurrent progestin administration each month, or intermittent use of both preparations. Common combinations include daily Estrace (1 mg) or Premarin (0.625 mg), with 5 mg of Provera the first 14 days of the month, or 10 mg of Provera given the first 10 days of each month. Alternatively, the patient can use the estrogen the first 25 days of each month and the progestin on days 12 through 25 (5 mg) or days 16 through 25 (10 mg) each month. No hormones are given the last 5 or 6 days of the month. Patients on this type of regimen can expect to have withdrawal bleeding during or after progestin use in each cycle. As long as a regular pattern persists this bleeding does not need further evaluation. Patients who have erratic bleeding on hormone replacement therapy need an endometrial biopsy or uterine curettage to rule out endometrial pathology. It is not necessary to perform these procedures prior to starting hormone replacement therapy unless some other indication is present. Patients must know that if they forget to take their medications or taken them erratically, they will have vaginal bleeding!

Treatment of Stress Incontinence

A wide variety of conservative treatment options can be offered to the elderly patient with stress incontinence. α-Agonists such as phenylpropanolamine (Ornade spansules), pseudoephedrine (Dexatrim, Sudafed), and other drugs are as effective in older as in younger women. When used, the patient's blood pressure should be monitored shortly after starting these medications, since α-stimulants can increase the tension in vascular smooth muscle and raise her blood pressure.

Pelvic floor muscle exercise programs are also useful, but not all patients respond equally well. Burgio achieved an 82% reduction in incontinent episodes using pelvic floor rehabilitation enhanced by biofeedback, and this success was maintained after 12 months follow-up. Tapp, on the other hand, found that physiotherapy was of questionable benefit in the treatment of stress incontinence in elderly women. The effectiveness of pelvic muscle rehabilitation depends to a great extent upon the enthusiasm and supervision of a dedicated instructor who can motivate her patients. Compliance with the exercise regimen appears to be a key factor in success or failure, and little progress should be expected until patients have been exercising for 3 months or more.

Other procedures, such as postural changes to improve control or suppress urgency (including crossing the legs, squeezing the thighs together, or bending over) should be discussed with the patient. Although many women have discovered these maneuvers by themselves, it is surprising how many patients do not make use of simple postural change to improve their bladder control. These techniques have been shown to reduce the volume of urine lost and most patients find them socially acceptable.

The criteria for deciding on surgery in the treatment of incontinence in the elderly female are the same as those for choosing surgical treatment in the younger woman. Is the problem surgically correctable? Do the risks of surgery outweigh the benefits? Are there overriding medical problems that cannot be overcome by careful pre- and postoperative management? Can conservative measures be used to improve a patient's condition to the point where she no longer wants surgery? Are there reversible causes for the incontinence that can be corrected, thereby making surgery unnecessary? An elderly patient must be given adequate information on which to base a wise decision. A reduction in incontinent episodes by 50% or a reduction down to one or two leaks per week may be a great improvement that makes surgery worthwhile for a patient. No woman should be denied surgery *on the basis of age alone.*

There are, however, special considerations involved in operating on elderly women. Regional anesthesia is often preferable, and in some cases local anesthetic may be used. Consultation with a geriatrician before surgery and in the immediate postoperative period will help provide optimum patient care, particularly as regards her medical status and fluid management. The choice of operation should be tailored to the needs of the individual patient, and no blanket recommendations can be made regarding the suitability of a particular operation for the older patient. Because elderly women are predisposed to postoperative urinary retention, nonobstructing operations are preferred and liberal use should be made of suprapubic catheters and clean intermittent self-catheterization. Prophylaxis against deep venous thrombosis (usually using pneumatic compression stockings) is recommended. The incidence of postoperative detrusor instability does not appear to be increased in elderly women undergoing bladder neck surgery compared to younger women.

Management of Urgency, Frequency, and Urge Incontinence

Neoplasia and chronic urinary retention should be excluded early in the evaluation of the urge syndrome in elderly patients. Once this has been done, the therapy for this condition is similar to that used in the treatment of younger women. However, because detrusor contractility may be impaired in this age group, and because special concerns exist regarding the side effects of anticholinergic medications in elderly women, pharmacologic treatment may not be the best first-line therapy for older patients.

Bladder retraining and behavioral modification are often as successful as drug therapy in elderly patients, and avoid the potential anticholinergic side effects of medications. The success of behavioral modification programs has been shown to vary in direct relationship to the motivation of both the patient and the health care provider involved. Patients who are treated with behavioral modification techniques should be selected carefully for their motivation, ability to learn, and willingness to complete a training program. Patients looking for a ''quick fix'' will probably not benefit very much from biofeedback training or bladder drill.

Instruction in fluid management is a key point in these programs. The patient should keep a frequency-volume chart which should be reviewed carefully with her to make sure she understands her current bladder habits and how they should be modified. Many elderly patients restrict their fluid intake severely in an effort to reduce their urinary frequency and incontinence. The highly concentrated urine which they produce under these circumstances may be even more irritating to their bladders than a larger volume of more dilute urine. Patients should be encouraged to drink at least 1500 ml of fluid each day. These liquids should be distributed evenly throughout the day, but drinking during the 3 hours before bedtime should be discouraged.

Instruction in bladder retraining should include both verbal directions given during the clinic visit as well as simple written instructions for use at home. When writing instructions for patients, write them at the *fourth grade level!* Written instructions that the patient cannot understand are useless! Patients who are given a specific timed voiding schedule may benefit from wearing a wristwatch with an alarm which can help remind them to use the toilet. Close follow-up and encouragement can be maintained by frequent telephone contact. The patient should keep a bladder chart periodically to document her progress and help pinpoint specific problems. Although younger patients may hope to achieve voiding intervals of 3 hours or longer at the end of bladder training programs, older patients will probably do better if they set their goals at achieving 2-hour voiding intervals.

Biofeedback techniques have been used in appropriately motivated older patients to help them learn voluntary bladder control. This type of training involves teaching the patient to control her bladder, sphincter, and intra-abdominal pressure by responding to a visual or auditory signal which is generated through the activity of an internal physiologic process. This signal can be obtained by measuring intravesical pressure with a pressure catheter, using a ''perineometer'' to evaluate pelvic muscle activity by surface EMG signals or pressure recordings from an intravaginal or intrarectal balloon, or by using weighted vaginal cones. Simple techniques which do not require elaborate or expensive instrumentation are obviously preferred. Although most physicians find the use of biofeedback techniques too time consuming for their practices, this therapy is cost effective when done by nurses or physical therapists.

Anticholinergic medications should probably be used in elderly patients after bladder retraining and behavioral modification have been tried and contributing factors such as drug effects and systemic disease have been evaluated. The dose of the drug used often must be reduced in elderly women because of impaired renal clearance and the possibility of producing urinary retention. Propantheline (ProBanthine) should be started in doses of 7.5–15 mg po TID and increased to higher doses or QID slowly, if at all. Oxybutynin chloride (Ditropan) should be started in doses of 2.5 mg po BID and increased slowly to TID or QID, or to doses of 5 mg at similar intervals. Dose titration of Ditropan may be improved by using it in syrup form. Because of its short half-life, Ditropan can be used episodically to help the patient remain dry for important events during the day or during the week. Patients are more willing to put up with its anticholinergic side effects on a short-term basis if they can remain dry for several hours while traveling, shopping, or visiting friends. Dicyclomine (Bentyl) also has a short half-life and can be used in doses of 10–30 mg po TID/QID. Hyoscyamine tablets (0.125 mg, Levsin) may be taken orally or sublingually, 1–2 tablets up to every 4 hours. Imipramine (Tofranil) is an attractive drug because it increases urethral tone due to its α-adrenergic stimulating properties and also relaxes the detrusor because of its anticholinergic characteristics and its effects on the central nervous system. It should be started in low doses (10 mg po TID) and increased carefully since it may cause orthostatic hypotension and cardiac arrhythmias in some patients. The calcium channel blocker terodiline (Micturin) has been used extensively in Europe and is currently being evaluated for possible release in the United States. It has been shown to be effective in treating urge incontinence due to both detrusor instability and detrusor hyperreflexia. Its major benefits include a long serum half-life (60 hours), which means that it can be given as little as twice (or even once) per day, and a lower side effect profile than other anticholinergic drugs. A few patients with pre-existing heart conditions have developed an unusual ventricular arrhythmia (torsade de pointes) while on this medication.

Anticholinergic drugs may cause mental confusion and drowsiness in the elderly. They may also precipitate acute urinary retention. Although narrow angle glaucoma is seen in only about 10% of glaucoma patients, it is associated with high intraocular pressures. The use of an anticholinergic medication may precipitate an acute intraocular crisis in such patients. Narrow angle glaucoma may be screened for quickly by shining a flashlight into the outer corner of the eye. If the light passes to the inner canthus, it is extremely unlikely that high pressure glaucoma is present. Constipation and dry mouth—two common side effects of anticholinergic medications—may be tolerated poorly by elderly patients. If these are problems, they may be overcome by liberal use of stool softeners and bulking agents to ease the bowels and sugar-free gum or lemon drops to help moisten the mouth.

Management of Urinary Retention or Overflow Incontinence

If the diagnosis of urinary retention or overflow incontinence has been made in an older person, the first step should be to review all medications (including over-the counter drugs) to see if this is the precipitating cause. It is not unusual to see significant urinary retention develop during the treatment of urge incontinence. Patients with suspicious neurologic histories or with (the normal) urinary residuals of 50–100 ml in this age group should be monitored carefully for the development of retention. It is a wise policy to recheck a postvoid residual in elderly patients within 1–2 weeks after starting or increasing anticholinergic medications, particularly if they have not improved or their condition has worsened. The drug responsible should be stopped until the situation corrects itself, and then may be reintroduced at a lower dose, with appropriate monitoring. If the patient's incontinence worsens while on anticholinergic medications, this is often a clue that urinary retention is developing.

Several voiding techniques may be of special benefit in the older age group. Because both urinary flow rates and detrusor pressure during voiding are diminished in elderly women, they may need to allow more time and more privacy for voiding. The sound of running water is often helpful in provoking a detrusor contraction in patients with hesitancy. Altered anatomy after surgery for pelvic relaxation sometimes makes it necessary for women to lean forward or stand up to void. This is especially true if they have undergone an obstructive operation for incontinence. Many clinicians believe that clean intermittent self-catheterization is too difficult for older women with chronic urinary retention to manage, but multiple studies have shown this is feasible therapy for the elderly if they are given careful instruction and encouragement. The use of intermittent catheterization is preferable to dealing with the complications of a long-term indwelling catheter. A patient's manual dexterity may be gauged by having her touch her index finger to the examiner's moving finger. As long as one hand is sufficiently dexterous to accomplish this task, the other hand can spread the labia to expose the urethral orifice. This is possible even if a significant tremor is present. A spouse or other family member can also be trained to perform clean intermittent catheterization if necessary.

The Incontinent Nursing Home Patient

Forty to 60% of nursing home residents suffer from urinary incontinence at least once per week. Such patients tend to be older and more infirm than community-dwelling elderly women, factors which predispose them to the development of incontinence. In fact, the development of incontinence is often the final factor which persuades families that they can no longer care for these women at home. Earlier medical intervention could probably have kept many of these patients in their own homes. Worse still, many nursing home residents are given permanent indwelling catheters as the only treatment for their incontinence, a situation which has resulted in urosepsis being a major cause of morbidity in nursing home patients. Although catheters are easy for nursing personnel to manage, avoid unpleasant smells, and prevent the breakdown of skin which is chronically exposed to urine, these goals can all be met without exposing the patient to the risk of infection from chronic catheterization.

Whenever a catheterized patient is encountered in a nursing home the question should be asked: Why does this patient have a catheter? Alternative attempts to solve the problem should be sought. Patients may be unable to get to the toilet on their own, but are reluctant to ask for help. Regular timed toileting will reduce incontinent episodes greatly in this group of patients. Patients should be prompted to urinate on a regular basis (at least every 2 hours) and should be encouraged to go whether they feel they urge or not. Absorbent pads and barrier creams can protect the skin and reduce the odor of urine. Clean intermittent self-catheterization (or intermittent catheterization by nursing personnel) may also be used. While the infection rates with these techniques are higher in nursing homes than in the home setting, they are still better than those which are found with chronic indwelling catheterization. It is perfectly reasonable to attempt to reduce the proportion of nursing home patients with indwelling catheters to 1–2%.

Geriatric patients—both those living at home as well as many in nursing homes—are frequently capable of much more than they are generally given credit for. When treated with the encouragement, respect, and dignity which they deserve, they can usually be helped to attain a much higher level of continence than they had before therapy was begun. Simple compassion demands that they be given the opportunity to prove themselves.

SUGGESTED READING

Reviews

Bavendam T. Geriatric female incontinence. Prob Urol 1991; 5:42–71.

Ouslander J (Ed). Urinary incontinence. Clin Geriatr Med 1986; 2:639–99.

Resnick N, Yalla S. Management of urinary incontinence in the elderly. N Engl J Med 1985; 313:800–05.

Epidemiology

Diokno A, Brock N, Brown M, Herzog A. Prevalence of urinary incontinence and other urological symptoms in the noninstitutionalized elderly. J Urol 1986; 136:1022–25.

Hu T. The economic impact of urinary incontinence. Clin Geriatr Med 1986; 2:673–87.

Hunskaar S, Vinsnes A. The quality of life in women with urinary incontinence as measured by the sickness impact profile. J Am Geriatr Soc 1991; 39:378–82.

Kunin CM, Chin QFC, Chambers S. Morbidity and mortality associated with indwelling urinary catheters in elderly patients in a nursing home—confounding due to the presence of associated diseases. J Am Geriatr Soc 1987; 35: 1001–06.

Starer P, Libow L. Obscuring urinary incontinence. Diapering of the elderly. J Am Geriatr Soc 1985; 33:74–76.

Etiology

Brocklehurst J. The ageing bladder. Br J Hosp Med 1986; 35:8–10.

Brocklehurst J, Andrews K, Richards B, Laycock J. Incidence and correlates of incontinence in stroke patients. J Am Geriatr Soc 1985; 33:540–42.

Castleden C, Duffin H, Asher M, Yeomanson C. Factors influencing outcome in elderly patients with urinary incontinence and detrusor instability. Age Ageing 1985; 14: 303–07.

Diokno AC, Wells TJ, Brink CA. Urinary incontinence in elderly women: Urodynamic evaluation. J Am Geriatr Soc 1987; 35:940–46.

Fantl J, Wyman J, Anderson R, Matt D, Bump R. Postmenopausal urinary incontinence: Comparison between nonestrogen-supplemented and estrogen-supplemented women. Obstet Gynecol 1988; 71:823–28.

Resnick N, Yalla S. Detrusor hyperactivity with impaired contractile function. An unrecognized but common cause of incontinence in elderly patients. JAMA 1987; 257: 3076–81.

Wells T, Brink C, Diokno A. Urinary incontinence in elderly women: Clinical findings. J Am Geriatr Soc 1987; 35: 933–39.

Diagnosis

Folstein MF, Folstein SE, McHugh PR. ''Mini-mental state: '' A practical method for grading the cognitive state of patients for the clinician. J Psychiat Res 1975; 12:189–98.

Hilton P, Stanton S. Algorithmic method for assessing urinary incontinence in elderly women. Br Med J (1982); 282:940–42.

Ouslander J, Staskin D, Raz S, Su H, Hepps K. Clinical versus urodynamic diagnosis in an incontinent geriatric female population J Urol 1987; 137:68–71.

Ouslander J, Leach G, Staskin D. Simplified tests of lower urinary tract function in the evaluation of geriatric urinary incontinence. J Am Geriatr Soc 1989; 37:706–14.

Resnick N, Yalla S, Laurino E. An algorithmic approach to urinary incontinence in the elderly. Clin Res 1986; 34: 832–37.

Resnick NM. Noninvasive diagnosis of the patient with complex incontinence. Gerontology 1990; 36(Suppl 2):8–18.

Treatment

Badlani G, Smith A. Pharmacotherapy of voiding dysfunction in the elderly. Semin Urol 1987; 5:120–25.

Bennett CJ, Diokno AC. Clean intermittent self catheterization in the elderly. Urology 1984; 24:43–45.

Burgio K, Whitehead W, Engel B. Urinary incontinence in the elderly. Bladder/sphincter biofeedback and toileting skills training. Ann Intern Med 1985; 103:507–15.

Burgio K, Engel B. Biofeedback-assisted behavioral training for elderly men and women. J Am Geriatr Soc 1990; 38: 338–40.

Burton JR, Pearce L, Burgio KL, Engel BT, Whitehead WE. Behavioral training for urinary incontinence in elderly ambulatory patients. J Am Geriatr Soc 1988; 36:693–98.

Castleden C, Duffin H, Mitchell E. The effect of physiotherapy on stress incontinence. Age Ageing 1984; 134: 235–37.

Creason N, Grybowski J, Burgener S, Whippo C, Yeo S, Richardson B. Prompted voiding therapy for urinary incontinence in aged female nursing home residents. J Adv Nurs 1989; 14:120–26.

Gillon G, Stanton SL. Long-term follow-up of surgery for urinary incontinence in elderly women. Br J Urol 1984; 56:478–81.

Hadley E. Bladder training and related therapies for urinary incontinence in older people. JAMA 1986 256:372–79.

Henderson J, Taylor K. Age as a variable in an exercise program for the treatment of simple urinary stress incontinence. J Obstet Gynecol Neonat Nurs 1987; July/Aug: 266–72.

Herzog A, Fultz N, Normolle D, Brock B, Diokno A. Methods used to manage urinary incontinence by older adults in the community. J Am Geriatr Soc 1989; 37:339–47.

Marron K, Fillit H, Peskowitz M, Silverston F. The nonuse of urethral catheterization in the management of urinary incontinence in the teaching nursing home. J Am Geriatr Soc 1983; 31:278–81.

Ouslander JG, Urman HN, Uman GC. Development and testing of an incontinence monitoring record. J Am Geriatr Soc 1986; 34:83–90.

Ouslander J, Blaustein J, Connor A, Pitt A. Habit training and oxybutynin for incontinence in nursing home patients: A placebo-controlled trial. J Am Geriatr Soc 1988; 36: 40–46.

Ouslander J, Sier H. Drug therapy for geriatric urinary incontinence. Clin Geriatr Med 1986; 2:789–807.

Tapp A, Cardozo L, Hills B, Barnick C. Who benefits from physiotherapy? Neuro Urodyn 1988; 7:260–61.

Tobin G, Brocklehurst J. The management of urinary incontinence in local authority residential homes for the elderly. Age Ageing 1986; 15:292–98.

Webb RJ, Lawson AL, Neal DE. Clean intermittent self catheterisation in 172 adults. Br J Urol 1990; 65:20–23.

Wells TJ, Brink CA, Diokno AC, Wolfe R, Gillis GL. Pelvic muscle exercise for stress incontinence in elderly women. J Am Geriatr Soc 1991; 39:785–91.

Whitelaw S, Hammonds JC, Tregellas R. Clean intermittent self-catheterisation in the elderly. Br J Urol 1987; 60: 125–27.

16   Urinary Tract Injury in Gynecologic Surgery

All gynecologic surgeons will injure the ureter or the bladder sometime during their careers. How often this happens and whether their patients will suffer a long-term injury depends upon their ability to recognize situations in which the urinary tract is at risk of injury, to identify the ureter and bladder during surgical procedures, and to recognize injury in the operating room once it has occurred. If proper precautions are taken, lower urinary tract injury should happen rarely and should never result in significant long-term disability for the patient. Even experienced pelvic surgeons will cause an occasional injury to the ureter despite having performed vastly more operations than the average practicing gynecologist. Therefore, when an injury does occur, the surgeon must not only feel confident that he has done all that he could to have prevented it, but must also feel confident that the injury can be detected quickly and that steps can be taken to repair it promptly.

Identification of the ureter is an acquired skill. It must be learned and practiced. The ureter is most difficult to find when the need to know its location is the most critical. It is easy to ignore exposing the ureter when the pelvis appears to be normal, but this means losing the opportunity to learn the anatomy of the ureter and to practice exposing it when the process is straightforward and without significant risk. The skills obtained in identifying the ureter under normal conditions will make locating the ureter much easier when the anatomy is distorted and the pressure on the surgeon is much greater.

Ureter During Abdominal Surgery

Ureteral injury occurs in 0.1%–1.5% of all gynecologic operations. Injury occurs less frequently during vaginal than during abdominal surgery, and is most likely to occur in patients undergoing radical hysterectomy. This is because cervical cancer expands into the parametrium and the need is therefore greater to dissect the ureter free from its surroundings during surgery for this kind of pathology. However, most ureteral injuries occur during routine simple hysterectomy, not the extensive surgery needed for malignant disease. Surgeons performing "routine" pelvic operations may develop a false sense of security which causes them to neglect the fundamental techniques and basic surgical principles that can prevent ureteral injury.

The ureter may be damaged anywhere along its course through the pelvis (Fig. 16.1). Injury may occur at the pelvic brim where the ureter is in direct contact with the infundibulopelvic ligament. It may occur along the pelvic sidewall when the ureter has become involved in invasive endometriosis or extensive pelvic infection. It may occur adjacent to the cervix where the ureter lies in the cardinal ligament, or at the point where the ureter passes into the bladder in the vesicocervical space. Injury occurs most commonly to the distal ureter, at or below the level of the cardinal ligament; but an injury at an unusual site is just as damaging to the patient—and just as preventable—as one occurring in a common location. Since the majority of pelvic ureteral injuries in the United States are caused by gynecologists, they should be the surgeons most knowledgeable about preventing these problems before they occur.

Several factors are critical if damage to the lower urinary tract is to be

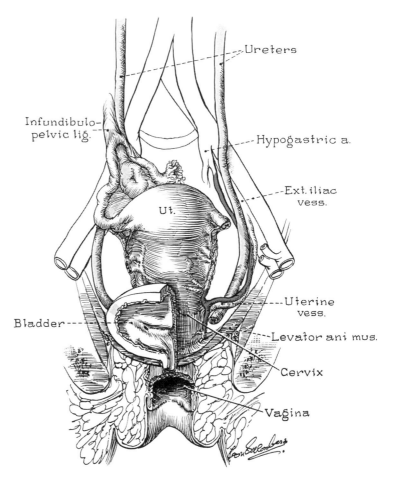

Figure 16.1 Normal anatomy of the ureters and their relations to other pelvic organs encountered in gynecologic surgery. (From Wharton, LR. In Ridley JH (Ed). Gynecologic Surgery: Errors, Safeguards, Salvage. 2nd ed. Baltimore: Williams and Wilkins, 1981, with permission.)

prevented. The most important of these is the surgeon's skill in identifying the bladder and ureter during the operation, *and the willingness to do this routinely.* Anatomical knowledge of the lower urinary tract and an understanding of the disease processes that can bring it in harm's way during a surgical procedure are prerequisites for avoiding intraoperative damage to these structures. Routine identification of the ureter during *all* pelvic operations will give the surgeon the confidence and skill necessary to cope with difficult situations when they arise. Since as few as one-third of ureteral injuries are detected in the operating room, a greater emphasis must be placed on confirming the integrity of the ureters before the abdomen is closed and the patient is awakened from anesthesia. Several techniques for doing this are available. All pelvic surgeons should be familiar with them so that ureteral damage can be detected and repaired promptly before renal function has been compromised.

Role of Preoperative Intravenous Urography

Will preoperative intravenous urography help reduce intraoperative urinary tract injury? Which patients should have such studies before surgery? Each surgeon has his own answer to such questions and these vary widely depending upon who is asked. Some surgeons advocate obtaining an excretory urogram on all patients with a pelvic mass; others feel that since the ureters will be identified during the course of the operation in any case, *routine* preoperative radiography is unnecessary and only serves to increase health care costs.

TABLE 16.1.   Indications for Preoperative Intravenous Urography

- Previous pelvic surgery that may have damaged the ureter (especially with ovarian remnant)
- Extensive or strategically located pelvic disease that may make identification of the ureter difficult
- Suspected anomalous development of urinary system
- Presence of a known genital tract anomaly
- Unusual urinary signs and symptoms
- Suspected ureteral obstruction
- Hematuria
- Presence of a unilateral pelvic mass suspected of being a pelvic kidney

The preoperative intravenous pyelogram (IVP) has four primary functions: (*a*) to demonstrate the presence of two functioning kidneys; (*b*) to reveal ureteral obstruction that has occurred as the result of disease or previous surgery so that it may be relieved during the operation; (*c*) to reveal any congenital abnormality such as complete or partial duplication of the collecting system or a pelvic kidney that may confuse the anatomical picture during surgery; and (*d*) to help determine the location of the ureter so that it may be identified more easily during the operation. This is helpful when the normal anatomy of the pelvis has been distorted. It must be understood, however, that the ureter is located in three dimensions in the retroperitoneal space and that its location is not fixed but is moveable. A two dimensional study such as an IVP will only be of limited value in determining the exact location of the ureter at any particular point in time. A preoperative IVP is not a substitute for intraoperative demonstration of the course of the ureter through the pelvis. Reasonable indications for obtaining preoperative urographic studies are given in Table 16.1. If in doubt, it is generally prudent to obtain the study.

Identification and Protection of the Ureter During Abdominal Surgery

The ureter has a length of about 25 cm, beginning at the renal pelvis of the kidney and ending in the bladder. The upper half of its course is abdominal, while its lower portion lies in the pelvis (Fig. 16.1). The pelvic half of the ureter is of particular importance to gynecologic surgeons. The ureter enters the pelvis where the common iliac artery bifurcates into the external and internal iliac (hypogastric) arteries. This is also the point at which the ovarian vessels enter the pelvis to form the infundibulopelvic ligament, a region which is visible radiologically because these intersections occur in the area of the sacroiliac articulation. The ureter and the ovarian vessels are normally in direct contact as they cross the pelvic brim, but upward traction on the uterus and adnexal structures during hysterectomy will pull the ovarian vessels anteriorly.

Ureter at the Pelvic Brim and on the Pelvic Sidewall

Once the ureter has crossed the pelvic brim, it lies on the medial leaf of the broad ligament. In normal situations, the ureter is visible here near the infundibulopelvic ligament. If it is looked for routinely during all laparotomies and laparoscopies it will become a familiar landmark. The ureter remains attached to the peritoneum of the medial leaf of the broad ligament when the retroperitoneal space is opened (Fig. 16.2). It is easy to see in this location until it reaches the dense connective tissue of the cardinal/uterosacral ligament complex, which obscures it from view in these regions. The surgeon should be particularly aware of the location of the ureter relative to the uterosacral ligaments and the cul-de-sac, since sutures placed in these areas may kink or obstruct it. This occurs most commonly during plication of the uterosacral ligaments or procedures to obliterate the cul-de-sac such as the Moschcowitz culdeplasty. A Halban-type culdeplasty, in which sutures are placed anterior-to-posterior in the saggital plane, is less likely to kink the ureter since the lateral peritoneum is not pulled medially during this type of closure.

Routine identification of the ureter during hysterectomy is a necessity. The location of the pelvic ureter can be determined in several different ways and gynecologic surgeons should become familiar with each of these techniques

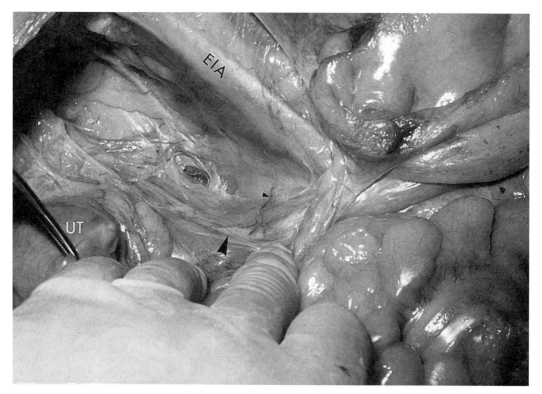

Figure 16.2   Intraoperative photograph showing the course of the ureter attached to the medial leaf of the broad ligament once the retroperitoneal space has been opened. The public symphysis lies to the left of this photograph, the sacrum to the right. EIA = external iliac artery. UT = uterus. The large arrow identifies the ureter, retracted medially. The small arrow identifies an accessory vessel supplying the ureter with blood.

since conditions will inevitably arise which will preclude the use of one or the other technique in specific situations. The ureter can usually be seen through the peritoneum, and its characteristic peristaltic motion can be elicited by compressing it with an *atraumatic* forceps. (This motion is referred to as *vermiculation* because it resembles the locomotion of a worm.) The ureter is often not visible through the peritoneum when the peritoneum has become distorted or inflamed because of extensive endometriosis or pelvic inflammatory disease, or in the presence of obesity. In these cases the retroperitoneal space must be opened and the ureter identified by dissection.

Retroperitoneal dissection to expose the ureter is usually done at the beginning of an abdominal hysterectomy after the round ligament has been ligated and divided. Once the peritoneum has been opened in this fashion, the incision can be extended lateral to the infundibulopelvic ligament, parallel to the midline, for a few centimeters. This opening can be expanded by placing traction on the cut ends of the round ligament, or through careful blunt dissection. As the peritoneum is separated from the pelvic sidewall, the ureter should remain attached to the medial leaf (Fig. 16.2). The ureter is generally most easy to find near the pelvic brim where it crosses the bifurcation of the common iliac artery into its internal and external branches. Once it is found in this location, it may be traced caudally towards the cardinal ligament as it courses deeper into the pelvis.

If the ureter is not immediately visible, it can often be identified by palpation. The characteristic ''snap'' of the ureter may be felt by placing an index finger in the cul-de sac, the thumb in the retroperitoneal space, and plucking the intervening peritoneum. As soon as the ureter has slipped through the examining fingers, the infundibulopelvic ligament can be grasped. This structure may then be clamped or ligated with the knowledge that the ureter is not within the ligature or clamp.

Several conditions can arise that increase the possibility of ureteral injury occurring at the pelvic brim or on the pelvic sidewall. Endometriosis may cause the ureter to become scarred to the peritoneum. Similarly, large ovarian or para-ovarian cysts can dissect into the retroperitoneal space and come into direct contact with the ureter. This situation is especially dangerous since lateral expansion of such masses may displace the ureter onto the anterior or medial surface of the cyst and change its location completely. If an attempt is made to remove the cyst without first identifying the ureter, the ureter may be damaged during the dissection. Large ovarian cysts may also displace the ureter into the area of the infundibulopelvic ligament. If the anatomy of this region is distorted, the vessels should not be ligated or transected until the ureter has been positively identified. This may require considerable effort, particularly when extensive endometriosis is present, but it is always justified. In patients with severe pelvic inflammatory disease or a tubo-ovarian abscess the pelvic peritoneum is usually so thickened that the only way to identify the ureter is by direct retroperitoneal dissection. Identification of the ureter then allows the surgeon to excise all of the affected ovary with confidence and will lessen the likelihood that an ovarian remnant will be left behind to cause problems.

Once the ureter has been identified, it must be determined whether the proposed surgery can be performed in the usual way without ureteral injury. If the ureter is adherent to some endometriosis or to a pelvic mass, it must be freed from these attachments. The ureter should be dissected in such a way that the blood supply on its wall is preserved. The ureter is surrounded by loose areolar tissue which allows it to move independently of the peritoneum. This cleavage plane should be used to separate the ureter from adjacent structures without injuring the ureter itself. Direct abrasion of the ureteral musculature may compromise its blood supply, leading to loss of peristalsis, stricture, or fistula formation.

Developmental anomalies of the kidney and ureter are common and they are often found in association with müllerian anomalies. When a müllerian defect is encountered, the surgeon should make special efforts to examine the kidneys, ureters, and bladder carefully. Among the anomalies which must be kept in mind are an abnormal location of the kidney (such as a pelvic kidney), partial or complete duplication of the collecting system, and the presence of a retrocaval ureter that descends from the kidney, passes around the vena cava and returns to the ipsilateral side of the pelvis. When the ureter is not found where it is expected, the dissection should be extended to identify it. This is often accomplished quickly by looking for the ureter at the pelvic brim and then tracing its course caudally into the pelvis. Once the round ligament has been transected and the peritoneal incision has been extended cranially, a narrow Deaver retractor may be placed under the peritoneum at the upper limit of the incision to expose a large retroperitoneal area above the pelvic brim. This opens a wide space for dissection and makes identification of the ureter much easier. Once the ureter has been located, it can be traced deeper into the pelvis as necessary.

Ureter at the Cardinal Ligament and Vesicocervical Space

As the ureter approaches the uterus, it enters the cardinal/uterosacral ligament complex. The uterine artery lies in the superior fold of the cardinal ligament and the ureter passes underneath it ("the water runs under the bridge") 1.5 cm lateral to the internal cervical os, after which it passes directly onto the anterior vaginal wall before entering the bladder. In order to propel urine through its lumen by peristalsis, the ureter must be free to move. It is therefore not fixed to the tissues of the cardinal ligament, but rather lies within a loose areolar sheath, independent of the surrounding tissues. This loose sheath forms a convenient cleavage plane when it is necessary to dissect the ureter in this area.

The ureter actually lies closer to the cervix and vagina after it passes the lateral margin of the cervix than it does at any other point. Here, in the vesicocervical space, it lies directly upon the anterolateral cervix and cervicovaginal

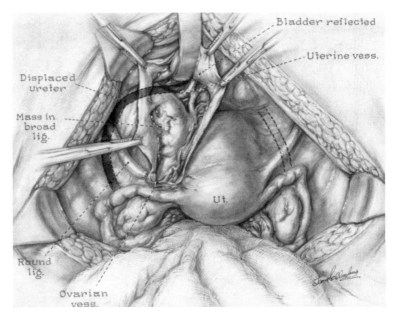

Figure 16.3 Displacement of the ureter due to a left adnexal mass. (From Wharton, L. In Ridley JH (Ed). Gynecologic Surgery: Safeguards, Errors, Salvage. 2nd ed. Baltimore: Williams and Wilkins, 1981, with permission.)

junction. This is a common location of ureteral injury. Relatively few clinicians appreciate the fact that the ureter lies in direct contact with the anterior vaginal wall, and that mobilizing the bladder off the cervix and vagina is important in retracting the ureter out of the operative field.

Ureteral injuries can occur in this area when the surgeon operates under the assumption that staying close to the cervix will protect the ureter. The anatomy of this region can be distorted by several common conditions. Direct identification of the ureter is often necessary if injury to it is to be avoided. The most common pathology distorting the anatomy in this region is a uterine leiomyoma. A fibroid tumor lying along the lateral aspect of the cervix can dissect into the broad ligament and come into direct contact with the ureter (Fig. 16.3). Cysts in the broad ligament, such as Gartner's duct cysts, can do the same thing. When the anatomy is abnormal, the ureter must be identified in the distorted area. Simply identifying the ureter at the pelvic sidewall is not enough.

The ureter may be palpated here by placing the fingers in the cul-de-sac and the thumb anterior to the cardinal ligament. By ''milking'' the tissue of the cardinal ligament between thumb and fingers from the base of the ligament toward the uterine artery, the characteristic snap of the ureter can be felt (Fig. 16.4). The ureter is easiest to feel in elderly individuals with atrophic connective tissue in the ligament. Once this is learned the ureter can be located easily, even in young women whose cardinal ligaments are more dense. The course of the ureter may be followed from the uterine artery to its entry into the bladder using these techniques.

The ureter must be dissected out of the cardinal ligament if the anatomy of this area is distorted by a leiomyoma, a broad ligament cyst, or other pathology. The technique for doing this is similar to that used during radical hysterectomy. The ureter should be identified on the pelvic peritoneum as it enters the ureteral tunnel in the broad ligament. The size of the tunnel should then be enlarged. This can be done by carefully spreading the tips of a hemostatic forceps placed into the tunnel, or by gentle dissection with a finger. Once this is done, the uterine artery overlying the tunnel can be identified, ligated, and transected to

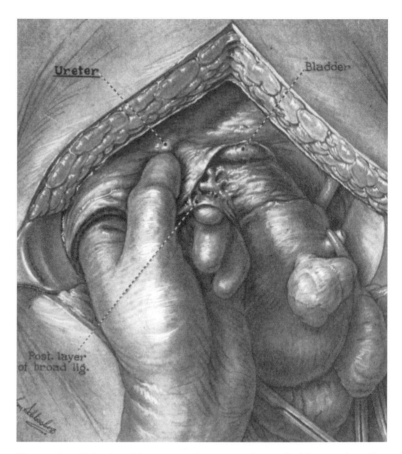

Figure 16.4 Palpation of the ureter as it traverses the cardinal ligament by rolling it between the thumb and index finger. (From Wharton, LR. Gynecology Including Female Urology. 2nd ed. Philadelphia: WB Saunders, 1947, with permission.)

Recognizing and Repairing Ureteral Injuries

How to Recognize Damage to the Ureter During the Course of an Operation

unroof the ureter. This process of ligating and dividing the tissue above the ureter should be continued until the anatomy is clearly defined. The uterus and its attached mass can then be removed safely. When a large myoma fills the pelvis and makes dissection difficult, it is sometimes easier to enucleate the mass to gain better exposure before attempting to remove the cervix; however, this should only be done after the ureter has been located. If the ureter cannot be identified during a difficult case, do not hesitate to ask for help! The assistance of another surgeon can help improve exposure in the operative field and another set of eyes will often help clarify a puzzling anatomic situation. Dogged persistence with an operation in the face of uncertain anatomic relationships will eventually result in ureteral injury.

Despite the use of all precautions, suspicion may arise that the ureter has been damaged during the course of an operation. Sometimes this is obvious: urine may fill the operative field or peristalsis may be seen at the end of a transected ureter. **Difficult cases should prompt the surgeon to *look* for possible injury, even though no obvious damage has been recognized.** When there is dense scarring in the area of ureteral dissection, when the ureter has been difficult to identify, or when a parametrial pedicle has come untied and re-establishment of hemostasis in the broad ligament has been necessary, the integrity of the ureter should be confirmed before concluding the operation.

If the ureter is dilated above the level of the operation, this indicates obstruction; however, absence of dilation does not ensure the absence of injury. The simplest test for determining ureteral patency is intravenous injection of 5 ml of indigo-carmine dye with observation of efflux of the dye through the ureteral orifice into the bladder. Methylene blue dye should *not* be given intravenously, since it can produce significant toxic effects, including methemoglobinemia. It usually takes 5–10 minutes for indigo-carmine dye to appear in the bladder, sometimes longer. If the ureter has been manipulated extensively during the course of the operation, its peristalsis may be reduced, prolonging the time necessary for the dye to appear. Sometimes intravenous injection of a diuretic such as furosemide will speed up the appearance of dye whose progress along the ureter has been delayed for this reason. The ureteric orifices can be observed directly through a large cystotomy or through a cystoscope placed either transurethrally or through a small cystotomy incision. The telescopic lens of a cystoscope or hysteroscope can also be inserted into the bladder through a small incision to look for the reassuring efflux of blue dye. The dye must be observed to spurt out of each ureteric orifice. Merely finding dye in the bladder is not enough, since only one ureter may be patent.

If doubt about ureteral patency persists following an attempted dye test, or if the location of a ureteral obstruction must be determined, a catheter should be passed up the ureter in retrograde fashion. This can be done using a 6 or 8 Fr pediatric feeding tube or using a small 3 or 5 Fr whistle-tip ureteral catheter. If this catheter passes easily all the way up to the kidney and there is free drainage of urine from the catheter, obstruction has been ruled out. If an obstruction is met or if the location of the catheter is uncertain, radiographic contrast dye can be injected through the catheter and x-rays taken to perform a retrograde pyelogram. Further dissection along the ureter while palpating the catheter running through it is also useful in determining the location of an obstruction. The surgeon must make sure that urine drains from the ureteral catheter. It is possible to pass a catheter without resistance through a defect in the ureteral wall and into the retroperitoneal space!

It must be emphasized that these procedures should be performed when there is any doubt about the presence of a ureteral injury. The desire to "get on with the next case" should be resisted until it is clear that no injury has occurred. Ureteral injuries have the best prognosis when they are recognized and corrected intraoperatively. A delay of several days means the development of progressive hydronephrosis, deterioration of renal function, and the possibility of severe infection—all of which can jeopardize the survival of the kidney.

Intraoperative Repair of Ureteral Injury

Several different types of ureteral damage can occur during surgery. The ureter can be kinked so that urine flow becomes more difficult, but not impossible. A ligature can constrict the lumen of the urethra without actually damaging it. This can occur without an actual needle injury to the ureter itself. More serious damage occurs if the ureter is crushed or torn. The most severe injury is complete transection of the ureter. Although meticulous dissection of the ureter will usually avoid this mishap, it will sometimes occur even in the most capable hands. If obstruction has occurred due to ureteral kinking, dilation of the ureter will often be found proximal to the point of kinkage. If this is recognized, the sutures which have caused the deformity can usually be removed, restoring the normal position of the ureter and allowing it to drain properly. If the ureter has been ligated with an encircling suture, the suture can be removed and the wall of the ureter inspected to see if it has been crushed. If it is healthy, exhibits peristalsis, and is devoid of injury nothing further needs to be done. If there is obvious damage to the ureter, surgical repair may be necessary. If the ureter is crushed or damaged, but not lacerated, placement of a ureteral stent for 4–6 weeks may allow it to heal. Unless the surgeon has significant experience in the evaluation and management of ureteral injuries, intraoperative consultation with an experienced urologist is advisable before making this decision. If the wall of the ureter has been lacerated, the decision must be made as to whether or not this laceration can be repaired without compromising the lumen, or whether the damaged area should be excised and a ureteral reanastomosis or reimplantation performed. If

TABLE 16.2. Indicators of Ureteral Obstruction

Flank pain
CVA tenderness
Unexpected fever or hematuria
Persistent abdominal distension or ileus
Lower abdominal mass suggesting a "urinoma"
Creatinine elevation >0.6 mg/dl above preoperative level

there is a small well-defined incision in the wall of the ureter, a direct repair should be carried out. Significant lacerations or complete transection require ureteral reimplantation or reanastomosis. Injuries occurring below the pelvic brim or within the distal 4–5 cms of the urethra are managed best by reimplanting the ureter into the bladder. Sometimes the reimplantation will be straightforward, but sometimes adjunctive surgical techniques, such as a Boari flap or psoas hitch, will be necessary in order to obtain the best possible result. Ligation of the ureter at the pelvic brim may require its reanastomosis, but ureteral reimplantation is preferred because it has a lower incidence of stricture and stenosis. Transureteroureterostomy, in which the damaged ureter is implanted into the unaffected ureter on the contralateral side, should be avoided in the primary repair of ureteral injuries. It is better to leave the contralateral ureter alone and avoid the possibility of impairing the drainage of the contralateral kidney. This may only make a bad situation worse.

It is not the object of this chapter to provide a comprehensive surgical discussion of ureteral injury and its repair, but all gynecologic surgeons should be familiar with the principles underlying these techniques. If a surgeon encounters a ureteral injury and is uncomfortable with its repair, he should get help from either a more experienced gynecologic surgeon or an experienced urologist.

Recognition of Ureteral Obstruction in the Postoperative Period

Prompt postoperative detection of a ureteral injury that was not recognized during an operation can prevent long-term renal damage. Injuries which are detected postoperatively will present with signs of obstruction or fistula formation. Necrosis of an injured ureter can lead to loss of urine through the vagina. This usually develops 1–2 weeks after surgery. Leakage from an injured bladder may either be immediate or delayed. Evaluation of the patient with vaginal urine loss following surgery is discussed later in this chapter.

Factors which may indicate the possibility of ureteral obstruction are listed in Table 16.2. A transient rise in serum creatinine may occur during the first 24–48 hours after a ureter has been ligated. Recent studies have shown that there is a transient rise in serum creatinine of 0.6 mg/dl or more after ureteral injury. This transient change in creatinine is best detected on the first postoperative day. Whenever ureteral obstruction is suspected an intravenous urogram should be obtained (Fig. 16.5). This is the most sensitive and specific test for detecting abnormalities. An ultrasound study may detect hydronephrosis which is suggestive of ureteral damage, but it will not detect a ureter that has been injured and is leaking into the peritoneal cavity, or one that is obstructed but has not yet produced calyceal dilatation. Patients who are allergic to iodinated contrast material may still be able to undergo a study using one of the newer noniodinated contrast media. If an obstructed ureter is detected, decompression of the kidney by placing a percutaneous nephrostomy tube may allow temporary relief of symptoms and help preserve renal function until definitive repair can be carried out. Since placement of this tube is done most easily while contrast is still in the calyces, the possibility that this may be necessary should be discussed with the radiologists at the time the initial intravenous urogram is obtained.

Management of Ureteral Obstruction Detected Postoperatively

The management of ureteral injury which is first recognized after surgery will depend upon the site of injury and its probable cause. Partial ureteral obstruction is often treatable by careful retrograde passage of a ureteral stent during

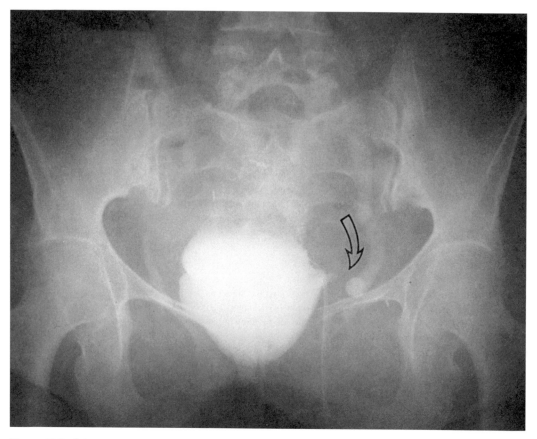

Figure 16.5 Intravenous urogram revealing an obstruction of the left ureter as a complication of a paravaginal repair operation for stress incontinence. The filling defect between the left ureter and the bladder indicates the point of obstruction (*arrow*). The bladder has filled with contrast through the unobstructed right ureter.

cystoscopy. In some cases it may be necessary to pass a stent in antegrade fashion via a percutaneous nephrostomy. The stent may then be left in place until the edema of surgery has resolved and absorbable sutures have resorbed. If a complete obstruction is identified, the first priority must be prompt decompression of the kidney to prevent renal damage. In the past this meant prompt return to the operating room for surgical restoration of ureteral patency, and this is still often the best policy. However, the development of percutaneous methods of renal decompression have meant that temporizing is possible in selected cases without undue risk to the kidney. If the obstruction is probably due to kinking of the ureter by an absorbable suture, for example, the kidney can be decompressed and observed to see if the ureter will open spontaneously as the suture dissolves. Ureteral patency can be checked by injection of radiographic contrast through the nephrostomy tube. If the ureter is still not patent after 8 weeks, surgical repair is indicated.

Some patients in whom the ureter has been transected and the injury has gone unrecognized will develop urinary ascites or peritonitis. This demands prompt surgical exploration. Renal decompression by percutaneous nephrostomy is not effective in these cases and does not play a role in their management. If urine leaks into the peritoneal cavity these patients will usually develop classical signs of ''chemical '' peritoneal irritation. Some patients, however, will develop a retroperitoneal accumulation of urine or ''urinoma.''

Postoperative Vaginal
Discharge of Urine

When urine is found escaping from the vagina postoperatively, a ureterovaginal or vesicovaginal fistula should be suspected. The first step in identifying the source of urine leakage is placing a dilute solution of methylene blue dye (5 ml in 1,000 ml of normal saline or sterile water) into the bladder to see if the fluid that escapes is colored. If it is colored then it probably is coming from the bladder. If the fluid is clear then it is probably coming from the ureter. If doubt exists as to whether or not the clear liquid is actually urine, a sample of the fluid may be collected and sent for measurement of creatinine. If creatinine is found in the sample in excess of the serum creatinine level, then the fluid is undoubtedly urine. Vaginal discharge does not contain creatinine. Careful inspection of the vagina may disclose the site at which the fistula has occurred, but often the only thing that is seen is a generalized ooze coming from the crevices of the vaginal apex after hysterectomy. Even if a vesicovaginal fistula has been found, an IVP should be performed to make sure that there has been no damage to a ureter. Cystoscopy will generally help identify the location of the fistula, and if indigo-carmine dye is given intravenously at the same time, ureteral patency can also be assessed. Vesicovaginal fistulas are discussed later in this chapter.

Bladder During Abdominal Surgery

Identification and Protection from Injury

The bladder lies directly adjacent to the anterior portion of the cervix and upper vagina. When it is distended, it covers the entire anterior surface of the uterus, as can easily be seen during any abdominal ultrasound examination. The empty bladder is a dish-shaped organ nestled within the bowl of the pelvis with the pubic bone anteriorly, the pelvic walls laterally, and the cervix and vagina posteriorly. It conforms to the shape of the structures that surround it. The anterior margin of the bladder is reflected onto the anterior abdominal wall, and is adjacent to the abdominal peritoneum. It projects onto the abdominal wall in the shape of a triangle, with the apex pointed towards the umbilicus. It is attached to the anterior abdominal wall by the remnant of allantois, the urachus. The posterior margin of the bladder lies on the cervix.

The bladder may be injured during surgical entry into the abdomen when the peritoneum is incised. Since the bladder extends cephalad furthest in the midline, it is best to enter the peritoneal cavity slightly to one side. The bladder should be drained, usually with an indwelling transurethral catheter, before the abdominal incision is made. Once the peritoneum has been opened, the bladder wall can be palpated to identify its upper margin and keep it free from injury as the peritoneal incision is extended. The upper margin of the bladder may also be identified by pulling up on the Foley catheter balloon and advancing the end of the catheter until it comes to rest against the uppermost margin of the bladder. The bladder often lies higher on the abdominal wall than the surgeon expects because of previous cesarean section or by being carried upwards by the growth of uterine leimyomas. Occasionally a patent urachus or a urachal cyst may be encountered, altering the anatomy of the bladder in this region. Once the peritoneum has been opened, the upper margin of the bladder can be felt as a distinct ridge if the tissue along the inferior margin of the incision is palpated between the fingers and thumb. If the peritoneum is elevated and transilluminated, the bladder will not permit the passage of light.

The posterior wall of the bladder lies on the uterine cervix and vagina. If the bladder is to expand when it is distended, the bladder wall must be free from the cervix and uterus. The loose areolar plane, called the vesicocervical space, allows this to occur. This cleavage plane also permits the bladder to be separated from the genital tract during hysterectomy or cesarean section. Because the peritoneum is less distensible than the bladder, a fold of peritoneum can be found on the cervix above the empty bladder. This is the fold that is lifted off the cervix as the bladder expands.

The vesicocervical space should be entered surgically in the area between the bladder and the top of the reflection of the peritoneum onto the uterus. The upper edge of the bladder can be protected from injury here by identifying it carefully before the peritoneum is incised. The bladder can be seen as a raised ridge on the surface of the uterus, and its upper margin can be palpated as a distinct ridge. If the position of the bladder is uncertain it can be filled simply by raising the drainage bag above the level of the Foley catheter, allowing the urine to drain back into the bladder and distend it. The end of the catheter can also be grasped through the bladder and pushed up to the top of the dome to determine its uppermost limit.

The incision in the peritoneal reflection should be made between the upper margin of the bladder and the top of the reflection. When this is done correctly, the peritoneum can be separated from the anterior surface of the uterus with ease because of the natural cleavage plane which exists in this area. The peritoneum above this region is densely adherent to the uterus and can not be elevated in this way. Once the incision has been made in this peritoneal fold, the bladder can be separated from the anterior surface of the uterus by spreading the tips of the scissors along the natural lines of tissue cleavage in this area or by using gentle dissection with a sponge or finger. Heavy-handed blunt dissection using a wadded gauze sponge on a ring forceps should be avoided. This technique may shear the tissue unnaturally, leaving part of the bladder adherent to the uterus. Many vesicovaginal fistulae are created during hysterectomy by improper separation of the bladder from the cervix and uterus. Special care should be used in patients who have undergone a previous lower segment cesarean section, since the bladder may be more adherent. If the bladder does not separate easily from the cervix, the surgeon must reassess the situation and decide whether or not the proper cleavage plane has been found. The anatomy should be properly identified before the operation continues.

Dissection is carried out best in the midline because this is the least vascular area. Once the bladder has been separated beyond the lower margin of the cervix, the space thus created should be widened to elevate the entire bladder off the cervix. This can be done by placing a finger from each hand in the midline space and separating them laterally. This not only elevates the bladder, but also carries the ureters laterally, out of the surgical field. This is critical if ureteral as well as bladder injury is to be avoided. It should not be overlooked. Since the blood vessels in this region run transversely from the pelvic wall towards the midline, lateral separation of tissue from the midline is better than dissection in a craniocaudal direction and is less likely to result in bleeding. In women who have had a previous cesarean section, the cleavage plan is often obliterated in the midline and can sometimes be found more easily by lateral dissection. Once the bladder is freed on each side it is usually easier to free the adherent area by sharp dissection.

The most common distortions of bladder position in this area are due to previous cesarean section. The upper margin of the bladder can be carried high on the surface of the uterus and can easily be injured if it is not carefully identified before the dissection is begun. Lower uterine segment leiomyomas may distend the uterus underneath the bladder, elevating its upper margin to an abnormally high position. Specific identification of the actual position of the bladder reflection prior to dissecting this area is the key to avoiding bladder injury.

Recognition and Repair of Bladder Injury

The surgeon must always be alert to the possibility of bladder injury. The bladder should be filled to look for leaks when the possibility of bladder injury exists. This should be done often enough that it can be carried out as a routine procedure without undue frustration for the operating room nurses. Simply filling the bladder with several hundred ml of sterile saline may be enough to confirm its integrity. If small defects are suspected another solution may be better. Sterile infant formula, such as Similac or Enfamil, is available in all hospital newborn nurseries and a supply should be kept in the operating room. Sterile milk does not stain tissues as do methylene blue or indigo-carmine. This can be a great advantage when the surgeon is attempting to find and repair small leaks in the

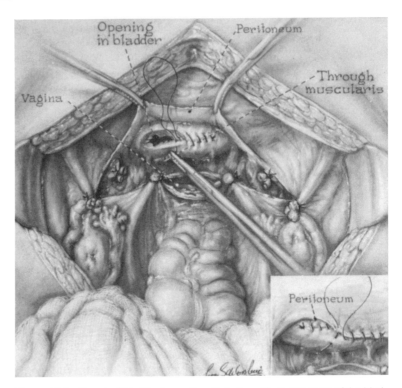

Figure 16.6   Repair of bladder laceration. Note the wide mobilization of the bladder to keep tension off of the suture line. (From Mattingly RF, Thompson JD (Eds). TeLinde's Operative Gynecology. 6th ed. Philadelphia: JB Lippincott, 1985, with permission.)

bladder. If dye or milk is not available do not hesitate to fill the bladder with saline. When in doubt, look! This can easily be done by connecting end of the transurethral catheter to the cylinder of a bulb syringe and pouring 200–300 ml of water into the bladder. A bag of cystoscopy fluid can also be attached to the Foley catheter and used to fill the bladder. If doubt still exists after bladder filling, the anterior wall of the bladder should be opened and its cavity carefully explored. This can be done easily by grasping the balloon of the Foley catheter, elevating it to the dome of the bladder, and then incising the bladder with an electrocautery blade or knife until the balloon is clearly seen and the interior of the bladder identified. When treated properly, the bladder is a very forgiving organ. With appropriate postoperative drainage, an anterior cystotomy in the dome of the bladder will heal uneventfully. The benefit of identifying and repairing an inadvertent cystotomy is worth the extra time and effort involved.

Once an injury has been identified, it must be repaired in a way that will assure complete healing and will avoid ureteral occlusion. Injuries to the dome of the bladder are usually simple and straightforward. When injuries have occurred near the base of the bladder, care must be taken to make sure that the ureters are not compromised by the repair. Once the defect has been identified, it should be elevated with Babcock clamps and carefully inspected around its entire circumference. All layers of the bladder must be identified (serosa, muscularis, and mucosa). Once this has been done the submucosa and mucosa can be approximated using a layer of fine chromic catgut suture (00 or 000) running from just beyond one lateral margin of the defect to just beyond the edge of the defect on the other side (Fig. 16.6). A second layer of stitches should be placed in the muscularis to imbricate the first suture line. Following the repair, the bladder should be drained with either a suprapubic or transurethral catheter.

Suprapubic catheters should generally be placed through a separate stab incision, rather than through the cystotomy, particularly if the injury was extensive. Drainage should be carried out at least until the hematuria clears, and most surgeons prefer to leave the catheter to open drainage for 5–10 days, depending on the location and nature of the injury. Because they lie in a dependent portion of the bladder, injuries occurring in the bladder base require longer drainage than do simple cystotomies in the bladder dome. Prolonged drainage for 7–10 days should be the rule if the defect is irregular or has occurred in an irradiated bladder.

If the injury occurs near the bladder base, closure of the defect can occlude one or both ureters. If ureteral patency cannot be assured before closing the bladder, the opening of the cystotomy should be extended away from the bladder base until it is large enough to see the ureteric orifices and insure that their integrity has not been compromised. This is done most easily by intravenous injection of indigo-carmine dye. If the repair is difficult, the dome of the bladder can be opened and catheters can be placed into the ureters to help identify their course and location.

Who should repair bladder injuries? As in the case of ureteral injuries this is more a political than a practical question. Most gynecologic surgeons have far more experience in operating on the bladder than in operating on the ureters, due to the need to mobilize the bladder during vaginal and abdominal hysterectomy as well as during cesarean section. When a simple cystotomy with clear surgical exposure has occurred, repair of the injury is straightforward. The patient is best served by an expeditious closure of the injury by the operating surgeon. If the cystotomy is in a difficult location or close to the ureters, or if the surgeon is uncomfortable with the repair, the help of a more experienced surgeon should be obtained. In no case is the patient served best by having a poor repair done by a surgeon with a false sense of pride.

Bladder and Ureter During Vaginal Surgery

Identification and Protection from Injury

Identification of the ureter during vaginal surgery is just as important as it is during abdominal operations. An excellent way to become familiar with the vaginal location of the ureter is to palpate it during a pelvic examination under general anesthesia prior to the start of the case. The ureters enter the bladder at the two upper apices of the urinary trigone. The lower apex of the trigone is occupied by the urethra. The distance from each ureter to the urethra is approximately 2 cm. The ureterovesical junction where each ureter enters the bladder is located 2 cm from the urethrovesical junction. The ureter lies immediately adjacent to the anterior vaginal wall in the upper one-third of the vagina, having entered this area just lateral to the cervix. The ureter can be palpated by placing an examining finger in the midline of the vagina just below the cervix and then moving both hands together towards the pelvic sidewall, milking the intervening tissue between opposing fingers (Fig. 16.7). The characteristic snap of the ureter can be detected when this is done. This is easiest to do on thin individuals, but the location of the ureter can be detected in most patients with practice. Another way of learning the location of the ureters is to palpate the anterior vagina during cystoscopy. The ureteric orifices can elevated by an examining finger under direct vision, and the position of the finger in the vagina can then be ascertained. An appreciation of how close the ureter lies to the vaginal mucosa will help the surgeon protect it during operations such as anterior colporrhaphy.

The location of the ureters is extremely important during vaginal hysterectomy. It is easiest to determine the position of the ureter after entry into the anterior peritoneal cul-de-sac. If a Deaver or Heaney retractor has been placed in the lateral vaginal fornix, the ureter can be palpated between the retractor and the surgeon's fingers as the parametrial tissues are examined. Knowing the position of the ureter helps prevent it from being injured both while the uterus is being removed as well as during subsequent procedures to help support the vagina in cases of severe prolapse. The cardinal and uterosacral ligaments can be shortened and then reattached to the vaginal cuff to help elevate and support

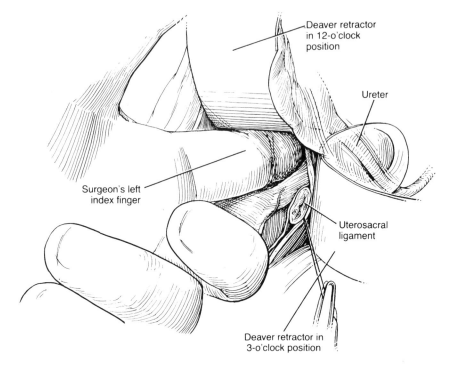

Figure 16.7 Palpation of the ureter during vaginal hysterectomy. (From Lee RA. Atlas of Gynecologic Surgery. Philadelphia: WB Saunders, 1992, p. 135, with permission.)

the vagina, but it is dangerous to do this without knowing where the ureters lie. The ureter can sometimes also be located if two fingers are placed in the posterior cul-de-sac and the peritoneum of the pelvic sidewall is palpated just anterior to the uterosacral ligaments.

Bladder injury during vaginal surgery is most likely to occur during anterior colporrhaphy and entry into the anterior cul-de-sac during vaginal hysterectomy. Identification of the bladder prior to performing a vaginal hysterectomy can be accomplished by exerting firm downward traction on the cervix while the anterior vaginal wall is palpated against it. The lower edge of the bladder can be felt as a slightly raised ridge along the anterior vaginal wall near the cervix where the smooth mucosa that covers the cervix meets the rugose vaginal epithelium. If the cervix is moved in and out, a line of demarcation which identifies the bladder can usually be seen between the vagina and the cervix.

The incision at the start of a vaginal hysterectomy should be made at the lower border of the bladder and carried deeply enough so that the vesicocervical space is entered, but not so deeply that the cervix itself is incised. This takes some practice. The proper plane of dissection in the vesicocervical space can be entered safely by elevating the loose tissue of the supravaginal septum and incising it with Mayo scissors. The tips of the scissors should be pointed down towards the cervix, not up where they might injure the bladder. If the scissors are held tangentially to the cervix it is virtually impossible to cut into the cervix too deeply. The loose tissue of the supravaginal septum that has been elevated by the forceps can be incised at the same time. Once the proper plane has been reached, the dissection can be carried out by gently spreading the tips of the scissors. Because this plane is composed of loose areolar tissue, dissection should be easy. If it is not, or if it is difficult to displace the bladder in this area the surgeon should be concerned that the dissection is in the wrong plane. Identification of the bladder is sometimes made easier by passing a curved sound through the urethra and into the bladder until it stops at the bladder edge between the vagina and the uterus. If a uterine prolapse is present, the surgeon's fingers can be inserted through a posterior colpotomy incision, brought over the top of the broad ligament lateral to the uterus, and hooked downward into the anterior cul-de-sac. This brings the peritoneum into view between the bladder and the uterus.

Recognition and Repair of Bladder Injury

Many surgeons empty the bladder after prepping the vagina for surgery but do not then place an indwelling catheter, allowing some urine to accumulate in the bladder. This helps to identify any inadvertent cystostomy. Once the anterior cul-de-sac has been entered successfully, an indwelling Foley catheter can be used to drain the bladder for the rest of the operation. If a cystotomy does occur, it will be recognized by the gush of urine escaping from the bladder as it is perforated. When this occurs, the edges of the bladder should be identified and their relationship to the ureteral orifices determined. During vaginal hysterectomy, cystotomies usually occur while entry into the anterior peritoneal cavity is being attempted. The perforation is typically located in the posterior bladder several centimeters above the level of the ureteric orifices, which can often be seen through the hole which has been made. If they cannot be seen, they can be palpated through the cystotomy with a finger, or located by cystoscopy. After the location of the laceration has been established in relation to the ureters, the opening can be repaired in two or three layers using absorbable sutures. The closure technique is similar to that described for repairing a bladder laceration during abdominal surgery. After the repair has been completed, the bladder can be filled with sterile milk or colored saline to test the integrity of the repair. Cystoscopy should be carried out to confirm the patency of the ureters after intravenous administration of 5 ml of indigo-carmine dye. The bladder should be drained until any hematuria clears. Usually 7–10 days of continuous postoperative drainage is advisable because the risk of fistula formation is greater with injuries of the bladder base as opposed to those of the bladder dome.

Bladder and Ureter During Retropubic Repair Operations

During dissection in the retropubic space it is important to be able to identify the bladder and the urethra as well as the ureters. Opening the space of Retzius requires retraction of the bladder away from the pubic bones and the pelvic sidewalls. This exposes the ventral surface of the bladder. The urethra is easy to palpate if a transurethral Foley catheter is in place. Pulling gently on the tubing will bring the catheter balloon down to the level of the bladder neck and will clearly identify the location of the urethra.

Because the space of Retzius is a potential, rather than an actual, space, it exists as a cleavage plane of loose areolar tissue between the pubic bones and the pelvic sidewall. This space is easy to open and expose by gentle blunt dissection in patients who have not had previous bladder neck surgery. As the dissection is carried laterally to the pelvic sidewalls, the obturator internus muscle and the white paravaginal fascia attaching to the arcus tendineus can be seen. Once these structures have been identified, the edge of the bladder can be easily identified by the dusky network of veins which run along its lateral margin, medial to the side of the pelvis. The lateral margin of the bladder can also be palpated in the space of Retzius. With one hand in the vagina and one hand in the retropubic space, the edge of the bladder will pop through the examiner's hands as they are moved laterally. The bulb of the Foley catheter can also be pushed up into the body of the bladder until it comes to rest at its lateral limits. Identification of the avascular fascial plane lying above the vaginal wall and lateral to the bladder is extremely important, because this is where the sutures should be placed during a Burch retropubic urethropexy or a paravaginal defect repair. If it is difficult to define the anatomy, the bladder should be opened and its lateral margins identified clearly.

The ureter can also be palpated in the space of Retzius. A hand in the vagina and a hand in the retropubic space can be used to palpate the intervening tissues in similar fashion to that seen in Figure 16.7. Starting in the midline near the cervix or the vaginal apex, the examining hands should be brought together and moved towards the pelvic sidewall, where the characteristic snap of the ureter can be felt.

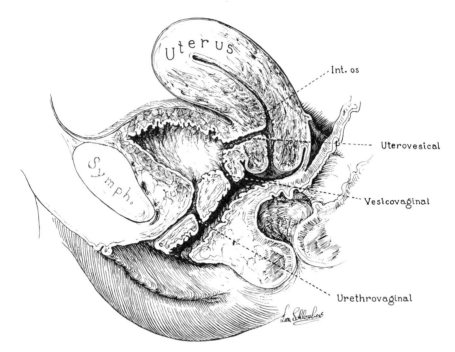

Figure 16.8   Types and locations of common genitourinary fistulae in women. (From Mattingly RF, Thompson JD (Eds). TeLinde's Operative Gynecology. 6th ed. Philadelphia: JB Lippincott, 1985, with permission.)

Injury to the bladder during retropubic urethropexy is most common in patients who have had a previous bladder neck operation. The bladder can be densely adherent to the inner surface of the pubic bone in such cases, and attempts at blunt dissection of the space of Retzius often results in a cystotomy. Where dense scar tissue exists, sharp dissection should be used to separate the bladder from the surrounding structures. This dissection is safest if it is kept right against the inner surface of the pubic bone. It is often possible to move laterally into areas which are not affected and scarred down. Freeing these areas first often helps to identify the anatomy better. Sometimes it is necessary to open the bladder in order to identify its location accurately. Do not hesitate to do this when needed. If an unintentional cystotomy occurs, do not hesitate to utilize it! Extending the opening in the bladder until all of the relevant anatomy can be seen can turn a maloccurrence into a temporary surgical asset. The bladder can then be left open until the end of the operation to help identify the appropriate anatomy and to allow for correct suture placement. Leaving the bladder open also allows the surgeon to see the efflux of indigo-carmine dye from each ureteric orifice after the suspension operation has been completed. It also makes ureteral catheterization easy if this needs to be done.

Postoperative Fistulae

The patient who has urine leaking from her vagina after surgery has a fistula until proven otherwise. Most commonly this is a vesicovaginal fistula, but cervicovaginal fistulae occur after cesarean section, and urethrovaginal vistulae may occur after excision of a urethral diverticulum (Fig. 16.8). The differentiation of a vesicovaginal from a ureterovaginal fistula has been discussed previously, but some aspects of the management of these conditions is appropriate here.

Vesicovaginal Fistula

The location of a postoperative vesicovaginal fistula can usually be determined through a combination of cystoscopy and physical examination with the bladder filled with colored saline or sterile milk. A plan for repair can then be made. Opinions vary as to the timing of the repair. Advocates of early intervention maintain that early repair is usually successful and avoids much of the suffering experienced by the patient who is waiting for her surgery. This is attractive to the surgeon responsible for the injury, as well as to the patient who is suffering total incontinence as a result of this injury. In uncomplicated straightforward cases, this is a reasonable approach. However, the surgeon should not be forced into an early repair under unfavorable circumstances. Advocates of delayed repair suggest placing an indwelling catheter to prevent overdistension of the bladder and to allow inflammation and induration to subside at the site of the injury. This will make surgical repair less difficult and may also allow a small fistula to close spontaneously. A period of 2 months should be adequate to see if this will occur. Cellulitis of the vaginal cuff should be treated vigorously. The patient should have adequate nutrition and proper care for other medical problems that may coexist.

If the fistula does not close spontaneously, then it must be repaired. The exact location of the fistula relative to the ureters should be identified prior to the operation. The Latzko partial colpocleisis operation produces excellent results using a vaginal approach for straightforward posthysterectomy vesicovaginal fistulae. This lessens the recovery time needed after the repair. Transabdominal fistula repairs tend to be favored by urologists, but they generally do not have a higher rate of success than a vaginal operation performed by an experienced fistula surgeon. Abdominal fistula repairs have a higher operative morbidity and should be reserved for complex cases. *Either* approach is better in the hands of a surgeon skilled in its performance than a makeshift operation done by a surgeon who is unfamiliar with the techniques of fistula repair. The surgeon who is confronted with a problem with which he is not comfortable should get help from a more experienced surgeon.

Ureterovaginal Fistulae

If a ureterovaginal fistula is suspected, its location should confirmed by intravenous pyelography. Ureterovaginal fistulae frequently appear several weeks after the operation because ischemia and necrosis from ureteral trauma often take some time before they disrupt the ureter. An episode of postoperative pyelonephritis often heralds the development of a ureterovaginal fistula. Once the problem has been identified, expert urologic consultation should be sought. The principles of management for patients with a ureterovaginal fistula are as follows. If the ureter is patent and its continuity can be demonstrated from the kidney to the bladder, then a period of expectant management may be undertaken in selected cases. The fistula may close spontaneously; however, it is also possible that healing will lead to stricture formation and obstruct the flow of urine. If expectant management is undertaken, an IVP should be obtained every 2 or 3 weeks to make sure that obstruction is not developing. If obstruction does develop, a percutaneous nephrostomy tube should be placed, or immediate surgical repair undertaken, to make sure that the kidney is not damaged. If spontaneous closure does not occur, then reimplantation or reanastomosis of the ureter should be undertaken as described above.

SUGGESTED READING

Identification of Ureters and Ureteral Injuries

Brudenell M. The pelvic ureter. Proc R Soc Med 1977; 70: 188–90.

Cruikshank SH. Surgical method of identifying the ureters during total vaginal hysterectomy. Obstet Gynecol 1986; 67:277–80.

Donovan AJ, Gibson RA. Identification of ureteral ligation during gynecologic operations. Am J Obstet Gynecol 1973; 116:793–94.

Duchin HE. Intraoperative evaluation of urinary tract integrity. In Slate WG (Ed). Disorders of the Female Urethra and Urinary Incontinence, 2nd ed. Baltimore: Williams and Wilkins, 1982:224–33.

Hofmeister FJ. Pelvic anatomy of the ureter in relation to surgery performed through the vagina. Clin Obstet Gynecol 1982; 25:821.

Kaye KW, Goldberg ME. Applied anatomy of the kidney and ureter. Urol Clin North Am 1982; 9(1):3.

Notley RG. Ureteral morphology: Anatomic and clinical considerations. Urology 1978; 12:9.

Piscitelli JT, Simel DL, Addison WA. Who should have intravenous pyelograms before hysterectomy for benign disease? Obstet Gynecol 1987; 69:541.

Sampson JA. Ureteral fistulae as sequelae of pelvic operations. Surg Gynecol Obstet 1909; 8:479.

Timmons MC, Addison WA. Suprapubic teloscopy: Extraperitoneal intraoperative technique to demonstrate ureteral patency. Obstet Gynecol 1990; 75: 137–39.

Urinary Tract Injuries during Pelvic Surgery

Benson RC, Hinmann F, Jr., Urinary tract injuries in obstetrics and gynecology. Am J Obstet Gynecol 1955; 70:467.

Eisenkop SM, Richman R, Platt LD, Paul RH. Urinary tract injury during cesarean section. Obstet Gynecol 1982; 60: 591–96

Everett S, Mattingly RF. Urinary tract injuries resulting from pelvic surgery. Am J Obstet Gynecol 1956; 71:502.

Kohler FP, Uhle CA, MacKinney CC. Urinary tract injuries incidental to gynecologic procedures. Obstet Gynecol 1966; 28:867–72.

Langmade CF. Pelvic endometriosis and ureteral obstruction. Am J Obstet Gynecol 1975; 122:463–69

Lee RA, Symmonds RE. Ureterovaginal fistula. Am J Obstet Gynecol 1971; 109:1032.

Major FJ. Retained ovarian remnant causing ureteral obstruction. Obstet Gynecol 1968; 32:748.

Mann WJ, Arato M, Patsner B, et al. Ureteral injuries in an obstetrics and gynecology training program: Etiology and management. Obstet Gynecol 1988; 72:82.

Newell QU. Injury to ureters during pelvic operation. Ann Surg 1939; 109:48.

Pettit PD, Lee RA. Ovarian remnant syndrome: Diagnostic dilemma and surgical challenge. Obstet Gynecol 1988; 71:580.

St. Lezin MA, Stoller ML. Surgical ureteral injuries. Urology 1991; 38:497–506.

Stanhope CR, Wilson TO, Utz WJ, Smith LH, O'Brien PC. Suture entrapment and secondary ureteral obstruction. Am J Obstet Gynecol 1991; 164:1513–19.

Symmonds RE. Ureteral injuries associated with gynecologic surgery: Prevention and management. Clin Obstet Gynecol 1976; 19:623.

Van Nagell JR, Jr., Roddick JW, Jr., Vaginal hysterectomy, the ureter, and excretory urography. Obstet Gynecol 1972; 39:784.

Wesolowski S. Bilateral ureteral injuries in gynaecology. Br J Urol 1969; 41:666.

Management of Injuries

Beland G. Early treatment of ureteral injuries found after gynecological surgery. J Urol 1977; 118:25.

Ehrlich RM, Melman A, Skinner DG. The use of vesicopsoas hitch in urologic surgery. J Urol 1978; 119:322.

Fry DE, Milholen L, Harbrecht PJ. Iatrogenic ureteral injury: Options in management. Arch Surg 1983; 118:454.

Hedgegaard CK, Wallace D. Percutaneous nephrostomy: Current indications and potential uses in obstetrics and gynecology. Literature review and report of a case. Obstet Gynecol Surv 1987; 42:671.

Kaplan JO, Winslow OP, Sneider SE, et al. Dilatation of a surgically ligated ureter through percutaneous nephrostomy. Am J Roentgenol 1982; 39:188.

Marmar JL. The management of ureteral obstruction with silicone rubber splint catheters. J Urol 1970; 104:386.

Shapiro SR, Bennett AH. Recovery of renal function after prolonged unilateral ureteral obstruction. J Urol 1976; 115:136.

Turner-Warwick R, Worth PH. The psoas bladder hitch procedure for the replacement of the lower third of the ureter. Br J Urol 1969; 41:701.

Witters S, Cornelissen J, Vereecken R. Iatrogenic ureteral injury: Aggressive or conservative treatment. Am J Obstet Gynecol 1986; 155:582.

17   Absorbent Products and Catheters

If the treatment of urinary incontinence and retention were completely successful, absorbent products and catheters would not be necessary. However, complete elimination of incontinence is not always possible for all patients. Reduction in the amount of urine leakage may greatly improve the quality of life for a certain individual, but the use of absorbent products and catheters may still be necessary for managing that patient's problem. Voiding techniques may help a woman empty her bladder during the day, but she may still need to self-catheterize at bedtime to ensure that her bladder is emptied completely at least once per day and to reduce her need to get up to urinate at night. Some patients will choose to continue wearing a pad, rather than undergo surgery or take medications with bothersome side effects. The physician who sees women with bladder problems must, therefore, be familiar with a wide variety of pads, catheters, and appliances.

Absorbent Products

Physicians and other health care workers tend to believe that surgery, behavioral modification, pelvic floor re-education, and drug therapy are the most common treatments used in managing urinary incontinence. In a postal questionnaire study of noninstitutionalized people 60-years or older living in the community, Herzog and co-workers found that the most common method for managing incontinence was actually wearing absorbent products (Table 17.1). Many women have been using absorbent products long before they consult a health care professional for treatment. This fact has not been lost on the paper products industry. According to figures from the Agency for Health Care Policy and Research, almost *half a billion dollars* was spent on absorbent products specifically designed for urinary incontinence in 1987. Women are accustomed to using pads for menstrual flow and often turn to these same pads to manage urinary incontinence. It is estimated that one-third of the menstrual pads sold in the United States are actually used for managing urinary incontinence rather than menstruation. The advertising campaigns for absorbent pads in magazines and on television depict attractive middle-aged women becoming president of the PTA or having romantic walks on the beach with their spouse while wearing a certain brand of incontinence pad, and perpetuate the myth that urinary incontinence can be hidden successfully by wearing a diaper. Those women who are too embarrassed to seek medical help for their incontinence often continue to hide their problem with absorbent pads and lose out on beneficial treatment. For these reasons it is extremely important that anyone considering the use of absorbent products for their urinary incontinence should receive information regarding the many therapies that are available. Absorbent incontinence products should be labeled so that patients understand that incontinence is a *symptom* with many possible causes and that many forms of help are available for this problem. Patients should be encouraged to seek medical advice rather than just hide the problem with a protective pad.

Despite the vast amounts of money spent on absorbent products, there is little information on how to select the appropriate pad for a given patient, especially for incontinent women who are living in a noninstitutional setting. Menstrual pads

TABLE 17.1. Management of Urinary Incontinence by Community-dwelling People over Age 60[a,b]

Absorbent pads	55%
Locating the toilet upon arrival	42%
Voiding manipulation	28%
Diet and fluid manipulation	16%

[a] Herzog et al. J Am Geriatr Soc 1989; 37:339–47
[b] More than one response was permitted

are actually not designed to absorb fluids like urine, so they may not actually be the best product choice for dealing with urine loss; however, they are clearly less expensive than pads specifically designed for incontinence.

In order of increasing size and protection, absorbent products include panty liners, full-length pads, combination pad-and-pant systems, diaper-like garments, and bed pads. Some of the commercially available absorbent products are listed in Table 17.2. Menstrual pads and panty liners may be appropriate for women with small, infrequent loss. Women who lose larger amounts of urine should try products made especially for incontinence. Specially designed products are often expensive, but in many cases free samples can be obtained from the company, allowing patients to compare products. Table 17.3 lists sources for these free products, current as of 1992. For women with large, frequent loss, there are special panty/pad combinations which facilitate fixing and changing the pad. Diaper-like products are bulky and are often visible under clothing. While infant diapers are less expensive than adult diapers, they do not have adequate leg room for adults. Improper use of absorbent products may contribute to skin breakdown and infection; therefore, medical supervision should be obtained for patients who are using absorbent products as long-term management. Considerably more research needs to be done into the efficacy and cost effectiveness of pad use.

Some of the most important factors to consider in choosing an absorbent product for incontinence are: security (freedom from fear of leakage out the side or back of the pad), odor, capacity, cost, comfort, and visibility—ideally pads shouldn't be seen under most clothing. Relatively minor considerations include things such as whether the pad makes noise when the patient is walking and how well the pad stays in place. Costs vary greatly from product to product. This should be considered when patients are comparing products with each other. For people on fixed incomes, the cost of some products may be excessive: Some women spend $100, $200, or $300 *per month* on absorbent products for their incontinence. This explains why some women try to extend the life of a single pad by lining it with such things as toilet paper, flannel, paper towels, or a second smaller pad. Washcloths are often used for this purpose and have the advantages of being reusable, relatively inexpensive, and comfortable. Washcloths also stay in place (compared to toilet paper and paper towels); however, they do soak through because they lack the protective plastic backing found on most pads. This plastic backing is the reason that stacking two pads of the same size together does not offer additional protection against incontinence. Capacity is another important consideration in recommending the type of pad to be used. Stress incontinent women who lose 10–50 ml do not need to wear large capacity undergarments, but a person who spontaneously empties 400 ml of urine from her bladder with an unstable detrusor contraction will find panty liners inadequate for her needs.

Most companies have rejected the idea of treating pads with chemicals designed to reduce the odor of urine: Some industry representatives say that women would rather change the pad. Nonetheless, elimination of odor is an important factor in wearing absorbent products, and changing the pad at frequent intervals is expensive. Treatment with calcium acetate can reduce the urine odor associated

TABLE 17.2.   Commercially Available Absorbent Products for Urinary Incontinence[a]

	Pros	Cons	Capacity	Cost($)
Nonconventional products				
1. Toilet paper	Available	Shifts, uncomfortable	<5 ml	N/A
2. Paper towels	Available	Shifts, bulky, uncomfortable	<5 ml	N/A
3. Washcloth	Comfortable, stays in place	Soaks through	20 ml	N/A
4. Baby diapers	Holds a lot	Bulky, shifts	200 ml	.20
Panty liners: All of these products stay in place, but sides may leak				
1. Carefree			5 ml	.06
2. Always			2 ml	.06
3. Stayfree Minipads			4 ml	.12
4. Kotex Light Days Oval			5 ml	.05
Full-length pads (the first four are menstrual pads)				
1. Kotex curved	Holds a lot	Sides leak, bulky	40 ml	.13
2. Stayfree Maxi		Sides leak, bulky	30 ml	.13
3. Kotex Ultra Thin Maxi	Thin	Back leaks	20 ml	.14
4. Sure and Natural Ultra Thin Super	Holds a lot, thin	Stiff, sides leak	50 ml	.13
5. Always Double Plus With Wings	Holds a lot	Back leaks, bulky	70 ml	.21
6. Always Maxi With Wings		Back leaks, bulky	40 ml	.17
7. Surety Shield Extra Absorbent	Holds a lot	Bulky, shifts, sides leak	150 ml	.37
8. Depends Shield Regular Absorbency	Comfortable	Noisy, poor adhesive	90 ml	.21
9. Tranquility Trim-Shield Regular Absorbency		Bulky, back leaks, too wide	120 ml	.39

Pad-pant combinations

The first three products are tailored for adult women and have a waterproof panel in the panty. These are used with disposable and/or reusable pads and liners. The price varies based on quantity. There are multiple reusable briefs available which are designed to hold reusable liners and pads. Also, mesh stretch briefs are widely available to hold pads in place: These may be cooler and more discreet than the reusable briefs for many patients.

1. Contenta-Swan
2. Free & Active
3. Undercare
4. Other: Confidentially Yours, Curity, Dignity, Maxishield, Suretys, etc.

Diaper-like products

These products are usually held in place by their own straps and can be worn without an incontinence pant. Elastic legs add safety, but may be uncomfortable especially in obese women.

1. Gards At Ease Shields-Super	Thin, comfortable	Back leaks	200 ml	.25
2. Depends Undergarment Regular		Noisy, bulky, sides leak	200 ml	.30
3. Serenity Guards Super		Bulky, shifts, poor adhesive, back leaks	200 ml	.64

4. Others: Attends, Suretys, Curity, Tranquility, Promise, Provide, Wings, etc.

Bed pads

Chux (J&J)	Available	Does not keep patient dry	

Other disposable underpads are widely available and have similar characteristics. Reusable cloth bed covers with waterproof backing are widely available through diaper or linen services, and are listed in the HIP Resource Guide.

[a] Modified from Bierwith. Urologic Nursing 1992; 12:75–77 and the HIP Resource Guide

TABLE 17.3.   Sources for Free Samples of Absorbent Products

Health Related Products, Inc. (Wings briefs and underpads)
   1-800-752-7914
Humanicare International (Free and Active regular and super pads)
   1-800-631-5270
Hospital Specialty Co. (Gards-at-ease shields, diapers)
   1-800-321-9832
Personal Products Co. (J&J) (Serenity guards)
   1-800-526-3967
Principle Business Enterprises (Tranquility shields, underpants, pads)
   1-800-843-3385
Proctor and Gamble Co. (Attends briefs, undergarments, underpads)
   1-800-543-0480
Scott Health Care (Promise pad/pants combinations)
   1-800-992-9939 (trial products must be obtained through representative)

These companies are listed by HIP as sources for absorbent products, but do not currently offer free samples of pads to patients (1993):

Kimberly-Clark (Depends shields, underpads, fitted briefs, undergarments)
   1-800-558-6423
ICD Products, Inc. (Surety shields, undergarments, and panties)
   1-800-262-0042
DRIpride/Weyerhauser (Provide briefs, pant/pad combinations, underpads)
   1-800-253-3078

with diapers. Chlorophyllin copper complex (Derifil, Nullo, PALS, Whoo Noz), taken orally, is excreted in the urine. This helps to reduce the odor which urine may produce.

Absorbent products are widely used in nursing homes, and account for *half* of the direct care costs of incontinence among nursing home residents. The AHCPR guidelines for using absorbent pads in nursing homes (Table 17.4) emphasize that these products should be considered *only* after there has been a basic evaluation of the patient's incontinence by health professionals. Early dependency on absorbent pads may delay or prevent definitive treatment, and carries the risks of skin breakdown and urinary tract infection. Nevertheless, these products are probably preferable to indwelling urethral catheters, but the patient must be examined regularly for skin problems.

Finally, providers of medical care need to be familiar with absorbent products to help guide patients in the proper selection of pads. Although sample products are available from various companies, advice on which category of pad to try should be based on the patient's degree of incontinence, fastidiousness, and social needs, in addition to her financial situation. Washable and reusable products can save greatly on costs for some patients. Setting up a display that shows the various types of absorbent products allows patients to examine them before they try to get trial samples.

Catheters

Indwelling Catheters

The use of catheters for postoperative retention and voiding problems has been discussed in Chapter 13, "Bladder Emptying Problems." Catheters are also often used in patients with severe incontinence for whom other therapies have proven ineffective. Indwelling catheters for women include urethral catheters (Foley, 5 ml or 10 ml balloon) and suprapubic catheters. The Bonanno, Stamey, and Cystocath suprapubic catheters are generally placed only for acute use, such as after surgery, and are too narrow for chronic use. Chronic use of a suprapubic catheter requires placement of a larger Malecot or Foley catheter. In general, suprapubic catheters are better than urethral catheters for any patient who needs urinary drainage for more than just a few days. Suprapubic catheters are easier to keep clean at the site of entry into the body, and appear to have less problems with infection. They are also considerably more comfortable than

TABLE 17.4. Factors to be Considered When Using Absorbent Products for Urinary Incontinence[a]

1. Functional disability of the patient
   Can the patient not get to the toilet in time, or is unable to undress in time? These patients may be helped by timed voiding with assistance.
2. Type and severity of incontinence
   Is this a type of incontinence which might improve with alternative treatment? Overflow incontinence may benefit much more from intermittent catheterization than from diapering.
3. Gender
   Although condom catheters are an external option for men, similar devices for women are uncomfortable and ineffective.
4. Availability of caregivers
   It may be less expensive to have a caregiver help with prompted voiding than to change multiple diapers each day.
5. Failure with previous treatment programs
   If other methods have failed, then a really good diaper can provide the patient with dignity and effective protection.
6. Patient preference
   Many patients may prefer absorbent products to the alternative of surgery or medications; the physician must be familiar with all of these options to help in this decision-making
7. Comorbidity
   Is use of absorbent products going to reduce morbidity, or increase skin breakdown? Is a community dwelling elderly person going to fall if she is running to the toilet in the middle of the night? Sleeping with a bed pad and diaper may be an option, although environmental considerations, such as a bedside commode, should also be considered.

[a] Modified from the AHCPR Guidelines, 1992.

a transurethral catheter which rubs over the sensitive urethral epithelium and a balloon which keeps pushing up against the bladder neck. Suprapubic catheters also allow patients to void without removing the catheter, and this makes management much easier for patients who will regain their voiding function, such as after bladder neck surgery for incontinence. Urethral catheters are easier to insert because they do not require special expertise or a full bladder. Unfortunately, urethral catheters are often inserted by default, such as when a nurse calls a physician to report that somebody has become incontinent. Once the catheter has been inserted, a false impression is created that the problem has been managed successfully since the incontinence has been channeled into a catheter and skin breakdown is not occurring. Given the choice between absorbent products and chronic urethral catheterization, absorbent products are preferable. Protecting the skin from exposure to urine may be needed if absorbent pads are used for long periods of time. This can be done by using sprays and barrier creams which protect even broken skin from the irritation of stool and urine. It must be emphasized that reversible causes of incontinence should be excluded before pads and catheters are used as primary management tools for incontinence. Occasionally it may be necessary to place a urethral catheter temporarily to allow healing of irritative skin conditions caused by chronic urine exposure.

Indwelling catheters are also placed sometimes to manage chronic urinary retention. Intermittent catheterization, performed either by the patient herself or by a caregiver, is a better option. Occasionally a permanent suprapubic catheter is inserted in patients with severely contracted, hyperreflexic bladders (e.g., refractory multiple sclerosis) or for patients needing long-term bladder drainage. Catheter leg bags should be changed and cleaned once a day, so these patients need to be provided with at least two bags. Enterostomal therapy nurses are good sources of supplies such as fixing straps and deodorizing sprays and are invaluable resources for taking care of these patients.

It is not known whether silicone, latex, or teflon is the truly the best catheter

TABLE 17.5.   Sources for External Devices for Women with Urinary Incontinence

Collecting devices
  1. Hollister (perineal cup connected to bag)
      1-800-323-4060
  2. Dale Medical Products (female voiding device)
      1-800-343-3980
  3. Mackie Medical Enterprises, Inc. (female urinal)
      1-800-426-4012
External adhesive device
  1. Advanced Surgical Instruments (adhesive "patch" worn over the urethra, currently being tested, 1992)
Finger cots for covering vaginal tampons
  Widely available in pharmacies without prescription

material. All have been associated with stone formation, urethral erosion, bladder spasms, and infectious complications. Catheters should always be fixed in two places to prevent inadvertent (and disastrous!) removal, and to prevent kinking of the catheter. Most indwelling catheters are replaced monthly, although this has not been studied well. Chronic suprapubic catheters are usually wide (18 Fr) Foleys or Malecots to prevent obstruction with mucus. Once the fistula tract matures, the catheters may be replaced without difficulty on a monthly basis. If infection occurs, the catheter and drainage system must be replaced in its entirety. Great care should be taken to assure that the drainage bag is always dependent in order to prevent retrograde flow back into the bladder with its attendant risk of contamination and infection. There is no evidence that routine bladder irrigation reduces infection. This practice should be discouraged except in the case of catheter blockage.

Any person with a chronic indwelling catheter should be evaluated periodically to see if it can be removed, and such patients should be followed regularly by a nurse or other specialized health care professional.

Some incontinent patients may continue to leak around their urethral catheters, or may leak through the urethra in spite of having a suprapubic catheter. The common response is to insert a wider catheter with a bigger balloon into the urethra. This makes no sense. The most common reason patients leak in this situation is from detrusor overactivity, not a urethral catheter that "doesn't fit." Use of progressively larger catheters and bigger balloons can destroy the urethra and bladder neck, resulting in total incontinence. Patients who by-pass their catheters and continue to leak need *evaluation*, not a bigger catheter! Pending evaluation, a better short-term solution may be use of absorbent pads or external collection devices such as those listed in Table 17.5. In general, external collection devices are much more effective in managing incontinence among male than among female patients.

Intermittent Catheterization

Self-catheterization catheters should be designed specifically for this purpose. Red rubber or Foley catheters are both expensive and floppy, requiring the patient to hold the catheter close to the end to make the catheter stiff enough for insertion. This often compromises clean technique. Patients are often very apprehensive about beginning self-catheterization, having the erroneous impression that this technique requires a high level of medical training and is "something only doctors and nurses do." For women, self-catheterization should be presented as similar to learning how to put a tampon in the vagina: It is easy once you figure out the correct opening and the correct angle for insertion.

The Mentor female self-catheter (Fig. 13.5) has a polished eyelet and round, smooth tip which makes insertion easy and comfortable; other manufacturers of self catheterization catheters are listed in Table 17.6. These catheters may be stored in a glass of soapy water kept in the bathroom; the patient simply rinses off the soap immediately prior to insertion. For travel, catheters can be stored

TABLE 17.6.   Other Useful Product Sources

Enuresis alarm (bed pad with built-in sensor which sounds alarm when wet)
Nite Train-r, Koregon Enterprises, Inc. 1-800-544-4240
Wet-no-more, Travis Industries, Inc. 1-800-437-9233
Vaginal cones
Dacomed Corp. Minneapolis 1-800-328-1103
Self-catheters (usually must write a prescription for these)
Mentor Corp 1-800-328-3863
Bard Home Health Division 1-800-526-4930
Baxter General Healthcare Division 1-800-423-2311
Perineometers
Biotechnologies, Inc. 1-800-537-3779
Hollister, Inc. 1-800-323-4060
Interactive Medical Technologies, Inc. (Gynos perineometer) 1-800-752-8333.
Surgical drapes
3-M TUR1000 (sterile perineal drape with hole for urethral catheter, vaginal con-
dom to permit placement of vaginal finger during retropubic procedures)
Catheter security
Mentor Corp (E-Z hold, adhesive/velcro device for securing catheter to abdomen
or leg)
Plastic Measuring Hats Physicians Supply 1-800-453-3040

in a plastic toothbrush holder or plastic bag, washed with soap and water and dried prior to storing them again. After hand washing, the catheter should always be grasped at the noninsertion end. Most women prefer to stand with one leg up on the toilet seat to self-catheterize, although sitting backwards on the toilet is also useful because there is more room to "aim" the catheter. The catheters do not need to be boiled and can be used for several weeks at a time. Self-catheters should be replaced when sediment remains after thorough cleaning. A prescription is usually needed to obtain the catheters through a pharmacist or medical supply house.

Other Useful Products

Table 17.6 lists product sources for enuresis alarms, urinary "hats," vaginal cones, and other products discussed in this book. Plastic urinary hats are extraordinarily useful for keeping a frequency/volume chart, and help patients in bladder training because there is immediate feedback on voided volumes. Hats with a sloping insert for graduated volumes are easiest to read; avoid hats with marks that jump from 50–200 ml, since this is the very range of voided volumes in which we have the most interest. Vaginal cones for pelvic muscle exercises were originally intended to be sterilized and reused by other patients, but they are now marketed in sets of 5 cones for individual use. The current (1993) cost is $90 to physicians, $110 to individuals. This expense is still much less than most perineometers. Because pelvic muscle exercises should be continued long-term, the expense is acceptable to most patients.

The most complete product guide available is the *Resource Guide of Continence Products and Services* available through HIP, Inc. (Help for Incontinent People). This guide is revised regularly and can be obtained by writing to HIP at P.O. Box 544, Union, South Carolina 29379 (Telephone 1 803-579-7900; FAX 1-803-579-7902). The current price to cover the costs of printing and postage is $10.00, a bargain for the information it contains.

SUGGESTED READING

Baker J, Norton P. Evaluation of commercially available absorbent products for urinary incontinence. Proceedings of the 21st International Continence Society, Halifax, 1992.

Bennett D, Diokno A. Clean, intermittent self catheterization in the elderly. Urology (1984); 24(1):43–45.

Bierwith W. Which pad is for you? Urologic Nursing 1992; 12:75–77.

Brink C. Absorbent pads, garments, and management strategies. J Am Ger Soc (1990); 38:368–73.

Givens C, Wenzel R. Catheter associated urinary tract infections in surgical patients: A controlled study on the excess morbidity and costs. J Urol (1980); 124(5):646–48.

Haeker S. Disposable vs. reusable incontinence products. Geriatr Nurs (1985); 6:345–47.

Herzog A, Fultz N, Normolle D, Brock B, Diokno A. Methods used to manage urinary incontinence by older adults in the community. J Am Geriatr Soc 1989; 37:39–47.

Jeter K. Managing intractable urinary incontinence with absorbent products, devices, and procedures. Problems in Urology (1990); 4(1):124–37.

Lapides J, Diokno A, Silber S, Lowe B. Clean, intermittent self-catheterization in the treatment of urinary tract disease. J Urol (1972); 107(3):458–61.

Norberg A, Sandstrom S, Norberg B. The urine smell around patients with urinary incontinence. Gerontology (1984); 30:261–66.

Shapiro J, Hoffman J, Jersky J. A comparison of suprapubic and transurethral drainage for postoperative urinary retention in general surgical patients. Acta Chir Scand (1982); 148:323–27.

Shepherd A, Blannin J. A clinical trial of pants and pads used for urinary incontinence. Nurs Times (1980); 76: 1015–16.

Starer P, Libow L. Obscuring urinary incontinence, diapering of the elderly. J Am Ger Soc (1985); 33:842–46.

Verdell L, Jeter KF, Brewer SA, Bouda JM. Resource Guide of Continence Products and Services. 5th ed.; Union, SC: Help for Incontinent People, 1992.

Wells T. Additional treatments for urinary incontinence. Top Geriatr Rehab (1988); 3:48–57.

18   Case Studies

It has been the authors' experience that there is often a significant gap between the way things are written in medical textbooks and the way they are encountered in clinical practice. This is not because the medical textbooks are wrong (although sometimes, in fact, they are), but because the ways in which individual patients present for care are unique. Individual cases often have their own special circumstances which may be quite different from the "classic" textbook description of the problem in question. The sharp edges of the textbook picture may get blurred when you are looking at "Mrs. Jones." This is why clinical medicine remains as much an art as it is a science. Skill in making clinical decisions comes only through practice.

The purpose of this book is to provide practical help in the management of women with lower urinary tract dysfunction. For this reason an annotated series of specific cases has been included to help bridge the gap between the textbook ideal and the reality that is encountered each day in clinical practice. A great deal can be learned from looking at specific patients, their evaluation, management, and outcome. Commentary has been provided to help illuminate the clinical decision-making process that took place in each case. The emphasis here is on illustrating *principles* of evaluation and management, rather than laying down unalterable dogma for the treatment of each condition. Other approaches might have attained an equally acceptable outcome for each patient. The purpose of these cases is to stimulate thought and to help clinicians formulate management strategies. We hope that this approach to problems helps this book achieve its ultimate goal—improved patient care.

Case 1

History. The patient is an 81-year old white female with a history of progressively worsening incontinence over the last 6 months. It is unclear from her history whether her urine loss is urge related or stress related. She denies any voiding difficulty, neurologic symptoms, or change in her medications over the last 2 years. She is generally healthy for her age except for diabetes, and has no history of neurologic disease. Her current medications include oral conjugated estrogens, insulin, and occasional ibuprofen for mild osteoarthritis.

Physical Examination. The patient has a normal neurologic screening examination. She is ambulatory and has normal mental status. Pelvic examination shows no evidence of genital prolapse and the urogenital region is well estrogenized for her age. Stress incontinence is not demonstrable in either the supine or standing position.

Investigations. Review of the patient's frequency/volume bladder chart showed spontaneous episodes of urine loss not associated with activity or provocative stimuli such as running water, etc. Her functional bladder capacity (largest voided volume) was 180 ml and her average voided volume was 50 ml. Virtually all of her voids were between 50–100 ml. Her 24-hour urinary output was 1200 ml. Urinalysis and urine cytology were negative. A cough stress test with a full bladder was negative. Her postvoid residual was 200 ml.

At this point a patient like this needs more complex urodynamic testing. The nature of her incontinence is still unclear, she has a significantly elevated postvoid residual urine, and she is elderly. Her diabetes should also be checked to see that it is in good control.

Subtracted cystometry was then carried out. After an initial void of 100 ml, the patient was found to have a postvoid residual urine of 250 ml. Her cystometrogram showed a cystometric bladder capacity of 350 ml. At capacity, she had an uncontrolled detrusor contraction that produced significant incontinence but did not empty her bladder completely. After refilling her bladder to 350 ml, she was able to void by relaxing her urethra and generating a low level detrusor contraction of only 5 cm H_2O, with a maximum flow rate of only 10 ml/sec. She voided 150 ml and again left a residual of 200 ml.

Diagnosis. Detrusor hyperreflexia with impaired contractility.

Detrusor overactivity in elderly patients probably has a neurologic etiology related to the effects of aging on the nervous system. In this patient diabetic neuropathy may also play a part; hence the use of the term "detrusor hyperreflexia." Her cystometrogram reveals uninhibited contractions which are powerful enough to cause incontinence, but which are not strong enough to empty her bladder completely. Although she can initiate a voluntary detrusor contraction during voiding, this contraction is also inefficient and does not result in complete emptying. Although her bladder will hold 350 ml, the chronic residual urine means that her functional bladder capacity is only 100 ml. This leads to urinary frequency, and may lead to chronic and recurrent urinary tract infections. Because she has uninhibited detrusor contractions at a volume of 350 ml, urinary incontinence is often a problem for her. This is a type of "overflow incontinence," but it is due to detrusor overactivity in the presence of a chronic residual urine; hence the term for this particular pattern is "detrusor hyperreflexia with impaired contractility."

Treatment and Outcome. This patient was begun on a program of clean, intermittent self-catheterization four times per day to eliminate the residual urine and increase her functional bladder capacity. With instruction and encouragement she managed this very well. Her incontinence decreased significantly, but she still had troublesome urinary leakage. She was then begun on anticholinergic therapy with oxybutynin (Ditropan) 2.5 mg po TID in addition to her self-catheterization regimen. Her incontinence resolved almost completely, but her catheterized residual urine volumes increased to between 400–500 ml as a result of the anticholinergic medication. As long as the patient continued this regimen, she was dry and happy. Measurement of residual urine was an important part of her initial evaluation. If her voiding problem had not been recognized (and it was, in fact, asymptomatic) treatment with anticholinergic medications would have increased her residual urine and would have made her incontinence worse.

Case 2

History. The patient is a 40-year old married white female, gravida 3, para 3, who complains of urine loss since the birth of her last child 3 years ago. She now leaks three or four times each day with sneezing, coughing, and other physical activity.

She also complains of pelvic pressure and chronic constipation. She denies any complaints of urgency, urge incontinence, or nocturia. She does have urinary frequency during the day and admits that this is because she empties her bladder at least every 2 hours to keep it as empty as possible so she will not leak. She wears a panty liner for protection at all times. There is no history of voiding difficulty, recurrent urinary tract infection, hematuria, or dysuria. She was instructed in pelvic floor exercises during childbirth preparation classes, but these have not been helpful. She has no other current medical problems and is on no medications. With three small children at home the patient is not currently interested in surgery, but finds that urine loss is affecting her lifestyle.

Physical Examination. Her general physical exam and neurologic screening examination are normal. There is demonstrable descent of the anterior vaginal wall to 2 cm above the hymenal ring when she strains. Her pelvic muscle tone is estimated at 2 on a scale of 0–5 by digital examination, and she can only sustain a muscle contraction for 1–2 seconds. Coughing in the standing position produces immediate urine loss. The patient confirms that this is the problem that bothers her.

Investigations. Her urinalysis was negative and she had no residual urine after a normal void. A frequency/volume bladder chart was kept for 2 days and showed a normal fluid intake of 1800 ml/day. Her functional bladder capacity was 500 ml according to her chart, with an average voided volume of 250 ml. She also recorded multiple episodes of urine loss associated with coughing, running after her children, and lifting.

Diagnosis. Stress incontinence.

The patient desires conservative management at this time. Since she had demonstrable stress incontinence, a normal neurologic exam, and no postvoid residual, she does not need cystometry before therapy is begun. It is possible that some of her leakage may be produced by detrusor overactivity, but in the absence of symptoms related to urgency or urge incontinence, and with a normal postvoid residual, she does not need further investigation. Conservative therapy poses almost no risk to this patient. If she does not improve or if she decides that she wants to consider surgery, simple or complex cystometry should be considered.

Treatment. The patient was taught pelvic muscle exercises using one-on-one instruction during a pelvic examination performed directly for this purpose. On return to the clinic 1 week later, she was found to be doing the exercises incorrectly. The proper technique was reviewed with her. Follow-up visits over the next 3 months showed that she had increased her awareness of these muscles and had developed a noticeable increase in their strength. She reported that wearing a tampon while taking hikes had also been helpful in reducing her leakage. Crossing her legs when she sneezed or coughed helped reduce her urine loss further. After 3 months of pelvic muscle exercises, she still had a problem with urinary incontinence with repetitive coughing or sneezing when she had hay fever. She was then given phenylpropanolamine in the form of Ornade spansules to use when she felt she needed it. This reduced her urine loss still further. She was now satisfied with urine loss occurring only occasionally with severe coughing or sneezing.

Case 3

History. This 30-year old female presents for help with urge incontinence which developed after she had meningitis at age 14. Her neurologic sequelae have been limited to the urinary tract and consist of severe urinary frequency, urgency, urge incontinence, and nocturnal enuresis. She was evaluated previously at a well-known urodynamic referral center, but finds that the anticholinergic medication originally prescribed for her is no longer helpful in controlling her symptoms. She is now voiding every 15–20 minutes trying to keep her bladder empty, and has to change bulky incontinence pads several times each day. She is incontinent each time she has sexual intercourse and is having two to three episodes of enuresis each night. She is unable to sleep with a man more than once because she wets the bed every night. Both her job and her social life have been seriously affected by her condition. She denies any other neurologic symptoms, voiding difficulty, recurrent cystitis, or pain. She has requested her past medical records several times but has never received them.

Physical Examination. Perineal sensation in sacral dermatomes $S_{2,3,4}$ is diminished symmetrically. Her anal wink reflex is absent. Her levator muscle tone rates only 1 on a scale of 0–5 and the contraction is not sustained. Her lower extremity reflexes and gynecologic examination are both normal.

Investigations. She has no urinary residual after voiding only 50 ml. Her urinalysis was negative. A frequency/volume chart revealed a reduced fluid intake of only 1000 ml per day. Her urinary output was recorded mainly as episodes of urge incontinence, occurring between 10 and 15 times per day, sometimes in sufficient volume to run down her legs. The voided volumes that she recorded ranged from 10–40 ml. Her bladder chart also confirmed several episodes of enuresis each night.

This patient has severe incontinence with known neurologic involvement. Although there appears to be no voiding difficulty, this patient may be at risk for upper tract damage because of high intravesical pressure. She needs a complex evaluation, particularly because she has failed "standard" therapy. Even if her earlier studies were available, her condition has worsened and she should be re-evaluated.

Her serum creatinine was normal. Because she was seen at a tertiary referral center, subtracted cystometry with simultaneous fluoroscopy and pelvic floor electromyography (videocystourethrography) was performed. On simple filling, without any extra provocation, the patient had a high-pressure detrusor contraction of over 100 cm H_2O at a bladder volume of 100 ml, which emptied her bladder completely. Despite her high detrusor pressure, no vesicoureteral reflux was demonstrated. The patient voided to completion with normal pelvic floor relaxation.

Most of the same information might have been obtained using the combination of a voiding cystourethrogram and a slow-fill subtracted cystometrogram with simultaneous pelvic muscle electromyography. In this case all of this information was obtained from a single study which encompassed both bladder filling and emptying.

Diagnosis. Detrusor hyperreflexia without voiding dysfunction. The etiology of her problem is neurologic damage from her childhood episode of meningitis.

Treatment. Despite her history of poor results using medical therapy, another attempt was made to treat her using several drugs at relatively high doses: oxybutynin (Ditropan) 10 mg po TID and imipramine (Tofranil) 25 mg po BID. In addition, she was placed on a regimen of timed voiding and bladder retraining. Although she improved, her incontinence remained a significant problem, and she wanted more effective therapy. Under general anesthesia she was found to have a structural bladder capacity of only 150 ml, and subsequently had an augmentation cecocystoplasty performed. This increased her bladder capacity and effectively "damped out" the pressure effects from her hyperreflexic bladder, making her involuntary contractions inefficient and restoring her continence. When last seen for follow-up she had a normal fluid intake and was voiding every 2 hours. She reported only rare episodes of urge incontinence, and no further problems with nocturnal enuresis or coital incontinence. She has married and is living a relatively normal life.

Case 4

History. A 35-year old white female, gravida 4, para 4, who works as a high school teacher, has been scheduled for a total vaginal hysterectomy and posterior colporrhaphy. She has been referred for preoperative urodynamic studies because of complaints of urgency, frequency, and occasional incontinence of many years duration. She reports an almost constant sensation of urgency, and finds it almost impossible to wait the hour between classes to void. Her episodes of incontinence are rare and are associated with increasing urgency when she tries to unlock her front door after getting home from school. She denies stress incontinence or voiding difficulty. She does not feel that her incontinence is severe enough to warrant surgery by itself, but she is extremely bothered by her prolapse. The rest of her medical and surgical history is unremarkable.

Physical Examination. On straining, her uterus descends to the hymenal ring, along with the posterior vaginal wall. A cough stress test with a full bladder is negative. A neurologic screening examination is normal. Levator muscle tone during a vaginal squeeze is good, rating 4 on a scale of 0–5.

This is a patient with significant lower urinary tract symptoms who has been scheduled for surgery. One strategy would be to treat her symptoms of urgency for 1–2 months to see what happens. If these resolved completely, surgery for her prolapse could proceed. However, this patient needed her surgery promptly, during the summer vacation from school. Her referring physician, who was uncomfortable performing simple cystometry, was planning to perform a urethropexy as part of the operation. Because of this a cystometric examination was carried out.

Investigations.   The patient kept a frequency/volume chart which showed frequency 12 times per day. Her functional bladder capacity was 300 ml with an average voided volume of 150 ml, and excessive daily fluid intake of 2500 ml per day. There were no episodes of nocturia or incontinence during the period in which she kept a bladder chart. Her urinalysis was negative and she had no residual urine after voiding.

A simple cystometrogram demonstrated no incontinence. Her first desire to void occurred at 150 ml, a strong desire to void at 300 ml, and a maximal desire to void at 350 ml. There were no discernible increases in bladder pressure during filling. A pessary pad test with her prolapse reduced demonstrated no urine loss with routine exercises and ambulation.

Diagnosis.   Sensory urgency and symptomatic genital prolapse.

This patient complains of urgency, frequency, and occasional incontinence, but there is no detrusor overactivity during simple single-channel cystometry. Her functional bladder capacity is also low.

Should a complex subtracted cystometrogram have been performed in the evaluation of this patient? This would certainly be acceptable. In this case, no diagnosis has been reached that would require surgery. Even if the patient has occasional motor urgency (urgency due to unstable detrusor contractions) it produces very little incontinence. She is a good candidate for bladder retraining. The referring physician understood that a urethropexy would not relieve any of her symptoms, but might rather produce new symptoms and voiding difficulty.

Treatment.   The patient underwent a total vaginal hysterectomy and posterior colporrhaphy for her pelvic relaxation. She decreased her daily fluid intake to 1800 ml, limiting her intake during school hours. Bladder retraining was successful and she now is able to void once every 2–3 hours without incontinence or significant urgency.

Case 5

History.   An 81-year old white female presents with four to six episodes of nocturia each night. Her family is concerned that she might fall on the way to the toilet and injure herself during the night. The patient is in fairly good health otherwise, except for mild congestive heart failure, mild hypertension, and adult onset diabetes which is controlled with an oral hypoglycemic agent. The patient refuses to use the bedside commode suggested by her social worker, and complains bitterly about the disruption of her sleep caused by her nocturia. During the day she voids every 1 1/2–2 hours. She has no history of neurologic disease and is not taking any medications which might be contributing to her problem.

Physical Examination.   General physical examination reveals only mild dependent edema in her lower extremities. Neurologic and gynecologic examinations are both normal for the patient's age.

Investigation.   A frequency/volume chart revealed voided volumes of 150–200 ml during the day and voids of 200–300 ml at night. Her daytime frequency was 5, with a nighttime frequency of 5 as well. Her functional bladder capacity was 350 ml. Her postvoid residual was 80 ml. Urinalysis was negative. The patient was drinking an average of 2000 ml during the day, but 1200 ml of her total urinary output was produced during the 8 hours in which she was trying to sleep.

Diagnosis. Postural diuresis.

Elderly patients already have an increased nighttime diuresis and this can be accelerated by the reabsorption and excretion of dependent fluids when the patient assumes a supine position at night.

Make sure that the patient's diabetes and heart failure are in optimum medical control. Make sure that her hypertension is not being controlled by a diuretic which she takes at bedtime. Make sure that the patient is not drinking fluids in the few hours leading up to bedtime and during the night when she gets up to void.

Treatment. Several treatment options exist once the considerations mentioned above have been explored. Taking a diuretic in the morning may be useful. Some patients are very successful in limiting the collection of edema in the lower extremities by wearing support hose and elevating their legs above the level of the heart early in the evening. An anticholinergic agent given at bedtime may improve bladder capacity and reduce the amount of nocturia in some patients. Finally, desmopression (a synthetic analog of ADH) has been used to reduce renal output overnight, restricting urine production. This should be used only after the other options have been tried and must be used under close supervision in elderly patients to avoid electrolyte imbalances and other metabolic problems.

Case 6

History. A 32-year old white female has been referred for evaluation of recurrent urinary tract infections. Her chief symptom is a 2-year history of progressively increasing suprapubic pain with bladder filling which is relieved (but only temporarily) by voiding. She now voids every 1/2 hour to relieve her pain. She denies dysuria, incontinence, or voiding difficulty. She has been diagnosed repeatedly with urinary tract infections and has been treated with multiple different antibiotics despite the fact that her urinalyses have shown no pyuria or bacteriuria and her urine cultures have all been negative. Not surprisingly, antibiotic therapy has not improved her symptoms.

Patients may report bladder pain as "I have another infection," which can be misleading. Patients also can be confused by the difference between pain and urgency. It is important to make this distinction because the therapeutic implications of an urge syndrome as opposed to a painful bladder syndrome are quite different.

Physical Examination. General physical, neurologic, and gynecologic examinations are all normal.

Investigations. Postvoid residual was normal. Urinalysis was negative. Urine culture, including culture for fastidious organisms, was negative. Urethral cultures for gonorrhea and chlamydia were both negative. Frequency/volume chart confirmed small voided volumes every 1/2 hour. Somewhat surprisingly, her first morning void was between 400–500 ml on successive days.

What else should be done to evaluate this patient? Urine cytology is often obtained, especially in older patients with these symptoms, to rule out a urinary tract malignancy. Cystourethroscopy is generally indicated. This can be done in the office to exclude the presence of foreign bodies or tumors. If the bladder capacity is normal in the office, it is unlikely that the patient has "classic" interstitial cystitis, but double-fill cystoscopy under general anesthesia (with bladder biopsy as appropriate) may be necessary to rule this out. The fact that this patient has a first morning void of 500 ml makes interstitial cystitis less likely. Urodynamic testing is sometimes useful in these patients to help rule out a low-compliance bladder or detrusor instability as factors contributing to their problem. This patient denies urgency as a significant symptom.

Office cystoscopy using topical urethral anesthetic revealed a normal bladder and urethra. Her bladder capacity at cystoscopy was 400 ml and filling to this volume reproduced her pain.

Diagnosis.   Presumed painful bladder syndrome, of unknown etiology.

Treatment.   The patient was put on a regimen of bladder training and fluid management. Since abnormal histamine release may be responsible for many symptoms in patients with painful bladder syndrome, she was given histamine receptor blockers in the form of cimetidine (Tagamet) 300 mg po TID and metoclopramide (Reglan) 10 mg TID. She had some improvement in her symptoms with this therapy, but wanted further treatment. She then underwent a series of bladder instillations using 50 ml of a 50% solution of dimethylsulfoxide (DMSO), a powerful anti-inflammatory agent, every other week for 6 weeks. After instillation the drug was allowed to remain in the bladder for 15 minutes each time, and was then voided out by the patient. This produced a moderate improvement in her symptoms. She is now coping with her painful bladder, but continues to have periods of intermittent bladder pain.

Case 7

History.   The patient is a 47-year old married white female, gravida 2, para 2, with a 4-year history of stress incontinence which has worsened significantly over the last 2 years. She also has complaints of urgency and some urge incontinence, but no symptoms of voiding difficulty. Two years ago she had a total abdominal hysterectomy and bilateral salpingo-oophorectomy for menorrhagia. Because she had complaints of stress incontinence, a Marshall-Marchetti-Krantz retropubic cystourethropexy was performed at the same time. She was dry after her surgery for 9 weeks, but when she resumed her normal activities she says her ''bladder fell down.'' Her incontinence returned and has worsened steadily since that time. She brought a copy of her operative report from her surgery with her to her visit. Review of the operative note shows that her bladder suspension was done with #2 chromic catgut suture. Her past medical and surgical history are unremarkable. She has taken estrogen every day since her hysterectomy.

Physical Examination.   General physical examination is normal. She is overweight, but not obese. Neurologic examination is normal. Gynecologic exam shows a mobile bladder neck with poor anterior support. Levator tone rates a 4 on a scale of 0–5. Copious stress incontinence is demonstrated with coughing. This is repeated several times and the patient confirms that this is her problem.

Investigations.   Her urinalysis was negative. Postvoid residual was only 10 ml, with a voided volume of 380 ml.

This patient has obvious stress incontinence; however, she also has less troubling symptoms of urgency and urge incontinence and a previous failed bladder neck suspension operation. Further urodynamic investigation of this patient is appropriate.

The patient forgot her bladder chart at the time of her urodynamic studies. Subtracted cystometry was carried out and showed a delayed first desire to void occurring at 370 ml, urgency at 440 ml, and a cystometric capacity of 575 ml. Compliance was normal. Copious stress incontinence was demonstrated with coughing during filling. There were no unstable detrusor contractions despite provocation. She voided normally with sustained detrusor contraction and a peak flow rate of 25 ml/sec, with a residual of 50 ml. Because of her previous surgery and her urge symptoms, this patient also underwent cystoscopy, with normal findings. There were no foreign bodies or sutures in the bladder.

Diagnosis.   Recurrent ''genuine'' stress incontinence after bladder neck suspension.

Patients who have failed an operation for stress incontinence generally should have a more extensive evaluation to see why they still have leakage. Sometimes this is due to the development of a new problem, such as detrusor instability or a fistula. In most cases, failed surgery is due either to initial misdiagnosis of the problem or a failure of surgical technique. In this case, the failure occurred due to inadequate support of the bladder neck. The patient was dry until shortly after surgery, when increased postoperative activity caused a support failure leading to the return of her incontinence. The chromic catgut sutures which had been used to support her bladder neck did not provide enough long-term support to permit adequate bladder neck fixation. Her incontinence worsened gradually during the intervening 2 years and was finally troublesome enough that she wished further treatment.

Treatment.   After discussion of possible treatment options, the patient underwent a repeat retropubic bladder neck suspension. This time she had a Burch colposuspension using permanent sutures. This provided good support for her bladder neck. At follow-up 1 year later, she was still dry, voiding normally, and very happy.

Case 8

History.   A 48-year old white female, para 3–0–0–3, presents for evaluation with complaints of repeated urinary tract infections and abnormal voiding following a total abdominal hysterectomy, bilateral salpingo-oophorectomy, culdeplasty, and Burch colposuspension for prolapse and stress incontinence 6 months previously. She has had three documented urinary tract infections since surgery in addition to frequent bouts of dysuria. Her infections responded to appropriate antibiotic therapy. In addition to recurrent infections, she also complains of hesitancy in starting her stream in spite of a feeling of urgency, and poor urinary flow which sometimes stops and starts. She no longer has any complaints of incontinence, but says her voiding "just doesn't feel right."

Her past medical history is unremarkable except for mild arthritis and a cardiac arrhythmia controlled by verapamil. She had a laparoscopic tubal ligation prior to her hysterectomy. Her only other medication is a transdermal estrogen patch for hormone replacement.

Physical Examination.   General examination is unremarkable. Her weight is 184 pounds, blood pressure 160/90. Her abdominal incision is well healed. Pelvic examination shows normal external genitalia. The cervix and uterus are surgically absent, the cuff is well healed and the vagina is well estrogenized. There is no rectocele or enterocele. The urethra is nontender, but the bladder neck has been elevated to a high position behind the pubic symphysis. She was examined with a full bladder and no stress incontinence was demonstrated.

Investigations.   Her urinalysis was negative and a repeat culture grew no bacteria. A bladder chart showed a normal daily urine output of 1650 ml divided among six voids, with a functional bladder capacity of 500 ml. The patient was able to void 250 ml with a residual urine of 20 ml. Cystoscopy was carried out under local anesthesia to rule out the presence of a foreign body or suture in the bladder. Her cystoscopic examination was normal, except for the high angulation of the bladder neck from her surgery. The patient subsequently had a complete urodynamic examination to characterize her bladder function more fully. Complex uroflowmetry showed a maximum urine flow rate of 10 ml/sec, with a voided volume of 140 ml and a residual of 55 ml. Filling cystometry demonstrated a sensory intact bladder of normal capacity and compliance. Her detrusor was stable during filling and stress incontinence was not demonstrated. The patient then had a pressure-flow voiding study. She achieved a peak flow rate of only 10 ml/sec with a detrusor pressure of 64 cm H_2O. She had a continuous flow pattern that was flat and prolonged. She voided 350 ml and had a residual of 75 ml.

Diagnosis.   Outflow obstruction following bladder neck surgery.

This patient has significant voiding difficulty following her bladder neck suspension for stress incontinence. Her surgery has cured her stress incontinence, but has replaced it with another problem which is just as troubling to her. The fact that she does not have a large residual urine does not rule out an emptying problem. Although her voiding function is normal (that is, she is able to generate a sustained detrusor contraction which empties her bladder completely), she must generate a high detrusor pressure in order to reach a very low rate of urine flow. If plotted along a nomogram, her peak flow rate falls well below the 5th percentile for her voided volume. This patient has surgically-induced outflow obstruction. This diagnosis can be reached with confidence only on the basis of pressure-flow voiding studies.

Several options exist for managing this patient. Since it has only been 6 months since surgery, expectant management with reinvestigation in another 6–12 months would be reasonable. Alternately, the patient could be taught clean intermittent self-catheterization to improve her voiding efficiency and followed closely. The use of intermittent antibiotic therapy or low dose suppressive therapy for her recurrent infections would also be appropriate conservative management.

Treatment and Outcome. The patient opted for expectant management, but her symptoms did not resolve. She continued to have frequent infections and difficulty voiding. Reinvestigation 18 months later confirmed her outflow obstruction and she underwent a takedown of her Burch colposuspension. Her bladder neck was repositioned using a vagino-obturator shelf procedure which resulted in improved voiding, the maintenance of continence, and a resolution of her recurrent infections.

Case 9

History. The patient is a 69-year old widowed white female, para 4–0–0–4, referred for evaluation with complaints of stress incontinence, frequency, urgency, urge incontinence, and nocturia. She leaks with coughing, sneezing, walking, lifting, bending over, or changing position. She has daily urge incontinence and wears heavy incontinence pads because of leakage that is severe enough to run down her legs and pool on the floor. She reports that her problems began after a urinary tract infection 8 months ago; however, 3 months prior to presentation she underwent a wide local excision of a carcinoma of the vagina with superficial groin node dissection, cervical conization, uterine dilatation, and curettage for a stage II squamous cell carcinoma of the vagina, and has subsequently received 5000 rads of whole pelvis radiation. She also has hypertension which is controlled with a combination of hydrochlorothiazide and reserpine. Other surgical operations include an appendectomy, varicose vein stripping, and left knee replacement.

Physical Examination. She is obese, weighing 260 pounds. Blood pressure is 130/70. Neurologic examination is normal. Pelvic examination shows an atrophic, excoriated vulva with marked radiation changes. The urethra and trigone of the bladder are tender to palpation. Levator contractions rate 2 on a scale of 0–5. The bladder is well supported, but copious stress incontinence is demonstrated with a single cough. The uterus descends halfway down the vagina with straining and there is a slight rectocele.

Investigations. Urinalysis was normal. Frequency/volume bladder chart showed 13 episodes of urination during the day and four episodes nocturia each night. The functional bladder capacity was 900 ml, with an average daily urine output of 3200 ml. Three incontinent episodes per day were documented on her bladder chart.

Immediately upon examining this patient's bladder chart it is apparent that part of her problem is increased fluid intake and poor voiding habits. She has a bladder capacity of 900 ml in midmorning after taking her diuretic, but multiple smaller voids throughout the day. This suggests that part of her problem is detrusor overactivity which she should be able to suppress.

Urine flow studies showed a maximum flow rate of 45 ml/sec, with a voided volume of 225 ml and a residual of only 5 ml. Filling cystometry was carried out and showed an early first desire to void at 75 ml, urgency at 140 ml associated with a high-pressure detrusor contraction which reached 60 cm H_2O and resulted in complete bladder emptying. She was refilled, and was able to hold 350 ml, but leaked copious amounts of fluid with coughing. Urethral pressure studies showed a maximum urethral closure pressure of only 12 cm H_2O. Cystoscopy showed chronic cystitis and radiation changes, but was otherwise unremarkable.

Diagnosis.   Mixed stress and urge incontinence.

This patient has incontinence due to two problems: unstable detrusor activity and stress incontinence. Her bladder chart shows that she can hold up to 900 ml during everyday activities, so a reduction in her bladder capacity from radiation therapy is not part of her problem, This also suggests that she is able to postpone voiding and suppress detrusor contractions when she makes herself do so. Some of her frequency is undoubtedly due to her fluid intake and her diuretic. Some of her stress incontinence may be due to bladder overdistension with large urine volumes. This patient has obvious factors which suggest she should be tried on conservative therapy before any surgery is considered: she is obese, she has hypertension, she has varicose veins, and she has had a gynecologic malignancy which resulted in radiation therapy. Therefore it seems prudent to try vigorous medical management to maximize her bladder function before further surgery is contemplated.

Treatment and Outcome.   The patient was instructed in fluid management and bladder retraining. She was also placed on imipramine 25 mg in the morning and 50 mg at bedtime because of this drug's dual effects on the bladder: increasing urethral tone due to α-receptor stimulation and decreasing detrusor contractility due to its anticholinergic properties. She was scheduled to be seen again in 4 weeks. At that time she had had a dramatic improvement in her symptoms, but complained of fatigue and sleepiness from the imipramine. The dose was then reduced to 25 mg twice per day. When seen again 1 month later, her improvement had continued. She had decreased her medication on her own to 25 mg at bedtime only and described herself as "100% improved." She desired no further treatment and maintained this level of control on follow-up.

Case 10

History.   The patient is a 66-year old white female, para 1–3–7–1, with incapacitating stress incontinence. Five months prior to presentation the patient underwent a modified radical vulvectomy with bilateral inguinal lymphadenectomies for a stage I carcinoma of the vulva. There was no metastatic disease and all surgical margins were clear. Prior to surgery the patient had no urinary tract complaints, but while hospitalized following her surgery she developed urinary incontinence. According to her, she now leaks "all the time." She complains of stress incontinence, urgency, frequency, nocturia, and some urge incontinence. Occasionally she reports urine loss during sleep. She leaks urine with coughing, walking, and simple change of position such as bending over or getting up out of a chair. Sometimes she loses urine for no obvious reason at all. She does have periods of dryness, but is wet more often than she is dry. She wears large incontinence pads which she changes four times per day. She has restricted her activities severely as a result of her leakage and rates her distress as "8" on a 10–point scale. A therapeutic trial of oxybutynin (Ditropan) 2.5 mg BID by her oncologist made no difference in her symptoms. In addition, the patient has chronic bronchitis and has smoked one pack of cigarettes each day for 53 years. She takes 300 mg of long-acting theophylline (Theo-Dur) each day, as well as occasional ibuprofen for mild osteoarthritis. Past surgical history includes an appendectomy, a left salpingo-oophorectomy, and a right ovarian cystectomy.

Physical Examination.   General physical examination is unremarkable except for diffuse crackles in the bases of both lungs and mild kyphosis of the spine. Neurologic examination is normal. Pelvic examination shows urogenital atrophy. The anal wink and bulbocavernosus reflexes are both absent. The vulva has been surgically removed. The urethra is heavily scarred and foreshortened. The external urethral meatus is reddened and the clitoris is absent. There is no fat pad over the pubic symphysis, merely a single layer of skin stretched directly over the pubic bone. The urethra and bladder base are nontender to palpation. The bladder neck is well supported and does not descend with straining. The uterus and cervix are normal and mobile, but well supported. Each time the patient coughs, urine pours out of the urethra.

Investigations.   Urinalysis was negative. Postvoid residual was 50 ml. The patient's frequency/volume chart showed five voids during the day and two episodes of nocturia at night. Her functional bladder capacity was 480 ml, with a daily urine output of 1790 ml. She recorded over nine incontinent episodes each day on her bladder chart.

This is a challenging patient. She has easily demonstrable stress incontinence and the onset of her incontinence is clearly related to her recent oncologic surgery. Her examination reveals a heavily scarred and shortened urethra, which nonetheless appears to have good support. Her bladder chart demonstrates frequent incontinence, normal voiding, and a normal capacity. Because of the sudden onset of her symptoms and her altered anatomy, a full urodynamic evaluation is prudent before instituting treatment.

Filling cystometry showed a delayed first desire to void at 410 ml, urgency at 480 ml, and a cystometric capacity of 500 ml. There were no unstable detrusor contractions during filling. Multiple episodes of stress incontinence were demonstrated during cystometry. Her maximum urethral pressure was 44 cm H_2O, with a maximum urethral closure pressure of 24 cm H_2O. Pressure-flow voiding studies showed a peak flow rate of 11 ml/sec with a maximum detrusor pressure during voiding of 34 cm of water. She voided with a sustained detrusor contraction and had no residual urine after voiding, but her flow pattern was poor and intermittent. She was able to interrupt her urinary stream during voiding and generated an isometric detrusor contraction of 38 cm H_2O. Cystoscopy revealed significant urethral scarring, but no other abnormalities.

Diagnosis.   Stress incontinence due to intrinsic urethral dysfunction.

This patient has incapacitating stress incontinence as an unfortunate consequence of her oncologic surgery. She reported no urinary tract problems prior to her radical vulvectomy, but this operation resulted in her losing most of her distal urethra and its supports. On examination the urethra and bladder neck were well supported but poorly functional, and copious incontinence was demonstrated. Her urine stream was poor, due primarily to urethral scarring, but voiding function was normal and she had good detrusor function. A "standard" incontinence operation, such as a Burch procedure, would not help this patient, since her problem is a defective urethra rather than one which is displaced during periods of increased intra-abdominal pressure.

Treatment and Outcome.   The patient underwent a suburethral sling procedure using fascia lata harvested from her thigh. A suprapubic catheter was placed at the time of surgery. A trial of voiding was started on the second postoperative day, but she had persistent large residual urine volumes throughout her hospital stay. She was discharged home with her catheter in place to continue her regimen of voiding and measurement of postvoid residuals. Two weeks after surgery she was voiding an average of 250 ml with residuals of 50 ml. Her catheter was removed and she was taught clean intermittent self-catheterization in case she developed acute retention or other voiding problems. At follow-up 2 months later, her stress incontinence was cured. The patient continued to have some voiding difficulty which slowly resolved over the next few months.

Case 11

History. A 59-year old white female, para 4–0–0–4, presents for evaluation with a history of stress incontinence during jogging, sneezing, coughing, or vigorous exercise. She has no symptoms of urgency, frequency, urge incontinence, nocturia, or voiding difficulty. Her symptoms began suddenly 6 weeks before referral and she was concerned that they would worsen and affect her active lifestyle. Her past surgical history was significant for a tonsillectomy, appendectomy, tubal ligation, and subsequent vaginal hysterectomy for refractory menometrorrhagia. Her medical history was significant for hypertension. She was taking 1.25 mg of conjugated estrogens and a total of 14 mg of prazosin (Minipress) each day (4 mg BID and 6 mg QHS).

In patients who present with a sudden change in urinary habits, look for precipitating causes. Items of particular importance include changes in medication and acute medical or surgical events.

Careful review of the patient's medical history showed that she had been on prazosin at a dose of 3 mg TID with poor control of her blood pressure approximately 6 months previously. Her medication had been switched to atenolol, but she developed unacceptable side effects. She had been switched back to prazosin at an increased dose of 14 mg/day 6 weeks before her referral. The onset of her symptoms coincided with this change in medication.

Prazosin is a potent α-adrenergic antagonist which is widely used in the treatment of hypertension. It works by decreasing peripheral vascular resistance through selective blockade of postsynaptic α-1 adrenergic receptors in vascular smooth muscle. This produces vasodilation. Because the bladder neck and urethra possess large numbers of α-adrenergic receptors, α-blockers can also reduce the tone of these areas and produce incontinence.

Physical Examination. General examination was unremarkable. The patient weighed 118 pounds and had a blood pressure of 160/88. Pelvic examination showed normal external genitalia with good support of the bladder and urethra. The tissues were well estrogenized. The cervix and uterus were absent and the vagina was well-supported. Significant stress incontinence was demonstrated during the examination.

Investigations. Urinalysis was normal. There was no residual urine after voiding. She did not keep a frequency/volume chart. Filling cystometry showed a first desire to void at 95 ml, urgency at 250 ml, and cystometric capacity at 310 ml. The detrusor was stable during filling and "genuine" stress incontinence was demonstrated. She voided 300 ml with a low flow rate of 8 ml/sec and a maximum detrusor pressure of 20 cm H_2O. Urethral pressure studies showed a maximum urethral pressure of 48 cm H_2O and a maximum urethral closure pressure of 30 cm H_2O. The functional urethral length was 1.8 cm.

Diagnosis. Stress incontinence, probably secondary to side effects of prazosin.

Treatment. The patient was advised that because of the sudden onset of her problem and its temporal association with her change in medications, it was probably related to her drug. Although she had been expecting to have to undergo surgery, she was advised to return to the care of her internist and be placed on another antihypertensive medication before considering an operation for her incontinence. She stopped taking the prazosin and was started on verapamil at a dose of 120 mg twice per day. Her incontinence resolved within 36 hours of the change in medication.

Follow-up urodynamic studies 6 weeks later were virtually identical to her

initial studies, except that her maximal urethral pressure had increased to 72 cm H_2O, her maximum urethral closure pressure had increased to 52 cm H_2O, and her functional urethral length had increased to 2.5 cm.

Case 12

History. The patient is a 31-year old widowed white female, para 1–0–0–1, with complaints of ''bad smelling'' urine, urgency, and difficulty voiding. She has a small amount of stress incontinence, but this does not restrict her activities. The patient reports having had normal bladder function until 3 years ago, when she underwent a radical hysterectomy with pelvic/periaortic lymphadenectomy for a stage IB carcinoma of the cervix. Her ovaries were preserved at the time of surgery. A suprapubic catheter was placed during her operation and removed 3 weeks after surgery. Because of persistent postoperative voiding difficulty, the patient was taught clean intermittent self catheterization, which she gradually discontinued. She reports voiding three to four times per day, and perhaps once per night. She has trouble starting her stream of urine and often strains to empty her bladder. Her stream is usually poor and often is interrupted. A persistent feeling of incomplete bladder emptying is present. She has had two urinary tract infections in the past year. Review of systems reveals chronic constipation, with only two bowel movements per week. Most of the time she must use a laxative or rectal suppository to effect bowel emptying. Past medical and surgical history is otherwise negative.

Physical Examination. The patient's weight is 144 pounds, blood pressure 116/70. General physical examination is normal. Neurologic examination is normal. There is a well healed transverse incision in the lower abdomen. The upper vagina is scarred, but the rest of the pelvic examination is otherwise normal considering her surgical history.

Although this patient has mild symptoms of urgency and stress incontinence, her symptoms are related mainly to voiding problems which started at the time of a radical hysterectomy. This is where the focus of her evaluation must be.

Investigations. She did not keep a bladder chart. Review of her records revealed that a urine culture sent by her referring physician 5 days ago was positive, but she had not been treated. The culture grew greater than 100,000 col/ml of *E. coli* and *Klebsiella pneumonia*. She was unable to void and had a residual urine of 250 ml. She was given a week's prescription of trimethoprim/sulfamethoxizole and scheduled to be seen again after completion of her antibiotics.

When she returned for her next visit, she still had not kept her frequency/volume chart. She voided 150 ml with a peak flow rate of 10 ml/sec, but had a residual urine of 150 ml. Filling cystometry showed a delayed first desire to void at 470 ml, ''fullness'' at 700 ml, and a maximum cystometric capacity of 750 ml. No incontinence was demonstrated. Bladder compliance was normal. Pressure-flow voiding studies showed a maximum flow rate of 14 ml/sec with a detrusor pressure of 34 cm H_2O at peak flow, assisted by significant abdominal straining. She was able to stop her urine stream, but had great difficulty in starting again. She was able to empty completely by voiding in a private toilet.

Diagnosis. Voiding difficulty and reduced bladder sensation secondary to surgical denervation injury.

Voiding difficulty is a common complication following radical hysterectomy. This generally occurs due to denervation of the pelvic nerve plexuses in the "web" of the cardinal ligament as the parametrial dissection is carried laterally from the uterus to ensure complete resection of the cancer. This patient had significant voiding trouble immediately following surgery, but was lost to regular follow-up since that time. Her urodynamic studies revealed significant loss of bladder sensation and intermittently elevated residual urine volumes. However, she is able to generate a detru-

sor contraction which, when combined with abdominal straining, is sufficient to empty her bladder, at least some of the time. She has had multiple urinary tract infections, most likely related to persistent residual urine.

Treatment and Outcome. A careful explanation was given to the patient regarding the nature of her problem and its etiology. She was instructed in double-voiding and the use of the Credé maneuver to help her empty her bladder, and placed on a timed voiding schedule every 3 hours. In addition, she was retaught how to perform clean intermittent self-catheterization and instructed to do so four times a day to evaluate her residual urine volumes. She was also placed on suppressive antibiotics each night using one regular dose trimethoprim-sulfa tablet as part of this initial regimen. On a timed voiding schedule with better voiding techniques her residual urines decreased to the range of 50–100 ml. Her suppressive antibiotics were stopped, and she was treated periodically with short courses of antibiotics for intermittent symptomatic infections.

Case 13

History. The patient is a 54-year old white female, para 2–0–2–2, with complaints of stress incontinence, urgency, and urge incontinence. The patient had undergone a total vaginal hysterectomy nearly 30 years previously for uterine leiomyomas. Six years later she had an anterior colporrhaphy for stress incontinence and a cystocele. This eliminated her symptoms for 5 years, at which time she underwent her second anterior colporrhaphy for recurrent stress incontinence. She now presents with a 2-year history of recurrent stress incontinence which has been worsening, accompanied by urgency and urge incontinence. Her local gynecologist has managed her with hormone replacement for menopausal symptoms and a vigorous program of pelvic floor muscle exercises. The combination of the these two therapies has produced a significant reduction in her urgency and urge incontinence. Stress incontinence remains her major problem. She works as a teacher in a community college and has been embarrassed on several occasions by urine loss during lectures when she has coughed while speaking.

Physical Examination. General examination is unremarkable. Her weight is 150 pounds, blood pressure 134/76. Neurologic screening examination is normal. Pelvic examination shows well estrogenized genitalia. There is significant scarring of the anterior vagina from her previous surgery. The bladder neck is hypermobile, but the vault appears to be well supported. There is no enterocele or rectocele. Marked stress incontinence is demonstrated with coughing. She confirms this as her major problem.

This patient clearly has stress incontinence on the basis of her history and physical examination. However, in view of two previous surgeries and a history of urgency and frequency, a more complete examination is warranted.

Investigations. Her urinalysis was unremarkable. A frequency/volume chart showed five voids per day with a functional bladder capacity of 475 ml, an average void of 300 ml, and a daily urine output of 1500 ml. She noted two to four episodes of incontinence each day. Uroflowmetry showed a maximum flow rate of 14 ml/sec, with a voided volume of 550 ml and a residual urine volume of 250 ml. The patient said that she was "nearly full to bursting" when she came in for her study. Filling cystometry showed a first desire to void at 200 ml, urgency at 600 ml, and a cystometric capacity of 650 ml. Marked "genuine" stress incontinence was demonstrated during filling when she coughed. The patient also developed detrusor contractions to a maximum height of 28 cm H_2O which caused some urgency but which did not lead to incontinence. She was able to suppress these contractions eventually. Pressure-flow voiding studies showed a maximum flow rate of 17 ml/sec with a voided volume of 525 ml and a residual urine of 125 ml. Maximum detrusor pressure during voiding was 46 cm H_2O.

Diagnosis. Mixed incontinence, with stress incontinence predominating, and an element of voiding difficulty.

This patient has three problems. She clearly has stress incontinence on the basis of poor bladder neck support in spite of two previous anterior vaginal repairs. Her detrusor instability has been significantly improved by behavioral modification and she is able to suppress contractions so they do not cause motor urge incontinence during cystometry. Activation of the pelvic floor muscles has an inhibitory effect on reflex detrusor activity, and this is undoubtedly why her Kegel exercises have helped her symptoms of urgency and urge incontinence, in combination with her estrogen replacement now that she has entered menopause. However, she has some voiding difficulty, with a relatively low flow rate and a moderately high detrusor pressure. Her postvoid residual following her initial urine flow study was elevated, but this was probably due to her overdistended bladder. Her second residual volume was still elevated, but not nearly as high.

Treatment and Outcome.   A full discussion was held with the patient regarding her diagnosis and the various methods of treating mixed incontinence. Because she had had two prior unsuccessful surgeries, she desired to try conservative management first, and was placed on bladder drill in combination with her pelvic muscle exercises and continued estrogen. In addition, she was placed on imipramine 25 mg twice a day. When seen for review 4 weeks later, she had not improved and wished to consider surgery. Her residual urine volume at that time was 75 ml. She subsequently underwent a retropubic bladder neck suspension (Burch colposuspension), with bilateral salpingo-oophorectomy, Moschcowitz culdeplasty, and placement of a suprapubic catheter. She was unable to void after surgery and was discharged with her suprapubic catheter in place to continue voiding trials at home. She was contacted weekly for review of her voided volumes and urinary residuals. After 3 weeks her catheter was removed and she was taught clean intermittent self-catheterization. Her voiding function gradually improved and she was able to catheterize only once per day or as needed. When seen for follow-up 3 months after surgery she was catheterizing herself only occasionally and no longer had either stress or urge incontinence; however, pelvic examination at that time revealed an enterocele descending approximately one-third the length of the vagina. The patient was informed that this was present, and would probably worsen over time. She returned 6 months later saying that it ''was time for more surgery.'' Pelvic examination revealed excellent support of the bladder neck and anterior vagina, but the patient had developed a massive pulsion enterocele distending the vaginal introitus to a diameter of 5 cm and bulging beyond it. This was subsequently corrected by an abdominal sacral-colpopexy, with excellent results. The patient had another suprapubic catheter placed at the time of her surgery, but was able to have this removed after a week. At further follow-up, her vagina remained well supported, she had no further problems with incontinence, and her voiding continued to improve.

Case 14

History.   The patient is a 28-year old female, para 1–0–0–1, who had an uneventful vaginal delivery of a 3220 g female infant. She presents at her 6 week postpartum visit saying that the has urinary incontinence whenever she coughs or sneezes. This is so bad that she must wear a perineal pad and change it up to five times per day. She is distraught and says this is absolutely intolerable for her and something must be done about it. She did not have any incontinence prior to her pregnancy, but developed some mild incontinence during this gestation. Her birth was easy, with a second stage of labor that lasted only 45 minutes and resulted in a spontaneous delivery over an intact perineum. She does not have any urgency or urge incontinence and can postpone the need to void until a convenient time and place. She has tried Kegel exercises, but says that they have not helped. Her past medical history is unremarkable.

Physical Examination. Her general physical examination is unremarkable. On pelvic examination, she has a cystourethrocele which extends 1 cm below the hymenal ring with straining. The cervix is 1 cm above the ring on straining. There is no rectocele. Contraction of the pelvic floor muscles rates 1 on a scale of 0–5. Stress incontinence is easily demonstrable on examination. It coincides exactly with the occurrence of a cough, and is repetitive with each cough. She identifies this as the type of incontinence that has been bothering her.

Investigations. Urinalysis is normal. Postvoid residual urine is 20 ml, with a voided volume of 350 ml. Her frequency/volume bladder chart shows voids of 300–450 ml, with an average daily urine output of 1750 ml.

Diagnosis. Postpartum stress incontinence.

Considerable trauma to the pelvic floor can occur even with otherwise uneventful vaginal delivery. Part of this damage is due to stretching of muscles and connective tissue, and part of it involves neuropraxia of the pelvic nerves. These factors all contribute to the development of postpartum stress incontinence. Pelvic neuropraxia probably influences both the strength of the striated urethral sphincter as well as the contractility of the levator ani muscles supporting the pelvic organs. Healing of this trauma is slow, but steady, and may take from 6–12 months.

Treatment and Outcome. The patient was reassured that her condition was not uncommon, and that it would improve over time with conservative management. She was given vaginal estrogen cream to use while breastfeeding to help prevent tissue atrophy during lactation. Her ability to perform pelvic muscle exercises correctly was confirmed during a pelvic examination. Periodic contact was maintained with her by the nursing staff for encouragement and to help maintain her motivation. Her incontinence was significantly improved by 4 months postpartum. At 6 months postpartum she had only mild leakage during periods of vigorous exercise.

The important point in this case is that childbirth may produce dramatic temporary changes in the pelvic floor. Significant prolapse and urinary incontinence may be encountered in the immediate postpartum period, but will resolve almost completely if they are managed conservatively. Intervention in these cases should be limited, allowing time to see what degree of recovery will occur spontaneously. Immediate postpartum surgery for stress incontinence can almost never be justified.

Case 15

History. A 64-year old woman, para 3–0–0–3, presents with the onset of urinary incontinence following the performance of a vaginal hysterectomy with anterior and posterior colporrhaphies for uterovaginal prolapse. Prior to her surgery she had mild symptoms of stress incontinence and she had been told that these would resolve after her cystocele was repaired. She also had a large protruding rectocele. Review of her operative note shows that reduction of her cystocele had been described, but there was no mention of any procedure to repair her urethral supports. She has typical symptoms of stress incontinence without associated urgency or urge incontinence. Her medical history is otherwise unremarkable.

Physical Examination. General examination is normal. Pelvic examination shows that the vaginal vault is well supported. There is no rectocele. Her genital tissues are atrophic. Stress incontinence is demonstrable each time the patient coughs, and there is associated descent of the urethrovesical junction. A Q-tip test shows 80° of urethral mobility. Careful support of the urethra using a ring forceps without compression or elevation of the bladder neck prevents further urine loss.

Investigations. Her urinalysis was normal. Her postvoid residual urine was only 20 ml after a void of 300 ml. She had a stable cystometrogram with a bladder capacity of 400 ml. Stress incontinence was again demonstrated during the study.

Diagnosis.   Iatrogenic stress incontinence after cystocele repair.

There are two ways in which this patient's surgery may have led to her stress incontinence. First, the cystocele which was present before her prolapse surgery may have masked an incompetent sphincter mechanism. Although it is not entirely clear how this happens, if a cystocele is repaired without steps to support the urethrovesical junction, latent stress incontinence can become manifest, and mild stress incontinence can sometimes become much worse. A second etiologic factor in this patient's problem may be that her rectocele may have helped occlude the urethra during coughing by providing compressive pressure from below. Repair of her rectocele may have removed this supportive cushion and unmasked her stress incontinence.

Prior to her operation, the patient should have been examined with a moderately full bladder with her prolapse reduced, and asked to cough. If stress incontinence could be demonstrated under these conditions, steps should have been taken to provide more durable urethral support at the time of her surgery. There is also a persistent misconception that the cystocele is responsible for stress incontinence and that repairing the upper portion of the vaginal wall under the bladder will cure the patient's urinary leakage. The specific supports of the urethra at the level of the urethrovesical junction are the structures which are important for maintaining continence. If proper urethral support had been achieved during her operation, this problem probably would not have occurred.

Treatment and Outcome.   The severity of her leakage was discussed with the patient. In such cases, if the incontinence is mild and the patient is not dramatically troubled by it, then a trial of estrogen cream and conservative management with pelvic muscle exercises for 3 months or so is justified. If the incontinence is significant, then surgical correction can be discussed. This patient chose to try vaginal estrogen and pelvic muscle exercises. Her symptoms improved somewhat, but she was still soaking two to three pads per day one year after her operation. She returned requesting surgical repair and subsequently had an uneventful retropubic bladder neck suspension which cured her incontinence.

Case 16

History.   A 45-year old woman, para 3–0–0–3, presents with a history of gradually worsening incontinence. She says that she wets herself when getting home from work with a full bladder, and also that she is incontinent when she coughs or sneezes. She wears a pad every day for protection, but it is usually dry when she changes it. Her past medical history is unremarkable.

Physical Examination.   General examination is unremarkable. Stress incontinence is demonstrable on examination and the axial mobility of her urethra is 45° during a straining Q-tip test. Careful support of her urethra with a ring forceps eliminates her stress incontinence. Her pelvic examination is otherwise normal.

Investigations.   A urinalysis was normal. Her postvoid residual urine was 10 ml after voiding 500 ml. A frequency/volume bladder chart showed a functional bladder capacity of 600 ml, with an average voided volume of 250 ml, and a daily urine output of 2100 ml. A cystometrogram showed a cystometric bladder capacity of 400 ml with no uninhibited detrusor contractions. "Genuine" stress incontinence was demonstrated during her study.

At this point in the evaluation of this patient it might appear that her problem is stress incontinence. However, when she is asked if the incontinence which is seen when she coughs is what bothers her, she clearly states that this is not her problem. She is concerned about the uncontrolled loss of urine which occurs when her bladder is full and she is racing for a bathroom. The stress incontinence does not trouble her because it is a rare event, usually doesn't cause visible wetting, and she can control it to some degree by emptying her bladder before she engages in exercise or by crossing her legs and tightening her pelvic floor before she coughs or sneezes. The presence of a stable cystometrogram (that is, a cystometrogram in which detrusor instability is not demonstrated) is not necessarily surprising since her unstable contractions occur during specific situations which may not be reproduced in a urodynamics laboratory.

Diagnosis. Mixed incontinence, with symptoms of urge incontinence predominating.

Treatment and Outcome. Since it is triggered by a specific situations, urge incontinence arising when a patient is near a bathroom with a full bladder does not always respond well to anticholinergic medications. Problems such as these are best treated initially by modification of bladder habits. The patient should try to make sure that she does not arrive home with an overly full bladder. Decreasing her afternoon fluid intake and voiding prior to leaving work are both useful suggestions in this case. She should make a habit of voiding at regular intervals and urinating before she is ''full to bursting.'' Some of her urgency may not be due so much to detrusor overactivity as to a weak sphincter mechanism that cannot keep urine in the bladder until a detrusor contraction can be suppressed. This explains, in part, why urge incontinence is so often associated with stress incontinence, and also helps explain why pelvic floor muscle exercises are often helpful for these patients.

On questioning this patient, it was discovered that she drank at least one to two cups of coffee during her last hour at work before leaving for home. She was instructed to empty her bladder on a regular basis, particularly before leaving work, and to cut down her coffee consumption. She stopped drinking coffee late in the afternoon, began emptying her bladder regularly, and had no further problems with ''key-in-the-lock'' incontinence.

Appendix A Useful Organizations and Publications

Patient Support Groups
Incontinence

HIP (Help for Incontinent People)
P.O. Box 544
Union, SC 29379
1–800–BLADDER; (803) 579–7900

This organization issues a regular newsletter, *The HIP Report,* focusing on the needs and interests of incontinent adults. The newsletter provides both patient education and self-help information. HIP has a wide range of educational materials for patients on a variety of subjects including bladder retraining, intermittent self-catheterization, types of surgical procedures, diagnostic tests, etc. An instructional booklet and audiotape on pelvic muscle exercises is available, as well a low cost videotape on urinary incontinence. A regular resource guide of commercially available products for incontinent patients is published. While no product comparisons are undertaken, they do not fear to berate the inferior and advertise the righteous!

The Simon Foundation for Continence
P.O. Box 815
Wilmette, IL 60091
1–800–23-SIMON
(In Canada, 1–800–265–9575)

This group issues a regular newsletter, the *Informer,* which is aimed at educating and providing emotional support for the incontinent patient. The Simon Foundation's mission is to remove the stigma attached to incontinence and bring the topic to public attention for discussion. Patient educational materials are also available. The group has put together a support program for incontinent patients called the "I Will Manage" program. A full syllabus and related course information are available from the Foundation.

Interstitial Cystitis

ICA (Interstitial Cystitis Association, Inc.)
P.O. Box 1553
Madison Square Station
New York, NY 10159
(212) 983–7620

This is a patient self-help group which organizes local meetings of patients and the families of patients coping with interstitial cystitis. The nature of the local groups ranges from supportive and innovative to angry. The Foundation has been instrumental in organizing patients to assist in several large-scale studies of interstitial cystitis. Publications include the *ICA Update* and brochures.

Commercially Available Books for Patients

Burgio K, Pearce L, and Lucca A. Staying Dry: A practical guide to bladder control. Baltimore: Johns Hopkins University Press, 1989. $12.95; 169 pages.

Gartley C (ed). Managing Incontinence: A guide to living with loss of bladder control. Ottawa, IL: Jamesson Books, 1985. $12.95; 138 pages. (Available from the Simon Foundation.)

Chalker R., and Whitmore K. Overcoming Bladder Disorders. New York: Harper and Row, 1990. $19.95; 338 pages.

Free Patient Guides

Agency for Health Care Policy and Research (AHCPR). Urinary incontinence in adults: A patient's guide. Center for Research Dissemination and Liaison, AHCPR Clearinghouse, P.O. Box 8547, Silver Spring, MD 20907. (1–800–358–9295.)

The United States Public Health Service has produced this brief educational pamphlet for patients. It covers simple anatomy and urinary physiology, the main causes and types of incontinence, as well as the diagnosis and treatment of incontinence.

Patient Educational Materials

ACOG Patient Education Pamphlet, "Urinary Incontinence," December, 1990. American College of Obstetricians and Gynecologists, 409 12th Street, SW, Washington, DC 20024–2188.

A brief overview of urinary tract anatomy and physiology, the symptoms and causes of incontinence, diagnostic tests and forms of treatment.

"Urinary Incontinence," Krames Communications, 312 90th Street, Daly City, CA 94015. (415) 994–8800. Discusses stress, urge, and overflow incontinence and the evaluation and treatment of these conditions. The artwork is good, but the publication needs updating. Costs vary with the number ordered; approximately $1.00 each.

Professional Organizations

American Uro-Gynecologic Society
401 North Michigan Avenue
Chicago, Illinois 60611–4267
Telephone (312) 644–6610
Fax (312) 527–6640

The American Uro-Gynecologic Society is a nonprofit professional organization dedicated to research and education in the field of female urologic dysfunction. The membership is composed mainly of gynecologists, but is open to medical professionals in all specialties. An annual clinical meeting is held. The organization also helps coordinate multicenter research projects in urogynecology.

International Continence Society

Paul Abrams, Secretary	**Werner Schafer, Membership Secretary**
Department of Urology	**Urologische Klinik der RWTH Aachen**
Southmead Hospital	**Aachen**
Westbury-on-Trym	**Germany**
Bristol B10 5NB	
England	

The International Continence Society is the main worldwide organization devoted to fostering communication and research in the field of urinary incontinence. Membership is open to professionals in all related medical fields and consists of urologists, gynecologists, geriatricians, biomedical engineers, and neuroscientists, as well as nurses and physical therapists. A large international meeting covering a wide range of interests is held every year.

Appendix B   Index to Case Studies in Chapter 18

Index

Page numbers followed by "f" denote figures; those followed by "t" denote tables.